INTERNATIONAL SEMINAR ON
NUCLEAR WAR AND PLANETARY EMERGENCIES
27th Session:

SOCIETY AND STRUCTURES: HISTORICAL PERSPECTIVES — CULTURE AND IDEOLOGY; NATIONAL AND REGIONAL GEOPOLITICAL ISSUES; GLOBALIZATION — ECONOMY AND CULTURE; HUMAN RIGHTS — FREEDOM AND DEMOCRACY DEBATE; CONFRONTATIONS AND COUNTERMEASURES: PRESENT AND FUTURE CONFRONTATIONS; PSYCHOLOGY OF TERRORISM; DEFENSIVE COUNTERMEASURES; PREVENTIVE COUNTERMEASURES; GENERAL DEBATE; SCIENCE AND TECHNOLOGY: EMERGENCIES; POLLUTION; CLIMATE — GREENHOUSE EFFECT; DESERTIFICATION, WATER POLLUTION, ALGAL BLOOM; BRAIN AND BEHAVIOUR DISEASES; THE CULTURAL EMERGENCY: GENERAL DEBATE AND CONCLUSIONS; PERMANENT MONITORING PANEL REPORTS; INFORMATION SECURITY WORKSHOP; KANGAROO MOTHER'S CARE WORKSHOP; BRAIN AND BEHAVIOUR DISEASES WORKSHOP

THE SCIENCE AND CULTURE SERIES
Nuclear Strategy and Peace Technology

Series Editor: Antonino Zichichi

1981 — International Seminar on Nuclear War — 1st Session: The World-wide Implications of Nuclear War

1982 — International Seminar on Nuclear War — 2nd Session: How to Avoid a Nuclear War

1983 — International Seminar on Nuclear War — 3rd Session: The Technical Basis for Peace

1984 — International Seminar on Nuclear War — 4th Session: The Nuclear Winter and the New Defence Systems: Problems and Perspectives

1985 — International Seminar on Nuclear War — 5th Session: SDI, Computer Simulation, New Proposals to Stop the Arms Race

1986 — International Seminar on Nuclear War — 6th Session: International Cooperation: The Alternatives

1987 — International Seminar on Nuclear War — 7th Session: The Great Projects for Scientific Collaboration East-West-North-South

1988 — International Seminar on Nuclear War — 8th Session: The New Threats: Space and Chemical Weapons — What Can be Done with the Retired I.N.F. Missiles-Laser Technology

1989 — International Seminar on Nuclear War — 9th Session: The New Emergencies

1990 — International Seminar on Nuclear War — 10th Session: The New Role of Science

1991 — International Seminar on Nuclear War — 11th Session: Planetary Emergencies

1991 — International Seminar on Nuclear War — 12th Session: Science Confronted with War (unpublished)

1991 — International Seminar on Nuclear War and Planetary Emergencies — 13th Session: Satellite Monitoring of the Global Environment (unpublished)

1992 — International Seminar on Nuclear War and Planetary Emergencies — 14th Session: Innovative Technologies for Cleaning the Environment

1992 — International Seminar on Nuclear War and Planetary Emergencies — 15th Session (1st Seminar after Rio): Science and Technology to Save the Earth (unpublished)

1992 — International Seminar on Nuclear War and Planetary Emergencies — 16th Session (2nd Seminar after Rio): Proliferation of Weapons for Mass Destruction and Cooperation on Defence Systems

1993 — International Seminar on Planetary Emergencies — 17th Workshop: The Collision of an Asteroid or Comet with the Earth (unpublished)

1993 — International Seminar on Nuclear War and Planetary Emergencies — 18th Session (4th Seminar after Rio): Global Stability Through Disarmament

1994 — International Seminar on Nuclear War and Planetary Emergencies — 19th Session (5th Seminar after Rio): Science after the Cold War

1995 — International Seminar on Nuclear War and Planetary Emergencies — 20th Session (6th Seminar after Rio): The Role of Science in the Third Millennium

1996 — International Seminar on Nuclear War and Planetary Emergencies — 21st Session (7th Seminar after Rio): New Epidemics, Second Cold War, Decommissioning, Terrorism and Proliferation

1997 — International Seminar on Nuclear War and Planetary Emergencies — 22nd Session (8th Seminar after Rio): Nuclear Submarine Decontamination, Chemical Stockpiled Weapons, New Epidemics, Cloning of Genes, New Military Threats, Global Planetary Changes, Cosmic Objects & Energy

1998 — International Seminar on Nuclear War and Planetary Emergencies — 23rd Session (9th Seminar after Rio): Medicine & Biotechnologies, Proliferation & Weapons of Mass Destruction, Climatology & El Nino, Desertification, Defence Against Cosmic Objects, Water & Pollution, Food, Energy, Limits of Development, The Role of Permanent Monitoring Panels

1999 — International Seminar on Nuclear War and Planetary Emergencies — 24th Session: HIV/AIDS Vaccine Needs, Biotechnology, Neuropathologies, Development Sustainability — Focus Africa, Climate and Weather Predictions, Energy, Water, Weapons of Mass Destruction, The Role of Permanent Monitoring Panels, HIV Think Tank Workshop, Fertility Problems Workshop

2000 — International Seminar on Nuclear War and Planetary Emergencies — 25th Session: Water — Pollution, Biotechnology — Transgenic Plant Vaccine, Energy, Black Sea Pollution, Aids — Mother–Infant HIV Transmission, Transmissible Spongiform Encephalopathy, Limits of Development — Megacities, Missile Proliferation and Defense, Information Security, Cosmic Objects, Desertification, Carbon Sequestration and Sustainability, Climatic Changes, Global Monitoring of Planet, Mathematics and Democracy, Science and Journalism, Permanent Monitoring Panel Reports, Water for Megacities Workshop, Black Sea Workshop, Transgenic Plants Workshop, Research Resources Workshop, Mother–Infant HIV Transmission Workshop, Sequestration and Desertification Workshop, Focus Africa Workshop

2001 — International Seminar on Nuclear War and Planetary Emergencies — 26th Session: AIDS and Infectious Diseases — Medication or Vaccination for Developing Countries; Missile Proliferation and Defense; Tchernobyl — Mathematics and Democracy; Transmissible Spongiform Encephalopathy; Floods and Extreme Weather Events — Coastal Zone Problems; Science and Technology for Developing Countries; Water — Transboundary Water Conflicts; Climatic Changes — Global Monitoring of the Planet; Information Security; Pollution in the Caspian Sea; Permanent Monitoring Panels Reports; Transmissible Spongiform Encephalopathy Workshop; AIDS and Infectious Diseases Workshop; Pollution Workshop

2002 — International Seminar on Nuclear War and Planetary Emergencies — 27th Session: Society and Structures: Historical Perspectives — Culture and Ideology; National and Regional Geopolitical Issues; Globalization — Economy and Culture; Human Rights — Freedom and Democracy Debate; Confrontations and Countermeasures: Present and Future Confrontations; Psychology of Terrorism; Defensive Countermeasures; Preventive Countermeasures; General Debate; Science and Technology: Emergencies; Pollution, Climate — Greenhouse Effect; Desertification, Water Pollution, Algal Bloom; Brain and Behaviour Diseases; The Cultural Emergency: General Debate and Conclusions; Permanent Monitoring Panel Reports; Information Security Workshop; Kangaroo Mother's Care Workshop; Brain and Behaviour Diseases Workshop

THE SCIENCE AND CULTURE SERIES
Nuclear Strategy and Peace Technology

INTERNATIONAL SEMINAR ON
NUCLEAR WAR AND PLANETARY EMERGENCIES
27th Session:

SOCIETY AND STRUCTURES: HISTORICAL PERSPECTIVES — CULTURE AND IDEOLOGY; NATIONAL AND REGIONAL GEOPOLITICAL ISSUES; GLOBALIZATION — ECONOMY AND CULTURE; HUMAN RIGHTS — FREEDOM AND DEMOCRACY DEBATE; CONFRONTATIONS AND COUNTERMEASURES: PRESENT AND FUTURE CONFRONTATIONS; PSYCHOLOGY OF TERRORISM; DEFENSIVE COUNTERMEASURES; PREVENTIVE COUNTERMEASURES; GENERAL DEBATE; SCIENCE AND TECHNOLOGY: EMERGENCIES; POLLUTION; CLIMATE — GREENHOUSE EFFECT; DESERTIFICATION, WATER POLLUTION, ALGAL BLOOM; BRAIN AND BEHAVIOUR DISEASES; THE CULTURAL EMERGENCY: GENERAL DEBATE AND CONCLUSIONS; PERMANENT MONITORING PANEL REPORTS; INFORMATION SECURITY WORKSHOP; KANGAROO MOTHER'S CARE WORKSHOP; BRAIN AND BEHAVIOUR DISEASES WORKSHOP

"E. Majorana" Centre for Scientific Culture
Erice, Italy, 18–26 August 2002

Series editor and Chairman: A. Zichichi

edited by R. Ragaini

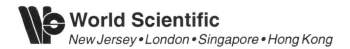

World Scientific
New Jersey • London • Singapore • Hong Kong

Published by

World Scientific Publishing Co. Pte. Ltd.
5 Toh Tuck Link, Singapore 596224
USA office: Suite 202, 1060 Main Street, River Edge, NJ 07661
UK office: 57 Shelton Street, Covent Garden, London WC2H 9HE

INTERNATIONAL SEMINAR ON NUCLEAR WAR AND PLANETARY EMERGENCIES 27TH SESSION: SOCIETY AND STRUCTURES: HISTORICAL PERSPECTIVES — CULTURE AND IDEOLOGY; NATIONAL AND REGIONAL GEOPOLITICAL ISSUES; GLOBALIZATION — ECONOMY AND CULTURE; HUMAN RIGHTS — FREEDOM AND DEMOCRACY DEBATE; CONFRONTATIONS AND COUNTERMEASURES: PRESENT AND FUTURE CONFRONTATIONS; PSYCHOLOGY OF TERRORISM; DEFENSIVE COUNTERMEASURES; PREVENTIVE COUNTERMEASURES; GENERAL DEBATE; SCIENCE AND TECHNOLOGY: EMERGENCIES; POLLUTION; CLIMATE — GREENHOUSE EFFECT; DESERTIFICATION, WATER POLLUTION, ALGAL BLOOM; BRAIN AND BEHAVIOUR DISEASES; THE CULTURAL EMERGENCY: GENERAL DEBATE AND CONCLUSIONS; PERMANENT MONITORING PANEL REPORTS; INFORMATION SECURITY WORKSHOP; KANGAROO MOTHER'S CARE WORKSHOP; BRAIN AND BEHAVIOUR DISEASES WORKSHOP

ISBN 981-238-361-1

This book is printed on acid-free paper.

Printed in Singapore by Uto-Print

CONTENTS

7. CONFRONTATIONS AND COUNTERMEASURES: PSYCHOLOGY OF TERRORISM

8. CONFRONTATIONS AND COUNTERMEASURES: DEFENSIVE COUNTERMEASURES

17. BRAIN AND BEHAVIOUR DISEASES WORKSHOP

OPENING SESSION

THE CULTURAL EMERGENCY

TSUNG-DAO LEE
Department of Physics, Columbia University, New York, NY, USA

KAI M.B. SIEGBAHN
Institute of Physics, University of Uppsala, Uppsala, Sweden

ANTONINO ZICHICHI
University of Bologna, Bologna, Italy; CERN, Geneva, Switzerland

Our scientific community watched in speechless horror, along with the rest of the planet, as hijacked civilian planes filled with passengers were crashed into skyscraper towers where tens of thousands of ordinary people were working. This is the reason for the choice of this year's topic: the Cultural Emergency.

Slaughter and massacres have been with us since the dawn of civilization, and witnesses and survivors always carry, ever after, a deep festering wound from having been involved in a horrible experience. We do not have to go back a thousand years to find dramatic examples of wanton manslaughter, all we have to do is look back at the last century. Then why is it that 9/11 had such an impact? September 11th is not "statistically" significant but it was the first time that billions could watch a large-scale massacre being perpetrated.

We are now faced with the Third Challenge. The two previous ones were perhaps easier to solve. We knew what we were basically facing: the Nuclear Holocaust in the eighties and, 10 years later, that of the risk of an Environmental Holocaust. N o o ne h ad predicted t he a rrival o f Terrorism e xcept i n E rice i n 1 996, during the 21st Session[1] of our International Seminar series.

Could Science contribute to understanding its roots, how to act and, first of all, what to do to overcome it? We should not forget the past: i.e. a few years ago when the world was ruled by two super-powers. Terrorism is the unexpected phase following the end of the bipolar world.

It was at the beginning of the eighties that Science at last decided to descend from its ivory towers to take part in the culture of our time with all its lucidity and determination. The future of the world was at stake. In their arsenals, the two

---

[1] See "High-Tech Terrorism as an Increasing Global Problem", Professor Karl Rebane, text annexed to Professor Rebane's current presentation.

superpowers (USA and USSR) had 60 thousand H-bombs and each of them had a destructive power 60 times higher than the one that destroyed Hiroshima. Ten thousand scientists of 115 nations signed The Erice Statement in which it was clearly stated that the armaments race was not the inevitable consequence of scientific progress but the evidence that political violence was spreading all over the world. The Erice Statement did not divide the world into good and bad but claimed for Science a source of good values, distinguishing it from the Use of Science (Technology). In this work of promoting Scientific Culture, Science found an ally of rare and exceptional value: John Paul II. Today, no one any longer confuses Science with bombs and Planetary Emergencies. In fact, the danger of the Nuclear Holocaust being overcome with the fall of the Berlin Wall, the Pope invited us to study the Planetary Emergencies carrying out the *scientific voluntarism*, which is *"one of the noblest forms"* says John Paul II, *"of love towards our fellows."*

Our response to the Second Challenge was to realise several dozens of pilot projects all over the world. One of which was related to the stopping of desertification. The pilot projects are listed in Annex A.The results yielded by our pilot projects represent the only concrete proof, brought to the attention of governments, that the 53 Planetary Emergencies could be overcome. Here we need to reflect a moment on the fact that, in none of our plenary, restricted or specialised sessions had we ever considered that Terrorism could be one of the new planetary menaces. We had discussed the dangers related to cheap weaponry such as those of Mass Destruction (WMDs), the chemical and the bacteriological bombs.

No one could foresee what occurred on September 11th and the subsequent developments, giving rise to the Third Challenge for Science, which will be the topic of our discussions during this 27th Session of the Erice Seminars. We are in fact convinced that scientific unity leads first to economic unity and then to political unity, thus stopping all conflicts. As Europeans, we can only ponder at the two nearly successful "suicide attempts" of the First and Second World Wars, and the state of Europe with 50 years of peace behind us.

It was the European scientists themselves who implemented, right after the Second World War, the basis of an effective scientific collaboration between the nations, which had been at war for centuries. Where there is scientific unity, there is no room for disagreements and political fights.

The Third Challenge will reside in finding out scientific and technological common grounds of interest to all: the rich (North) and the poor (South). It is beyond dispute that the developing Countries (5 billion people) cannot and must not repeat our mistakes: our Civilization is in danger. The problems of "sustainable development" must be discussed and studied without any conflict, in an atmosphere of rigorous knowledge of the problems, mutual trust and effective collaboration. The roots of Terrorism must be understood thoroughly since the first enemy of humanity is emerging in all its clearness, and it is Ignorance.

We need to open the doors of our scientific laboratories to the best intellectual energies without ideological, political, or racial barriers.

Scientific, medical and technological problems must be addressed inside an international collaboration in order to determine if Science can contribute to the solutions required by the Third Challenge.

After believing, throughout the twentieth century, that we had finally entered the age of enlightenment, our whole planet suddenly realised that it was sick. A sickness of the soul that our doctors cannot cure. Nor can our politicians reassure us with a spectrum of attitudes going from extreme posturing to total apathy. A sickness that our community identified, 20 years ago, as the Cultural Planetary Emergency.

Since 1986, the World Federation of Scientists has confronted – as mentioned above – many Planetary Emergencies and has proved, by conducting pilot-projects, that they could be mitigated or eradicated, provided there is a political will. In terms of our fight against the Cultural Emergency, we have been trying to educate the media on the difference between Science and Technology, and the necessity for objective and measured reporting of scientific and technological discoveries. Up to now, little has been done since the solutions were, and still are, in the hands of non-scientists.

We have to ask ourselves how we can avoid a Cultural Holocaust if we don't come up quickly with concrete proposals. The Cultural Emergency, unlike other Emergencies, is entirely fuelled by mankind. It has now proved to all that it could devour our civilisation if left unattended. We believe that the time has come for us to play a significant role in the mitigation of the Cultural Emergency.

For those of you who participate in our Meetings for the first time, and who might think we are "poets and dreamers," let me tell you why we believe we can contribute to the solution of what has become the most important of all Planetary Emergencies. We are the largest international "no strings attached" scientific community of volunteers. We can call on thousands of scientists the world over, who all achieved the highest responsability in advanced research activities, covering all fields of Science and Technology. Let me recall that 22 years of activity in project implementation and the results, shown in Annex A, represent our best source of self confidence.

Sometimes, through some of our members, our conclusions and recommendations have been heeded at the highest political levels. This was the case during the Nuclear War Seminars, prior to the ratification of the Salt II Treaty, with the Erice Statement which stimulated a series of actions from Deng Xiao Ping, Mikhail Gorbachev, Olaf Palme, Sandro Pertini, Ronald Reagan, Pierre Trudeau and John Paul II.

Scientists are, by definition and by training, rational in their approach to a problem and used to solving complex and involved issues. By reviewing and analysing the problems at hand, with the help of eminent specialists in the relevant domains, we can arrive at certain conclusions and propose solutions, which can then be disseminated throughout our community, worldwide. During this Seminar, participants will be able to discuss conflicting views with a wide selection of factions, both officially during the debates and unofficially outside the lecture halls.

During the first days of the Seminar, some of our very eminent colleagues in various disciplines will describe the conflict situations, point out the determining factors and try to unravel the intricacy of measures and countermeasures. On the third day, we will split up into four Groups: while most of us continue hearing reports on other Emergencies in this very Hall. The following three Working Groups will convene elsewhere:

Society and Structures – Group A – chaired by William Shea, on:
"Culture – Ideology – Human Rights – Freedom & Democracy"
Society and Structures – Group B – chaired by K.C. Sivaramakrishnan, on:
"Economy – National and Regional Geopolitical Issues"
Confrontations & Countermeasures – chaired by R.A. Mason, on:
"Present and Future Confrontations–Preventive and Defensive Countermeasures".

The Working Groups will deliberate for a full day and each is expected to produce a written summary, synthesising the main issues of its Emergency subtopics and their probable consequences. The summary should contain a series of proposed recommendations for their mitigation, through actions to be undertaken by the international scientific community in general and the World Federation of Scientists in particular.

On 23 August, during the Debate and Conclusion Session, each group representative will present his report to the General Assembly, following which, we hope to be in a position to draft a proposal for concrete steps to be taken by the scientific community worldwide.

ANNEX A

PROJECT IMPLEMENTATION WORLDWIDE

THE 55 IMPLEMENTED PILOT–PROJECTS which demonstrate how to avoid an environmental holocaust

The World Federation of Scientists has implemented 55 projects in 50 developing countries. Its scientific achievements are highlighted hereafter:

1. *A programme on desertification* has shown that this process is in fact foreseeable and can be halted and even induced to revert.
2. *Mathematical models to predict droughts and floods* were developed and shown to be effective for long-term, large-scale predictions.
3. *The damming effect of mountain ranges* on the pattern of monsoons and its consequences on the extent of droughts have been demonstrated.
4. *The forecast of extreme, localised meteorological events* by using inexpensive hardware and software was developed for application in the Mediterranean Basin and made available to developing countries world-wide.
5. *An advanced seismological network to detect seismic events* in the Mediterranean basin has been completed. In addition, three regional seismic networks were installed in seismic-prone developing countries. The data collected are not only of immediate use by the beneficiary countries but are also centralised for detailed analysis in Rome, in order to determine models for predicting seismic events.
6. *A system for forecasting and controlling the rise in the water level* of the Yellow River basin has been implemented. This system will prevent a loss of human life numbered in millions and regulate the serious problem of sedimentation.
7. *The psychological, social and economic consequences of deafness* in pre-school children can now be avoided.
8. *The scientific proof of a new ambulatory method of caring for babies* born prematurely in developing countries, where access to incubators is limited, has been demonstrated and implemented in Latin America, Asia and Africa.
9. *Within the context of research efforts to discover an AIDS vaccine,* the World Laboratory's world-wide network against AIDS established Research Centres in East and West Africa.
10. *Numerous bright young scientists* from developing countries have been able to take part in experimental programmes at the forefront of scientific research in high-energy physics at CERN.
11. *Detectors employing highly sophisticated technology* have been developed for the accelerators of the future.
12. *Spectroscopy equipment* for environmental research, based on laser ablation of *bio-molecules,* were developed to detect minute quantities and record molecular weights up to one million Daltons, and amino acid sequences in proteins.
13. *A World Laboratory Nuclear Fusion Centre* has been set up in China to train young physicists from Southeast Asia.

14. *A research, development and application programme* on renewable energy sources is being undertaken in the field of photovoltaic and nanocrystalline cells.

15. *A new approach towards promoting interaction between industry and university research* has been implemented in Buenos Aires.

16. *An epidemiological survey of heart diseases* was conducted in Kenya and 2 research centres were established in East Africa.

17. *A new source of protein* has been developed based on the cultivation of a variety of bean.

18. *An extensive training programme in advanced biotechnologies* has been implemented and three research centres established in China

19. *Scientists from 10 countries of the Mediterranean basin* were trained in meteorological and oceanographic modelling and three research centres have been established in the Mediterranean area.

20. *Thanks to the different research programmes of the World Laboratory, some 1,200 man-years of scholarships* have been granted to young scientists from 39 different developing countries, thereby allowing them to participate in research work at the very highest scientific level and under the direct supervision of eminent scientists.

2. SOCIETY AND STRUCTURES: HISTORICAL PERSPECTIVES — CULTURE AND IDEOLOGY

SMILE AND FEEL SECURE, GOD IS WITH THE BELIEVERS:[1] RELIGION AND THE CAPACITY FOR GLOBAL TERROR

EDA SAGARRA

Irish Research Council for the Humanities and Social Sciences, Dublin, Ireland

God has been on 'our' side for as long as the world's great monotheistic religions have seen politics as the spread of divine truth by other means. As long as they have, in a word, confused faith with forms of colonial imperialism. Which most, if not all, have done at some point in their history, and some still do today. The deadly slogan of my title, which allegedly legitimized the Twin Towers Massacre, only echoes the words of other religious fanatics, such as the thirteenth-century papal legate who, when ordering the burning alive of the 'heretical' citizens of the Cathar city of Beziers, is quoted as having declared: 'God will recognise His own.'[2] And even those religions which no longer hold to such practices have left behind them a potentially lethal legacy: namely, the notion of messianic conversion plus an arsenal of manipulative rhetoric, which other faiths and indeed many secular regimes have proved eager to adopt and exploit.

We are all of us gathered here as scientists, using the term in the inclusive sense that all but native English speakers employ. Our numbers include (I quote from our seminar programme): 'eminent economists, decision makers, defence specialists, political analysts and sociologists.' Cultural historians seem also well represented among us. Scientists come with impeccable credentials. They are children of the Enlightenment, seekers after Truth in the service of the betterment of humankind. (There have been a few blips in past times, to be sure, as the Harvard biologist Richard Lewonthin, among others, has highlighted,[3] but they count as nothing by comparison with the record of monotheistic religion in human history.) The modern theologian, on the other hand, has no such ease of conscience. The Christian theologian, in particular, carries a burdensome heritage. He and his kind may be said to have contributed at least as much to human wretchedness as to human happiness, as much to conflict as to its resolution, to have contributed more to dividing humanity rather than uniting it. And if tolerance is in evidence in Christian discourse in many parts of the world nowadays, could this not be seen simply as a desperate strategy, a panic reaction to the irrelevance of belief in the western world?

Tolerance, moreover, tends to appeal to officers more than men, to those who are secure more than to those who are vulnerable. World-wide, the appeal of the comforting certainties of religious fundamentalism is winning far more converts, not just to Islam, but also to certain forms of Judaism and to the ranks of fundamentalist Christians who view society and the political process through the intolerant spectacles of a literal creed. Their contempt for critical self-reflection makes them unattractive partners for scientific discourse. And how, a reasonable scientist may ask, can you engage with someone who disputes your right to be?

How do you deal with the dilemma of Hilaire Belloc's ditty:

Pale Ebenezer thought it wrong to fight
But Roaring Bill, who killed him, thought it right

Roaring Bill apart, it is a characteristic of modern western secular thought, from which our system of international relations derives, to have particular difficulties with systems of belief, thought and behaviour which blur or negate the distinction between politics and religion. And so we fail to engage with them. But can we afford not to? Surely, the singularity, peculiarity and deadly power of the 'asymmetric warfare'[4] unleashed on the West last September, derive from the total blurring of that distinction. Some cultural analysis of the phenomenon would seem relevant to a discussion on modern global terror.

I propose in this short paper to look at how theologians associated with that rather unique institution, the Irish School of Ecumenics, have engaged with the issue of faith and violence as exemplified in the Northern Ireland conflict. And, secondly, how they are attempting, at the level of praxis, often as behind-the-scene pastoral mediators, and through engagement with theologians and scholars of different disciplines across the world, to contribute to its resolution. The efforts of ecumenical theologians do not win general approval, either with their own authorities, who see them as potential religious or moral relativists, or with orthodox theologians, who mistrust what they see as their political agenda. And certainly not with the fundamentalists, with whom they seek to reconcile. Irish ecumenist theologians offend all sides with their focus on what they identify as 'the hermeneutics of suspicion.'[5] And suspicion of the Other is, in Northern Ireland, in the Middle East, in parts of Pakistan and India or the North American Bible Belt, a key element in the armoury of moral certitude. Ecumenical theologians, then, are seen as subversive, as 'rocking' the boat. Which is what they largely intend. The modern theologian is, as is not always understood, both philosopher and cultural critic. A key feature of ecumenical academic enquiry is the general recognition of the need to understand cultural difference, and especially the cultural and linguistic character of doctrinal statement. He or she -and today it is quite often a 'she' -are remarkably close to those eighteenth-century enlightened advocates of *'sapere Qude,'* whose 'dare to know' constituted the first effective nail in the coffin of Christian and religious orthodoxy. Moreover, in challenging the values of that once so conservative society, that of Ireland, theologians have worked with civil rights activists,[6] to be a little-publicised but nonetheless profound influence for change.

What has all this got to do with 'global terror' or at least with 'faith and violence?' Quite a lot. For the resistance to the Other, self-definition *ex negativo,* the self-righteous rejection of any claim to truth on the part of the Other and the belief in the permissibility of violence to 'defend' the 'true faith' are all at least as entrenched in the Northern Ireland conflict as in anywhere else in the world. The dogmatic slogan: 'Error has no rights' which would legitimate in the eyes of the perpetrators and their leaders the killing by a few 'martyrs' of 4000 innocent people of sixty nations, has long since found a chord in the hearts of northern fundamentalists who attack the religious services and sacred places of the 'other' Christian community. The blurring of the spheres of politics and religion in both cases is absolute. Ecumenism is about changing that but also changing, through reflection, the language, and particularly the metaphors, that people inhabit.[7] Hermeneutics, the de-construction and re-construction of identity, of ethnicity, of memory, as of history, are central areas of enquiry for the modern ecumenical theologian. Small wonder that many of them have a particular attraction to modern Ulster lyric poets, such as John Hewitt or Seamus Heaney, whose work so subtly explores the way in which the 'acrimonious dead' shape these issues in Northern Ireland.[8] Small wonder too, that they should draw the venom of those they would help, often in the colourful language of Old Testament rhetoric absurdly pressed into the service of one's own prejudices. As a fundamentalist Protestant cleric phrased it in a student debate on the subject I once chaired: 'Ecumenism', he roared, 'is the thin end of the Scarlet Woman.' Ecumenical enquiry, as pursued by theologians, cleric and lay, in the Irish School of Ecumenics, focuses on the theologies of the conflict and how these determine social behaviour, often in areas far removed from matters of doctrine or belief. Theologians of all Christian confessions recognise theology as always having been an essential part of the problem. In the North of Ireland, as in other religious conflicts, the churches have provided a theology to act as an 'interpretative framework' for each side. Thus, Republican nationalist theology has long defined itself as victimhood, the native nationalist population seeing themselves as the victim of colonial imperialism, identifying their sufferings with the crucifixion of Christ and favouring the resurrection metaphor to encapsulate their vision of future successful revolution. That the 1916 Irish Rising was an 'Easter Rising' made it all the more potent. Northern Protestant Unionist theology, by contrast, embraces a doctrine of Covenant: the confiscation of the land of the 'barbarous' native Irish Catholics by the seventeenth-century British authorities and its planting with Scottish and English Protestant settlers came to be interpreted as a God-given mission, a Covenant with the Almighty to which the settlers and their descendants must hold fast. They must remain faithful under attack, in a land in which they were the rulers, but a permanent minority. The siege mentality is as powerful in certain Northern Protestant circles today as ever it has been.[9] Memory, re-enacted as religious and political ritual in the annual marching season and inscribed in the discourse of the politicians, assures the lethal potency of that Covenant and sense of siege. The Irish nationalist funeral commemorations, an equally dogged ritual, ensures the survival of the ancient sense of victimhood among the Catholic community. Analogies will not be hard to seek in other such religiously-informed conflicts.

Elizabeth Bowen nicely encapsulates the acrimonious difference of the two theologies in her line about 'we,' that is, the propertied, those of us secure in the comfort of our beliefs and possessions, having everything to dread from the 'dispossessed.'[10] As scientists we need a nuanced understanding, at intuitive as well as cognitive level, of the compensatory role of religion in vulnerable people's lives, in those who have lost, or believe they have lost, social hope.[11] And vulnerability comes in many guises. To a Northern Ireland Roman Catholic today, long conditioned to a sense of second-class citizenship in his or her native place, defined for more than a century as 'Ulster: a Protestant state for a Protestant people', it is hard to accept present-day Unionists in the role of 'vulnerable' But they are. That the Northern Ireland education system, brilliantly exploited by the nationalist minority, i.e. by the 'victims', aided by the religious teaching orders, has now created a vibrant and successful middle class from among the former unskilled classes, exacerbates the sense of siege. This is particularly true in those working-class Protestant areas whose skill base and higher standard of living/conspicuous consumption has been destroyed by the second industrial revolution, by the collapse of the ship building, textiles, steel industries in Belfast. Oddly enough, Catholic nationalists, much more than Protestants, have favoured the new technological industries. Moreover, demography is on the side of the nationalists. Even the British government seems to be. An elite faced with the loss of traditional power *is* vulnerable as well as being more prone to violence. And the nationalist community at every level must learn to understand this. To understand and accept the 'Other,' while yet being able to disagree with his or her beliefs, is just as important for the Roman Catholic nationalist as for the Protestant Unionist who believes that to be a Roman Catholic is not to have the right to call oneself a Christian. This is but one of the things ecumenicists in Ireland are seeking to work through at community level.

This is one of the reasons why in every project, the Irish School of Ecumenics tries to translate the findings of research into practical application, as in continuing education and training, community, youth and schools projects. This is also why in every initiative, there are always partners from different, and traditionally opposing Christian dispensations working together. Probably the most ambitious has been *'Moving beyond Sectarianism'*. Here models of facing and dealing with the quite extraordinarily bitter and deep-rooted sectarianism which is part of the daily life of Northern Ireland, have been developed and tested with diverse groups such the police, school children, community workers, clergy, paramilitaries etc. The directors of the six-year research project, *Moving Beyond Sectarianism,* Joseph Liechty and Cecelia Clegg come from very different dispensations, the one an American Mennonite historian, the other a Roman Catholic nun, psychologist and theologian. Like all such ecumenical partnerships, they do not share each other's beliefs, but they honour their authenticity. For ecumenism is *not* a kind of 'spiritual esperanto'[12]. Many of their insights, such as the role of 'idolatrous loyalty to the nation' in religious belief and practice, of the role of the clergy as 'tribal chaplains' are sharpened by reference to other types of politico-religious conflict, such as the Serbo-Croat.[13] What might well be of interest to those involved in conflict resolution, is their chapter on what they call 'mitigation.'[14] By 'mitigation' they mean a situation of negotiation where 'non-negotiables' (of which monotheistic religions have many) are 'mitigated' by the parties' (initially of course, the facilitators') concentrating on lessening or even eliminating negative outcomes of a belief, a commitment, or an action. They do so by appealing to resources from within that tradition, or, at least resources not in conflict with that tradition. The Bible, which is such a doughty weapon in the hands of Christian fundamentalists, they note ironically yet in deadly earnest, 'is a treasury of mitigating principles' (237), – even including for Roman Catholics the issue of women priests.

It is perhaps necessary for secular science to appreciate that religious belief is anything but monolithic, and that religion, like theologians, has an astonishing capacity to re-invent itself - sometimes for better, sometimes for worse. The radical re-thinking of what is known as Christian mission in the last forty years is an example of the former. What was once the object of such mission, i.e. 'conversion' and 'proselytising,' is now seen as a form of colonialism, a sort of religious 'scramble for Africa.' In place of the old medieval papal ecclesiology: *'extra ecclesiam mila salus,'* Christian missionaries recognise the authenticity, if not necessarily the validity, of the world's great religion; many, through their work on religious pluralism, have come to believe in: *'extra humanum mila salus.'* The 'scramble for Africa' has been replaced by an ethos of *'dunamis'* in the original sense of the word: to be able, or 'letting be.'[15] Christian 'missionaries' teach and try to practice or promote solidarity, self sufficiency, resistance to injustice. Latterly, agriculturalists, geneticists, primary health care workers or peacekeepers in NGOs are as likely to be the new missionaries as those in clerical garb. Of course they have an agenda. But it is surely one that can allow itself to be rated in terms of human betterment.

The relevance of all this for our present seminar is perhaps that secular modernist intellectual enquiry can, after all, derive benefit from the work of contemporary theologians and their forebears. Such work can help to give due recognition to the force religion still constitutes in certain parts of the world. It can throw light on the contribution of religious socialisation to value systems, and remind us of religion's capacity, often underestimated today, for the cultural conditioning of communities, including those who are not, or are no longer, active believers. It can also, perhaps, provide sophisticated instruments of dialogue, as for example in the area which, following the example of South Africa, has established itself on the international political agenda: forgiveness in conflict resolution.

Certainly, a number of modern theologians, who use the tools of modern cultural criticism, who are themselves, or work closely with, philosophers, psychologists, linguists, historians, political and social scientists, have made a contribution which is worth listening to, to the great policy debates of our times, including the one which indirectly gave the title to our seminar, the age-old problem of conflicting religious cosmologies, and the melancholy satrap of the monotheistic religions: violence.

REFERENCES

1.   From an anonymous document, found, it is alleged, in the possession of three of the seventeen perpetrators of the Twin Tower Massacre. Quoted by Noel Dorr in an unpublished paper (January 2002) to the Irish School of Ecumenics from

Kanan Makiya and Hassan Mneimneh, *Manual for a Raid* in *New York Review of Books* XLIX, no.1, 17 January 2002, pp. 18-21. I am grateful to Ambassador Dorr, who was Secretary General of the Department of Foreign Affairs at the time of the Belfast Agreement negotiations, for the many insights of his paper and permission to quote from it.

2. Stephen O'Shea (2000) *The Perfect Heresy: The Life and Death of the Cathars.* London Profile Books. p. 131.

3. 'Biology as Ideology,' in Eda Sagarra and Mireia Sagarra (eds) (1993) *The Dancer and the Dance.* Trinity Quatercentenary Symposium. Dublin. pp. 55-64, especially the section on sociobiology, p. 61.

4. Dorr, p. 19.

5. Some, such as the Reverend Terence P. McCaughey, Presbyterian minister and author i. a. of the influential *Memory and Redemption: Church, Politcs and Prophetic Theology.* Dublin 1993, are both.

6. See, for example, Joseph Liechty and Cecelia Clagg (2001) *Moving beyond Sectarianism. Religion, Conflict and Reconciliation in Northern Ireland.* Dublin. p. 351.

7. See the Augustinian Gabriel Daly's incisive and deeply ironical discussion of what he sees as classical Christian theology's occasional, and potentially fateful penchant for seeking univocation in metaphor: driving' a fine and evocative metaphor on to the rocks of deficient sensibility' in: 'Forgiveness and Community', in Alan D. Falconer and Joseph Liechty (eds): *Reconciling Memories.* Dublillf 1998, p. 197. Conversely he would see post-Enlightenment theology as tending in the opposite direction, towards equivocation and semantic drift in its use of metaphor, particularly in soteriology.

8. The phrase comes from Edwin Muir's poem 'The Wheel' in *Collected Poems.* London 1960, p. 105.

9. Alan D. Falconer (minister of the Church of Scotland, ISE director 1990-5 and current Secretary of the World Council of Churches): 'Remembering' in *Reconciling Memories,* p. 13. See also his 'The Reconciling Power of Forgiveness," pp. 177-194. Also Natalie Zemon Davies on the long association between religious ritual and rites of social violence in *Society and Culture in Early Modem France.* Cambridge 1987, pp. 152-187, here pp. 152f.

10. Bowen's (1984) *Court and Seven Winters.* London. p. 455.

11. See Duncan B. Forrester, 'Politics and Reconciliation', in Michael Hurley SJ (ed.), *Reconciliation in Religion and Society.* Belfast 1994, p. 111-122, here 122.

12. Trevor Smith, Vice-Chancelllor, University of Ulster in Hurley (1994), p. x. Similarly, Pope John Paul emphasised on the occasion of his invitation to representatives of twelve of the world's religions to join him in a day of prayer at Assisi in January 2002, that 'the day of prayer is not meant in any way to indulge in religious syncretism'. Quoted in *The Tablet,* 26 January 2002, p. 26.

13. The authors emphasise the particular relevance to their enquiry of the work of the Croat theologian, Miroslav Volf (1996) *Exclusion and Embrace: A Theological Exploration of Identity, Otherness, and Reconciliation.* Nashville.

14. *Moving beyond Sectarianism*, pp. 226-239.

15. The phrase is from John McQuarrie, (1977) *Principles of Christian Theology.* London. quoted in Falconer, p. 184.

THE CULTURE OF TERRORISM

FARHANG MEHR
University of Boston, Boston, MA, USA

DEFINITION OF TERRORISM

The events of September 11th in New York and the resulting horror and damage to life and property, as well as the after-effects on the U.S. economy, have assigned terrorism to the list of planetary emergencies. However, so far no comprehensive or universally accepted definition of terrorism exists. For the purposes of our present discussion, we can refer to the definition of terrorism as "a strategy of violence designed to promote a desired outcome by instilling fear in the public at large" (M.S. Bassiouni and others). This definition differentiates between freedom fighting and terrorism; while freedom fighters must work within the constraints of conventional means; terrorists operate with no such restraints. Should freedom fighters resort to a strategy of violence and the killing of innocent people, they acquire a terrorist identity.

Given the diversity of terrorist groups, the forging of an exclusive definition seems out of reach. Terrorist groups differ in their origins, their goals, their targets and their tactics. They differ in their size and structure and are committed to engaging in different levels of violence. While some operate secretly, others seek the support of different governments or factions within governments. Emphasizing these political ties, the U.S. State Department has defined terrorism as "pre-meditated, politically-motivated violence, perpetrated against non-combatant targets by substantial groups or clandestine state agents normally intended to influence an audience."

Combining elements of these two definitions, we can characterize an act of "terrorism" as one that is associated with violence, is premeditated by a group or an individual connected with a group, is addressed to the public, intends to instill fear in the public, and is aimed at changing the political, social and/or economic status quo in a non-conventional manner. Victims of a terrorist act are usually incidental to the terrorist's objective. The assassination of a political or a law-enforcement figure with the view of exhibiting the vulnerability of the regime is an exception to this rule.

The assassinations of Emperor Francis Ferdinand, Martin Luther King, Indira Ghandi, Rajiv Ghandi, John F. Kennedy, Anwar Sadat and Hassan Ali Mansoor, to name a few, were terrorist assassinations aimed at removing the leader of a country or charismatic figures of a given political movement from a position of power and creating public fear. The reward of such assassinations would be relatively minimal if the momentum of the chaos and fear was not sustained. We refer to such assassinations as acts of "private terrorism." While private terrorism involves an act of violence against an identified victim, "public terrorism" which we commonly refer to as "terrorism", involves an act of violence without regards for the identity of the victims.

Private terrorism is an old phenomenon, dating back to the time of Adam and Eve, when Cain killed Abel. As mentioned earlier, assassinations or attempted assassinations of leaders of governments and movements continue to this date. Recorded instances of public terrorism start perhaps with the Zealots and the Sicarii groups who in the first century A.D. launched terrorist attacks against their Roman occupiers. Later, from the 11th to the 13th century, the Assassins engaged in acts of terrorism against Seljuks in Iran and Mesopotamia.

DRIVING FORCES BEHIND TERRORIST ACTS

An act of terrorism may be motivated by one or several factors. Terrorist groups have diverse ideological backgrounds; communist, socialist, religious radicals, religious fundamentalist, Nazi/Fascist, anti-autocratic and nationalistic with de-colonizing or separatist aspirations. Terrorism may be home grown or imported. When imported, it is often modified to incorporate the historical and cultural values of its new host group/movement.

In examining the driving force behind terrorism, insight into the psyche of the individuals engaging in acts of terror becomes important, both as a means of preventing a given terrorist act from unfolding and as means of deterring future terrorist attacks. Thus far, psychologists and researchers in related disciplines have not identified a prototype or particular form of psychological or personality deviation in terrorists. Studying the psychological profile of terrorists is difficult given the secrecy of terrorist projects and the unavailability of the terrorists, who are either in hiding or killed as a result of their act of terrorism. These theories are therefore based on the analysis of the wills and diaries of terrorists, the court records of their collaborators and other second-hand sources.

Based on these sources, psychiatrists and psychologists have made tentative suggestions concerning pathological traits and urging impulses in would-be terrorists. One of the common characteristics of these individuals is that they have never integrated the good and bad parts of the "self." They split out the evil part of the self and project it onto others. They suffer from self-idolization and polarization of people (that is, the adopting of an "us" vs. "them" perspective). All those who think and act differently from the terrorists are viewed as evil and responsible for the misery and injustice they have identified. In contrast, the terrorists and members of their groups are good and righteous, committed to finding a remedy to the injustice and rectifying the situation despite the conventional obstacles in place. Many terrorists feel marginalized and are subjected to humiliation. Their situation has created within them a sense of frustration and desperation.

Aggressive, action-oriented with a desire for revenge, jealous as well as adventure seeking, and excitable are other characteristics mentioned as driving forces for terrorists.

These conclusions are clearly tentative and need further research. Regardless, in the absence of a uniform psychological and emotional identifier, terrorists should be considered ordinary people with needs, grievances, complaints, hopes, aspirations and aims. Where they differ is in their values, that is, whether they view the means used as justifying their ultimate objective.

THE ROLE OF SOCIAL, ECONOMIC AND POLITICAL FACTORS

As discussed above, dissidents turn to terrorism when they conclude that non-violent or conventional opposition methods have failed and will never succeed in bringing about their desired objectives. Terrorism is therefore the weaponry of the weak and the disadvantaged. Individuals feeling isolated from society at large, whether due to religious or ethnic persecution or lack of political equality and social mobility, exhibit an added frustration and sense of desperation and become easy converts to terrorist movements. Terrorist organizations give such individuals a sense of belonging and empowerment, hope for implementing changes and removing the injustice they see around them as well as a sense of purpose. At least initially, many of these organizations also provide their new recruits with higher income. New recruits often believe that they are advancing the interests of their family and their community in the long run. Acceptance within the hierarchical structure of terrorist groups provides the recruits with a sense of accomplishment and advancement, particularly as they gain greater status within the group.

The social, political and economic conditions of a given society clearly affect the rise of terrorism within that region. Political autocracy and oppression often result in injustice and humiliation. People longing for freedom, equality, fairness and justice strive to bring about change. When change within a system appears unlikely, revolt becomes the viable option. Covert movements to overthrow the government and change the social and political status quo are established. Economic deprivation in conjunction with either a perceived or truly oppressive social and or political climate encourage terrorist movements. After all, the disadvantaged within a society are the ones lacking economic, social or political power. Terrorist actions involving drug traffickers however is an exception to this rule. In those cases, the terrorist acts against political leaders, judges or law-enforcement officers are aimed at preserving the economic well being of the criminal groups.

THE MEANS AND WEAPONS OF TERRORISM

The tactics used by terrorists and their application depend on the availability of resources, including technological expertise, and the objective of the terrorist act itself. Terrorists share a collective logic which is based on a cost-benefit analysis of the given act: The cost of the operation in terms of human sacrifice (both for the terrorist members and their victims), publicity, and the financial cost on the group is weighed against the potential benefit. Often the potential benefit is the extent to which the terrorist act shatters the authority of the government or movement that is being targeted and highlights the cause of the terrorists. Other times, it is more concrete and involves the freeing of prisoners or receipt of funds.

The weapons of terrorists have changed since the days they attacked their victims with swords and daggers. By 1879, the Russian terrorist had graduated to guns for assassination. By the early 1900s, the invention of dynamite and the use of bombs allowed terrorists a greater arsenal of weapons with which to achieve their objectives. Recent advances in science have unleashed the threat of nuclear and biological terror.

Terrorism has also evolved in terms of the tactics being used by various terrorist groups. This evolution can be demonstrated in the history of many terrorist groups. In the 1950s, the Peoples Liberation Front for Palestine (PLFP) declared war on the economic and strategic interests linked to the state of Israel. The tap line in the Syrian Golan and the pipeline linking the Haifa refinery to the port of Kishan in the Mediterranean were targeted. After the explosion, both targets were repaired and it became clear that the PLFP's objective was not realized. Undeterred, terrorists linked to the Palestinian movement murdered Israeli athletes at the Munich Olympics. Faced again with a failure to meet their political objectives, the terrorists redirected their tactics to hostage-taking, plane hijackings and barricade seizures of embassies. The 1983 suicide car bombings of the U.S. embassy and marine headquarters in Lebanon added a new momentum to the terrorist movement, as it successfully resulted in the U.S. withdrawal from Lebanon. As surveillance and anti-terrorist training against this type of destruction became more sophisticated, a more sinister and creative use of the destructive force was sought, culminating in the events of September 11th. Similar changes in tactics for terrorism can be traced in various other terrorist groups including the IRA, the Tamil Tigers of Sri Lanka, the Mojahedin in Algeria, as well as the terrorist movements in Kashmir and Chechnya.

The number of innocent victims in terrorist acts is haunting. In 1977 in Iran, the Islamic radical terrorists burnt a cinema building in Ahwaz that caused the death of over 300 people. This had been preceded by assassination of political figures and several American military advisers in Iran. In 1983, 350 people were killed and more than 250 were wounded as a result of a suicidal car-bombing of the U.S. embassy and the U.S. marines' headquarters in Lebanon. A similar attack on the French paratroop headquarters in Lebanon resulted in 58 dead and 15 wounded. Timothy McVeigh's bombing of the Oklahoma federal building, the bombing of the Pan Am flight over Scotland and finally the events of September 11th have resulted in the death of over 3000 innocent people.

THE CULTURE OF TERRORISM

The culture of terrorism stems from the national, historical and religious culture of the people. It is shaped by prevailing socio-economic and political conditions, the innovative characteristics, ambitions and aspirations of the terrorist group leaders. It is indigenous, even though, as mentioned before, the group adopts parts of the culture of other terrorist groups. This is particularly true of ideological and religious terrorist groups. Individuals who join terrorist groups may receive recognition at the initial stage, but have to give up their individuality in favor of the group identity. The leaders of the groups are as ambitious and interested in survival and image maintenance as the leaders of the governments or movements they oppose. Members of most terrorist groups cannot challenge the leaders' decision and do so only at the risk of being eliminated.

The culture of terrorism is fortified through education and indoctrination by parents at home, teachers and peers at schools, as well as writers and artists working from within the community and abroad. Pressure by peers may take the form of reproaches for cowardice and a non-patriotic attitude. Indoctrination is a mission-oriented education that leads to fanaticism. The textbooks in ideological and theocratic states, as well as schools set up or sponsored by terrorist groups, teach hatred of the "enemies" and focus on the legitimacy of their own ideology or religion. Globalization and the ready access to televisions, satellites and, in some instances, the Internet, have increased the influence of writers and the media on public opinion.

The number of incidences involving religious terrorism throughout the world is increasing. This may be in part due to the religious radicals' emphasis on the difference between 'believers' and 'heretics.' The terrorist events in Gujarat between Hindus and Muslims, in East Timor, the Philippines, Egypt, Sudan and Nigeria between Muslims and Christians, in Pakistan between the Shi'ite and Sunni sects of Islam, and in China where Tibetan monks have been subject to acts of violence, show that religious terrorism is not a phenomenon peculiar to the Middle East, and in particular the Arab-Israeli conflict. However, the complexity of the situation in the region and the fact that it has been the subject of much recent debate makes it an interesting point of focus for our discussion.

For the Jews of Israel and Zionists, self-revelation that Israel is the Promised Land to which the Israelis should return after slavery and oppression is of crucial importance. Orthodox Jews therefore maintain that all of Palestine and Jerusalem belongs to them. After initially immigrating to the Promised Land, Zionist Jews resorted to terrorism to reclaim and establish their own state. In 1939 the Jewish terrorist group 'Irgun' began an attack on public gathering places, British administrative buildings and law enforcement officers in Palestine. In 1944 the Israeli terrorist group 'LEHI' (Fighters for Freedom of Israel) assassinated Lord Moyne, the British deputy minister of state for Middle East affairs in Cairo. In 1949, the same terrorist group assassinated the UN mediator, Count Folke Bernadotte of Sweden.

The Muslims who had lived in that geographical area since the time of Salaholdin Ayoubi consider it a land belonging to Uma (the Islamic community). Muslims also believe that the followers of other religions in Dar al-Salam or the "Zone of Islam" should remain subordinate to Muslims. Palestinians, after being displaced from their homes in the twentieth century, began a movement to oppose the existence of Israel. Terrorism was seen as a legitimate means to reclaim the lost land. During this period, Palestinians organized numerous groups, some of which were terrorists. These groups sometimes cooperated under the umbrella of FATAH or PFLP, and at other times fought independently as they did not always agree on the means for accomplishing their goals. As mentioned earlier, in the 1970s, resort to new techniques such as hostage-taking and plane-hijacking gave the terrorists the opportunity to bargain and secure concessions from governments. This was followed in the 1980s with a wave of suicidal car-bombings and individual suicide bombings, the latter being used more frequently today. The recent wave of suicide bombings raises questions as to whether the Palestinian terrorist groups are engaging in a long-term evaluation of the viability of their tactics which are now, literally, self-destruction and the reduction of their numbers. Unfortunately, the uncompromising attitude on the part of both Israelis and Palestinians, has not resulted in the restoration of peace.

In examining religious terrorism, it is important to examine the religious ideology that has been used to justify it. Again, focusing on the Arab-Israeli conflict reveals some interesting theological arguments for the methods used by religious terrorists.

In Islam the concept of nationality does not exist. Muslims in totality form the Uma. This fraternal position makes the Palestinian cause that of all Uma; and all Muslims are duty-bound to help Palestinians both financially and physically, in their fight against Israel. That is why the governments of Iran, Syria, Lebanon and some other Muslim states have, in different ways, supported Islamic terrorist groups like Hamas, Hezbollah, and the Mojahedin.

Also, the mounting suicide-bombings by Muslims in recent years has prompted some to argue that Islamic principles, or the Quran justify or even encourage suicide. A number of chapters in the Quran state that Muslims must sacrifice their property and the life both to defend and promote Islam. The history of Islam and its spread throughout the Middle East and Northern Africa provides evidence of this idea. A Muslim who dies for Islam becomes a shahid (martyr) and goes to Heaven to enjoy all the bounties and blessings that are there.

On the other hand, going strictly by the Quran, the act of suicide is considered a sin. Based on this reading of the Quran, suicide bombers have come under attack by some moderate Muslims. The radical Muslims try to justify the religious terrorist acts in Israel by arguing that there is a distinct difference between "readiness for death" and "seeking to die." In car-bombings, after all, there is the likelihood of escape. Furthermore, Islamic radicals argue, in a suicide bombing the decision-maker and decision-performer are different people hence the act does not amount to suicide. At most it may be considered 'attempted suicide'. Interestingly enough, in Judaism, too, suicide is a sin and those who commit suicide must be buried not in the community's cemetery but outside its wall. It must be emphasized that suicide, as a tactic, has not been limited to terrorists in the Middle East. In 1982, Bobby Sands and a group of eleven Catholic followers died as a result of a hunger strike started to protest the events in Northern Ireland.

PREVENTION AND CONTROL OF TERRORISM

Given the complex nature of terrorism, its prevention and control are problematic. One suggested response to terrorism has been to increase the cost of terrorism to the terrorists. As terrorists look for cost-efficiency, the argument is put forth that by making terrorism more costly for them, we could deter them from opting for terrorism. The Israeli government has adopted this principle and implemented a policy of destroying the homes of suicide terrorists or suspected terrorists. This often means destroying the home of their family, that is their parents and close relatives. Recently the Israeli court denied a motion by Palestinians requesting a 48-hour notice before the military destroys the home of a terrorist or suspected terrorist in the occupied territories. The continuation of the *Intifada* and the escalation of suicide bombings have called into question the success of this policy. The mounting criticism by the international community, particularly in Europe and Asia, has also raised questions about the success of this policy for the Israeli campaign on the public opinion front.

Another tactic encouraged by many and used by the Israeli government has been the deportation of the suspected terrorists. In 1993, the Israeli government deported suspected Hamas members and Islamic radicals to Southern Lebanon. A backlash of public opinion convinced the government to allow the vast majority of them to return to Israel. Recently, the Israeli government has re-employed that tactic, exiling Palestinians suspected of planning terrorist activities or aiding terrorists to the Gaza. The success of this tactic is questionable.

A second suggested response to terrorism has been to use more efficient intelligence to prevent terrorist attacks. This solution is costly and its success uncertain, particularly given the unpredictability and secrecy inherent in terrorist acts. In light of globalization and with that, the ease of transportation, it is virtually impossible to detect where, when and how one of the numerous terrorist groups in the world will launch an attack on the U.S. or Western interests. As the multitude of suicide bombings in Israel have demonstrated, this is difficult even in a limited geographical area.

A third proposed response is to counter terrorism with terrorism. In other words, engage in acts of private terrorism, which target terrorist leaders and eliminate their sanctuaries. As terrorism in all its forms is against international law and may involve the death of many innocent people, public opinion is unlikely to sanction such acts of violence, even when the evidence on which it is based may be questionable.

The best alternative is somewhat idealistic and by all means, the most difficult one to implement. The overriding motive for terrorism is a real or perceived sense of injustice. Autocratic governments and despotic rulers with regimes that disallow non-violent methods for expressing grievances create the social, political and often economic conditions that plant the seeds for terrorism. Desperation and frustration of the disadvantaged ensure the growth of discontent and strengthen terrorism. Terrorist behavior is not a norm; it is neither a *sui generis* plague appearing from anywhere, nor an explicable random strike against humanity. The conflicts should be resolved through dialogue among governments, cultures and people. The conflicts that are conducive to terrorism are an aspect of the present clash of cultures, the economic and power gaps within particular societies as well as among different nations. Strengthening of the United Nations (UN) is imperative to this effort. Only when the UN frees itself from: (i) the influence and threats of the world powers; and (ii) the power created as a result of the alliances of weaker nations who group together for ethnic/religious reasons and economic self-interest alone, regardless of the impact of their actions on other countries or peace in the region; can the United Nations meet its objective effectively.

The resolution of terrorism requires us to understand what creates it. This requires patience for meaningful dialogue. Only through dialogue can we begin to address and remove the cynicism, fear and mistrust of the would-be terrorists. Some recent events reveal that this goal is achievable. In the last two months the IRA has publicly apologized to the relatives of the innocent victims who died in their act of violence. In addition, those involved in the assassination of Anwar Sadat declared that assassination of the president of Egypt was "un-Islamic." Albeit slowly, it seems that terrorists are realizing that violence does not pay. One hopes that the governments and powerful nations will also realize that terrorism cannot be eliminated by sheer force.

REFERENCES

1. Walter Reich (ed.), (1998) *Origins of Terrorism*. Washington, DC, Woodrow Wilson Center Press.
2. Charles D Smith (1996) *Palestine and the Arab-Israeli Conflict*. 3rd ed. New York, St. Martin's Press.
3. Michal C. Hudson (ed.) (1990) *The Palestinians: New Directions*. Washington, DC, Center for Contemporary Arab Studies.
4. Pierre Terzian (1985) *OPEC: The Inside Story*. London, Zed Books Ltd.
5. Soroosh Irfan (1983) *Revolutionary Islam in Iran*. London, Zed Books Ltd.
6. George Sale (trans.) (no date) *The Koran*. London Frederick Warne.
7. The Bible.
8. *Boston Sunday Globe*, July 4, 2002, p.1.

ISLAM AND MODERNITY: IDEOLOGY AND VIOLENCE IN THE MIDDLE EAST

KAMRAN TALATTOF

The University of Arizona, Tucson, Arizona, USA

The West spent much of the twentieth century encountering communism through the cold war, the arms race, and vigorous ideological scuffles. The ideological challenges to communism, especially by western intellectual liberal Marxists, proved effective in its demise. This historical precedent leads us to question the current situation regarding another threatening ideology: Islamic fundamentalism. Why have the West, western intellectuals, and western media not effectively engaged in an ideological dialogue and debate with Islamic fundamentalism? There are two explanations for this shortcoming. First, before the demise of the Soviet bloc, the West found an ally in Islamic fundamentalism. Second, until September 11, Islamic fundamentalist violence unfolded in certain regions in Asia and North Africa and not on American soil.

The end of the cold war and the events of September 11 have changed the notion that Islamic fundamentalist violence is solely an eastern problem. It is now a global peril, and requires not only aggressive containment and security and military measures but also, and perhaps more importantly, ideological and cultural treatment. In the latter regard, we have to recognize the significance of Islamic liberalism in its ideological struggle against fundamentalist interpretations of Islam. Islamic liberalism should be perceived as a natural ally of the West, and our foreign policy should indeed be constantly aware of this discursive conflict in the Middle East.

Islamic liberalism is an ideological and cultural reality in existence since the mid-nineteenth century in the Middle East, North Africa, and South Asia, where liberal Muslim thinkers have attempted to promote the idea that Islam and western models are compatible. For more than a century, liberal Muslims have advocated a softer, more tolerant, and more democratic version of Islam. The history of this internal debate between Islamic liberalism and Islamic fundamentalism is uneven, yet lively. Throughout history, the two contrasting trends have been outspoken and confrontational, and have at times even resorted to deadly clashes.

Islamic modernism was especially dominant during the late nineteenth and early twentieth centuries but has reemerged in places like Iran in recent decades. Prominent theologians and scholars who critically scrutinized the orthodox Islamic concepts and methods to develop new notions of jurisprudence and Islamic theology advanced this discourse. This new theological discourse resulted in a paradigmatic shift comparable to the nineteenth-century Enlightenment. Prominent Muslim thinkers from Egypt and India-Pakistan were among the advocates of this discourse. They lauded western accomplishments, such as technology, the Newtonian conception of the universe, and Darwinian evolutionism, and western styles of living. They came to believe that Islam was also capable of adapting itself to modern times and its rationality and civic order.[1]

Islamic modernists in Egypt, such as al-Afghani, through his philosophical and political writings; Muhammad Abduh, through his modern interpretation of Quran; Farid Wajdi, through sociological and political writings; Qasim Amin, through his presentation of women's issues; and Abd al-Raziq through his works on the concepts of state and polity, addressed all aspects of modernity and their implications for their own society. They strongly believed that it was through the development of these ideas that the progress of European civilization was made possible. Indian Muslims presented similar issues and arguments in the mid-nineteenth century. Sir Sayyid Ahmad Khan presented a natural theology, Chiragh Ali wrote about modernity, Shibli Nu'mani wrote hagiographies, Amir Ali defended rationalist approaches toward history, and Mumtaz Ali defended women's rights. In Iran, Islamic modernists supported the Constitutional Revolution (1905-11), which was the first major attempt to modernize the country.[2] Shiite leaders such as Ayatollah Naini defended the legitimacy of constitution-making in that country on rational grounds.[3]

An article that appeared in Aligarh Institute Gazette in the mid–nineteenth century in India exemplifies the way modernists presented their arguments:

> This union of Religion with social customs and juridical laws has done the most serious injury to the Muhammadans in every part of the world; and unless soon and timely dissolved there is every probability of the Muhammadan name becoming a by-word and the Muhammadan races a laughing stock among civilized nations... That this inability to break through the union of Religion and Law is really the cause of our decline may be proved from the history of the Christian Religion. For those nations who were able to assert and maintain the Liberty of Private Judgment have made continued progress in the arts and sciences and in civilization in general; while those nations that were unable to assert the Right of Private Judgment and succumbed to the authority of the Popes, the Bishops, and the Inquisitions have not only made no progress but have on the contrary considerably declined in civilization and power, although they won for themselves, and for a time preserved, extensive empires and almost overpowering political and military prestige among the other nations of Europe.[4]

In Egypt, the modernist Farid Wajdi by referring to European scientific amplifies the way these liberal Muslims advanced their arguments:

> In this article, we will limit our discussion to the strongest refutations against religion and their weaknesses as based on the sayings of famous European scientists. This is with the intent that our reader understands the direction that

European scientific thought has taken and becomes certain, after we cite the basics of Islam, that it is truly the destiny of souls and the grace of spirits.[5]

As mentioned, Islamic liberalism has made a second strong emergence in Iran and their confrontation with fundamentalism is no less passionate than that of their ancestors in the nineteenth century. The reformist movement in Iran impatiently seeks democracy, freedom, the assurance of human rights, and friendly relations with the West.

Islamic fundamentalism appeared with the decline of liberal-nationalism before and during the 1950s, and in the case of Iran in the late 1970s. And it appeared in an autocratic situation and in competition with other militant ideologies such as Marxism. Islamic fundamentalists categorically rejected the western capitalist model. Hasan al-Bana and Sayyid Qutb from Egypt; Abul Ala Maududi from Pakistan; Mustafa as-Siba'i from Syria; Abbasi Madani, Shaikh Nahnah, and Ali Belhaj from Algeria; Ayatollah Khomeini, Ayatollah Motahhari, and Ali Shariati from Iran all promoted absolute loyalty to a politically focused Islam and rejected non-Islamic sources of learning.

Ayatollah Khomeini, for example, presented a theory of the Islamic State based on the rule of jurisprudence and Sharia as interpreted by sanctioned clergy and applied by councils of religious leaders who were either voted into or assigned to their positions. In reciprocal degrees of fastidiousness, the democratic nature of the state and the insoluble and ultimate rule of the Supreme Muslim leader were to be secured. The inherent contradictions of this model are becoming clear with every election in Iran. But fundamentalists did and do appeal to large numbers of destitute, disenfranchised, and disillusioned Muslims. Ali Shariati, a French-educated sociologist with great influence on Iranian youth, wrote in the mid-1970s:

> *Economism* is the fundamental principle of the philosophy of life in Western industrial capitalist society, where, as Francis Bacon put it, "Science abandons its search for truth and turns to the search for power." ...Humanity is every day more condemned to alienation, more drowned in this mad maelstrom of compulsive speed. Not only is there no longer leisure for growth in human values, moral greatness, and spiritual aptitudes, but this being plunged headlong in working to consume, consuming to work, this diving into lunatic competition for luxuries and diversions, has caused traditional moral values to decline and disappear as well. ...Democracy and Western liberalism — whatever sanctity may attach to them in the abstract — are in practice nothing but the free opportunity to display all the more strongly this spirit and to create all the more speedily and roughly an arena for the profit-hungry forces that have been assigned to transform man into an economic, consuming animal.[6]

As for fundamentalist terrorists, we may describe them in several ways. From a political point of view, they are dogmatic and repressive. From a psychological point of view, they border on insanity. Culturally, they may be perceived as backward and reactionary. From a sociological point of view, their agenda is determined by the state, the colonial power against which they are fighting, the political model they have borrowed, and their stance against liberal reformist Muslims in their societies. However, these descriptions, while often true, do not explain an entire group's resolution to commit violent acts.

The problem lies in the fact that in autocratic societies and dictatorial regimes there is no room for disagreement and opposition: dissenting voices are violently extinguished. The opposition is always forced to work clandestinely, hide activities, and attract attention through planned and often violent outbursts, a process that results in internal decay. This process happens quickly if the opposition is suppressed harshly and left without any hope for freedom of expression. The rise of fundamentalism is the product of these conditions in numerous countries in the Middle East. Such movements often arise after western-supported coup d'états. In Middle Eastern countries where there is some room for oppositional political activities, fundamentalism has grown the least.

Fundamentalists commonly oppose some aspects of western civilization and what they perceive as imperialist oppression. They criticize the West for the economic and technological backwardness of their own societies and the western support of repressive regimes in the region. They adamantly defend Palestinians' rights to a nation, an issue that once symbolized Arab nationalism but is quickly becoming the aphorism of Islamic fundamentalism, and similarly they condemn the United States' unconditional support for Israeli actions and, over the last decade, the treatment of the Iraqi people. Of course, many people in the United States and the rest of the world discuss and debate these issues. What makes fundamentalists' treatment of these topics distinct is that they use these issues to promote a fictional universal ideology that is extremely incompatible with the real aspirations of the people in their societies.

What does explain the rise of Islamic fundamentalism? Previous approaches to the study of the two radically different versions of Islamic thought in this century have not been cogent in explaining the rise of Islamic fundamentalism. For example, class analysis seeks to explain the emergence of Islamic fundamentalism in terms of certain traditional middle-class interests in Middle Eastern societies. This includes the views of Middle Eastern leftist groups and the contentions of some prominent scholars of Middle Eastern studies who refer to this ideology as the "Islam of the Oppressed"[7] or the ideology of some deprived traditional middle class.[8] The Iranian Revolution clearly proved that social groups embrace fundamentalism across class divisions. Historical analyses, such as those of John Esposito and Du Pasquier, see the seed of this movement as having taken root in an early period of Islam and explain the contemporary movement in terms of early emergence of oppositional theologies.[9] This approach does not take into consideration the very modern concerns of Islamic fundamentalists, such as issues of state, women, and the West. Some scholars, however, have more successfully explored this dichotomy with regard to the questions of modernity and the West.

As noted, the West and modern concepts and the western roles in the region have had a central significance in these debates, giving rise to two distinct viewpoints on the relations between Islam and modernity. Indeed, I argue that these two discourses are responses to two contemporary western ideologies: liberal capitalism and Soviet

Marxism. Muslim responses were paradigmatic; that is, when the Islamic paradigm comes into contact with other ideological and social paradigms, it responds by producing a similar ideology in terms of socio-political agendas, rituals, and figurative language. More specifically in modern times, these responses include liberal Islam as a response to western influence and fundamentalist Islam as a response to Marxism. Each of these paradigmatic responses has its own form, characterization, and figurative language. They borrow concepts as well as metaphors from the discourse to which they are responding. The first uses liberal rationality and discursive arguments, and the second resembles the Soviet Marxist polemical style.

Like Marxists, fundamentalists are concerned with ideology, the rational sciences, and a response to the production of knowledge and science. This position is most obvious in the debates between Muslim fundamentalists and modernists over Islamic jurisprudence. Both Marxists and fundamentalist Muslims are concerned with linking their ideology with politics to devise a form of government that serves and protects their ideological and social precepts. Both have a binary notion that the world must be perceived as two camps. In the case of the fundamentalists, the camps are the dar al-Islam (the Islamic world) versus the dar al-Harb (the world of war, or the world of the infidel). For Marxists, of course, the two domains were the Soviet bloc versus the West. Each has formulas about nearly all aspects of life, including the role of women and gender relations, lifestyle, and proper behavior in various settings. Islamic fundamentalists, however, reject the notion of significant or swift social evolution and portray the West as solely an aggressive, exploitative, and materialistic force. They promote Islam as a state ideology that stands diametrically opposed to development through liberal capitalism.

However, because all religious manifestations of Islam remain faithful to the principles of the faith, and because both liberals and fundamentalists adamantly promote the acceptance of God's unity, the Qu'ran as His word, Muhammad as his prophet, and the pillars of Islam, there is reason enough to believe that both of these Islamic trends belong to the same paradigm. Yet modernist and fundamentalist Muslims provide two accounts of and two different responses to the issues facing Islamic society. They promote two different styles of life. They produce two different types of literary works. And they resemble two different modern ideologies: western liberalism and Marxism, respectively. All of these resemble each other in their appeal for universalism. All this means that assuming that the religious Islamic discourse as a whole is responsible for the promotion of violent activities is tantamount to isolating the resourceful and progressive ally in Islamic liberalism in Muslim society. It also means that just as the ideological challenges to communism were taken seriously, the significance of the debates between Islamic liberalism and Islamic fundamentalism should also be acknowledged.

Therefore, in addition to supporting Islamic liberalism, the western ideological challenge to the fundamentalists should include promoting the idea that the West has many positive things to offer: freedom, democracy, education, growth, and peace. Terrorists have none of these. Addressing cultural as well as socio-political conditions in which such violent ideologies thrive will deprive the terrorists of any possible constituency. The foreign policies of the western powers is the place to start dealing with all these issues. And to that, these foreign policies should become part of the culture of the election campaigns. Traditionally, the candidates for the parliament and the leadership of the house are well versed and skilled in local and national issues and use these issues to compete with their rivals. However, once they are in office, they face the task of handling a foreign policy that affects the lives of millions in other countries.[10] I believe that issues of foreign policy must become subjects of election campaigns and debates.

REFERENCES

1. Mansoor Moaddel and Kamran Talattof (2000) *Contemporary Debates in Islam: An Anthology of Modernist and Fundamentalist Thought* (New York: St. Martin Press), pp. 1-21.
2. Ervand Abrahamian (1982) *Iran Between Two Revolutions* (Princeton, N.J.: Princeton University Press), and Janet Afary (1996) *The Iranian Constitutional Revolution, 1906-1911: Grassroots Democracy, Social Democracy, and the Origins of Feminism* (New York: Columbia University Press).
3. Ibid.
4. Anonymous Mu'tazilite Muslim. "The Present Economical Condition of the Musalmans of Bengal," Aligarh Institute Gazzette, Vol. 12, nos. 73, 74, 75, 77, and 79 (1877-1880) in *Contemporary Debates in Islam*.
5. Farid Wajdi (2000) "Islam and Civilization," excerpt from *Al-Madaniyah wa al-Islam* [Islam and Civilization] in Mansoor Moaddel and Kamran Talattof. *Contemporary Debates in Islam: An Anthology of Modernist and Fundamentalist Thought.* New York: St. Martin Press, pp. 135-143.
6. Ali Shariati, "Modern Calamities" in Mansoor Moaddel and Kamran Talattof. *Contemporary Debates in Islam,*, pp. 315-316.
7. Juan R. Cole and Nikki Keddie, Eds, (1986) *Shi'ism and Social Protest* (New Haven: Yale University Press).
8. Misagh Parsa (1989) *Social Origins of the Iranian Revolution* (New Brunswick: Rutgers University Press).
9. John Espisito (1988) *Islam: The Straight Path* (New York: Oxford University Press), pp. 117, and Roger Du Pasquier (1992) *Unveiling Islam* (Cambridge: Redwood Press), pp. 137.
10. For example, it is imperative for the candidates to know that according to many surveys, the Israeli-Palestinian conflict has become the most important personal and social concern to Arab identity and Arab nationalism and cannot be dealt with simply through traditional lobbying efforts. Tens of polls have been conducted by as many international organizations to discern how significant the Israeli-Palestinian conflict is to people both inside and outside the Middle East. Example Gallup Polls on this subject, taken in the United States, can be found at USA Today. (online) "USA Today/CNN/Gallup Poll Results" Nation section.

Available at http://www.usatoday.com/news/nation/2002/04/08/usat-poll-mideast.htm. Accessed: August 12, 2002 And also USA Today. (online) "Latest Gallup Poll" World section.

At http://www.usatoday.com/news/world/2001/02/2001-02-06-poll.htm. Polls of the Palestinians themselves can be found by searching the site of the Center for Palestine Research & Studies, Nablus. Palestinian Center for Policy and Survey Research (PSR): Index of Polls. http://www.pcpsr.org/survey/index.html.

VIOLENCE AND STRATEGIC CHOICES: THE CASE OF ISLAMIST MILITANCY

IBRAHIM KARAWAN

Middle East Center, University of Utah, Salt Lake City, UT, USA

Much has been written since September 11 in particular about the threat posed by Islamist militancy and strategies to confront it. Like other groups that rely on violence to pursue their political objectives, militant Islamist groups that have been active on national and international levels refused to make any distinctions between the combatants and noncombatants, military and civilians, those who are likely to be guilty and many who are decidedly innocent. Creating a climate of gripping fear and uncertainty to paralyze their opponents through violent means has become the key objective for such groups.

Like other violent groups, they are keen to justify their strategy and actions under the category of the "absence of alternatives." In essence they insist that those in positions of power and dominance on the level of states as well as on the level of the international system will never really respond to peaceful marches, legal petitions, political practices, humanitarian appeals, or merely eloquent statements. They have to be eradicated through a violent or insurrectional approach. For them, the fundamental feature of the setting in which their "struggle" is launched is not the abundance of options but the utter absence of alternatives to violence.

However, a successful strategy of confronting Islamist militancy that came to the center of international attention lately requires understanding the defining characteristics and logic of strategic action by these militant groups. The fact that they claim to act in the name of religion does not mean that analysts should look for clues primarily in religious texts. Such search for the so-called essence of Islam or "essentialism" regarding that religion itself, I would argue, is an exercise in futility. Arguments about whether this or that political or militant action belongs or does not belong to a certain essence of Islam is beside the point and I am surprised that many have devoted so much time and effort in hashing and rehashing such arguments.

The truth is that "Islamic arguments" can be used to justify and also to critique diametrically opposed positions. Islam has in fact generated over many centuries a vast body of religious texts, scholarship, and authoritative judgments through which anyone can search and find support for contradictory positions on war and peace, violence and co-existence. Militant groups use parts from the *Qur'an* to legitimize their actions in their own societies, but as to be expected, their stands are contested by other Islamist thinkers as misguided and distorted. More important than looking at some religious texts for explanations of militant actions, one should examine the strategic beliefs and choices of the leaders of such movements regarding notions of time, reliance on small numbers, fronts of action, and counting on the adversary to overreact to violence in ways that may ultimately produce political quagmire and defeat. Let me look briefly at these points.

FIRST, THE LOGIC OF SHRINKING TIME

Even though militant Islamists share with other Islamists the objective of gaining political power and building Islamic states, they use violent means in a way that reflects their sense of the urgency of direct confrontational action. They have a particular sense of time (which can be found in the statements of Sayyid Qutb, Ayman al-Zawahiri, and Usama bin Laden among others) that sees Islam as facing a great danger both from within and without, cultural and political, economic marginalization, identity distortion, as well as political subordination.

According to the militant perspectives, if these trends are allowed to continue, the menace they pose to Islamic beliefs and values is going to be enormous and the repercussions can be catastrophic. It is the image of five minutes to midnight, an image that requires not incremental action, but radical rage for god or as they put it in the Arabic term *ghadbatun lil lah,* a rage for God. From such a perspective, the option of doing nothing under these conditions is like the gradualist option of working within the existing systems of domination and is a non-starter. Even if militant action did not produce its intended results, its success in generating a climate of fear and utter unpredictability is highly desirable according to their strategists.

Political Islamists by contrast have a different assessment of the time dimension as it relates to their strategic choices. In fact, they believe that time has worked in their favor and that Islamist reliance on violence is unwarranted and counter productive. Nasir, Bourgiba, Ataturk, and the Shah of Iran tried to weaken the social and political influence of Islamic movements in their societies, but they failed. However, militant Islamists insist that the main criteria of success for them is to seize state power in a decisive manner because short of doing that, the passing of time poses grave threats to Islamic beliefs and interests.

SECOND, THE LOGIC OF SMALL NUMBERS

Most of the well known militant Islamist groups in the Middle East are composed of small numbers of cadres relative to the size of military and security institutions which they confront. Clearly, one has to take into consideration that while the actual cadres that implement acts of violence represent a very tiny minority, some others are involved in the process in the areas of planning, intelligence gathering and training, among the activities necessary for the functioning of these groups. But even with taking that dimension into consideration, memoirs of militant leaders and estimates by security agencies agree that their overall numbers have been very small at least if compared to those available to the other side. In most cases these groups are not willing to trust potential recruits whom they might suspect of being infiltrators associated with their adversaries.

Militant groups find in their small numbers other evidence of the correctness in their ideological cause as a "believing minority" or "a Quranic generation of a new type" in the image of early Muslims during the foundation period. This vanguard, as described by Sayyid Qutb, a leading ideologue of Islamic militancy, has to be composed of a select few who know what nobody else knows. It is a vanguard that directs the struggle not according to what the masses may want at a given moment in time, but in pursuit of what they ought to have wanted always, but did not. Such a vanguard is a tiny minority that can be trusted to be the true Muslims who act as the combative fighters at this stage in which "westoxification" has spread in Muslim societies.

Small numbers are not only ideologically correct, but they also provide certain strategic and tactical advantages. They can hide in a sea of millions and tens of millions. It may be difficult for states to strike at them with a very significant degree of precision and when they miss they can pay a heavy political price. And small numbers of militant cadres and their own handlers can inflict heavy human and economic losses on their opponents, as September 11 and the cases in Algeria and Egypt have demonstrated.

THIRD, THE LOGIC OF SHIFTING FRONTS

Militant Islamist groups can move from national contexts to international targets based on expediency or reassessment of the strategic situation they face. Let me cite an example from the Middle East. During the period of 1979-1982, the hopes of the militants increased as acts of Islamist violence escalated in Saudi Arabia, Egypt, and Syria. Other cases of militancy had materialized in Jordan, Iraq, Yemen, and Algeria over the following two decades. But the dominos that were expected to fall into the hands of militant Islamists did not do so. The states targeted by these militant campaigns proved to be more resilient, more cunning, and more repressive than many had anticipated. The regimes that were expected to collapse "in the short term" are still with us, and if they happen to disintegrate, there is no compelling reason to conclude that militant Islamists will be their inheritors. Militant roads to power through assassination, military coups, and armed insurrection have a vast record of failures in achieving their objectives as shown in Egypt, Algeria, and Syria.

When many militant Islamists found their paths to power to be blocked, they then began to develop a few alternative strategies. Some sought to reach ceasefires with their regimes to deal with political and organizational losses as well as with internal divisions. Others have fled their home countries and switched from the domestic level to the global level or from the national to the international domain. The attacks against American targets starting in 1996 reflect that shift which culminated thus far in the attacks on the symbols of American economic and military power in New York and Washington DC. The groups behind these attacks hoped to return to their home countries later with two messages. To the masses there, this was the message: "Why are you afraid of America? America is a paper tiger!" And to the regimes, this was the message: "If America could not protect its most secure military institutions from our long arm, why should you or anyone else think that it will be able protect you?!"

FOURTH, THE LOGIC OF PROVOCATION

The last component in the strategic calculations of the militant groups is what may be called the logic of provocation. Militant leaders tell us and their followers that their main objective is to shake what they deem to be the state's basic foundation, namely its *hybah* or the sense of awe and invincibility it engenders among the masses. This is to be accomplished by demonstrating the state's utter failure to protect its leaders and key institutions. In response, states are not expected to simply do nothing. Doing nothing under such conditions may amount to committing political suicide. The militants engage in deeds that the state cannot afford to ignore with the aim of provoking it to strike back and to do that so indiscriminately that the resentment of emergency laws, widespread arrests, restrictions on movement, mass searches, heavy-handed repression and casualties would create opportunities to weaken the legitimacy of the state in the eyes of segments of society or credibility of its policy on the international level. This applies to the case of September 11. Will the policy of the U.S. prove that the four logics of militant Islamist action might work?

3. SOCIETY AND STRUCTURES: NATIONAL AND REGIONAL GEOPOLITICAL ISSUES

CONFRONTATION AND COOPERATION IN SOUTH ASIA

K.C. SIVARAMAKRISHNAN
Centre for Policy Research, New Delhi, India

I would like to make it clear at the outset that this paper is just an introduction and an overview of South Asia's recent history, its troubled present and its uncertain future. Numerous theses and books have been written about the region and the countries by many scholars of national and international repute. For this paper of limited scope and intent I have drawn substantially from several of these accounts. At the end of this short paper, there is a list of references for those who wish to know more about the South Asia region. I hope that the present paper will serve at least as an introduction to those unfamiliar with the region. From those who are better informed I can only ask for indulgence.

The assistance of A. Shankar and Sarala Gopinathan in preparing this paper is gratefully acknowledged.

INTRODUCTION

South Asia is not one political entity but a congeries of communities with strong religious, socio-economic and cultural ties. At times, much of South Asia has also emerged as a political unit, such as during the time of Asoka (250 BC) or the Mughal Emperor, Akbar (1605 AD). However it is the British who fashioned over 300 years a reasonably coherent geographical and political construct for India. As of 1939 at the beginning of the Second World War, India consisted of two major parts; one was British India directly administered in the name of the British Crown by the Viceroy; the other comprised over 600 princely states each with a ruler of its own but subject to the paramountcy and control of the British. Invariably in each of these states there was a Resident or Administrator chosen or appointed by the Viceroy.

PARTITION

The Great Divide of 1947 split British India into two parts- India and Pakistan. Pakistan inherited about 23% of the landmass of undivided India and about 18% of its population which at that time was about 345 million. The 600 plus princely states were free to join either India or Pakistan as may be decided by their rulers, irrespective of geographical continuity. Theoretically, these princely states could also choose to remain independent on their own since the British paramountcy ceased. Some states indeed chose this alternative for a few days or a few months creating significant problems for all concerned.

There are several authoritative accounts about the genesis of the partition of India. The events leading to it have been adequately chronicled. The creation of Pakistan was based on what is called the 'two-nation theory.' According to this theory the Hindus and Muslims of India constituted two separate nations. This itself was a rather contrived notion prompted more by politics rather than other factors. For several centuries the Indian sub-continent had been multi religious, multi-ethnic and multi-lingual. Of the 345 million people in undivided India about 65% were Hindus, 30% Muslims and the rest belonged to other religions. While the Muslim population was to be found in all parts of the country, it was in a majority in the western province of Punjab and nearby areas, as well as in the eastern province of Bengal. Pakistan, it was decided, would comprise a part of Punjab, Sind, Baluchistan and north-western Frontier, as well as a part of Bengal to be called East Pakistan. The rest would remain as India. The two parts of Pakistan, West and East, would be separated by 1200 miles of Indian Territory.

Through much of recorded history, the communities of the sub-continent have lived and worked together and traded with each other. At times they also had clashed on minor and major issues. None of these disputes were long or sharp enough to tear the fabric of the society. A major reason was that the State itself, particularly during the British period, was by and large neutral and kept the peace. Given their large numbers, the majority of the Hindus and Muslims had also found ways of co-existence and co-operation in most of the country for most of the time. The history of pre-independence and numerous analyses by scholars confirmed that the people in general, whether Hindus or Muslims, did not want partition. Yet their leaders either allowed themselves to be pushed by events and political compulsions or advocated the dismemberment of the country as the only way to independence. What was dormant and containable in any pluralistic society became sanctified by politics and eventually became the organizing principle of one of the largest political re-arrangements in recent human history.

The impatience of the political leaders as well as the inclination of the British Empire to withdraw, culminated in partition. The division of Punjab and Bengal and the demarcation of new boundaries was entrusted to a Commission headed by Cyril Radcliffz, Vice Chairman of the Bar Council of England whose qualification for the job appears to be that he had never set foot in the sub-continent. What took the British 300 years to put together was severed in seventy days.

THE CARNAGE

Contrary to the hopes of political leaders, as well as captains of the departing British Empire, partition created a serious divide, particularly in Punjab and Bengal. It affected every village and town, every street and neighborhood. Mistrust and fear exploded to the surface. The carnage of partition began more than one year before the event with the great Calcutta killing, and lasted for another year thereafter. At least half a million people lost their lives. By the middle of 1948 about 5 million Hindus moved from West Pakistan to India. A similar number moved from India to Pakistan. In East Pakistan it was expected that Hindus sharing Bengalee as the common language with Muslims would stay on as minorities. But these hopes were also belied. At least a million people are estimated to have come to India as refugees from East Pakistan in the first two decades after partition.

THE AFTERMATH

Of the 600 princely states almost all acceded to India or Pakistan based mainly on geographical contiguity. As mentioned before, a few states held out, such as Junagadh, Hyderabad and Kashmir. Others were resolved, but the ruler of Kashmir wanted to keep all his choices open till the last minute and even after the appointed day of 14th August 1947. The ditherings of the ruler, the expectations of the Indian and Pakistani leaders, the role of Mountbatten who was Viceroy till the 14th and Governor General of India after the 15th, armed intrusion into Kashmir and other circumstances contributed to a controversy and conflict which have remained intractable to this day. The problem of Kashmir is dealt with in a subsequent section of this paper.

But Kashmir, highly visible as it is, is not the only confrontation that has afflicted South Asia. The emergence of Bangladesh which came about by exploding the two nation theory, the ethnic conflict in Sri Lanka which has claimed more than 60,000 lives, rising Maoist insurgency in Nepal, separatists and sectarian movements in West Pakistan and India's north east are all part of the South Asian reality now.

BANGLADESH

The two-nation theory seeking separate nations for Muslims and Hindus was proved false by the emergence of Bangladesh. At the time of partition, West Pakistan had about 55 million people and East Pakistan 75 million. It was separated by 1200 miles of Indian Territory. Unlike Punjab, Hindus remained a significant minority in East Pakistan comprising about 20% of the population. In West Pakistan the population was principally Urdu and Punjabi speaking; in the east, the predominant language for both Muslims and the Hindu minority was Bengali or Bangla. The disregard for Bangla and its very rich cultural and literary traditions became a sore point in the West and East Pakistan relations from the beginning. In 1948 students of East Pakistan led a widespread popular movement in favour of Bengali and in protest against Urdu becoming the state sponsored language. In 1952 the draft constitution declared Urdu as the national language. The protest demonstrations in which some student leaders died in police firing marked the beginning of the end of Muslim league in East Pakistan.

In 1958, Pakistan came under Martial law and Ayub Khan. The 1962 Constitution proposed by Ayub Khan was not accepted. In 1969, Yahya Khan succeeded Ayub Khan as the Military Dictator and proposed a National Assembly of 330 members. East Pakistan was to have 169 members. In the elections held in December 1970, according to rules laid down by Yahya Khan, the Awami League won 167 seats. The National Assembly was to meet in March 1971 and Yahya Khan promised to transfer power to an elected government. However, Zulfikar Ali Bhutto of the Peoples Party of Pakistan who had won 88 plus seats in West Pakistan was not prepared to concede Pakistan government to Mujibur Rehman of east Pakistan only on the basis of the majority of seats. The talks between Yahya Khan, Bhutto and Mujibur failed. Eventually Mujibur Rehman proclaimed independence of Bangladesh. In the armed struggle that followed, the Bangladesh freedom fighters composed largely of the former Pakistan army and aided by the Indian army defeated Yahya Khan's forces and an independent Bangladesh emerged later in 1971. The two-nation theory was buried when Hindu-India and Muslim-Bangladesh joined forces to defeat Muslim Pakistan.

SRI LANKA

Around 1948 when Ceylon became Independent from British rule, its population was about 7 million. Out of this about 65% were Buddhists, mostly speaking the Sinhalese language. Hindus were about 19% who were also Tamil speaking. Muslims and Christians accounted for about 16%. Ceylon or Sri Lanka as it is now called has been populated mainly by migrants. The Sinhalese themselves are descendants of migrants from north and eastern India. The early kingdoms of Sri Lanka were established around 500 BC. Buddhism was introduced in 300-250 BC. Due to its close proximity with south India, migration was also significant from the coastal and other areas of south India. From the third century BC until about AD 1017 Anuradhapura flourished as the capital of Sri Lanka. From the 7th to the 11th century AD, the politics and culture of South India and the Chola and Pandya kingdoms dominated Sri Lanka.

When the Portuguese came to the island seeking cinnamon and spices, there were 3 kingdoms in Sri Lanka – two Sinhalese and one Tamil kingdom in Jaffna, in the northern part of the island. By then the island's economic and social interaction with south India and immigration from there were pronounced. The Sinhalese and Sri Lankan Tamils became the significant populace of the island. After the Portuguese and the Dutch came the British. Plantations for tea, rubber and spices were developed and large numbers of cheap labour were imported from south India to work in these plantations. They were called 'Estate Tamils' as a category distinct from Sri Lankan Tamils.

In 1948 Sri Lanka adopted a Westminster type parliamentary democratic system. It lasted for 30 years but representation and participation of the various ethnic and linguistic groups did emerge as contentious issues. While the Sinhalese were a majority in the country, the Tamils constituted about 65% of the population in the north and eastern provinces. Regional autonomy emerged as an important cause for these areas. There was also the feeling that labour imported for the plantations were birds of passage and should return to India. The government structure was eventually replaced by a Presidential form.

In the mid 60s under an India-Sri Lanka accord, several thousands of the 'Estate Tamils' were repatriated mostly to Tamil Nadu. In 1972, Sinhalese was made the official language and Buddhism the state religion. Around the same time the government also made some efforts to settle Sinhalese people in areas traditionally occupied by Tamils. From mid 60s to the mid 70s various negotiations were held between the Tamil minorities and the Sri Lankan government. For much of this period, the Tamil groups had remained largely peaceful and non-violent. However, the settlement of Sinhalese people in Tamil areas and the inability to reach a negotiated settlement led to a hardening of attitudes on both sides. By the end of the 1970s various Tamil political groups had begun asking for a separate homeland for themselves to be called Eelam in and around the northern and eastern parts of the island. In 1976, the LTTE (Liberation Tigers of Tamil Eelam) was born as a militant outfit committed to secure Eelam. In 1981 the Jaffna Library, well known as a repository of Tamil culture was burnt down. In 1986, LTTE declared the defacto independence of Jaffna. Since then terrorism and bloody conflicts between the Sri Lankan armed forces and the LTTE have alternated without either side winning or loosing.

Inevitably the conflicts in Sri Lanka have had their impact on the society and politics in the Indian State of Tamil Nadu. The LTTE cadres often used Tamil Nadu as a base for their operations. This in turn strained Indo-Sri Lanka relations and also helped encourage insurgent elements elsewhere. Under the Rajiv Gandhi-Jayawardane Pact, India agreed to provide a peace keeping force to disarm the LTTE and enable reconciliation between the Tamils and the Sinhalese. The Pact largely failed. Rajiv Gandhi, initially hailed as a friend and saviour of Sri Lankan Tamils was himself assassinated in an LTTE suicide attack in 1991.

In 1994, Chandrika Kumaratunge, daughter of former Prime Minister, Bandaranaike who had himself been assassinated by a Buddhist Monk, became the President. Since then various attempts have been made to resolve the conflict by both negotiation and military resolve. Mediators like Norway have also tried to work out an agreement. The conflict has continued and terrorism has remained, claiming both politicians and civilians. Though conflict in Sri Lanka began with a religious overtone, differences became acute mainly because of the failure to accommodate linguistic differences. Attempts to eliminate dissent have threatened the very existence of a country, otherwise blessed with a stable population and an internationally acclaimed record of gains in literacy and health care. Its economy, which held much promise, continues to be under severe strain.

KASHMIR

It is not usually known that the state of Jammu and Kashmir until mid 1800s was not one state. The area covering about 140,000 sq. miles comprised six regions with distinct geographical, ethnic, religious and linguistic features. Jammu and Poonch in the south were contiguous to the Punjab plains, partly uplands and had a majority of Hindus. The valley of Kashmir had a Muslim majority. Baltisthan and Ladakh comprises mainly Buddhists who are ethnically akin to Tibetans. The mountainous Gilgit area was populated by various tribal people. The composite state of J & K was brought about by a series of conquests, negotiations and purchases all prompted by British imperial and security considerations because of Kashmir's proximity to Russia. Mahsarajah Hari Singh was the last ruler of the State who inherited it in 1925. By all accounts his rule, unlike some of the large princely states of India, was an autocracy. The British kept the peace and made sure that the different regions of the state did not cause too much trouble.

When the time came to choose between India and Pakistan Hari Singh dithered. The partition riots, which had already begun to burn in Punjab, had their impact in Poonch and Jammu. As the clashes spread, 15th August 1947 came and went. Hari Singh continued to vacillate though there were attempts, diplomatic and otherwise, from both India and Pakistan to secure a decision. One part of Kashmir declared itself independent to be called Azad or Free Kashmir. A mixture of mercenaries, armed tribesmen and regular soldiers raided the valley early in October and were within striking distance of Srinagar, the state capital. On the 26th of October, Hari Singh signed the Instrument of Accession to India and sought Indian military help to deal with the raiders. On the 27th October a massive airlift of Indian forces took place. The raiders were pushed back but the regulars of the Pakistan army joined the conflict under the banner of Azad Kashmir. Oddly enough, the commanders of both the Indian and the Pakistan army were still British though the Governor Generals were different - Mountbatten in India and Jinnah in Pakistan. The first Kashmir War was brought to an end on 27th July 1949 with a cease-fire line and an agreement brokered by the UN for the resolution of the conflict. About half of Kashmir to the north and north-east was on the outer side of the cease-fire line and became Pakistan controlled Azad Kashmir. The other half comprised much of the valley. Ladakh, Poonch and Jammu areas were with India. To this day the defacto line of control has remained.

Between the first war and the second, which occurred in 1965, various attempts were made through and outside the UN, towards a resolution. Different forms of referendum and plebiscite were considered. Within India and Pakistan the domestic political scene changed. Ayub Khan became military dictator in Pakistan. Jawaharlal Nehru died. In 1962, the Chinese crossed a traditional boundary in the north east of India to claim the state of Arunachal Pradesh and then withdrew. In 1963, Pakistan in an agreement with China ceded about 2000 square miles of Kashmir's territory to China. The second Indo-Pakistan war, triggered by a series of border clashes, which occurred in 1965 and ended with the Tashkent agreement between Ayub Khan and Indian PM Shastri on 10th January 1966. The very next day Shastri died unexpectedly. Apart from agreeing that Kashmir was a dispute between India and Pakistan, the agreement achieved little. The main point of this Agreement, that both armies withdraw to the 1949 cease-fire line, was implemented by February.

In the next five years Bangladesh's liberation was a momentous event in the sub-continent. The war was not limited to the east of India. As part of countering the conflict in the east, Pakistan opened a front in the West. In the event Bangladesh became an independent country, the Indian armed forces prevailed and a large number of Pakistani forces taken as prisoners. Eventually the Simla agreement of July 1972 between Mrs. Gandhi and Pakistan's Prime Minister, Mr. Bhutto, reiterated the agreements of the past and affirmed the line of actual control as of Dec. 1971. Yet another war, yet another agreement, but there was no peace even thereafter.

Between 1972 and 1989, for a period of 17 years, the line of control held, by and large. However, significant political changes took place both in India and Pakistan. Within Kashmir itself elections were held to the State legislature. The political groupings within the state became many. Terrorism emerged as an important means of securing political decisions. India's complaint which continues till today is that these terrorist acts were largely organized by camps in Azad Kashmir and aided by Pakistan. Pakistan argues that these are not terrorist acts but popular uprising by the people of Kashmir against Indian 'occupation.' In February 1999, the Indian and Pakistani Prime Ministers met again in Lahore and reaffirmed their intent to solve the bilateral problem peacefully. But later that year in the severe and inhospitable altitudes of Kargil north of the valley, Pakistan and Indian forces clashed again with heavy casualties. The race for military supremacy has continued with both India and Pakistan acquiring nuclear capabilities. Kashmir has cast a permanent shadow on the relations between the two countries.

The demand for an independent Kashmir is as unacceptable to Pakistan as it is to India. Pakistan cannot take Kashmir from India only on the ground that the valley of Kashmir has 4 million Muslims. After all, there are nearly 130 million Muslims in India which is only slightly less than Pakistan's 137. However, Pakistan leadership cannot give up because Kashmir is an important issue in its national position and politics. The two-nation theory, which emerged as an issue in the prelude to independence, first divided the country and then created the basis for an Islamic state. Jihad, which has been variously interpreted from intellectual quest to wars for religious liberation, has found it possible to acquire political acceptance in such a state. Jihad is now enmeshed with terrorism. In the meantime, the sub-continent continues in a state of near permanent tension.

COOPERATION

However, the story of South Asia has not been only of confrontation. The Indus Waters Treaty of 1960 between India and Pakistan allocated the main Indus river and two tributaries for Pakistan's use while the other three tributaries were kept for India. A permanent Indus Water Commission monitors the treaty, which has held till this day in spite of the wars between the two countries. On the eastern side of the sub-continent, the accord between India and Bangladesh in 1996 has provided for the allocation of the Ganga waters between the two countries. Similarly the Mahakali Treaty between Nepal and India concluded in the same year has enabled basin development under the aegis of a Mahakali Commission. Both these treaties have made it possible for the integrated development of the Ganga-Brahmaputra basin, one of the largest river basins in the world and home to 600 million people in Nepal, India and Bangladesh. Beneath the din of political controversy, much spadework and planning have also been accomplished for an Asian highway and transport network. The South Asian Association for Regional Cooperation was created 12 years ago by the Governments of India, Pakistan, Nepal, Bhutan, Bangladesh, Sri Lanka and Maldives. The SAARC commissioned a group of eminent persons from these countries to prepare a blue print for South Asian cooperation. The Agenda for 2000 and beyond envisages a South Asian free trade area, a South Asia economic union, flow of investment within the region, the development of infrastructure and various collaborative schemes for poverty eradication, environment, education, health care and empowerment of women.

While the agenda awaits a more opportune movement, the fact remains that it reflects the real needs of the large majority of the people in the sub-continent. The basic needs of the people in most of the countries of the region are largely unattended. In each there is a mismatch between political priorities and public needs. Military expenditures continue to receive a higher allocation than education and health care. Population planning has received some attention but the present rates of growth are still unsustainable. Poverty and inequality continues to be high in most of the South Asian countries. In spite of some spectacular examples of individuals rising to the top, the position of women in most political positions in some of the countries continues to be unsatisfactory. Overall the Human Development Report of 2001 places the South Asian countries within the lowest third of the list. The Maldives and Sri Lanka are slightly better at the 77th and 81st places but India is 115, Pakistan 127, Nepal 129 and Bangladesh 132.

SOME POSITIVE FEATURES

One positive feature is democracy. India took the conscious decision to adopt a parliamentary form of government based on universal adult franchise. In spite of religious, ethnic and linguistic diversity within the country, this democratic system has endured. As many as 13 general elections have been held in the country and over 100 state elections. The electoral system and machinery in India has emerged as a robust and independent institution. In 1990, Nepal adopted a system of constitutional monarchy and parliamentary democracy. Elections have been held twice for the Parliament. Local Government reforms and decentralization have also been pursued. However, the political system is under severe stress to cope with the divisive political culture and rising maoist insurgency. Sri Lanka too has struggled hard to keep its democratic system. Bangladesh, after a period of initial distress, is now showing signs of increasing acceptance of a democratic system. In contrast, for much of its 50 years Pakistan has been under a military rule. Despite efforts to the contrary, the Judicial systems in the South Asian countries have managed to retain a fair measure of respect. Decentralization is another common endeavor. Local rural and urban governments are slowly becoming important political entities.

The ethnic diversity and the cross border flow of labor and refugees are both a challenge and an opportunity for South Asia. Labor from Nepal moves into the border districts of India as well as Sikkim and Bhutan. With limited land resources, migrants from Bangladesh move to adjoining parts of India as well as elsewhere. Refugees from Sri Lanka are significant in Tamil Nadu. The conflict in Kashmir has also resulted in considerable displacement. Whilst the free movement of goods and investments between the South Asian countries is discussed and encouraged, the movement of labor is consciously discouraged. This is not unusual because most of the countries in the world adopt similar positions. Yet, in the South Asian region, the population pressures will not allow ethnicity to be confined within the so-called national borders. It is also a fact that cross border migration has provided a source of cheap labor, and migrants, like everywhere else in the world, work hard to better themselves, and in the process also contribute to the economy. Dealing with diversity is both a national and a regional issue for South Asian countries.

Civil society organizations are a visible factor in many South Asian countries. One manifestation of this are the several unofficial dialogues between Pakistan and India, India and Bangladesh as well as regional discourses. Compared to the variety and magnitude of the problems, the scale and frequency of these dialogues admittedly is limited but still they represent an assertive aspect of the civil society in these countries. Another manifestation of the civil society is the fact that several individuals from the region command the status of world citizens. Mahbub Al Haq of Pakistan who established the Human Development Report in the UN has a more relevant and credible system of monitoring the progress and performance of countries is one such person. Manmohan Singh of India who ushered in many of its economic reforms is another. Mohammad Yunus of Bangladesh or Ella Bhatt of India who clearly demonstrated the creditworthiness of the poor and their ability for self-improvement are other examples. Yet, the fact remains that the perception, values and status of these world citizens are in sharp contrast with the realities in their respective countries. But these are voices that cannot be stifled and indeed they are spreading and being emulated widely.

However, a robust civil society depends very much on the structure of the society itself. The South Asian countries have had a feudal past. Inequities have been pervasive and discrimination widespread. In the struggle for independence these issues were both submerged in some cases and addressed in some others. The emergence of the market place as the arbiter in daily life has partly aggravated some of the issues. Respect for human rights in a western jurisprudential sense is very recent but tolerance has been an important aspect of the South Asian faiths. Religions extremism has definitely undermined that. Like the sorcerer's apprentice, some efforts are now being made to put the Jinn back in the bottle.

The South Asian countries have made noticeable gains in new areas of technology. Information technology and the strident advances that some countries in the region are making is one example. Communication technology is another. Governments are no longer the monopoly of information flows. Scientific research and application are also receiving increasing levels of attention and respect. These point to the fact that the South Asian societies have indeed begun to shed their traditional inhibitions. Their doors are more open than before. When doors are opened there is little merit in keeping the windows shut for short-term political gains.

REFERENCES

1. Alastair Lamb (1972) *Kashmir, A Disputed Legacy*, Oxford University Press, Karachi.
2. Anand Verma (2001) *Reassessing Pakistan – Role of Two Nation Theory*, Centre for Policy Research, Delhi.
3. B G Verghese (1999) *Waters of Hope, From Vision to Reality*, Centre for Policy Research.
4. B G Verghese (2001) *Reorienting India*, Centre for Policy Research.
5. Ian Talbot (2000) *India and Pakistan – Inventing the Nation*, Arnold, London.
6. Ian Tabolt (1998) *Pakistan – A Modern History*, Oxford University Press, Delhi.
7. Lawrence Ziring (1992) *Bangladesh from Mujib to Errhad*, Oxford University Press, Karachi.
8. *Perspectives on South Asia* (Pai Panandikar and Navnita Behera – Editors), Centre for Policy Research, Delhi, 2000.
9. Patrick French (1997) *Liberty or Death – India's Journey to Independence and Division*, Harper Collins.
10. Rajmohan Gandhi (1999) *Revenge and Reconciliation, Understanding South Asian History*, Penguin Book.
11. Sunil Khilnani (1997) *The Idea of India*, Hamish Hamilton, London.
12. Subhas Chandra Nayak (2001) *Ethnicity and Nation Building in Sri Lanka*, Kalinga Publications, Delhi.
13. SAARC, (1999) *Vision beyond 2000*, South Asian Association for Regional Cooperation.

NEUTRALITY AND THE ARAB-ISRAELI CONFLICT

DAN V. SEGRE
University of Lugano, Switzerland

For the purpose of this talk, I define neutrality as non-interference in other peoples' affairs and I define modern neutrality as an internationally recognized, institutionalized system of non-interference in other peoples' affairs.

This basic political and moral type of behavior in international relations was specifically mentioned in the Hebrew Scriptures as a condition for the political survival of the Jews. However, it has never been practiced by them in the past or in the present. Like most other nations their leaders have relied on power politics.

My purpose is to try to show why a reconsideration of the old Jewish principle of political neutrality – combined with the study of modern experiences of institutionalized mechanisms of self-control – could provide a constructive new approach to the Middle East crisis.

Let me start by qualifying my position concerning the historical value of the biblical message. With the exception of a few events like the siege of Jerusalem by the Assyrian king Sennachebir, in the year 701 BC, the Old Testament cannot validate historical facts.

Therefore, when I mention various forms of past Jewish sovereignty, I do not claim that they are interchangeable with modern political institutions, but that they can be a source of inspiration and religious legitimization for modern political ideas.

In the course of their history, Jews produced several original political ideas, such as that of the constitution of a people under God, the universality of mankind, prophecy as legitimate opposition to royal authority. Neutrality is one of these original Jewish ideas. It was conceived not only as a most appropriate system of foreign policy for a Jewish commonwealth, but as an expression of Jewish national identity.

Curiously, political neutrality has never been put into practice by past Jewish rulers who, like modern Israeli ones, have followed the path of power politics. This is surprising, since neutrality is an intrinsic part of the character of the Jewish people, which the Old Testament defines as a "kingdom of priests and a holy nation" destined "to dwell alone and not be part of other nations" (Ex. 19/6; Num. 23/4). Even more surprising is the fact that such an idea, strongly defended by Jewish prophets (Jer. 22:13, 17-19; Isaiah 31; Ezk. 17:15) as the only strategy capable of safeguarding the independence of the ancient Jewish states, has not been articulated in the immense Jewish rabbinical literature.

As I have argued elsewhere (Segre, 1994 and 2000), at the core of the ME crisis is the Arabs' refusal to accept the existence of a non-Arab, non-Muslim polity in their midst. This refusal combines the virulence of a nationalistic struggle by two peoples for the control of the same land with the passions of ancient judeophobia and modern antisemitism.

The distinction between these two forms of hostility towards Jews goes beyond the purpose of this presentation. I will limit myself to noting that Judaism has always represented a challenge to existing values – religious, social, moral, economic. Well before the surge of modern anti-Semitism, it created a situation of antagonism with other cultures, which resentfully reacted to, and/or adopted parts of the Jewish monotheistic moral and social credo. Judaism caused deep religious-political lacerations in the ancient Hellenic and Roman world. which led to wars against the Jews, to their revolts, followed by their political subjection and dispersion. It caused a theological and social conflict with Christianity that only very recently seemed to disappear.

After centuries of relative peaceful coexistence of Judaism with Islam – albeit in a situation of personal inequality and absence of sovereignty – the emergence of a powerful Jewish state in Palestine, physically dividing the Arabs of the West from the Arabs of the East, challenging both their national unity and their political renaissance, has created a trauma in the Muslim consciousness. It has produced a situation of fear and hostility out of all proportion to the territorial and demographic dimensions of the conflict itself. It has developed a new type of "judeophobia." It took 20 centuries for the Church to mature to the point of no longer feeling it is necessary to kill Jews in order to affirm its faith. How long will it take for Islamic societies to accept equality with different political and religious identities?

The Middle East crisis has also become a symbolic clash of cultures, refractory to normal diplomatic efforts. Attempts of this kind, made in the course of half a century, have exacerbated tensions rather than reduced them. Can the idea of neutrality offer a better approach to the conflict?

This is not the place to discuss the juridical intricacies of neutrality, nor to debate whether neutrality is an anachronism in modern, globalized society. I will only point out that a state can be neutral *and* a member of the United Nations – as Switzerland will shortly be. Turkmenistan, of all nations, was unanimously accepted as a neutral state by the UN General Assembly in October 1995. Whether or not the final form of the relationship between Israel, Palestine and the Arab states turns out to be one of classical neutrality, the idea of neutrality is relevant to the ME crisis because it befits the particular character of a Jewish state, of a demilitarised Palestinian state, and could benefit the Arab countries and the international community alike. Let me consider Israel first:

On one hand, the Zionist idea of creating a new type of Jew through their return to the land of their ancestors, and living in the first secular community in their history, has proved an illusion. Zionism, in its effort to solve the Jewish question, has added to it an Israeli question, which a century of conflict with the Arabs is turning more and more into a new Jewish question.

On the other hand, Israel is rapidly reaching the point of becoming the largest Jewish community in the world. At that moment, Zionism will have fulfilled its declared aim to re-establish a majority group of Jews in the land of Israel. But Zionism's triumph will not be complete if it does not free Israeli Jews from its original sin: that of being the only national movement born *not* from the desire of a people to achieve political independence but from the *unachieved* desire of Jewish westernised élites to be assimilated as equal partners in the host nations and cultures.

Whether or not the Jews wanted, in the past, to be part of a Jewish state, a strong Jewish political national consciousness exists today. It is supported by a state which not only considers itself Jewish, but which has become a major military and industrial power, something which past Jewish states were unable to achieve.

After the experience of the Holocaust, the Moslem insistence on eliminating the Jews as a sovereign entity in their midst, and the Arab efforts to "reduce Israel to its proper size," the Middle East crisis may become a theatre of massive destructive retaliation. It must bring both Jews and Gentiles alike to reflect not only on the cost of a new war against the Jews, but also on the contribution that a Jewish state, in peace, could make to civilisation.

This is not the place to debate the nature of Judaism. I shall limit myself to note that today the Jewish question concerns a very small people, faced, as never before, with the challenge to prove whether a Jewish identity exists by virtue of its own values or by external pressure, as Sartre, among others, believed.

Whether one considers the singularity of the Jewish fate to be a mystery, like Jacques Maritain; or a poison like Voltaire; or a deadly bacillus like Himmler; or a cancer like Nasser; or a "blessing for all the nations," as the Old Testament claims, Judaism represents, and will continue to represent in the future, a disturbing presence in human society. Therefore, if the Jews cannot be eliminated from the face of the globe (as their enemies have so often tried to do in the past, and would like to do in the present), some way must be found to promote their coexistence with the rest of the world, if not for the sake of historical justice, then in the interest of international stability. This means establishing a framework of relationships in the Middle East capable of accepting the *singularity* of a Jewish state.

Jewish particularism finds its earliest expression in the two passages of the Scriptures, already mentioned, which suggest that the best way for Jews to prosper as a state is "to dwell alone and not be part of other nations." Such aloofness, combined with a high standard of private and public morality, represents the basic tenet of political Judaism.

Translated in terms of modern politics, the declared willingness of Israel not to meddle in its neighbours' affairs, could be the first step on the road leading to the reduction of fears and suspicions toward it in the Arab world. It would also help to change the mystifying view that the Palestinian crisis is a kind of proxy representation of all the conflicts of the globe: a war of poor nations against the rich ones, of theocracy against democracy, of nationalism against tribalism, of the West against the East, of modernisation against tradition, and so forth. A symbolic struggle of this kind is indeed insoluble.

A situation of internationally recognised neutrality could, on the contrary, grant the Israelis the physical security and peace of mind necessary for devoting themselves not only to the material development of their land, but to the revival of the message of Judaism for a modern, multicultural, society.

In a time of diminishing ideological nationalism, of increasing political ethnicity and individualism, the Jewish right to integrate without being forced to assimilate in a part of a global society, cannot be seen as an anti-historical, sinful cosmopolitanism. There is no longer justification for the French revolutionary cry: "to the Jews, everything; to the Jewish nation, nothing." The long, tragic Jewish struggle for equal acceptance, without forced loss of collective identity, could be an example for other minorities striving for international coexistence based on reciprocal self-respect.

Inborn Jewish aloofness should no longer be considered an expression of arrogant, religious "chosenness." Voluntarily accepted boundaries – the fundamental element of neutrality – are already accepted facts in non-conventional armaments, agreements, in those banning anti personnel mines, protecting the environment, supervising the exploitation of zones of world interest, such as the Antartic, not to speak of the international co-operation developed in the conquest of space. Even Europe has finally abandoned its *machtpolitic* in favour of what British senior diplomat Robert Cooper calls "a post-modern system" *(The Observer*, April 7, 2002), based on self enforced rules of behaviour

At present, there is little evidence that Israel appreciates the advantages of a constructive policy of self-control, befitting a small people carrier of a great heritage. Yet, an echo of the validity of political non-involvement could already be found in Theodor Herzl's 1902 book, *Altneuland.* Another echo is traceable to the late Moshe Sharett, Israel's first foreign minister, in his maiden speech at the UN in 1949, in which he called for a policy of nonalignment for his country. Twenty years later, Nahum Goldmann, president of the World Jewish Congress, published in *Foreign Affairs* an unheeded but remarkable article on "The future of Israel" advocating non-identification with any ideological block.

Strangely enough, given the myriads of proposals which have been put forward as possible solutions to the Palestine conflict, the word neutrality has not found its way into the ME debates. This is surprising, since neutrality would not limit Israel's defence capability, while the obligation of impartiality towards, and non-interference in, the affairs of neighbouring states could benefit Israeli internal politics, by favouring a climate of restraint between the secular and the orthodox Jewish sector, and between the Arab and Jewish citizens of Israel.

In fact, by accepting the principle of neutrality, secular Jews who uphold territorial compromise and civic justice, as a condition for the security of the Zionist national home, would have a moral weapon, based on biblical law, with which to confront the expansionist claims of many religious nationalists. Similarly, religious Jews who believe that the Scriptures legitimize the Jewish claim to the Holy Land, would have a rationale for opposing military strategies that contradict the moral and political logic of biblical neutrality.

Is Israel capable of developing modalities through which the state could conform to the principles of aloofness and Jewish political morality? Hard to say. But if in the past, political realists could claim that tension with the Arabs was a powerful unifying element for a nation of immigrants like Israel (the Arab boycott was certainly one of the main causes of Israel's industrial development), the first and second Intifada and terrorism have shown both sides that wars cannot be constructive any longer.

A Palestinian state, whatever its future dimensions and internal structure, will also be "singular" in its own way, by virtue of its historical development, and by the vicinity of Israel. It will be very different from the rest of the Arab states. The acceptance by the Palestinians of the idea of internationally recognised institutions, based on reciprocal Israeli-Palestinian self-control, might serve Palestinian interests better than their constant appeal to "historical justice" and vengeance. Furthermore, the acceptance by the Palestinians and the Israelis of elements of neutrality, would benefit those Arab states to which Israel poses military, political, psychological and ideological threats, not to mention the internal instability created in these states by the Palestinian question.

Uncommon situations call for unorthodox solutions. Even if past and present models of neutrality cannot be applied directly to the Palestinian-Israeli case, placing intractable problems in a different framework may reduce animosity, fanaticism, and the suspicions involved. The idea of neutrality, if properly presented, could become a constructive approach to the conflict. At least, it could help to develop that "reluctant tolerance," suggested by Isaiah Berlin, which neither party would like to respect, but none of them would hate, strongly enough, to scuttle.

I am grateful to Josef Agassi and Athanasios Moulakis for reading drafts of this paper and making many useful suggestions.

SCIENCE AND TECHNOLOGY TO ADVANCE REGIONAL SECURITY IN THE MIDDLE EAST AND CENTRAL ASIA

ANDREW F.B. TOMPSON, JEFFERY H. RICHARDSON, RICHARD C. RAGAINI, RICHARD B. KNAPP, NINA D. ROSENBERG, DAVID K. SMITH, DEBORAH Y. BALL
Lawrence Livermore National Laboratory, Livermore, CA, USA

INTRODUCTION

This paper is concerned with the promotion and advancement of regional security in the Middle East and Central Asia through the development of bilateral and multilateral cooperation on targeted scientific and technical projects. It is widely recognized that increasing tensions and instability in many parts of the world emphasize – or reemphasize – a need to seek and promote regional security in these areas. At the Lawrence Livermore National Laboratory (LLNL), a national security research facility operated for the U.S. Department of Energy, we are pursuing an effort to use science and technology as a "low risk" means of engagement in regions of strategic importance to the United States. In particular, we are developing collaborations and cooperative projects among (and between) national laboratory scientists in the U.S. and our various counterparts in the countries of interest.

HOW CAN SCIENCE AND TECHNOLOGY IMPROVE REGIONAL SECURITY?

First and foremost, scientific cooperation is often recognized as a means of mitigating conflict.[1] Scientific collaborations can address meaningful problems that could otherwise lead to destabilizing tensions in some regions of the world. Because science and technology have become the dominating factor in the global economy, they can either close or exacerbate the economic gap between rich and poor countries. Science and technology use a common language that transcends state and cultural boundaries, offer a positive and benign process for engaging governmental and civilian organizations, and involve participation from military, academic, ministerial, private organizations and other important stakeholders. As a result, scientific cooperation may be come an important facilitating factor among nations in conflict. Specific and targeted science and technology projects can make a tangible difference by improving the indigenous capacity and standard of living and providing tools to respond to real and critical regional problems.

They are a powerful process for collaboration and can lead to collateral economic, educational, and public health benefits.

OUR APPROACH

We are using a three-step process to foster the development of scientific collaboration and cooperation in two areas of the world important to the United States national interest – the Middle East and Central Asia.

Over the past five years, for example, we have (i) conducted several fact-finding technical missions to these regions in order to develop scientific contacts, meet government officials, visit important non-governmental organizations and academic institutions, and otherwise gain a sense for important technical problems affecting the regions, especially those that are congruous with our own technical capabilities.

Following these visits, we have (ii) developed a prioritized group of projects through a series of regional workshops involving American and regional scientists. In general, the projects we develop are fully collaborative, bilateral or multilateral in nature, and are, of course, science and technology based. These projects must provide an opportunity for engagement in the region of interest, for addressing real problems in the regions, and, if possible, also promote the improved education and welfare of the local population.

Ultimately, (iii) funding for the projects is sought, both for participants in the regions as well as for the U.S. counterparts. It is important to emphasize that we are not developing a "blind" or unidirectional program of aid and grants, but, rather, establishing real and lasting cooperative ventures on a bilateral or multilateral basis. Although many projects may involve small amounts of funding or require short turn around times, the scientific relationships created in this process can be continuing and lead to more involved interactions in the future.

The Middle East and Central Asia
In the Middle East, for example, the need for engagement among various parties (Israel, The Palestinian Authority, Jordan, and Syria, among others) has long been recognized as an important aspect of the peace process and overall progress toward regional security. More recently, the growth of international terrorism in Central Asia and the potential trafficking of nuclear materials and drugs is being recognized as a threat to the emerging economies in the region – e.g., the development of important energy resources. This has revealed a stronger need to promote broad-based regional cooperation in a number of areas, especially with respect to the resolution of the disposition of shared water resources and the elimination of regional environmental threats.[2]

COOPERATIVE PROJECT SUBJECT AREAS

As a result of our fact-finding trips and regional workshops, we have pursued a number of science and technology collaborations in the area of environmental threats in both the Middle East and Central Asia.

The environment provides an obvious topic for regional engagement, as most environmental issues are either intrinsically regional (e.g., transboundary river basins, groundwater aquifer management, air pollution, etc.) or are replicated on a regional basis (e.g., water salinity problems, industrial pollution of surface and groundwater, Soviet era radioactive material legacies, etc.). The U.S. Central Combatant Command (U.S. Military), whose are of responsibility includes Central Asia and portions of the Middle East, has recognized and endorsed this concept, making "environmental security" a key part of its engagement strategy.[3] Although there has been considerable debate as to whether environmental degradation or regional competition for scarce water resources can lead directly to violent conflict, there is general agreement that these factors exacerbate existing conflicts and can be regarded as a vehicle to stimulate broader regional cooperation.[4-6]

Engagement focused on environmental issues (e.g., water quality and quantity) includes characterization and simulation to first define environmental threats, rapidly engineered upgrades to proactively manage environmental issues affecting public health, the economy and state stability, and regional technical and government networks to coordinate solutions. Coordinated emergency response planning and exercises addressing potential environmental disasters (e.g., floods, earthquakes, and terrorist attacks) promote regional cooperation and develop indigenous capacity and infrastructure. These are meaningful issues that can be translated in to substantive actions on the ground in these countries. In the following sections, a summary of some of the projects underway or under consideration by our organization will be provided.

Middle East

Experiential Education in Groundwater Hydrology: Bridging the Technical - Policy - Populace Gap.
This is a small bilateral project being conducted between LLNL and several partner organizations in Jordan under the sponsorship of the Bureau of Educational and Cultural Affairs of the U.S. Department of State. The project involves two principal activities that are being coordinated with the Jordan University of Science and Technology (JUST), the Royal Society for the Conservation of Nature (RSCN) and the Jordanian Ministry of Water and Irrigation (MWI).

The first part of the project involves a series of educational activities with all partners to educate primary-aged children, laypersons, academic, government, other technical professionals, and farming communities on basic groundwater issues – its production, depletion, movement, pollution, and recycling as part of the hydrologic cycle. This is particularly relevant in Jordan where water shortages are acute, reliance on renewable groundwater is significant, and, as in most places, the general awareness or recognition of groundwater as an important resource is limited. The lack of reliable water supplies in Jordan and the region as a whole can threaten the kinds of economic development that are often seen as necessary ingredients for long-term peace and stability in the region.

As part of this activity, we are constructing a series of two-dimensional physical groundwater models for use by RSCN, JUST, and MWI. RSCN, in particular, will utilize these models in their Azraq Wetlands Visitors Center for demonstration and educational purposes. Although such physical models may be used for education of school children (Fig. 2), they will also be used and replicated in the university environment at JUST, as well as for public awareness and outreach purposes at the MWI.

The Azraq wetlands are located in the middle of the Azraq basin in central Jordan (Fig. 1) and exist now only because of a small restoration effort that has been implemented by RSCN. What exists now is only a remnant of a vast and thriving oasis that existed in this location for thousands of years as a resting point for animals, waterfowl, and desert travelers alike. The death of the wetlands was created by large-scale, unsustainable production of groundwater from the Azraq aquifer – underlying the oasis – and the subsequent lowering of regional groundwater levels. The Azraq aquifer extends from Syria to Saudi Arabia and has been largely used to provide water to the capital city of Amman. Aquifer management is complicated by numerous illegal and undocumented wells, complicated geology, and an inability to effectively understand or predict the nature of increasing salinity in much of the aquifer's water.

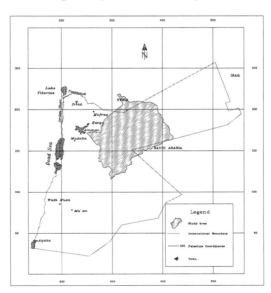

Fig. 1. Location of the Azraq groundwater basin in Jordan.

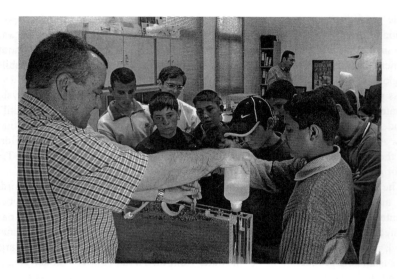

Fig. 2. Demonstration of physical model to schoolchildren at the Azraq Wetlands Visitors Center in Jordan.

A second part of this project involves technical exchanges, primarily with JUST and MWI, regarding the use of new LLNL computer-based groundwater simulation models. In this part of the effort, we are developing an application of an LLNL-developed model to the Azraq aquifer (Fig. 1). The model is intended to provide an improved basis for aquifer management in much of Jordan.

Solar Powered Desalination and Pumping Unit for Brackish Water
In many parts of the Middle East, including both Jordan and the Palestinian territories, there are numerous small villages populated by indigenous nomadic or semi-nomadic people that rely on remote – and often brackish sources of groundwater for human and livestock consumption. The relatively high salinity levels in this kind of water (~3000 – 8000 parts per million) are not acceptable over the long-term from human health perspectives.

The overall technical objective of this type of project is to develop expandable, portable, and remotely powered systems to supply desalinated water to small communities (less than 2000 people) and their associated livestock. Such a system should be able to deliver at least 100-200 m^3/day, be powered by renewable (photovoltaic) energy sources and be portable enough to be transported in a small truck for nearby communities.

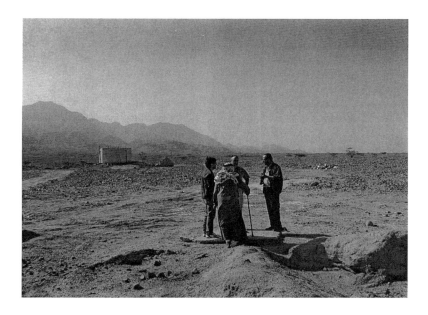

Fig. 3. *Visit to Qatar, Jordan on April 12, 2002. Project participants confer with village leader (rear facing, front) on top of a new 50 m-deep well from which a new solar-powered desalination unit will draw brackish groundwater. Treated water will be delivered to the recently completed cistern for the village, several meters in the background.*

A prototype effort has recently been initiated by the National Renewable Energy Laboratory (NREL) of the U.S. Department of Energy, in collaboration with the Middle East Regional Cooperation program of the U.S. Agency for International Development, the Jordanian Ministry of Water and Irrigation (MWI), and the Royal Scientific Society of Jordan. In this project, a portable, solar-powered desalination unit developed for the U.S. military was procured and is being shipped to the small village of Qatar, 35 km north of Aqaba, in southern Jordan (Figs. 1 and 3). Although the village has access to brackish groundwater in a series of newly developed wells, it relies nonetheless on freshwater delivered by truck each week from Aqaba. At this time, additional units are being considered for other locations in Jordan and in the neighboring Palestinian territories.

<u>Central Asia</u>
Radionuclide Contamination at the Ulba Metallurgical plant
The Ulba Metallurgical Plant (UMP) is situated in Ust-Kamenogorsk, in eastern Kazakhstan. In its 50-year history of continual operation, the facility has dominated the industrial base of the city through the production of processed uranium and specialty

metals such as beryllium, tantalum, and niobium. By the mid 1950s, commercial processing of beryl ores at UMP allowed the large-scale production of high-purity beryllium oxides, alloys, and ceramics for a wide variety of atomic defense (including nuclear weapon) and industrial applications. Since this time, tantalum and niobium have also been regularly produced as metal powders and ceramics. Uranium production also began in the 1950s and evolved toward the production of low-enriched uranium during a period when the former Soviet Union was developing large-scale applications of nuclear power. UMP produced significant quantities of propulsion fuel for the nuclear navy fleet of the Soviet Union and, subsequently, Russia. From 1976 and continuing to the present, the plant has produced fuel pellets for nuclear power plants on a commercial scale.

Accompanying the production of these metals is a significant amount of liquid waste residues, which have been, and continue to be generated and disposed of in several retention basins adjoining the facility (Fig. 4). The engineered containment barrier underlying one of the basins has failed and allowed accumulated liquid wastes in the basin to percolate into groundwater and pose a significant threat to nearby potable groundwater supplies in Ust-Kamenogorsk. Although this basin is no longer used, precipitated and other solid forms of the wastes remain in the basin, are entrained in accumulated rainfall and snowmelt, and continue to be discharged into the local groundwater as a persistent and lasting source of contamination.

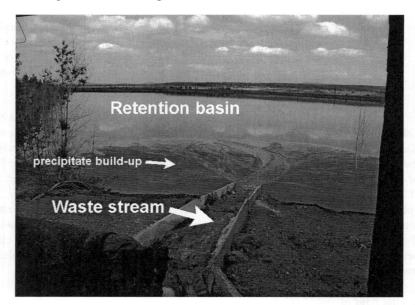

Fig. 4.   One of three actively used evaporative retention basins at the UMP plant in Ust-Kamenogorsk, Kazakhstan, showing existing mixed waste discharges and the build up of precipitate wastes.

The overall objective of the project–which is still in its planning stages–is to develop a conceptual and numerical model of groundwater flow and chemical transport that can be used to analyze the migration of contamination in the water supply aquifers underlying the UMP disposal basins. The model will be applied ultimately as a means to protect local groundwater quality by facilitating the remediation of existing contamination and the stabilization and control of contaminant discharges from liquid waste ponds at the plant. In addition, the model will also be used, in its initial stages of development, to determine the need for, and guide the acquisition of additional characterization and model calibration data, and later in the design of groundwater monitoring strategies. The importance of this project is underscored by the importance of the UMP plant itself as a productive economic enterprise for all of Kazakhstan.

Assessment of Radionuclide Migration in Groundwater at the Semipalatinsk Test Site
The Semipalatinsk Test Site (STS) in northern Kazakhstan was one of several areas used for the testing of nuclear weapons by the Former Soviet Union. Of a total of 456 nuclear tests carried out at STS, 340 were conducted in underground shafts or tunnels, 30 others were exploded on the ground surface, and the remaining 86 were detonated in the atmosphere. Within the STS, underground testing occurred within tunnels bored into the Degelen Mountain complex (209 tests) and within vertical shafts at the Balapan (109 tests) and Murzhik (26 tests) areas (Fig. 5).

Although there has been considerable interest in the distribution and impacts of residual radionuclides produced by the atmospheric testing (e.g., radiologic fallout and dose), there has been far less scrutiny of the fate of residual radionuclides from underground tests and, in particular, their potential to contaminate and migrate in groundwater and other drinking water supplies in the STS area.[7] Existing efforts have largely concentrated on monitoring programs in wells, rivers, and precipitation discharges from tunnels, and have not focused on examining the future potential for additional contamination or understanding more completely the interconnected processes that lead to such contamination.

The overarching rationale for the project – which is still in its planning stages – is based upon the need for preserving the integrity and quality of groundwater resources in Kazakhstan and, in particular, for understanding the nature and magnitude of specific threats to these resources posed by the legacy of underground nuclear testing. Based on the hydrologic setting and nature of the nuclear tests conducted, our

Kazakhstani colleagues have identified the Balapan site within the STS for the development of a hydrologic flow model and the smaller Zarechny site located within Balapan for the development of the initial radionuclide transport model (Fig. 6). The models will be used to study the release of radionuclides from one or more underground nuclear tests conducted below the water table and to examine the potential for their eventual migration in groundwater away from the testing areas.

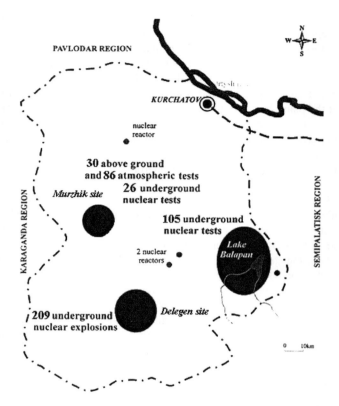

Fig. 5 Schematic of the Semipalatinsk Test Site in Northern Kazakhstan with the Balapan area highlighted.

Specifically, the overall project will emphasize:

- The nature of radionuclide releases from underground nuclear tests into groundwater, and their subsequent migration in groundwater, to be better quantified and understood;
- Better and more informed perspectives on these problems to be developed such that existing monitoring data may be better understood or such that future monitoring operations may be better planned;
- Improved understanding of the risk posed from groundwater contaminated with test-related radionuclides, better management practice for remediation or other reclamation activities, and in general, development of decision-making tools to better evaluate or otherwise modify groundwater use practices in contaminated areas; and

- Similar analyses to be undertaken at other testing areas within the Balapan area or the STS in general (Figure 5), or to manage other radionuclide contamination problems not associated directly with underground nuclear testing.

The project will parallel similar endeavors that have been initiated at the U.S. testing areas at the Nevada Test Site[8] and at the French testing areas in the South Pacific.[9]

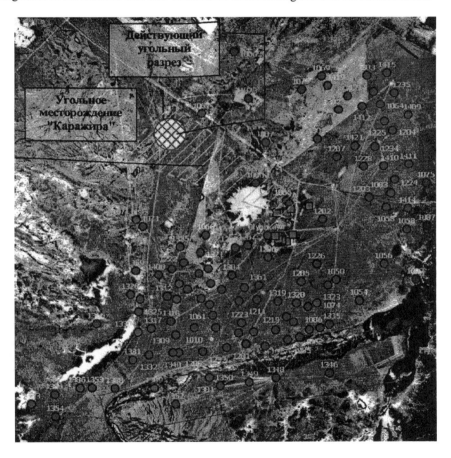

Fig. 6. Areal photo of the Balapan area in the Semipalatinsk Test Site in Northern Kazakhstan showing red "military" shafts and green unused boreholes. The smaller Zarechny site is outlined in the bottom (courtesy: S. Subbotin).

Protecting Yssyk-Köl from Radioactive Contamination and Preserving Kyrgyzstan's Economic Future

This project has been developed to eliminate a significant radioactive threat to Yssyk-Köl in eastern Kyrgyzstan – one of the world's largest mountain lakes – and to preserve what is widely believed to be this country's key economic resource. Central Asia has emerged as an area of extreme strategic interest since 11 September. The war in Afghanistan has accentuated the region's ethnic rivalries, the slow growth of democratic regimes, the collapse of regional economies, and the rise of fundamentalist Islam. Compounding these social and political conditions is an environmental legacy from the Soviet nuclear weapons program – the Kaji-Say radioactive uranium tailings pile – that threatens to destroy assets fundamental to any economic recovery.

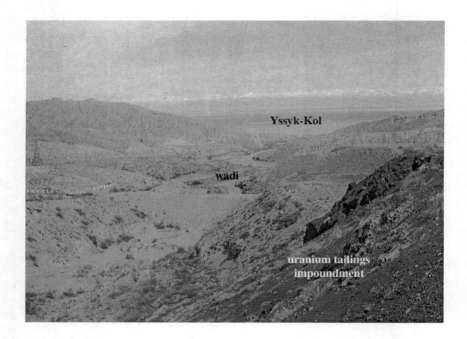

Fig. 7. A photograph of the precarious lake-side bank of the Kaji-Say radioactive tailings pile. Looking to the North, Yssyk-Köl is approximately one kilometer away. The snow-capped Tien Shen mountains can be seen in the distance. The dry stream bed (wadi) in the background floods during rainstorms and threatens to sweep the uranium pile downstream into the lake.

The Kaji-Say tailings pile is precariously poised on the banks of a wadi (dry, ephemeral streambed) approximately one kilometer away from Yssyk-Köl (see Fig. 7).

The tailings pile has a volume of about 150,000 m³ and has been swelled by the continual addition of debris, some of which is radioactively contaminated equipment. Although though the precise contents of this pile are not available, spot exposure readings as high as 800 µR/hr have been recorded; the limiting exposure standard in Europe is 60 µR/hr.

The hazard at Kaji-Say is the catastrophic collapse of the uranium tailings pile, its incorporation into a flash flood, and the subsequent transport of radioactive sludge to Yssyk-Köl. Rain storms in this arid climate are infrequent (less than 300 mm of rain per year) but severe and intense. The position of the pile and its unstable slopes make it wholly susceptible to collapse and transport. This project, recently funded by the U.S. Department of State, will involve:

- Relocating uncontained uranium tailings from below an existing retention dam to above the dam,
- Rehabilitating and armoring the existing retention dam to prevent radioactive debris from reaching Ysyk-Köl,
- Conducting erosion control operations at the base of the uranium tailings pile,
- Repairing the existing tailings cover,
- Installing a specialized fence with appropriate signage
- Development of a series of monitoring wells along the axis of the wadi to assess whether (or to what extent) underlying groundwater has been contaminated from uranium leached from the tailings piles.

Situated at an altitude of 1,620 m, Yssyk-Köl is analogous to Lake Tahoe in the United States, although it has more than 12-times greater surface area (~ 6,220 sq. km). It reaches a depth of 702 m, is slightly saline, and is ice-free in winter. No motor craft are allowed on the lake in an effort to preserve its water quality. Yssyk-Köl is well known throughout the Eurasian continent as a popular Soviet-era vacation destination. Collapse of the Soviet Union was accompanied by a collapse in tourism. Any radioactive contamination of Yssyk-Köl would be quickly reported through-out the Eurasian continent (and perhaps world) and would jeopardize this as an economic resource for generations.

This project will provide a technological and science-based strategy for mitigating the threat of radionuclide contamination cross the entire region. It is a demonstration project that produces a trained workforce, a sound scientific approach, and the appropriate analytical tools to interpret results.

SUMMARY

This paper has been concerned with the promotion and advancement of regional security in the Middle East and Central Asia through the development of bilateral and multilateral cooperation on targeted scientific and technical projects, especially those that that focus on the resolution of important regional environmental threats. Although several prototype projects developed by the authors and their regional colleagues have been described, they by no means represent the full spectrum of problems, nor the range of Western organizations involved in collaboration and solution efforts. For example, the U.S. Agency for International Development, through its Middle East Regional Cooperation Program, has developed a significant cooperative program involving the sue and management of groundwater in the West Bank and Gaza[10]. In Central Asia, for example, there are numerous and significant environmental problems surrounding the Caspian and Aral Seas. We are considering several new collaborations on the Caspian Sea, which will complement the work of the Caspian Environment Programme[11]. Several other regional cooperative efforts with European organizations are also being focused on the Aral Sea[12,13].

ACKNOWLEDGMENTS

This work was conducted under the auspices of the U. S. Department of Energy by the University of California, Lawrence Livermore National Laboratory under contract W-7405-Eng-48.

REFERENCES

1. C. de Cerreno, A.L. and A. Keynan, eds. (1998), *Scientific Cooperation, State Conflict: The Role of Scientists in Mitigating International Discord*, Annals of the New York Academy of Sciences, Vol. 866, NY.

2. IGC (2002), Central Asia: Water and Conflict, ICG Asia Report No. 34, International Crisis Group (http://www.intl-crisis-group.org), Osh/Brussels, May.

3. Hughes, E.L., K.H. Butts, B.F. Griffard, and A.L. Bradshaw, Jr., editors (2001), *Responding to Environmental Challenges in Central Asia and the Caspian Basin*, Center for Strategic Leadership, U.S. Army War College, PA.

4. Homer-Dixon, T., (1999), *Environment, Scarcity, and Violence*, Princeton University Press, Princeton NJ.

5. Wolf, A.T. (1997), "International Water Conflict Resolution: Lessons from Comparative Analysis," *International Journal of Water Resources Development*, 13, 3.

6. McMelis, D. and G.E. Schweitzer (2001), "Environmental Security: An Evolving Concept," *Environmental Science and Technology*, 35(5), 108A

7. IAEA (1998a), *Radiological Conditions at the Semipalatinsk Test Site, Kazakhstan: Preliminary Assessment and Recommendations for Further Study*, International Atomic Energy Agency, Vienna (STI/PUB/1063).

8. U.S. DOE (1997), *Regional groundwater flow and tritium transport modeling and risk assessment of the underground test area, Nevada Test Site, Nevada*, U.S. Department of Energy, Nevada Operations Office, Environmental Restoration Division, Las Vegas, NV (DOE/NV--477).

9. IAEA (1998b), The radiological situation at the atolls of Mururoa and Fangataufa. Technical report, Volume 4. Releases to the biosphere of radionuclides from

underground nuclear weapons tests at the atolls. International Atomic Energy Agency, Vienna, Austria (IAEA-MFTR-4).

10. http://www.usaid.gov/wbg/program_water.htm
11. http://www.caspianenvironment.org/
12. http://www.aral.uz/
13. http://www.environmonument.com/Aralsea.htm

HIGH-TECH TERRORISM – A RAPIDLY GROWING, GLOBAL PROBLEM

KARL K. REBANE
Department of Physics, University of Tallinn, Tallinn, Estonia

High-tech terrorism (HTT) is not a disaster of casual nature. HTT is the unavoidable result of the development of technology and society; a result of "progress". HTT is one of the most dangerous and persistent threats to mankind in the near future. The three pillars for HTT are:

1. "valuable*" goals* have been created;
2. *means* to attack *efficiently* have come into existence and are available;
3. the progress of the means of attack has been always faster than that of the means of defence. Nowadays the gap in favour of attack has become tremendous and is continuing to grow rapidly.

The three trends became very strong at the end of the last century. The situation and means of attack became highly efficient and thus the birth of HTT became inevitable. This engendered the forecast that the first large-scale HTT attacks, many orders of magnitude more destructive in lives and property than the earlier ones, were to come around the turn of the century.[1]

One of the potentially dangerous future developments is the attraction for losers' to clandestinely use HTT to support their interests in international relations. (If war is the continuation of politics with other means (Clauzewitz), then HTT is the continuation of (conventional) war with other means and moralities.)

Democracy and terrorism are related to quite an extent in the same way as the measurement of co-ordinate x and momentum p in quantum mechanics (via the Heisenberg's relation of uncertainty: $\Delta \leftarrow \Delta p$? h, where Δ shows the accuracy of measurement):

$$T \, ?D \cong constant.$$

Here T is the strength of counter-terroristic measures, D – the "measure" of democratic freedom. The equation is to show that strengthening of counter-terrorist measures inevitably brings along some losses in democratic freedom. Below are a few examples:

1. An effective measure against terrorism is to keep an accurate list of permanent and transient inhabitants for each local community (support and reward neighbourhood watch and local police duties).
   That system was strictly and effectively implanted everywhere in the Soviet Union. It helped quite a lot against criminal activities and terrorism. On the other hand, the detailed control of the population served as a powerful tool to support the Soviet regime, including its antidemocratic deeds and atmosphere.
2. Control the flow of information, Internet in the first place. Introduce restrictions.
3. Control the flow and concentration of financial, natural, military, human resources and know-how.
4. Keep lists of potentially "valuable" objects for HTT and control and very considerably improve their measures of defence.
5. Establish broad, sensitive and effective international control over those organizations, including governments, capable of terrorism and suspected of helping terrorism.
6. Implant informers, networks of them. Pay very well.
7. Treat relatives and friends of the terrorist, especially those of suicidal executors, as guilty. Punish them. Absolutely inhuman but effective: in many cases this can be and has shown to be historically, including in recent history, effective, and sometimes the only measure that really works to influence a devoted fighter (also a political enemy in history).

One basic premise of terrorism is that it is very difficult, desperately difficult for the losers or potential losers to accept defeat. This causes terrorist dreams, and sometimes leads to their realization as terrorist actions.

To help the losers overcome the difficulties – political, mental, economic, cultural, nationalistic – is an effective measure to decrease the sources nurturing of terrorism.

In the sphere of relations between common people, the rules of reasonable behaviour for the prevention of violence and keeping down trends towards dreaming of terrorist actions, have been well formulated in the Ten Commandments Moses brought down from Mount Sinai.

In general, the role of religion must not be ignored.

HTT is a global problem and, as for other global problems (planetary emergencies), can only be properly managed by a body authorized by the wide international community to control and command at the global level adequate technological, economical, military and natural resources, technological and scientific know-how, improve education, and further better understanding of the realities of the world we live in.

70

REFERENCES

1.	Karl K. Rebane. "High-tech terrorism as an increasing global problem," in *Science and Culture Series, Int. Seminar on Nuclear War and Planetary Emergencies*, 21-st Session, "E.Majorana" Centre for Scientific Culture, Erice Italy, 19-24 August 1996. Series editor and Chairman: A. Zichichi, edited by K. Goebel. World Scientific, Singapore, 1997, pp. 231-234.

HIGH-TECH TERRORISM AS AN INCREASING GLOBAL PROBLEM[*]

KARL K. REBANE
Department of Physics, University of Tallinn, Tallinn, Estonia

INTRODUCTION

High-tech terrorism (HTT) is terrorism of the kind that uses high-tech knowledge and weapons for the destruction of people, property, vital know-how and information systems or that threatens to use that kind of destruction.

Nowadays about 500 organizations worldwide are either using terrorism or considering the possibility (effective, even justified) of using it.

So far there have been no HTT actions. The recent use of Sarin dispersed in Tokyo marks a start and displays a trend.

Two features make high-technology terrorism dangerous and an urgent global problem. Firstly, the potentially destructive power of HTT is many orders of magnitude greater than that of the conventional terrorism mankind has faced up to now. Secondly, the current technological, political, economical, and environmental situation has prepared all the necessary conditions for HTT to be used on quite a large scale in the near future. In the other words, characteristically short times for growth (frequency and magnitude of actions) and changes (various means and ways) of applications are to be expected.

If I were asked to give some figure as an approximate estimate, I would say that the probability of the first HTT action (real damage or large scale threat) in the years remaining in this century constitutes as much as 80-90%. I hope that my estimate turns out to be entirely wrong, because it seems to so pessimistic, but, today, I cannot give a more optimistic forecast.

In this paper I do not discuss:

1. The definition of terrorism;
2. The borderline between pure, i.e. definitely criminal terrorism, and terrorism which to some extent could be interpreted and justified as part of a struggle for freedom, for civil or human rights, against injustice, etc. by some people.

---

[*]Originally presented at 21st Session in 1996.

Items 1 and 2 can be analysed by political and social scientists with much better expertise.

3. Any list of possible ways and means for HTT actions both now and in the near future which will, to a certain extent, be dependant on the availability of know-how of HTT.

HTT is one more very sensitive point of modern life in which a completely free flow of knowledge could be disastrous and must certainly be controlled.

REMARKS

The means for HTT are provided by current technology, based on the great achievements of physics, chemistry, biology (molecular and other), medicine, military, environmental and space sciences, computer science, on the misuse of this knowledge and know-how which is useful and crucially necessary to mankind.

The Internet provides information on manufacturing not only gun powder, but also napalm. What if the Internet opens a home page for HTT know-how and instructions: the means, technology and ideology, the planning, action design and relations with the mass media, etc.?

Scientists and engineers provide the basic knowledge of HTT and thus they carry considerable responsibility. Direct responsibility lies with those involved in the activities of producing and delivering the means for HTT.

(Conventional) terrorism has definitely played a role in the history of civilization.

The impact of HTT is going to increase by several orders of magnitude and will probably become as great as that of nuclear weapons in the post World War II policy.

Terrorist organizations are often rich in resources such as money, property, and the provision of privileges. They also have much more freedom to manage their resources than legal institutions.

There are always people in science and technology who are dissatisfied with their position, salaries and career prospects. Quite a number of them would be disinclined to reject work for HTT if they had better working conditions.

The other and very effective means to obtain the necessary work force is to put terrorist pressure on them. The Farnesine declaration says that poverty can destroy dignity. Terrorism can do the same.

Thus the realistic conclusion is to assume that the labour power for HTT can be provided and, in fact, already is being provided.

The dissolution of the Soviet Union has greatly enriched the high-tech labour market.

It is difficult and expensive to dismantle nuclear warheads and destroy chemical, biological, etc. weapons. The possibility of them leaking into terrorist hands exists.

Civilisation's general trend of creating more and more powerful, sophisticated systems and concentrating them at one site - this is also valid for vital global networks, etc. - is also creating "valuable" targets for terrorism. The targets are very difficult to defend against conventional terrorism (a well organised terrorist unit can easily conquer or destroy a nuclear power station). They are impossible to defend against HTT actions (e.g. guided missiles against nuclear power stations or computer viruses in the networks vital for the control of nuclear weapons).

Conventional terrorism, when backed further and further into a corner will be strongly inclined to use HTT.

CONCLUSION

It is very difficult, if not almost impossible, to stop the rising wave of HTT. The general situation and development trends make it difficult to fight terrorism and almost impossible to stop HTT.

Offensive weapons are always developed faster than the means of defence (sword versus shield compared to nuclear and biological weapons versus what? Nothing?) The gap between offensive and defensive potentials continues to increase.

Due to the above, defence is now being based on the threat of attack (not only counterattack!). Mutually Assured Destruction is actually mutual HTT threat at government levels!

Morals, ethics, the hierarchy of human values proved unable to keep up with the fast growth of technology in manipulating natural (and human) resources. Building on them might be more practical, wiser, safer and more useful than fighting terrorism.

We have to rely strongly on the fact that almost impossible is fundamentally different from impossible. We must try hard because there is hope.

- We should place high-tech terrorism on the "Planetary Emergencies" list;
- A group and a project on HTT could be established within the World Federation of Scientists;
- Advise the governments to strengthen Interpol into some kind of Super-Interpol, to whom a very considerable part of significant control functions and rights to realize them is delegated.
- Initiate the updating of the UN Constitution with the aim to delegate real responsibilities and the corresponding rights and real power to execute them to this large and strong international organisation. One of the most internationally important objectives has to be HTT.

We must admit that the present Constitution of the United Nations, accepted fifty years ago, was written in view of regulating the problems between states. Today very difficult problems exist inside historically established states, between nations and groups that have ethnical and religious differences (e.g. the former Yugoslavia, Soviet Union). The other source of serious problems is the illegal activities at both the national and international levels (e.g. narco-business and terrorism). UN has few legal rights and too little power by far to decisively contribute to the solution of these problems.

- In the long run the only hope lies in education, the understanding of global problems, the improvement of moral standards and high personal and collective responsibility.
- Cooperation with religion (faith in general) should not be ignored. Terrorism kills morals and is thus especially dangerous.
- The objective has to be to delay the advent of HTT, at least its most destructive activities. That is the same task that the governments of nuclear states have being contending with and have succeeded in controlling for over half a century with regard to both nuclear weapons and other weapons of mass destruction.

4. SOCIETY AND STRUCTURES: GLOBALIZATION — ECONOMY AND CULTURE

GLOBALIZATION AND CULTURE

AHMAD KAMAL
Senior Fellow, United Nations Institute of Training and Research, New York, NY, USA

Globalization is such an important and pervasive word in our current vocabulary, that it has almost become the flavor of the day. Despite its wide use, it remains a confusing concept in many ways. Like Aristotle's analogy of the candle, the more you know about it, the more you become aware of how little you really know.

Essentially, globalization is about a *shrinking* world, a world shrinking both in space and in time.

The fact that the world is shrinking geographically is nothing new. The world has been shrinking for thousands of years. This began when the first humans, who originated in what we now call East Africa, traveled north first, and then into Asia and Europe in the one direction, and to Siberia and then into the Americas in the other direction. Migration was thus the first human experience in globalization, one that placed the whole world on a single stage. Then came the age of travel, when courageous individuals like Marco Polo and Columbus, started expanding the parameters of the European experience by traveling and exploring, driven partly by curiosity, partly by a search for spices and silks, and partly by a simple desire to find out whether the earth was flat or round. Following this era of travel came trade, when people became aware of how much you could gain by exchanging goods, or even by exchanging ideas and cultures. Still later, you have the sad story of colonial empires, which imagined that they spanned the globe, and could boast of a sun that never set. Each colonial power perceived the world through its own blinkered perspective of a self-centered-stage, as one single space to be exploited. Fortunately, the sun never rises now on some of those arrogant empires.

So these historical shrinkages in space are not new. We must then ask, wherein lies the difference today? There are two obvious points to be considered. Firstly, there is this phenomenal increase in the speed of communications. Whereas an idea in a letter could take weeks or months to reach an addressee in another country, the same idea in an email can now cross the world instantaneously. Secondly, there is greater awareness. We are much more aware now of what is happening around the world, due in part to the CNN syndrome, and in part to the greater level of mutual dependency.

Trans-national corporations were the first to realize the opportunities inherent in this new game, in which the world is a single stage. Their successful and ruthless exploitation of these opportunities is what has created a real sense of doubt and despair.

People are not at all sure that they are happy with these developments. That is why you now have wave after wave of protest, with tens of thousands of people coming out onto on the streets of major North American cities, and repeat crowds in many other capitals of the world. Part of thus unhappiness arises from a sense that while we talk of globalizing opportunities, we are actually globalizing poverty and inequality. Globalization has been a one-way street only.

With all the happy talk of globalization of opportunities, the gap between rich and poor is growing. If you compare the average income-per-head of the top 25% in the developed states with that of the bottom 25% in the developing states, the ratio between those two is currently around 90:1; interestingly, if you go back 30 years you will find that it was only 40:1. So this gap is not just unacceptable in absolute terms, it is also doubling and getting worse.

It is inevitable to conclude then that globalization has widened the gap between peoples in the world. Let us look at four indicative examples.

Firstly, human rights and migration. A respect for human rights is of course a vital part of all the spiritual under-pinnings of society. However, this principle has assumed far greater importance over the past few years. It is this increased focus on eliminating serious human rights violations that underlies the progressive erosion of the erstwhile inviolate principle of "sovereignty" and "exclusive domestic jurisdiction," which was once seen as entitling a nation state to act as it liked within its borders. Nowadays, this "chastity belt" of Article 2.7 of the United Nations Charter has lost much of its sanctity, and countries or rulers that violate human rights can no longer claim that their actions are nobody else's business. In other words, the walls that enabled countries to seal themselves off have fallen down before the onslaught of human rights concerns, and clearly this is a most positive development.

Unfortunately, this erosion of these hermetic walls of sovereignty works in one direction only. If respect for human rights implies a respect for the desire of peoples for a better and more decent life, and an elimination of obstacles, then people from poorer countries should also be able to cross those walls in the other direction also in their search for a better life. Alas, they cannot do so. In fact, in many ways, the barriers to free movement are higher than ever before, with progressively tighter restrictions on immigration. So you have a fundamental inequality here – one part of the world can criticize the other with impunity for human rights violations, but people from the countries that are most often criticized cannot migrate towards the richer countries in their search for a better life. So while we talk glibly of an open world of opportunity, we are actually doing our utmost to prevent this world from really opening up. This is a sad one-way street indeed.

Secondly, trade. Trade has visibly emerged as a major engine of growth. The assumption of the open and competitive market then was that barriers of all types would be progressively dismantled, for the general benefit of all. Only the "competitive edge" would rule. Yet protectionism is rampant, particularly in relation to the exports of poorer countries, which stand lower down on the scale of industrial sophistication. The tariffs on textiles (an item of great interest to developing countries), for example, are a full ten times higher than the tariffs on industrial goods (which are of interest basically to developed countries trading among themselves).

Protectionism is only the one side of the coin. On the other side, we have subsidies, which prop up the relatively inefficient agriculture of the developed countries at immoral levels. The OECD countries are spending roughly a billion dollars a day today on such subsidies, seven times as much as the total aid that is given to the developing countries. It is these massive subsidies that create the glut that lowers commodity prices, and ensures that the poor of the world will not be able to pull themselves out of the morass of abject poverty.

So, in general, while we may talk about a level playing field in trade at the world level, it is nevertheless a field in which the "weight" of the richer countries is so heavily skewed in their own favor, that the results are foregone for the developing countries. Efforts to insert respect for the principle of Special and Differentiated Treatment in favor of developing countries have lost ground with the establishment of the World Trade Organization. Imagine the consternation of the Nike worker in Indonesia who realizes now that he would have to work for 100,000 years to make what the chief executive of Nike makes in just one.

Thirdly, the environment. The environment is the perfect globalizer, as it has no respect for nationalities and passports and borders. We see its impact every day, as environmental events in one part of the world produce effects in other parts of the world, frequently with devastating results.

Once again, these effects are unevenly distributed. Some see no evil in their over-exploitation of finite fossil fuels and inordinate pollution of the atmosphere, while others in far corners of the world suffer consequences in health and economic well being. One-fourth of the total gashouse emissions that we pour into the atmosphere come from a single country alone.

Fourthly, the Internet. Of course, the Internet offers great opportunities for those who can use it, allowing anyone with access to it to draw upon as much of the data-base of universal knowledge as the richest or most powerful. In that, it is one of the major milestones in human history, ranking with moveable type, or the mass-produced paper back, as a great and democratic equalizer. But just as a sizeable part of the world has neither access to safe drinking water nor to electricity, the vast majority of the peoples of the world do not, and will not, have access to the Internet in any foreseeable future. Just to take one example, in sub-Saharan Africa, 90% of the connections to the Internet are in just one country, a former bastion of colonialism of the worst type. So, the tool exists, but it cannot be used by those who need it most. And yet, in it lies perhaps the only chance for the future. Where an effort has been made, the internet and cell phones have helped rural villages get connected to the rest of the world, helped women in developing nations become entrepreneurs.

A major problem with the Internet arises from the predominance of English as a language of choice. Language is not just a neutral tool for communication; it also embodies culture, and defines the parameters of our thinking processes. It would be a very sad day indeed if one single culture were to spread and dominate all others. Homogenization may be good for milk, but it is not necessarily good for the rich diversity of cultures in the world, many of which are an endangered species now.

To sum up, globalization is doubtless an opportunity, but regrettably it has only served the interests of the few so far. The real beneficiaries have either been corporations, most of whom are based in the West, or governments, also in most cases from that same part of the world. The latter have often been able to utilize the forces of globalization to impose their model upon other cultures and civilizations, many of which are far older and culturally far richer.

Globalization clearly puts the state and the peoples of the world under pressure, and in so doing it creates the tensions that we have seen on the streets of so many countries.

Where then do we go from here? The answer lies perhaps in an exchange of cultures and a dialogue between civilizations, rather than in a one-way belief in cultural superiority. Cultures need to be respected in their diversity, and nurtured in their differences, and not forced into the mold of a lowest common denominator. Since globalization appears to be moving forward inexorably, we need to ensure that it becomes a process whereby the citizens of the world can be more integrated, and yet more different, in a shared world. Only if we achieve that unity in diversity will history judge us kindly.

Who can do that? Certainly not the governments, who are mostly lost in a self-constructed wilderness of questionable politics. Certainly not the international financial institutions, which are highly susceptible to the policy interests of member governments, and subject to criticism about their own poor governance. Certainly not the private sector, whose primary responsibility has to lie inevitably in the profit motive, as called for by their share-holders.

That leaves the burden to be borne by the citizens of the world, the peoples, the think-tanks, the academia, the community organizations, or what is normally referred to as Civil Society. It is Civil Society alone that realizes that the cultural diversity of ideas and principles is part of the nuance and color of the world, and which can muster the competence and commitment to understand that that the objective of globalization should be mutual benefit, mutual enrichment, mutual happiness, and mutual responsibilities, if we are to move forwards.

Unfortunately, or fortunately, even the best of organizations and institutions and movements need leadership to give them vision and purpose. Without such leadership, Civil Society is likely to disperse its energy into diffused directions, and along unfocused paths. That is where this meeting in Erice assumes its importance, as a lighthouse on a Sicilian hill, which can help in directing the ships of Civil Society safely across the uncharted waters of Globalization.

DEFENDING AGAINST MASS-CASUALTY TERRORISM: TECHNOLOGIES ENABLING STRATEGY AND TACTICS FOR ROBUST DEFENSE

DR. LOWELL WOOD

Lawrence Livermore National Laboratory, Livermore CA; Hoover Institution, Stanford University, Stanford CA, USA

"We have nothing to fear but fear itself." — Franklin D. Roosevelt

TERRORISM

"Politics by other (quite different) means"

◆ Classic David vs. Goliath confrontation
  – Small, light-&-agile against huge, heavy-&-slow
  – Terrorists aim to defeat adversary's <u>policy</u>, not adversary forces *per se:* banditry writ large – or war writ small?
    · <u>Nobody</u> attacks Western forces in this, the latest Western Century
    · *Attack <u>where defenses aren't</u>,* to frighten people and humiliate governments – to coerce behavior "innovatively"
    · *Except for crucial Bonaparte-Lenin <u>system-destroying</u> case*
      – E.g., threat-enforced, prolonged evacuation of cities

◆ Not <u>worth</u> defending against, in conventional geo-politico-military cost-exchange terms
  – <u>Mass-casualty</u> damage expectancy is (typically) negligible
    · *On national scales* – micro- to (at worst) milli-"RISOP units"
  – Defensive costs will be large, effectiveness (at best) moderate
  – Defensive efforts concede many basic advantages *ab initio* to mass casualty-oriented terrorist-adversaries
    · $\geq$$10^{11}$ expenditures to avert 10^9 - 10^{10} damage-expectancies?

STRATEGIC ASYMMETRIES

◆ Slight imperfections in <u>first-time</u> serious exercising of counter-terrorism defenses impose real costs
  – Intelligent terrorists select softest "point" for attack
    • In space, in time, in target-parameters, . . .
    • e.g,. civilian airliners and ships, embassies, small troop outposts,...
  – <u>Nobody</u> does something demanding very well on the first attempt
    • It's *practice* that perfects – for both the offense <u>and</u> the defense
  – Fundamental competence of government readily called into question by terrorism success – *starkly*
    ◦ *"...to provide for the common defense,"* – U.S. Constitution, Preamble
    Bonaparte-Leninist scenarios enabled – ultimate political catastrophe

◆ Terrorists can be <u>exceedingly</u> serious-in-preparation – while democracies cannot
  – Strong democracies don't rise to non-visible threats
    • Not 'easy prey' for demagogues – or heeding of "DEWs"
  – "Show me the bodies" attitude prevalent in U.S. Congress
    • A stance as old as Periclean Athens

BASIC DEFENSIVE STRATEGIES

◆ Leverage West's strengths and terrorists' weaknesses
  – <u>West's advantages</u>: economic and scientific/technological wealth; geographic de-coupling; huge security 'plant'-in-being
  – <u>Terrorists' disabilities</u>: covertness requirements; high-tech demands; logistics & lengthy lines-of-communications; cash-starvation; 'first time' clumsiness; intellectual/cultural limitations; moral odium

◆ De-leverage West's weaknesses and terrorists' strengths
  – <u>West's disadvantages</u>: openness; extensive civil liberties; innocence presumption; "faint at sight-of-blood" syndrome; 'fearlessness'
  – <u>Terrorists' capabilities</u>: ever-longer technological levers; cultural barriers; language-shields; superpower stockpile 'leakage'; fanaticism; long-range planning & armor-chink exploitation; covert state sponsorship; "stampede generation" options

◆ Implement *and* test *<u>layered</u>, high-integrity* defenses
  – <u>Independently-functioning, high-capability</u> layers
  – Both *active* and *passive* features <u>which are *known-to-work*</u>
    • Akin to anti-submarine warfare – where *stealthiness* is of the essence
      – Reliable defeat of stealthiness is a sufficient condition for victory

· Only 'live' exercises demonstrate-&-validate *actual, real* capabilities

OPERATIONAL STRATEGY

♦ <u>Deter</u>, by making plausible attempts at terrorism dauntingly difficult – and appallingly expensive
   – *"Our doubts are traitors, and make us fail, by fearing to attempt."* – W. Shakespeare
   – <u>Only</u> ubiquitous shield for West's most-exposed assets

♦ <u>Detect</u>, <u>disrupt</u> and <u>destroy</u> attempts underway, far from target-areas – and publicize successes
   – Fight on *their* territory, not *ours* – <u>and</u> on *our* terms

♦ <u>Defeat</u> serious attempts *passively*

♦ <u>Deny</u> success to most serious attempts *actively*

♦ <u>Attribute</u> attacks reliably-&-swiftly, and <u>retaliate</u> *memorably* and multi-axially

"DAUNTINGLY DIFFICULT"

♦ Impose long-term-unendurable stresses on terrorist *personnel security* systems
   – <u>Very</u> few recent instances of "solitary malignant polymath"-as-terrorist
     • <u>Terrorists come in teams</u> – which *always* have a weakest member
     • "Unbearably attractive-&-eminently credible" offers to weakest terrorists nearly always succeed
       – Powerfully leverages the economic strength of the West
       – Surpassingly easy to implement – at remarkably low cost
         • <u>Zero</u> marginal cost, until/unless used – and then cheap
       – Amply precedented in recent law-and-practice
         • $5 M bounty offered for African embassy bombers
         • $25 M offered for senior al Qaeda leaders
     • Attractiveness and plausibility features: bounty size, terms, reliability-of-payment, minimization of personal risk, . . .
       – E.g., great enough to effectively <u>compel</u> desired behaviors
       – E.g., Witness Protection programs, for target-and-family

♦ Impose great and <u>continuous</u> stresses on *terrorist communications* systems
   – Means for stressing traditional (broadcast-type) adversary comm systems are notably effective
   – Means for *effectively* and *reliably* stressing new (e.g., Internet-based, encryption-leveraging) comm technologies need to be developed-&-deployed *urgently*

- Terrorists talk to each other; the West must be *listening* – and *hearing*, and *acting*
  - Present-day deficiencies in all three areas
  - Not only are we "going deaf," but we're not aptly *interpreting* what do we *hear*, or *acting* on what we *know*!
    - E.g., modernization of domestic intelligence practices is urgently needed – most date from the pre-Internet era
      - "The Constitution isn't a mutual suicide pact!"
      - But West-defining civil liberties can't be compromised, either

- Impose continuous, multi-axis stresses on terrorist *lines-of-communication* (LOCs)
  - Terrorists must eat, sleep, dress, wash, travel, procure supplies-&-equipments, prepare packages-of-nastiness...
  - Each of these is detectable-&-exploitable, e.g.,
    - Tagging of terrorists so as to detect at points-of-entry
    - Tagging of terrorist vehicles, for tracking-from-afar
    - Tagging of terrorist explosives, for trip-wire screens
    - All done covertly – so that tags' existence is unknown
  - Terrorists tend to be technologically naïve, except in terrorism-specialty areas – and thus are surprise-prone
    - "Any sufficiently advanced technology is indistinguishable from magic." – A.C. Clarke
    - Nazi reactions to apparent *Enigma*-cracking are instructive

  Paranoia is terrorism's occupational disease–exploit it!

- Interact closely-&-creatively with the international terrorism sponsorship network
  "Follow the money trails, and you soon will understand everything else."
  - Crucial to understand *who* funds terrorism, and exactly *how* – & even *why*
    - With contributions-in-kind, as well as money
    - A "Distant Early Warning" system that almost never fails
  - Statutory prohibitions against entrapment probably don't protect international terrorists – or their sponsors
    - Most-effective-possible way to spend funds
    - The rodents must be taught to fear readily-available cheese...
      - ...and thus there will be fewer of them

TECHNOLOGIES: DETERRENCE

- Facilitation of information *procurement*
  - Make it easy to sell pertinent information to governments.
  - International toll-free numbers, risk-minimized meeting arrangements, data sieving-&-analyzing automation,...

– A complete <u>system</u>, with multiple fail-safe features

◆ Facilitation of information *acquisition*
  – Modernization of classical ways-&-means
  – *Internet*-directed, fiber optic-focused, automatic processing-&-<u>action</u>
    • Enabled by modernized, technology-updated statutory specs
    • Crucial to not hobble ourselves by our technical dominance
  – Supplemented by special techniques-&-technologies
    • Terrorist-focused: e.g., quick-reaction; single-event fail-safe
  – Enormously expensive
    • Gov'ts. pay the basic bills anyway; anti-terrorism is collateral

◆ Facilitation of terrorist facility penetration
  – This *isn't* the "<u>hard</u> underground facility" problem
    • Non-State-sponsored groups lack the funds to dig, button-up
  – E.g., covert emplacement of pickups
    • Exploit classical techniques/technologies of high utility
      – E.g., sweep-resistance, data exfiltration requirements relaxed
    • 'Reduction of present problem to a previously-solved problem': "baby-sitting" juvenile delinquents who grew old

◆ Facilitation of tracking of terrorists-&-gear
  – Tags, tags and tags – *exceedingly* high efficacy gambit-set
    • *Body*, *equipment*, *vehicles* and *materials* tags
    • Emphasis on covertness, long-range detectivity, low false-positive rates; leveraging of full set of existing Western assets
    • <u>Rich</u> set of technological options – little-exploited yet
      – Extensive public discussion attenuates operational effectiveness
    • West-accessible choke-points become strongly leveraged
      – Tripwire capabilities may be deployed over most of the world
  – Key issue: what types of tags are policy-permissible?
    • E.g., most effective body-tags may pose peculiar issues

"DETECT, DISRUPT & DESTROY"

◆ Akin to harrying flights of bombers all the way to their targets – <u>and</u> all the way back to their bases
◆ Enlist *everyone, everywhere*, as part-time anti-terrorism agents
  – Offer *huge*, standing rewards for "information leading to the arrest-&-conviction…"
    • Akin to bounty-<u>packages</u> offered to weakest terrorism team-members – but offered to the *general public, world-wide*

– Spend *pennies* buying information from those that have it, versus *dollars* on hordes of Western civil servants who (probably) don't
- "Transform your life, reliably, with a single phone-call!"
- *Failure to offer such incentives* is an unmistakable message about Western seriousness regarding terrorism
  – Saving a major Western city is worth less than a single California Lottery jackpot (>$125 M)?!?
  – Spend <u>billions</u> to (thinly) armor embassies, but only <u>millions</u> to discover their attackers?!?

Terrorists are thereby forced to regard *everyone, everywhere* as a potential police agent <u>aimed at them</u>

◆ Scan continually for terrorism-in-transit at <u>all</u> major points-of-entry – <u>all</u> kinds of tripwires, *everywhere*
  – Overtly, at friendly points; covertly, at others

◆ Have <u>practiced</u> Standard Operational Procedures for *<u>robust</u>* interception of terrorism-underway
  – <u>Statutory</u> authorization for (creative) use of "all necessary means" against *<u>mass-casualty</u>* terrorist threats
    • E.g., sabotage of mass-destruction weaponry in terrorist hands
      – 'Lesson taught' in sponsor's 'backyard'
    • E.g., intensive (plausibly-deniable?) harassment of terrorist camps
    • E.g., (remote?) deception-detection systems
    • Eliminate delays-&-ditherings
      – Formal, legalized Declarations of War against mass-casualty terrorism
      – Akin to the U.S. campaigns against the Barbary pirates, 2 centuries ago
  – Exercised by specialized teams, supported by the full spectrum of Western means
  – Extensively rehearsed-&-drilled – formidable 'Red Teams'

'D, D & D' TECHNOLOGIES

◆ Tripwires at checkpoints (e.g., ports-of-entry)
  – Document-inspectors, body-scanners, explosive-sniffers, gamma-ray detectors, . . .
    – active <u>and</u> passive probing for terrorists and their equipment-&-materials
    • Mostly seeking covertly-implanted tags
      – Both active and interrogated – body, equipment, materials, …
    • But also natural emissions of terrorist-peculiar materials
      – E.g., gamma-rays from SNM; vapors from organic compounds;…
    • And signals 'actively elicited' from contraband
      – E.g., gammas from N^{15}, Cl, U^{235},…
      – *Image* and *process*, as well as *detect*, to attain low false-alarm rates

- Leveraging modern sensor and DSP technologies
- Two <u>quite</u> different technology *families* of tripwires
  - Only the friendly-deployed one is known to exist…
  - Differences in packaging, power supply, data-return
    - But comparable underlying sensor technologies

"DEFEAT SERIOUS ATTEMPTS"

- ◆ *Exponentially-higher* barriers, as terrorist threats approach their Western targets, e.g.,
  - Comprehensive, concealed sets of tripwires at all points-of-entry and intra-West LOC 'choke-points'
    - Seeking SNM, N^{15}-in-HE, Cl-in-LE, chem/explosive vapors, . .
    - <u>Continually</u> looking for {personnel, materials, equipment} tags
    - Supported by cellphone-telemetry, real-time processing, quick-response (e.g., heli-transported) squads – 'civilian Rangers'
    - Rich spectrum of technological options currently available
      - Low cost of mass-produced high-tech (e.g., GPS/cellphone hybrids) supports <u>massive</u> proliferation of high-effectiveness tripwires – phones bearing Si-based sensors
      - $1 B buys 100,000-1,000,000 mass-produced tripwires ($1-10 K ea.)
        - E.g., 1,000 robust tripwires covering <u>each</u> of 100 largest cities
  - (Far) larger incentives offered for information
  - Robust, <u>active</u> search/detection means employed
    - E.g., long-range, high areal sweep-rate probe-beams for SNM, chemical explosives, e.g., airborne probe-detector systems
      - Look for characteristic signatures in 'echoes' from probing
    - E.g., near-real-time, extensively field-deployed advanced bio-agent sensors – exquisitely sensitive and fast-reporting

'SERIOUS ATTEMPTS' DEFEAT TECHNOLOGIES

- ◆ Long-range/high-speed nukes-in-transit detection
  - Gamma-ray 'color' imaging systems
    - Deployed (covertly) on bridges, airport runways, docks, …
    - Large detector areas <u>and</u> high angular resolution confer high detectivity <u>and</u> fine localization of gamma-sources
      - E.g., see nukes at >100 meter ranges, while flying overhead
      - Preclude cities from being emptied by a single nuke-as-threat
    - Small, dense (highly-proliferated!) versions for imaging materials in luggage, crates and other close-proximity items
      - In their own emissions – or via elicited (interrogated) emissions
      - Detect/defeat truck-borne ~0.1 kT chem super-explosives in cities
        - Preclude 'easy' near-term Leninist-Bonaparte scenarios

◆ Near-real-time bio-agents-being-dispersed detection
  – Addressing the issue that empirical chemical formulae aren't bio-agent revelatory – residue *sequences* are crucial
    • Only empirical chemical formulae can be readily 'read' from afar
  – E.g., fly-able PCR-centered micro-scale bio-labs probing suspicious particulate plumes-in-air
    • Results in minutes – perhaps before plume 'touches down'
  – Near-real-time analysis for aero-toxins, e.g., high-P LCC
  – Both leveraging small RPV and LIDAR technologies

"DENY SUCCESS TO THE MOST SERIOUS ATTEMPTS"

◆ Maximally strenuous, across-the-spectrum damage-limitation efforts, e.g.,
  – *Real-time* detection-&-defeat of nukes, chem/bio agent-dispersing platforms
  – *High-rate, large-scale,* highly-automated clean-up of chem/bio-contaminated areas-&-volumes
  – Prompt <u>rescue</u> *en masse* of otherwise fatally-damaged civilians with advanced, *ad hoc* biomedical means
  – Super-high-rate mass-immunization and –prophylaxis

◆ Executed by pre-deployed equipment and intensively-exercised personnel, utilizing <u>highly-proliferated pharmaceutical mini-depots</u>, . . .
  – "Acting as in time of war" – e.g. 'block wardens'
  – Leveraging the huge logistics advantages of the defense

SUCCESS-DENIAL TECHNOLOGIES

◆ Turn off nukes *as they detonate*
  – Near-speed-of-light particle beams induce neutronic pre-initiation *<u>after</u> HE detonator action is detected* remotely and beam is aimed – *nuclear yield precluded in predictable manner <u>after</u> the device is fired*
    • Leverage existing storage ring/beam-projection technologies
    • A *known-to-work* gambit – <u>implementation</u> is the challenge
    • Also useful for <u>robustly</u> disarming pre-emplaced nukes

◆ Neutralize chem and bio-agents with high fluences of UV-C light from megawatt-class beam projectors, for swift clean-up of large areas
  – Photo-oxidize neurotoxins and fatally photo-damage the DNA of *all* pathogens, at high areal sweep-rates
    • 100-1000 Watt-sec/m^2 sterilization fluences <u>always</u> suffice
      – Megawatt system <u>definitively</u> cleans up 1,000-10,000 m^2/second
    • Leverage existing UV-C curing systems industrial base

- ◆ Prompt, *en masse* rescue of attacked, (otherwise) fatally-damaged people
  - − Self-injectable 'high biology' toxin-scavengers
    - • Competitively sequester toxins from circulating serum
      - − Designer macromolecules targeted on specific compound-classes
    - • Early endotoxin examples now in Phase II trials
      - − Modify molecular structures to target military (neuro)toxins
        - • Act to raise LD50s of agents by 2-3 orders-of-magnitude

- ◆ Super-high-rate mass immunization and pathogen-prophylaxis, for the pre- & recently-infected
  - − <u>Today:</u> sustained-release anti-bacterial/-viral antibiotics supplementing mass (preferably, oral/nasal) vaccination
  - − <u>Tomorrow:</u> panspectral contra-pathogen/-toxin (e.g., D(A-S)/RNAi-generating) human epi-chromosomes
    - • Hosts made *exceedingly* inhospitable to all military pathogens and toxins – for a few weeks until epi-chromosomes are lyzed
    - • Key features are timely R&D exploitation and leveraging of the logistics superiority of the defense

- ◆ Passive defense against ionizing radiation fields
  - − Sulfhydro/disulphide compounds-based prophylaxis

"ATTRIBUTE AND RETALIATE"

- ◆ <u>Crucial</u> aspect of deterrence

- ◆ Far more important to be right than quick, but swift-&-sure retaliation upon attack-attribution is the most effective
  - − *Disproportionate, comprehensive* retaliation is indicated
    - • *Incalculable* pain for <u>all</u> participants – <u>not</u> just immediate actors
      - − But oblige the martyrdom-inclined <u>only</u> if unavoidable
    - • Maximize pre-attack uncertainty in actors <u>and</u> sponsors
      - − E.g., incentivize "weakest link" to betray attack, to avoid response
  - − <u>Never, ever</u> quit the *vigorous, active* pursuit of the guilty
    - ◦ The Mossad-Eichmann paradigm: "We'll hunt you down, wherever you hide, as long as it takes, whatever it costs."
      - − Technology *strongly* favors the hunter over the hunted
    - • *Behavior-compelling* incentives proffered for information
      - − Even 'religious fanatic' groups have their weakest member
        - • 'Prisoner's Dilemma' incentive-structure aids the Good Guys

- ◆ Attribution: necessary-&-nearly-sufficient for success
  - − Citizenry <u>demands</u> identity of the guilty – forestalls panic

- Enabled by either technical means or an "impossible to refuse" offer to buy information – preferably, both
    - Again, leverage West's economic strength by <u>purchasing</u> the required information – <u>and</u> sufficient supporting evidence!

RED TEAMS AND 'LIVE' TESTING

- ◆ Crucial to have innovative, independent, competent crews whose full-time job is to "Think Red"
    - Identify, document & 'advocate' chinks-in-armor
    - Design and supervise "practice attacks"
    - Evaders of "Red Team-ing" are bureaucratic frauds
        - Yearn to be paid to erect-&-preside over 'Potemkin villages'
        - Untried/untested defenses almost invariably fail-when-used
- ◆ <u>Essential</u> to exercise <u>often</u> against <u>'live'</u> threats
    - <u>No</u> advance information provided about timing, nature, direction,…of "practice attacks"
        - Must be realistic – mustn't mislead re actual capabilities
        - No 'magic wand' defenses, e.g., "The nuke is located <u>here</u>"
            - Too many exercises have some basic "magical" characteristics
            - And Tinker Bell assuredly won't be there when we really need her!
    - Frequent "attacks" needed, to keep <u>everyone</u> practiced, <u>everywhere</u>, against <u>all</u> types of problems
        - <u>Metrics</u> employed comprehensively; realistic 'grades' given

"THE IMPORTANCE OF BEING EARNEST"

- ◆ *"You can't have a credible ballistic missile defense with cardboard radars."* – F. Dyson, ~'72

- ◆ Deterrence arises from *credible capabilities* and *undoubted will* to exercise them
    - Potent means, realistically and continually exercised
    - Supplemented by "scalps hanging from belt" from real-world anti-terrorism successes

- ◆ The West must be perceived by cold-eyed folks abroad to be truly serious about suppression of terrorism – or "They <u>will</u> come!"
    - "You talk the talk, but do you walk the walk?!?"
    - *"You Americans are very powerful, but you quickly run short of breath."* – Syrian Foreign Minister, 1984

PERTINENT ELEMENTS OF WESTERN SERIOUSNESS

- ◆ Statutory declarations of purpose
  - With specifics, teeth, comprehensive authorization,. . .
    - Including "...all necessary means are authorized" – the moral equivalent of war, so *everyone's* on-notice, at home *and* abroad
- ◆ "Whatever it takes" budgeting for advanced means
  - "Do the job, and send us the bill" – ~$100 B/yr.
  - Over-and-above the *status quo ante* ~$10 B/yr.-in-U.S.
    - Now, semi-vigorous exercising of "classical" capabilities
    - "Incrementally improve iron lungs" vs. "develop polio vaccines"
- ◆ Bureaucratic gridlock swept away
  - Before: 101 U.S. agencies competing-for-turf, -budget,...
  - After: Single *unified* U.S. program in EOP, under a *plenipotentiary* "czar" with impeccable credentials
    - Obviating much of the "new wine in old wineskins" nonsense
- ◆ Heads-of-states make "call to arms" to all Westerners
  - E.g., FDR's summons in '40 to defend West and its values

SUMMARY

- ◆ Good News: *Intelligently-designed, thoughtfully-implemented, continually-exercised* defenses against mass-casualty terrorism can succeed
  - Shields-&-barriers can be made so durable-&-high that only *readily-attributable state-level attempts* could possibly break through
  - "Standard Gambit" of throwing huge amounts of money and advanced technology at national security problems *can work* in this area, as well
  - "Classic luck" *probably* will hold, in that smaller-scale mass-casualty terrorism will appear in "vaccination quantities" long enough before really large-scale threats, so we'll have "Distant Early Warnings" followed by "clear and present dangers" only after usefully-long intervals
    - The first kilodeath adequately long before the first megadeath

- ◆ Bad News: Likely Western efforts fall far short of our potential – *qualitatively* and *quantitatively*
  - *Commitment*, not material resource-level, now is the limiting factor – and it's severely limiting
    - Westerners can't focus *effectively* on less-than-crisply-defined threats – and "terrorism" is currently too ill-defined
    - New batches of smallpox vaccine delayed a decade?!? Modern anthrax vaccine only in the indefinite future?? No antidotes to advanced neurotoxins *even in*

prospect?!? No long-range/high sweep-rate nuke detectors?!? No high-rate/high-efficacy chem/bio agent area clean-up means in prospect?

- Hordes may be hired to march-in-place, but the brightest-&-best won't play until the Western gov'ts. get serious
  - 'Faster pace' recommendations (e.g., '97) largely ignored
  - Agencies <u>all</u> covet the gov'ts.' mandate; <u>none</u> will pay-to-play
    - "Not within <u>our</u> current mission-envelope" attitude is pervasive today
    - No "executive authority" for recent & current U.S. "coordinators"
  - Mediocrity of present efforts is <u>*manifest*</u> – "Potemkin defenses"
- Since overall governmental seriousness isn't yet (!) in sight, serious *planning* is the best realistic option
  - *And* tech-base development, and prototype RDT&E, and ...
    - Best prototypes may have significant "operational legacy" for exploitation in first major emergencies

- ◆ <u>Lots</u> of potentially useful terrorism-suppression technologies are waiting in the Western tool-kit, e.g.,
  - Tiny, exquisitely sensitive silicon-based sensors
  - 10 billion operations/second digital signal processing chips
  - Thumbnail-scale GPS receivers
  - Rationally-designed, swiftly-synthesized biomolecules with reliably-predictable properties
  - 10% wallplug-to-UV/C high-brightness light sources

- ◆ <u>What's missing</u>: systems design, component integration, packaging-for-applications – the 'heavy lifting' to secure the West's anti-terrorism future via advanced capabilities
  - Sporadic/unfocused "tech base" expenditures; little prototyping or T&E of advanced systems
    - Myriad programs 'execute,' but <u>very</u> little comes out the pipe-end
  - Talent-intensive, resource-<u>un</u>demanding, quickly-executed work – through prototyping/field test-&-evaluation
  - Unlikely to be done, until gov'ts.' seriousness is evident
    - Required talent is 'bought' for gov't. programs only with difficulty
      - Presently pre-occupied, e.g., making money in the 'New Economy'
    - But streams into government service in times of emergency

The best defense is a top-notch offense
  - Fighting in the <u>Bad Guys'</u> strategic depth is *the* way-to-go

CONCLUSION

- ◆ <u>Take-Home Message</u>: The West <u>can</u> beat terrorism – handily! But we *likely* won't <u>start</u> to do so *seriously* until we've been significantly hurt.

- ◆ *Getting prepared* to <u>start</u> winning is the current business
  - – By means compatible with Western 'style,' way-of-life
  - – To minimize lost time/waste motion, once we're serious
  - – E.g., create enabling statutory frameworks, executive arrangements, chief-of-governments' funding-reserves,...
  - – E.g., greatly-improved *pertinent* intelligence capabilities
  - – E.g., tech-base advances; prototype-oriented RDT&E...
    - • *We're not <u>really</u> trying, thus far*
    - • *The West's brightest-&-best scientists and technologists aren't engaged* – they don't <u>even</u> recognize that a *<u>real</u>* problem exists

- ◆ Essential to be clear-sighted about what we're <u>not</u> doing
  - – E.g., so as to minimize panic of citizenry when first *<u>major</u>* losses occur – to obviate Bonaparte-Lenin *coups d'etat*
    - • *<u>Strategic</u> targets*: Western cohesiveness; citizen confidence in governments.; commitment to civil liberties

- ◆ <u>Must</u> have balance between defense and offense

OIL POLICIES AND TERROR: GETTING OFF OIL

WILLIAM FULKERSON
Joint Institute for Energy and Environment, University of Tennessee, Knoxville, TN, USA

I am pleased and honored to be asked to give this presentation[1] that derives from one person's brooding over September 11. What makes Islamic extremists hate the United States enough to target New York City? Is there anything we can do beside protecting ourselves and punishing the perpetrators? How is the United States perceived and why?

Dr. Perez Hoodbhoy, professor of physics at Quaid-e-Azam University in Islamabad reflected on these questions in a dark but revealing essay that was presented in the Nautilus Institute Special Forum #43: in December 2001. The following is a quote from that essay that I like.

"...Now is the time to ask why. Like clinical pathologists, we need to scientifically examine the sickness of human behavior impelling terrorists to fly airliners filled with passengers into skyscrapers. We also need to understand why millions celebrate as others die. In the absence of understanding there remains only the medieval therapy of exorcism, for the strong to literally beat the devil out of the weak. Indeed, the Grand Exorcist (the United States), disdainful of international law and the growing nervousness of even its close allies, prepares a new hit list of other Muslim countries needing therapy: Iraq, Somalia, and Libya. We shall kill at will is the message."

Dr. Hoodbhoy concluded:

"...If the world is to be spared what future historians may call the 'Century of Terror,' we will have to chart the perilous course between the Scylla of American imperial arrogance and the Charybdis of Islamic religious fanaticism. Through these waters, we must steer by the distant star towards a careful, reasoned, democratic, humanistic, and secular future. Else, shipwreck is certain."

So, Hoodbhoy says the United States is perceived as "imperial and arrogant."

He further observes that modern technology has made it possible to wreak havoc on thousands through the efforts of a few, sometimes a very few, particularly if those few

---

[1] This talk derives from a paper of the same title with the number JIEE 2002-03. It is available on the web at http://www.jiee.org/pdf/2002_03Oil.pdf. The paper contains documentation and more information than is included here.

are willing to sacrifice themselves. This is why the war on terrorism can last a long time unless we do something about the root causes.

Because I am an energy nut, my brooding caused me to ask these questions for which I do not yet have complete answers:

Does oil have anything to do with the U.S. being a target?

How can U.S. policies in the Middle East be freed of oil influence?

Can the U.S. substantially reduce its oil dependence?

How could it be done, how long would it take, and how much would it cost?

Would the benefits to the U.S. and the world be worth the effort and cost?

With respect to Sept. 11 we know who did it, and we know why. At least, we know what bin Laden wrote about his motives.

Osama bin Laden's reasons for declaring war on America:

U.S. Occupation of Saudi Arabia (U.S. troops permanently stationed in Saudi Arabia to protect the House of Saud from its enemies internal and external and the fleet in the Persian Gulf.).

The Gulf war and follow on sanctions and the misery inflicted upon Iraqi people (a million killed?).

U.S. support of Israel in persecuting Palestinians.

Persecution of Muslims around the globe (Lebanon, Tajikistan, Burma, Cashmere, Assam, Philippines, Somalia, Chechnya).

Two of these reasons, the first two, derive in part from U.S. dependence on oil. They are what I call oil policies. To some considerable extent U.S. policies in the Middle East are held hostage to our demand for oil, especially inexpensive oil.

So, I began to ask how could we free our Middle East policies from being held hostage.

Oil is a very difficult enigmatic commodity. The United States has been trying to solve the enigma for more than a quarter of a century (since the Arab oil embargo of 1973-74) with only limited success.

Oil involves politics, the economy, the environment, and its products are used by everyone and for essential needs.

At a cost, oil use can be reduced. The U.S. has done it before, but why should we want to do it now? I have mentioned one reason to liberate U.S. policymaking and maybe reduce the risk of terror. Three other reasons are just as important.

These three are:

Mitigating climate change and reducing urban pollution

Increasing energy or oil security (by reducing the effects of oil supply curtailments).[2]

Husbanding oil for the developing world.

---

[2] It should be noted that to the extent that world oil prices are inflated by Cartel manipulation, oil importing countries pay a premium that is equivalent to wealth transfer to the producing countries. Some of this excess profit may find its way into support for terror.

If done cleverly reducing dependence could be supportive of all four reasons. I am going to assume that that is what is wanted.

This last reason is important to me. The United States should not be perceived as using more than its fair share of an essential resource. As the world's only super power the U.S. should see as enlightened self-interest an obligation to help the 2 billion people of the planet who are so poor they have no means for a reasonable life. One step could be for the U.S. to lessen its draw on world oil resources. Today the U.S uses 25% of world oil production.

Suppose the United States decided to reduce its dependence on oil over a number of decades to low levels, how might it be done?

Two Policies to reduce oil dependence may be sufficient if they are practiced over the long term. They are:

Efficiency standards applied to all vehicles and ratcheted up with time. These may be accompanied by incentives and incentives could be used to accelerate the scrappage of polluting and less efficient vehicles as well; and

Flexible taxes on oil products sufficient to stimulate substitution.

An implicit third policy in this strategy is support and encouragement of R&D to produce technologies that reduce the costs of the transition.

Taxes may be sufficient without efficiency standards (or R&D), but I am skeptical, so I suggest employing all three policies.

We know how to improve the efficiency of light duty vehicles by a factor of at least 100 %. This improvement can be cost effective on a life cycle basis particularly if external costs are taken into account. Much more may be possible in time if fuel cells and hydrogen pan out as many hope and expect. Standards should be applied to all vehicles including SUV's and light trucks. It may eventually be necessary to apply standards to heavy trucks and aircraft as well, but the first target should be the light duty fleet.

Taxes could be raised sufficiently that substitute fuels can compete. For example, ethanol derived from cellulosic raw materials could compete today if gasoline were taxed at about $0.5/gal (equivalent to about a $20/bbl tax on crude oil). Corn ethanol is subsidized at $0.53 today, and making it as a gasoline additive is profitable, and production is increasing.

Taxes could be flexible and driven up when world oil prices are low and down when world oil price spike. In this way oil price shocks can be avoided, and the consumer will see a more or less steady, albeit high price for petroleum products. Tax revenue should be returned to the public and used to fund infrastructure changes to promote substitution and RD&D.

Taxes should be designed to encourage substitution for oil products by other fuels and energy sources that are indigenous, are cleaner in production and use and emit less greenhouse gases.

Figure 1 shows the major substitution possibilities for petroleum in transportation, none of which are very easy.

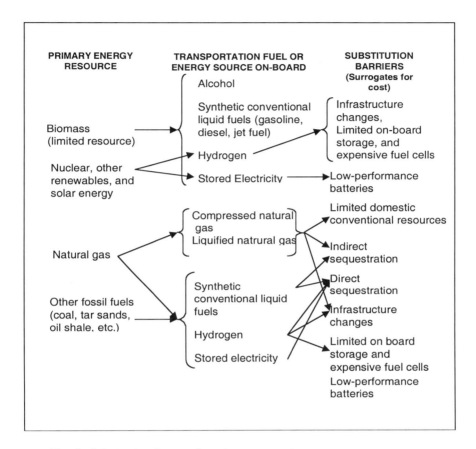

Fig. 1. Substitution for petroleum in transporation.

Here I have tried to identify the primary energy sources (left column) that can produce various on-board energy options (center column). Then I have tried to indicate the barriers to each possible substitution in the right column. These barriers are a surrogate for cost that is the principal barrier.

The fact is that there are no substitutes that are economic competitors with petroleum. The closest we have is natural gas that can be used directly to power vehicles and stored on board in compressed or liquid state.

The beauty of natural gas is that, on a life cycle and full energy cycle basis, it will emit less carbon and less pollution, and it is the most economical substitute as long as the price of natural gas remains in the range projected by the Energy Information Administration in its reference energy scenario. The trouble is that the price will not likely be as low as EIA projects as more and more is used for fueling vehicles. Also natural gas emits carbon dioxide emissions when it is burned. It may eventually be necessary to convert natural gas to hydrogen and sequester the CO_2 produced.

Biomass can provide fuels that are carbon neutral if the biomass fuel system is run in a sustainable manner. Biomass suffers because it is a limited although substantial resource. It could be adequate to fuel heavy trucks and aircraft, for example.

Non-fossil energy sources such as nuclear power and other renewables can be used to produce hydrogen and electricity to power vehicles. These sources produce no carbon and minimal other emissions. Electricity and hydrogen are hard to store on-board in practical and safe ways, however, and hydrogen requires a new infrastructure.

Hydrogen is an attractive possibility in the longer term. It can be made from many sources; it burns clean without carbon emissions. It can be produced from non-fossil energy sources. But it is hard to store, and developing a hydrogen infrastructure will be a formidable and expensive proposition.

Other fossil fuels can be used to produce substitutes ranging from conventional liquids to hydrogen or electricity. In a greenhouse-constrained society their use would require successful sequestration of emitted carbon.

So, there is no silver bullet or magic elixir.

My favorite transportation system, free of oil products, would use natural gas at first with a transition to hydrogen and biomass derived fuels for trucks and aircraft. It would be ultra-efficient.

If the United States adopted this oil dependence reduction strategy what would be the impact on the world oil market? If it is implemented gradually, producing say a decline of 1-2% per year in oil use, the impact should not be great. World oil resources would be more available for use by the rest of the world perhaps allowing more for developing countries who need it most. Of course, reduced U.S. demand will dampen world oil prices somewhat, but not much. That is not a bad thing.

Since the policies are directed inward they should have limited impact on producing and exporting countries. They would have major impact on the downstream part of the U.S. oil industry, but not on the upstream part. Gradually, U.S. production would be exported.

What do I conclude (my opinion only)?

There are four good reasons for the United States reducing its oil dependence to low levels. The new one is mitigating terror and freeing our policies from oil.

Such a transition will take decades to accomplish, and it will cost a lot money, effort and unswerving dedication. It will require some sacrifice by the people of the U.S.

Would the benefits be worth it? I don't know, but the issues should be studied and debated.

If the United States embarked on reducing its oil dependence, it would be giving something important back to the world. The gesture might be a step toward reducing the impression that the U.S. is imperialistic and arrogant.

ECONOMIC FACTORS OF CONFLICT AND VIOLENCE: THE ECONOMICS OF ARMED CONFLICT

PETER LOCK

European Association for Research on Transformation, Hamburg, Germany

The economies sustaining, if not causing current armed conflict have slowly moved to the centre stage of research in recent years. Important multipliers in this evolving debate have been the macro-quantitative studies of Paul Collier, a high-ranking economist at the World Bank and a comprehensive book, "L'économie de la guerre civile," edited by Jean/Rufin (1996), two French scholars with a background in humanitarian work. In spite of the differences in their methodological approaches the diverse authors in this academic discourse unanimously report illegal economic transactions of some kind as a pervasive feature of the current forms of armed conflicts. These transactions link the current wars with the global economy, though often the economic and financial tracks start in shadow-economic spheres and emerge only in later stages in the regular economy. Nevertheless these wars are not sustainable without external economic collaboration, either legal or illegal. Though the coverage in the media is regularly dominated by discourses of identities, of ethnic or religious strife. These ideological discourses are identified as a major, if not the dominant stimulus of strategies of violent conflict resolution leading to internal wars. Unfortunately these views often guide the political reactions to on-going armed violence in the international arena as well. However, the recognition of underlying economic patterns necessarily linked to the global economy would enforce a radical rethink of the ways the international community should react to countries engaging in armed conflict. It will be argued in this paper that from this perspective the current approaches of the major actors in the international system towards on-going conflicts must profoundly change if policies of conflict prevention and resolution are to be effective.

The conceptualisation of armed conflicts as manifestations of economic processes weakens many idiosyncratic explanations which often dominate the rhetoric of actors involved in violent conflict. It facilitates an analytical tool allowing to decipher the logic of seemingly irrational violence and atrocities as strategies of economic dominance, in which the market is replaced by violence or the threat thereof. In the process of internal wars the economic logic often turns war fighting into a self-perpetuating "mode of production." In such circumstances the task to build peace becomes extremely difficult because the agents of war have long since learnt to pursue their interests at the level of media presentation and to adjust their fighting strategies accordingly. In some cases acts of war resemble a stage setting to extract support from international actors. With hindsight it has become evident that the script of the war in Bosnia was full of staged events while the parties to the war had engaged London-based public relations agents in order to favourably influence the public opinion throughout the world. The reading of the underlying logic is complicated by the fact that violence is not only orchestrated to exclude the "enemy" from access to resources, but it also serves to prop up the absolute control the respective political entrepreneurs wield over "their" group. In the post-Dayton Bosnia this pattern led to a fragmented society dominated by organised crime deliberately nurturing rhetoric of ethnic and religious identity as a cover. The political entrepreneurs in former Yugoslavia who enforced the confrontation of identities as a means to stay in or gain power were certified by the Dayton agreement and have consolidated their position in spite of the presence of the UN-administration.

The argument elaborated in this text is not that armed conflicts are mono-causal events. But the economic dimension is of singular importance because it offers hitherto largely neglected possibilities of outside leverage. It also highlights structures of tacit, not always intended support through global economic networks, which operate within the political domain of industrial countries.

GLOBALISATION AND SOCIAL POLARIZATION

The social reporting of various agencies, currently waving the neoliberal flag, such as, among others, the World Bank and the United Nations Development Programme, whose task is to contribute to the regulation of economic globalisation, cannot obscure the fact that at present, in large sections of the world, globalisation is marked simultaneously by economic growth and state collapse, coupled with social polarization within societies and between states and entire regions. In a situation of tension such as this, armed conflicts and zones of all-out violence begin to take shape within societies. This dynamic then radiates into the globally intermeshed black market as violent actors aim to resupply their arsenals and most importantly wash their revenue.

It has long been a matter of controversy within the social sciences whether the violent escalation of conflicts into internal social wars is attributable to social inequities and grievances or to the greed of a handful of actors. The answer to this question determines what measures the international community, and in particular humanitarian and development aid organizations, might reasonably take in order to proactively counter all forms of armed violence. Social inequity and greed are not, of course, mutually exclusive as causal factors. But on the basis of our present knowledge, it is the greed of a few actors that would appear to be the driving force in many internal wars. What fosters the formation of black economies, in which economic exchange is ultimately regulated by recourse to violence, is not absolute poverty but aggressive competition for internationally marketable resources and the prospect of handsome, though unlawful profits.

In a social situation of absolute poverty, the actors involved have only minimal opportunities to acquire the instruments they would need to enforce a redistribution of income and chances. They do not have sufficient income for such a strategic investment, nor do their very small-scale activities on the informal markets generate the quantities of hard currency needed to be able to arm themselves. If a member of the poorest of the poor within a society can be identified as an armed actor in internal social conflicts, the obvious question to be asked is who invested in this actor or for whom the arming of such an individual serves as a means to an end. The child soldiers, a pervasive feature in internal armed conflicts in many countries, are cases in point. There must be an entrepreneur in the background who invests his dollars in the purchase of automatic guns which are exclusively traded in convertible currency and arms child soldiers. We will only understand such atrocious scenarios if we can design a simulation showing why this particular investment appeared to the respective entrepreneur as his "rational" choice of investment.

If these problem-areas were confronted with a 'watertight,' legally operating global economy, the criminal business-operators would have no chance to succeed, no chance to earn hard currency and in turn to operate as buyers on the illegal small-arms markets to resupply armed conflicts. In fact, however, globalisation is made up of three interconnected spheres which facilitates a broad range of unregulated transactions.

The normal, legally operating economy
This is the only entity considered in the study of national economy (the traditional German terms are Nationaloekonomie or Volkswirtschaft). Only in this sphere taxes are raised, but taxes, it should not be forgotten at any time, form the basis of statehood. Neoliberal doctrine has transformed national economy into a global financial market that is beginning, in its turn, to undermine the state-based nature of national economies and societies.

The informal economy
This is the space where the majority of the world's population organizes its survival. This half of the world's population lives in a state of constant legal and physical insecurity. The state monopoly of the legitimate use of force offers them no protection. Security has to be organized on a private basis, often against corrupt state officials. The monopoly on force is usurped by criminal forces at local levels. The informal economy, in the shape of economic migration and migration for the purpose of survival (refugees), is proving to be one of the most dynamic factors within the current process of globalisation. Migration is operating on a huge scale in the twilight areas of all societies and has created labour markets which are illegal, but have become an indispensable segment in the host society.

The openly criminal economy
The criminal economy can be described as an unknown number of globally operating, violence-based rather flexible networks. They are constantly reaching parasitically into the normal economy and are extorting protection-money in the informal economy among others. Drugs are perhaps the major driving-force of global networking in the criminal sphere. Experts estimate the global gross annual 'criminal' product to amount to at least

1500 billion US dollars. The diffuse global financial markets provide the operational medium for the activities of the criminal economy whose actors ultimately aim at washing their unlawful profits.

The present global economy can be schematised as *a circularly escalating process embracing neo-liberal globalisation, social fragmentation and polarization amd shadow globalisation.* Internal armed conflicts articulate themselves in this environment and display the economic features observed, namely the necessary involvement in the global shadow economy. But the connectedness to the global shadow economy is not restricted to countries suffering armed conflict on their territory. In many other countries spheres other than the regular economy prevail as well without causing armed conflict to emerge.

VIOLENCE AND ECONOMIC REGULATION

As a further step in the analysis, based on evidence from a large number of countries, I propose to expand the analysis of societal violence to include forms of armed violence other than internal war as well. One might describe the transformation of the organisation and the forms of armed violence from war-like confrontations towards seemingly diffuse manifestations of violence as a consequence of social fragmentation and polarization which opens spaces for violence-based imposition by criminal actors. The ensuing homicide rates often exceed the balance sheet of violence in "wars." The post-conflict murder rates in El Salvador would be case in point. Conceptualising broader armed violence is a precondition for effective policies aiming at reducing the appalling number of casualties related to one or the other form of "economic regulation" whether they occur in the context of a war or in the context of a failed state. I suggest that our state-centric perspective, permanently reinforced by the redundant literature on the paradigm of "democratic peace," hinders us in accounting for the on-going transformation of the forms of violence and, even more importantly, the nature of the territoriality of conflicts.

War, as hitherto defined, is possibly being replaced by more targeted and decentralised acts of violence. In order to initiate this debate I would like to draw attention to the fact that the recent transformation of political regimes towards democracy appears to be associated with dramatic increases of homicide. The context is similar in all cases. The paradigm of liberal globalism delimits economic development strategies governments can pursue. The new democratic regimes regularly do not manage to reduce social fragmentation and polarisation. Brazil,[1] South Africa,[2] Nigeria,[3] Russia[4] as well as post-conflict countries[5] are cases in point. The doubling of homicide rates, not officially documented in all cases, point in this direction. These situations easily exceed the casualty rates in many enduring "wars," Colombia[6] appears to represent two cases in one: For many years an internal war lingers on, but Colombia remains a democratic country according to internationally accepted standards. But homicides not related to the internal war are clearly the dominant form of violence. There can be no doubt that these appalling homicide rates represent gun-related casualties. The pervasive diffusion of small arms and not proliferation is instrumental for the emergence of such massive violence. The largest share, though certainly not all of this violence, represents "regulatory violence." It is employed to enforce economic and financial transactions at different levels, including protection, theft and illegal trade. In this respect this seemingly diffuse violence resembles many features of what has been identified as "economies of war" in many current conflicts, but with respect to its territoriality and perseverance this armed violence is distinct.

M. Duffield[7] has introduced the concept of "network war" into the debate. This paradigm points in a direction which might be helpful in understanding the distinct territoriality of violence in cases such as South Africa and Brazil, where violence regulates large spheres of the economy without escalating into forms which would classify as war. Integrating "network warfare" into the schematic representation of the current globalisation process as schematised in this text possibly brings us closer to an understanding of the transformation of violence as (among other functions) a tool of competing strategies of violent economic regulation of the global shadow economy from war towards seemingly chaotic forms. The increasing emergence of transnational identities as a result of the current shadow globalisation which nurtures migration also point towards a deterritorialisation of potential conflicts.

Conceptualising globalisation as three antagonistic and at the same time symbiotic or at least interdependent dynamic spheres allows us to understand the different meaning of territoriality for the networks which constitute the three spheres. As already explained the three spheres can be identified as the regular economy, the informal and the criminal sphere. In the context of the currently dominant paradigm of liberal globalism all three spheres can be described as webs of interconnected networks with global reach. Hence the application of violence or the threat thereof as a means to impose the economic interest of the respective network does not create a territorial front. The need to apply "regulatory violence" may occur in geographically disparate locations. A network of drug traders may require the application of "regulatory violence" at any link of the chain from the plantation to the consumer in any of the markets around the globe. Traditional warfare about territorial control does not pay off for global networks operating in the shadow economy. They defend their operational space which may be quite flexible, if required under the circumstances, with targeted violence and even terror. The operational space is distinct from territorial control. It may amount to full territorial control, but the latter is not a necessary condition. Generating a certain level of insecurity may already provide for an optimal operational space, because every criminal network depends on the availability of a sphere and a location facilitating the symbiotic exchange with the regular economy.

A similar logic possibly applies to the global players among the transnational corporations. They require safe operational spaces which are often provided by private security firms in otherwise violent environments. In some cases transnational corporations contract even the armed forces for the special protection of their assets.

As a concomitant trend of fragmentation under global liberalism the privatisation of security enhances the separation of social spheres. It is a response to the pervasive, in some cases deliberate weakening of the state which can no longer provide security as a free public good. The private security industry is globally one of the fastest growing economic sectors. If security is turned into a commodity, an intra-societal protection race ensues, continuously enlarging its territorial range: It further enhances social fragmentation by creating peripheries where people lack the resources to purchase their security and fall prey to criminal rackets for their "protection."

Such spaces emerge not only in the context of "withering states." In continuously spreading spaces the state deserts its role as holder of the monopoly of legitimate violence. Instead private agents either provide security on a contractual basis or as is often the case impose "security" on those who cannot afford to buy their security in the legal market. As social fragmentation surges in the footsteps of "liberal globalism" growing numbers of territories are controlled by local strongmen who vie for the monopoly of violence. However, often different networks operate on the same territory making such constellations highly instable.

However it is important not to focus exclusively on "failed states" or the Third World in general. By implication not only weak or failed states comprise large informal and criminal economic spheres, developed industrial economies have assimilated large informal as well as criminal networks. In Germany, the presence of these largely invisible networks is reflected in posters decorating the entrance of post offices and many chain stores which inform the "invisible actors" in ten carefully selected languages that 'the safe cannot be opened by the personnel.' Certain services are a domain of illegal qualified labour, health care in private homes for example. In Spain prostitution generates an estimated 12 billion € per year, at least two thirds of the workforce in this sector are illegal immigrants from Central and Eastern Europe. Economists argue that during the recent boom in the United States inflationary pressures were significantly delayed because of the availability of illegal labour in large, almost unlimited supply. These examples should suffice to justify a systematic study of the global dynamics of the shadow economy which mirrors the current configuration of liberal globalism in the regular economy.

In many countries undergoing systemic transformation and a good number of developing countries, the economy is dominated by informal sectors and criminal actors. This goes hand in hand with the implosion of state structures. Those who form part of the state apparatus become highway-robbers to civil society. Their greed stifles any entrepreneurial initiative aimed at self-help. If a society has got itself into a situation where the façade of state authority, appropriated by the forces of economic criminality, and the protagonists of that authority, produce a feeling of generalized insecurity, the regulatory systems of civil society dissolve and are replaced by structures based on self-defence. Rival militant identities take shape, mostly based on the notion of the exclusion of others.

Mass flight and emigration—generally by the most productive individuals—are the rule in such situations, and they further blight the chances of overcoming the all-enveloping informalisation and criminalisation of economic activity. The diasporas that quickly take shape in the wake of crises, and which initially live mainly in illegal conditions, ensure survival in the crisis regions by providing support. Examples of this are: the Lebanon (all groups), Kosovo (Albanians), Sri Lanka (Tamils), Chechnya (Chechens). At the same time, however, the diasporas provide a human infrastructure for lucrative illegal transactions of every kind. It is the diasporas that regularly fill the war-chest in cases of armed conflict. This is the case, for example, in Northern Ireland (Catholics) and in Nagorno-Karabakh (Armenians).

All over the world, crises and civil wars have led to the formation of transnational human-resource networks, some of which have already achieved global scope. In each case, only a tiny elite secures legal status in the diasporas. The total number of people involved is difficult to estimate. The United Nations High Commission for Refugees gives the total number of displaced persons and refugees in the world as approximately 50 million. But the number of people living illegally in foreign countries, hoping to secure survival or a better life, is much greater than this. The total very probably runs into the hundreds of millions. These people constitute an important blackmailable resource for managing the grey or criminal spheres of the globalisation process—spheres that have long since ceased to be confined to traffic in drugs and human beings. Even in states governed by the rule of law, these people often live in the shadows, beyond the scope of the law. In most cases, their precarious existence is dominated by hierarchies underpinned by violence. The state monopoly on force operating in the host country has no impact on their sphere of existence. Economically, they form a solid part of the relevant national economy, but they are excluded from political participation.

Whether it be ghettos of socially dependent minorities in the metropolises of the industrial nations, the huge poverty-stricken zones that surround every large city in the Third World, or abandoned industrial centres in the former Soviet Union: the experience which the inhabitants of these places have of state authority is essentially that of living in a collapsed state. In these 'exclaves of economic and social apartheid,' parallel social structures take shape. The monopoly on force is held by territorially organized gangs, which—like nation-states—settle border disputes by armed force. Protection money replaces taxes. People living in such precarious circumstances are a resource for, amongst other things, arms and drugs trafficking and other risky activities in demand in the black economy. Anyone who is poor has no choice and accepts criminal risks.

INTERGENERATIONAL APARTHEID

As all of this were not bad enough the current globalisation produces a social fragmentation which I describe as "intergenerational apartheid." Historically, the present time will probably be described as an age of mass youth unemployment. The economic (dis-)order that is currently unfolding in line with the neoliberal paradigm has nothing to offer the majority of the world's young people when they reach working age. There is no role for them, either in the present-day 'regular' economy or in traditional rural structures. These latter are in the process of disintegrating all over the world. The modern sector cannot absorb the up-and-coming generations into the labour force: it is part of the logic of global competition that rationalized, capital-intensive production-methods and marketing strategies should ultimately triumph on the markets.

All over the world, a large part of the rising generation of workers is thus being involuntarily driven into the no man's land of informal economies and is thereby becoming an inexhaustible resource for any and every kind of (economic) criminal. A clear example of this dilemma is provided by the present situation in Algeria. Algerian society, like many societies in the Third World, is a very youthful one. About half the population is less than 15 years old. It is estimated that at present about 60 per cent of those looking to enter the job market for the first time are unemployed. There is no prospect of any improvement. The young people in question (if male) are known as hitistes ('those who prop up/lean on the wall'). They are always on the look-out for a chance to do a good deal on the trabendo circuit—casual smuggling, mostly with France—or to bolster their identity, and thus also their existence, by some other means, mostly within the grey area of the informal economy or through services to criminal circles. In their life time liberal globalism for all its growth prospects is unlikely to provide a workplace in the regular economy. And increasingly young people in various countries understand their situation.

In many countries, more than half of all young people belong to this excluded group. In situations such as this, devoid of any prospects, having the use of instruments of force such as an automatic rifle becomes an extremely attractive proposition: with a weapon in his hand, for the first time in his life a young man has the experience of being respected by others—even if the sentiment in question is actually sheer terror on the part of the person under threat, perceived as respect. Force exerted through an automatic rifle becomes the means of resisting social exclusion. Force promises access to the world of industrial mass consumption—to which there is constant media exposure, even in the furthest corners of the world.

Following the end of the so-called liberation movements and the almost total disappearance of the concomitant utopian ideas of social equality, it is now almost exclusively young males that figure as violent protagonists in armed conflicts and armed violence. This is probably due in part to the fact that economic modernization brings with it a radical devaluation of those roles in the production process that were previously assigned exclusively to men. As a reaction to this, and in the absence of cultural-emancipatory and economic alternatives, male identity is construed in terms of acts of violence that give a feeling of superiority and autonomy. The lost position in the production process is replaced by participation in the social production of violence. This logic is also reflected in the crime figures of developed states and the prison population in developed countries where young males belonging to a discriminated minority form the majority. Offences involving firearms are overwhelmingly the preserve of young men.

Political wheeler-dealers with criminal economic interests who operate in civil-war scenarios make cynical use of the impulsive urge of young men to take up arms to defend themselves against exclusion from the legal production-sphere and from society. Hence, at bottom the phenomenon of the child soldier in the Third World has more in common with youth-gangs in highly industrialized states than the mostly separate discussion of these two social pathologies would suggest.

The never-ending civil wars and the pervasive "regulatory" violence elsewhere are fuelled, amongst other things, by the total exclusion of the rising generations in the context of state collapse and of whatever economic catastrophes underlie the particular situation. The best way young men can participate in society is as 'soldiers.' Moreover, the chances of survival are probably much greater than in the chaos of the civil societies paralysed by the war. Working as a 'soldier' is therefore not just highly attractive to rootless young men; in the jargon of modern economics, it is also a 'rational choice.'

FINAL REMARK

This text reflects an on-going research. I started out with identifying general features observed in the context of war economies. These features were modelled as part of the globalisation process which I stylise in three antagonistic and at the same time symbiotic spheres. However, when testing the findings it turned out that the economic features identified in the context of war economies were also present in many countries not affected by armed conflict. This was not entirely surprising since every illegal transaction geared to garner convertible currency (i.e. dollars) is bound to penetrate into global markets outside the conflict region either directly or via a chain of "shadow" traders. At the same time crime statistics and other information suggest that it will be possible to diagnose a dramatic increase of homicides in countries characterised by extensive informal and criminal economic sectors. Presently I am engaged in searching reliable data to validate this correlation, it is not an easy task and will still require some time.

Though the correlation between shadow economy and violent crime led me to hypothesize that the pervasive fragmentation and social polarisation developing in the footsteps of liberal globalism represented by the so-called Washington consensus manifests itself in a broad variety of forms of "regulatory violence": This violence is crowding out the market as a regulatory mechanism because the "failed" and weak states can not any longer protect markets protected by law as the mechanism of economic regulation. Thus, armed conflict is only the tip of the iceberg of "regulatory violence." Studying globalisation as a system of interacting networks in all three spheres leads to the hypothesis that "regulatory violence" used to protect the functioning of shadow-economic networks both internally and against competing networks requires acts of violence in distant geographical locations belonging to the operational space of the respective networks. It follows, as a trend at least, that we might expect a deterritorialisation of "regulatory violence", in other words social violence in form of internal warfare with traditional geographical fronts is likely to be replaced by seemingly chaotic, but growing levels of "regulatory violence" which should be measurable in growing homicide and crime rates.

The dynamics of shadow globalisation are self-perpetuating because the reproduction of the state depends on taxes which can only be extracted from the regular economy. In order to identify countries were the informal and criminal spheres actually dominate the economic activities it is important to look at the trends in tax collection. Because without tax there is no accountable state, instead there are only political entrepreneurs who have appropriated the state in order to pursue their business in the shadow economy.

As this is a note reflecting on-going unfinished research I apologise for the rather approximate explication of my exploratory ideas about the current direction of globalisation. I will eventually post a more elaborate version of my research on my website: www.Peter-Lock.de.

REFERENCES

1.   Angelina Peralva (2001) "Perspectives sur la violence brésilienne," in: *Revue Tiers Monte*, t.XVII, no. 167, Julliet-Septembre 2001, pp. 537-554.

2.   Mark Shaw (2002) *Crime and Policing in Post-Apartheid South Africa, Transforming under Fire*, London (Hurst & Co.); Jonny Steinberg ed. (2001) *Crime Wave, The South African Underworld and its Foes*, Witwaterstrand University Press.

3.   Human Rights Watch, Nigeria The Bakassi Boys The Legitimization of Murder and Torture, May 2002, Vol. 14, Number 5.

4.   *International Study of Firearms*, United Nations 1998.

5.   For El Salvador see: Human Rights Watch; for Liberia see: Human Rights Watch

6.   See: Peter Waldmann, Der anomische Staat Über Recht, öffentliche Sicherheit und Alltag in Lateinamerika, Opladen (Leske + Budrich) 2002, Chapter 11.

7.   Mark Duffield (2001) *Global Governance and the New Wars, The Merging of Development and Security*, London (ZED Books).

5. SOCIETY AND STRUCTURES: HUMAN RIGHTS — FREEDOM AND DEMOCRACY DEBATE

WHEN IS A SUPERPOWER WELCOME?

WILLIAM R. SHEA
Committee for the Humanities, European Science Foundation, Strasbourg, France

With the fall of the Berlin Wall in 1989 a new era of lasting peace seemed finally possible. After two world wars, the 20th century ended with Germany and Russia having become democratic nation-states. The Western political value of the rule of law legitimised by democratic consent now seemed assured. But whereas peace had rested on a balance of powers in Westphalia in 1648, in Utrecht in 1713 or in Vienna in 1815, what characterised the new order was not so much the triumph of democratic values as the overwhelming and apparently unchallengeable power of the United States with its supremacy in the weapons systems created by nuclear and information technology, its enormous wealth, and the universal attraction of its popular culture. America's European allies were at best subordinate and dependent associates. This, it was hoped, would be a unipolar world of a kind not seen since the fall of the Roman Empire and, like the Roman Empire, it would be based on the rule of law.

The new international order over which a form of hegemony would be exercised could be seen as the outcome of five developments:

1. The recognition of human rights within all states, regardless of their internal laws. This criterion was developed during the struggle against totalitarianism.
2. The widespread development of nuclear weapons that render the defence of borders ineffectual.
3. The existence of global threats that transcend borders. These include famine and disease, but also environmental problems, or the population explosion with the resulting pressure on migration.
4. A world economic regime that ignores borders in the movement of capital investment.
5. A global communication network that penetrates borders electronically and threatens languages, customs and cultures.

This new political order would tend to conform to the economic order of the dominant State, namely to views such as these that can be presented as a new Decalogue:

1. Capital markets have to become less regulated in order to attract capital investment.

2. Capital has to become more global in order to achieve maximum return on investments.
3. Labour markets have to become more flexible in order to compete with foreign markets and keep jobs at home.
4. Access to **all** markets has to be assured, and trade has to become less regulated, if the world economy is to grow.
5. Government subsidies, spending, and welfare programs have to be managed in order to permit more investment in infrastructure, and to allow greater private saving (which will lower the cost of investment).
6. Tax policy has to provide incentives of growth in order to attract enterprises and maximise innovation and entrepreneurship.
7. Without incentives for capital formation and capital retention, domestic investment will not take place or it will flee along with foreign investment.
8. If investment goes elsewhere, then innovation and productivity go with it.
9. As a consequence, the products of other states will be cheaper and better. Jobs will be lost and therefore tax revenue will fall, and unemployment and welfare costs will become unbearable.
10. Higher taxes will produce even lower revenues.

Disregard of this Decalogue would produce its own punishment:

1. The State that resists liberalising its labour markets in order to protect high-wage jobs will end up with no jobs to protect.
2. The State that resists cutting back on welfare will find that it has to cut back anyway when revenues fall, and that it will have to pay even larger welfare bills.

The new Orthodoxy could nonetheless be played out in several competing formulations:

A. In Washington: State intervention will continue to be anathema and the reason given will remain the same: the State can never adjust prices as quickly and as efficiently as the market.
B. In Tokyo: Protection of domestic industries will remain a priority.
C. In Berlin: Insuring social and economic equality among citizens will continue to be emphasised.

To makes this clearer, let us compare Berlin and Tokyo:

Berlin	Tokyo
Public funding of Education	Education: financed privately
Low savings	High savings
High currency value	Low currency value
High interest rates on corporations	Low interest rates on corporations
Low interest rates on consumer loans	High interest rates on consumer loans
Higher quality of personal life (maximising freedom of individual choice)	Personal sacrifice (maximising the freedom of society as a whole)
Leisure consumption	Long working hours

So much for the scenarios. But they can only be realised if peace and security are maintained world-wide. To be safe for trade, the planet has to be policed. We cannot allow dissident groups to perpetrate acts of defiance on the scale of the disaster of the eleventh of September 2001. Neither can we stand by and let conflicts become endemic, and violence and the thirst for revenge escalate.

There are doubtless many reasonable and rational ways of dealing with these international problems. We are here in part to examine some of them. I will merely draw your attention to one that is receiving increasing attention in the scholarly and not so scholarly literature. Witness the cover page of the Summer 2002 issue of the distinguished American political review published by the Woodrow International Center for Scholars. Or, at a more popular level, the *Harvard Magazine* that is mailed to Harvard University Graduates to keep them in touch with the concerns of their Alma Mater.

THE ROMAN EMPIRE

The Greek historian Polybius (about 200-120 B.C.) wrote a universal history in the second century B.C. to explain how Rome, "succeeded in less that fifty-three years in imposing their form of government on nearly the whole inhabited world." Between Hannibal's campaign that began in 220 B.C. and the defeat of the Macedonians at the battle of Pydna in 168 B.C., Rome made itself the Master of the World.

Polybius and perhaps as many as one thousand young officers and civil servants were brought to Rome and detained in Italy. In a sense, Polybius was the equivalent of a graduate student or a postdoc in Rome for fifteen years. He saw that Roman power was both inevitable and irresistible and he asked himself why. He also asked himself how to explain the harsh new realities to his Greek-speaking compatriots. He argues throughout his book that what formed the basis of Roman domination was manpower, military skill and might, intimidating toughness in adversity, and moral seriousness often compounded with self-deception. It also had much to do with applying Roman law everywhere (whether this suited other people or not) and even more with preventive strikes.

I urge you to read Polybius' *History*. You will find it topical.

HOW FREELY SHOULD MONEY FLOW?

ALFRED GREIDER
Bank Julius Baer & Co. Ltd., Lucerne, Switzerland

Before we can address this question properly we have to define what money really is. In the strict academic sense it means a method of payment to purchase goods or services. But of course in today's world we know that the use of money plays a much bigger role. To start with I would like to differentiate between physical money and "virtual" money.

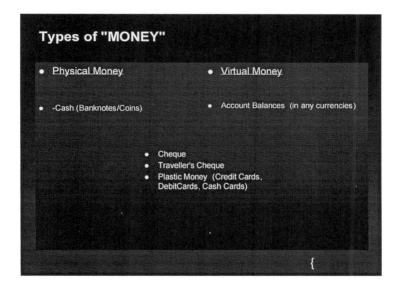

With this differentiation we have also made a clear distinction of how the flow of money can be controlled by governments, tax authorities and crime prevention units.

It is quite obvious that the control of physical money is mainly conducted at the border of a country in random checks of the incoming people. But very often those checks are made well inside the country and you can imagine that you need a lot of explaining to justify your possession of $100,000 in cash in almost any country. Before we go to the virtual money we have to look at the payments which are made in both circles. I am talking about credit cards and cheques which are physical money in the form of plastic or paper but the settlement is virtual and here the detection can take place in both areas. The random border checks not only discover cash but of course they would also look for foreign credit cards and cheques.

For the real "virtual" money however the story becomes much more complicated because the money transfer is made by electronic devices and is therefore much more difficult to detect.

Let me explain how a wire transfer works today:

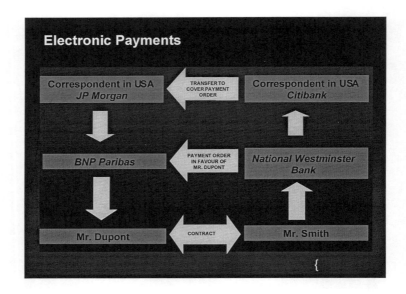

Mr. Smith owes his supplier Mr. Dupont an amount of U.S. $700,000. Let's assume that Mr. Dupont is located in France and Mr. Smith in the UK, but still the amount in question is in U.S. $.

Mr. Smith is giving his Bank, the National Westminster Bank the instruction to pay U.S. $700,000 to BNP Parisbas in France in favour of Mr. Dupont. National Westminster Bank knows that BNP Parisbas has a correspondent in the USA which is different to the correspondent they are using. National Westminster therefore sends an electronic message to BNP Parisbas saying that they should credit the account of Mr. Dupont with $700,000 and that they will receive the cover through their correspondent JP Morgan Chase in the USA. National Westminster Bank then will send another message to their correspondent, the Citibank to debit their account with the same amount and pay to JP Morgan Chase in favour of BNP Parisbas as a cover for a direct payment order.

What can we learn from this transaction? First of all, "virtual" money never leaves the country of origin. U.S.$ can only be paid in the USA, Swiss Francs only in Switzerland and so on. Even if the U.S. authorities are able to find this payment, they still do not know who has given the instructions and who is going to receive the money. All they would know is that there was a direct payment from National Westminster to BNP Parisbas. This method of payment is by far the most efficient and most widely used system for international payments. The name of this system is S.W.I.F.T. and all banks of a certain standing are members of this organisation. I have been told that the security of this system is very high and so far no cases have been reported whereby anybody got access to this system and has used information out of it.

But coming back to our initial question: how freely should money flow? It seems from my previous explanations that the flow of money is pretty free, so why do we talk about this subject at all? It is quite obvious that most countries in the world are worried about criminal activities being funded with anonymous "free" payments.

Another big worry to some countries is tax evasion where certainly Switzerland is one of their prime targets. I will come back to the role of my country later on in my speech.

It is therefore clear that everybody would want a free flow of money around the globe but at the same time to ensure that criminal acts can be detected. We all know that it is impossible to fulfill both requirements and therefore we have to compromise. In looking a little bit closer at this whole subject, we immediately find out that the big problem is that different countries have different rules and regulations regarding the free flow of money. In some countries the amount of cash you can bring into the country is limited to a certain amount, or at least has to be reported, when a certain limit is exceeded. For electronic transfers, some countries require a notification to their central bank and probably to their tax authorities as well when a certain amount is exceeded. In other countries no reporting takes place at all. Some countries require the name and address of the ordering party and anonymous payment orders are not accepted. So we see that in almost every country there is a different set of regulations which of course makes it easier for criminals to channel their money through countries with few restrictions.

Now let's come to the role of my country in this whole context. Switzerland has been known for centuries to be the safe haven for international investors. This is still the case today. A recent study shows that of the money which is invested outside their home country, roughly 1/3 is invested through Switzerland. We are, therefore, the biggest international banking center in the world.

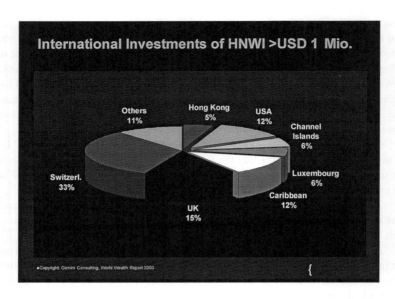

If however we look at the same question from an institutional investor's viewpoint, we find out that Zurich is far behind the other big financial centers.

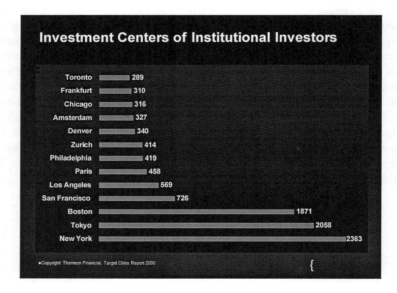

The reason for this is that most of institutional money is invested in the home country and since Switzerland is a very small country it is quite normal that we do not have a top spot in this field.

But how is it that Switzerland is such an attractive place to invest money? Most will say that this is because of the Swiss Bank Secrecy, which certainly plays a role. But I believe there are other reasons as well. Switzerland has been a safe haven during the two world wars of the last century and maybe even more important: Private Banking is an old industry in my country since sophisticated services for private customers have been provided by our banks for over 100 years. That is also one of the reasons that the famous private banks in Switzerland were all founded in the 18th and 19th century. What is the role of the Swiss Banks today?

In Switzerland, tax evasion is not a criminal offence, therefore if you get caught evading taxes you never go to jail in my country. This situation applies to all foreign nationals who invest their money in Switzerland. It is therefore impossible for us to help any foreign country to detect a person who has possibly evaded taxes in his home country. This however does not mean that Swiss Banks do everything to help their foreign customers to evade taxes. On the contrary, Swiss Banks have very strict rules to identify their customers properly, so we really do know our customers. In addition to that, no Swiss Bank will help any foreign national to bring money into Switzerland or back to his home country. The customer has to do this at his own risk. Interestingly enough, we see a clear tendency towards properly taxed money being invested more and more in Switzerland and this is proof to me that we seem to do a good job in investing money and are able to provide an excellent service. I believe these are the real strengths of the Swiss Banks. Another field where Swiss Banks have an advantage is that many foreign nationals decide to retire in Switzerland, mainly for tax reasons. I think it is therefore useful to have a look at the tax burden in different countries.

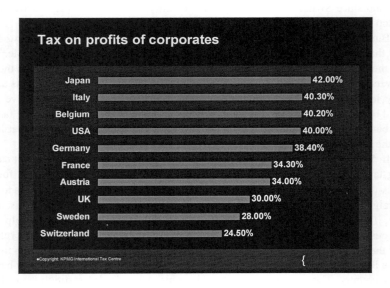

You see from this chart that the corporate tax rate is quite reasonable and therefore it is no surprise that often international companies have their holding company in Switzerland.

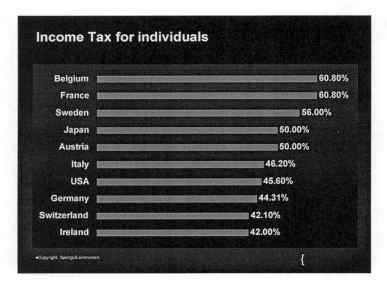

On the personal tax front however, the differences are definitely smaller and it is certainly true that there are many more reasons than purely taxes to move to Switzerland such as security, health care, geographical location, beauty of the country and so forth.

I know that the discussion on the Swiss Bank Secrecy is mounting mainly within the E.U. As a Swiss Banker, my position is very clear. I see no reason to abolish the bank secrecy because we have nothing to gain. But this is a very egotistical viewpoint, I agree. Therefore let's discuss what can be gained for the world if Switzerland gives up their bank secrecy.

Quite obviously the Swiss Banks would lose large amounts of their non-taxed customer money. This would flow elsewhere. At the same time we would have too many bank employees so there would be severe job losses. But do you honestly believe that people owning non taxed money would declare it and pay their penalty on those amounts? Certainly not to a large extent. This money would be invested in other, more exotic locations and the only result of this would be that the importance of Switzerland would disappear. Is that the only reason to abolish the bank secrecy?

I very much believe that we should look at the whole situation from a different angle and please let me come back to my initial question: How freely should money flow?

Switzerland has a very efficient system to identify customers who try to use the bank secrecy for criminal activities. This does not mean that we will never be used by criminal organisations, but the controls are so strict that we are confident that it is very unlikely that such money goes through our country. I have already mentioned that we do know all our customers. I can assure you that I personally know all my customers very well, I have often visited them at their home and I do know other family members. We also always know where the money which is to be invested comes from, and how it has been created. It is quite obvious we do not want to become the bankers of the criminal world but for our customers who want to keep their privacy. At the end of the day, if bank secrecy no longer exists, this would mean that the governments would know a lot more about their citizens. But let me ask you honestly, are governments more trustworthy than Swiss Banks?

I do not want to list the different scandals which have occurred on different government levels, it would take too much time. But I do believe that the change from bank secrecy to government knowledge would be a bad deal for everybody. Already today we know that governments all over the world have access to e-mail communication, phone conversations and much more. Do we really need to fulfill Orwell's predictions about a tightly controlled world? We are well on the way to that and when it has happened we wonder how it ever came about and reflect on how beautiful the good old times were. I am therefore very grateful to all of you if you use your influence to make sure that the government has time to concentrate on its duties and leave the honest citizens alone.

COMBATING TERRORISM: AN EVENT TREE APPROACH

RICHARD WILSON
Department of Physics, Harvard University, Cambridge, MA, USA

INTRODUCTION

This talk was first presented at the Global Foundation Conferences at Chatham House, London on December 5th 2001 and again at Fort Lauderdale, FL on December 12th 2001. Also at the Probabilistic Safety Analysis and Management meeting (PSAM6) in San Juan, Puerto Rico on June 24th 2002. Some suggested modifications have been included. As I prepared it I realize that it is not enough to discuss how industries may be made immune from terrorist attacks: they cannot be absolutely immune. We need what was called in the nuclear industry "defense in depth" and we need to analyze the relative importance of different steps by an "event tree analysis." I find that the actual attack is the last step in the event tree. As with more conventional uses of event trees the earlier in the chain of events that there is intervention, the easier it is, and the more effective. So I start by analyzing my immediate personal reactions to the problem. Then I discuss the problems and paradoxes of extending widely the immediate response of Americans, including myself, to the act. This includes a discussion of the way in which terrorism is defined and in which different people perceive it. This then leads to an approach which is essential; a multifaceted approach to combating terrorism of which I discuss three facets; the avoidance of world situations that breed terrorism; the containment of the terrorist; and the difficult task of limiting the damage that a terrorist might cause. This in turn may be broken up into parts with a risk analysis approach. Finally I try, very briefly, to consider how it can all be put into perspective. It will be seen that I build primarily on my own experience and studies over a period of years.

SUPPORT FOR PRESIDENT BUSH'S AIM TO STOP TERRORISM

After the September 11th terrorist attack on the World Trade Center and the Pentagon, I, like most Americans, had very complex feelings. Like the vast majority, I felt the animal reaction, "let us get the guy who did this." This is difficult, because in the very nature of a suicide attack the person directly responsible is dead. I agree with President Bush that the person who plans such activities is a person we want to catch and punish. But therein lie the complications. How do you find the planner? And what is a terrorist? When is a man a terrorist and when is he a freedom fighter? Is a terrorist a coward if he blows himself up? Moreover, merely rooting out existing, known terrorists is a reactive approach rather than a positive approach of making society somewhat safer and/or reducing the number of terrorists.

I also am much more aware than most Americans that the destruction of September 11th 2001 is far from unusual in the world. What is unusual, is that 3,500 people were killed in a short time, and by terrorist action. It has been said that everything changed on September 11th. But not so much for me. On September 1st, 1939, I left home on my bicycle, leaving London, Great Britain, not knowing whether I would see my parents again. 2 million children left London that day expecting imminent air raids. 15 months later the center of London looked worse than New York did after the collapse of the World Trade Center. I tend to take a long-term view. Supposing that we catch the guy responsible (maybe Osama Bin Laden) what is to stop Osama Bin Laden's associates from taking over the organization, and worse still, what is the to stop others, not yet known, becoming terrorists? Thus I very quickly realize that one must address terrorism in many different ways of which the first and most important is to address the root causes of terrorism or as many of them as we can. This then leads me to think about the whole issue intellectually, and I find that there are many areas in which Probabilistic Risk Assessment can be very relevant.

WHAT SHOULD A PHYSICIST DO?

Firstly a physicist will define the problem. In this he will try to ensure that the language he uses is the same as the language his associates use so that he is properly understood. Definitions are all important. Secondly he tries to break the problem up into manageable parts. Hopefully these parts are uncorrelated with each other or at least have as few correlations as possible. In safety engineering these correlations are called "common mode failures" The analyst's skill comes in choosing the parametrization to ensure this independence as much as possible. My colleague, the late Ed Purcell, thinking of how best to design his experimental equipment so that it could be easily adjusted, used to call this "the orthogonality of knobs." As I do this, I first notice an important scientific revolution going on in society which inevitably influences everything we try to do.

THE REVOLUTION OF GLOBALIZATION. GLOBALIZATION AND ITS CONSEQUENCES

We are developing a Global Economy. Indeed globalization seems inevitable. Globalization is more than a globalization of markets, although we know that can bring increased economic prosperity – often my avoiding the middlemen and traditional traders. The protesters at Seattle, and Genoa, and even the NGOs at Durban, understood this better than the official delegates to these conferences seemed to do. But even they failed to realize that globalization is simultaneous with, and may be a partial consequence of a major scientific revolution. There are scientific developments in three fields that have already begun to influence us and together they will make enormous changes. I do not think we can stop these changes even if we want to but we should be prepared for them even though no one knows the full extent of the revolution that they are causing. They are in:

1. Communication technology
2. Biology and
3. Physics.

The new communications technology – itself deriving from applications of physics – ensures that anyone in the world with minimal equipment can be full aware of everything that is happening. All that he needs is a laptop computer with a satellite telephone line. Moreover that line will be more reliable than the existing local telephone service. We have, and use, technology to watch each other. It is hard to hide. Even 30 years ago a photograph of Moscow from a satellite 100 miles in the sky enabled me to count the number of people in line to enter Lenin's tomb. There is an inevitable openness that creates an inter-dependence which will affect all of our lives.

We have sequenced the human genome. This will bring the opportunity to cure or to kill. Biological weapons are true weapons of mass destruction and must be controlled if the human race is to survive. We will probably soon synthesize cocaine substitutes which can be made cheaply and in facilities that are harder to identify than the poppy fields just as we manufacture amphetamines now very easily. That will make the international cooperation on the "drug war" even more important. Anthrax is in the news today. But many more people have been killed by our failure to control drugs such as cocaine than by anthrax. On the other hand we can also wipe out pests – such as locusts – that eat our crops. But only if nations cooperate. When Ethiopia had a civil war, cooperation was suspended and the effect on the neighbors – an increase of locusts – was pronounced.

Physics has brought us in the last 50 years nuclear medicine, nuclear powered electricity but of course the atomic bomb. The world has fortunately recognized the supreme importance of keeping nuclear weapons in check. More nations have signed the non-proliferation treaty than any other treaty. By signing this treaty each state gives up some sovereignty and becomes dependent on the others. None of us would support self-determination if that included a right to make atomic bombs and threaten the rest of the world.

In another respect, globalization brings us few options. It is no use saying "stop the world I want to get off." But in addition to the economic benefits it brings the world troubles closer - and makes global terrorism, as distinct from local terrorism, inevitable. It will be now with us forever so we had better understand it. Which terrorists are evil?

Almost 100% of Americans, including myself, supported President Bush in his aim to capture Osama Bin Laden and his followers. Although we might not use the word ourselves, we all agree that their actions and the men themselves are evil. Most other Governments in the world so agree also. Although the bombing in Afghanistan seems to be justified by the events of the week of November 11th 2001, in spite of many peoples' forebodings, there is still room for questioning the overall U.S. war on terrorism. President Bush has called Osama Bin Laden "evil." Also evil, and with more serious consequences, was

Adolph Hitler. Bertrand Russell, a prominent pacifist in World War I, publicly stated that fighting Adolph Hitler and his Nazi gang was different from the German Kaiser in World War I since Adolph Hitler was evil. There is less international support for Mr. Bush's war on terrorism when the aim is widened to include all terrorists. It then becomes necessary to understand who is a terrorist. There can be terrorists on both sides of a dispute. In such a case the world (probably through the UN which was set up for the purpose) might have to place itself in the middle with a risk of loss of life of personnel. Getting rid of Hitler took six years and 70 million lives. Hopefully the world can get rid of evil men a little more simply now.

The Chinese regard the Japanese Emperor Hirohito as evil, especially for his direct involvement in, if not ordering of, the rape of Nanking in which 300,000 Chinese were massacred. Although I was aware of this massacre as it occurred, it was far away, and Europe had more local matters to consider. I was also unaware until recently that the Emperor was personally aware of the massacre and could have stopped it, and that the hero of the 50 odd westerners in the Chinese capital who tried to limit of the massacre was the head of the Nazi party in China. Surely this tells us that one can find heros in most unlikely places. The American acceptance of the Emperor after 1945 was very puzzling to many people – especially to Chinese.

Some people regard Saddam Hussein as evil. But far fewer than regarded Hitler as evil. Nonetheless I remember a telephone call at the start of the Gulf War from a friend with an Iraqi diplomatic passport. "There are a lot of bright people in the world," he said. "Can't one of them find a way of getting rid of that man?" But the world could not get rid of Hitler easily either.

Hitler, Hirohito and Hussein had in common their stated aim of a greater Germany, a more powerful Japan and dominance of Iraq respectively. To western minds, Bin Laden has only negative aims – wanton destruction of society. But I am in a western society and maybe he appeals to those who want to replace our western society with an eastern one that we in the west barely understand.

To go further I now turn to the more traditional role of a physicist, particularly an academic one to define the problem.

DEFINITION OF A TERRORIST

I like to go back to the Oxford English Dictionary. As I do so I will ask a set of questions. The reader will surely notice that I have many questions but few (if any) answers. Indeed I do not expect anyone to agree with me, or each other, on answers to all of them. But they should be pondered by us all.

The first use of the word discussed was applied to the Jacobins in the reign of Terror in the France of 1795. "The terrorists, as they were justly denominated, from the cruel and impolitic maxim of keeping the people in implicit subjugation by a merciless severity."

Another use was to the extreme revolutionary society in Russia and the implication of important people was known in 1905 "Several notables are believed to be more or less implicated in the acts of the Terrorists."

It was also applied (in 1866) to those in Ireland objecting to British rule: "Miss G...., daughter of a Wexford terrorist, directed many of the tortures which were so extensively practiced."

And in 1805 there were the religious terrorists: "some book of the religious terrorists which tended to infuse the alarm of foul perdition."

These uses of the word terrorist all in some way apply to a person or people, individual or governmental, which terrifies people. How did President Bush use the word terrorist in his speeches? How did we hear it? Mr. Bush seemed to consider it applies solely to those who oppose the policies of governments or entities whom America (Mr. Bush) dislikes. In parlance today, as formerly, the word was used against any people, or a government that one did not like. The President of Pakistan took care to explain that he opposes terror in all its forms – by which I assume he includes oppression of a people by its government or an occupying government. I suggest that we all heard it in the way we wanted. However most people in the USA use the word only to describe actions we and our government do not like, and by extension actions another government does not like. But that leads to problems. I list a number of conundrums which list is, unfortunately, very far from complete.

1. Was Hitler and his Nazis a gang of terrorists even though they were the legitimate government of Germany, originally elected by the people? Were opponents of Hitler terrorists? Especially Colonel Von Stauffenburg who tried to assassinate Hitler with a bomb in a brief case?

2. Were the Hutus in Ruanda terrorists even though they were (as we know) supported by the legitimate government in their slaughter of the Tutsis?

3. Were the Young Turks terrorists when they victimized the Armenians in 1916? Or were the Armenians terrorists because they were not model citizens of the Ottoman Empire and would not be slaughtered quietly?

4. Again, were (and are) the opponents of British rule (or Protestant rule) in Ireland (or part of it) terrorists? Has the situation changed since partition was generally agreed in 1922?

5. Is the government of Russia guilty of terrorism against the people of Chechnya (who have as much voting power as other residents of Russia) or are the radical Chechens guilty of terrorism against Russia? Or both?

6. Is the government of Sri Lanka acting like the Jacobins against the Tamils of the north, or are the Tamils a bunch of terrorists to be tamed?

7. Were the French fighting a terrorist group, Greenpeace, when they sank the ship in a New Zealand harbor? Or were they terrorists themselves?

8. Was Oliver North a terrorist? He was arranging the financing of the Contras, a group opposing the legitimate Government of Nicaragua, for his own ideological reasons, and contrary to the explicit instructions of the elected U.S. Congress.

9. When does a government using excessive force against a dissident group become terrorist themselves? Were the actions against the dissidents in WACO Texas,

terrorist activities in the Jacobin sense or were they fighting terrorists? At least one American (Timothy McVeigh) thought the former and became a terrorist himself in response.

10. Was General Custer fighting a band of Indian terrorists as he made his last stand, or were the Indians fighting an oppression worse than the French had experienced in 1795? I note that at the time most Americans believed the former. Nowadays it is politically correct in some circles to believe the latter. It is safe to do so, since the Indians are dead or cowed, and it costs nothing to do so.

11. Was Castro a terrorist or a freedom fighter when he opposed the government of Batista? Are the people who oppose him terrorists, whether they live in Cuba or Florida? What about those branded by Castro as terrorists to whom the USA has given citizenship? The U.S. supported Castro's overthrow of Batista and supported those who tried to overthrow Castro. Is the U.S. government merely against any Cuban (or Carribean or...) government, which doesn't toe the U.S. line?

12. Finally, I mention an issue that arouses more emotion and interest in the USA than most others. However a professional must not duck difficult issues. It is here that his professionalism can be most useful. Is the government of Israel a terrorist government because with respect to the Palestinians they follow (to quote the description of the Jacobins) "the cruel and impolitic maxim of keeping the people in implicit subjugation by a merciless severity?" Or are the Palestinians all terrorists because they belong to an organization opposing the present government of Israel and its policies and particularly in its early days, to drive them into the sea? Although they believed that Israel imposes a ruthless occupation upon them? Are the Israeli actions justified because of Palestinian terrorism (or resistance) or unjustified because (according to many people) even the Israeli presence is contrary to U.S. Security Council resolutions? One man's terrorist is another man's freedom fighter.

The expression "freedom fighter" has been used by those who argue that a particular group is fighting for the freedom of his country against foreign domination and oppression, and that this somehow justifies any otherwise unpleasant act that he or she performs. This phrase needs definition more than most others but the definition is inevitably subjective.

A leading theoretical physicist Professor Victor Weisskopf once (in my presence) corrected a Russian interpreter for referring to the October revolution of November 1917 as a rebellion. Rebellion according to OED is organized armed resistance to the ruler of Government of one's country. But when the rebellion succeeds, it becomes a revolution: "the complete overthrow of one's government." Likewise when a terrorist succeeds in his objective of overthrowing the established order, he is regarded as a freedom fighter.

Clearly Jefferson, once a rebel, became a freedom fighter. (Most people would not call him a terrorist because he did not engage in violence, although he indirectly urged it. However Jefferson did not, in his writings condemn terrorism.) In contrast, Monachem

Begin was definitely a terrorist organizer in 1945 when he organized various activities such as the blowing up of the King David Hotel in Jerusalem. But he later became leader of his country (Israel), which had become free and independent. Bourgiba was jailed as a terrorist by the British in Cairo, but later went on to become the first President of his country (Tunisia). Syria, Iran and Iraq were on a short list of States that the U.S. State Department accuses of encouraging terrorism. Yet Syria supported the USA in the Gulf war and now has a seat on the UN Security Council. Has Syria thereby stopped being a terrorist country? Or were we wrong in thinking it was one before?

In addition to the present bombing in Afghanistan, Americans have to look back at their own history to grasp the complications of such a simplistic distinction.

"Single acts of tyranny may be ascribed to the accidental opinion of the day; but a series of oppressions, begun in a distinguished period and pursued unilaterally thro' every change of ministers, too plainly prove a deliberate, systematical plan of reducing us to slavery."

As I read these words aloud, a listener thought that these might be the words of Gerry Adams – the leader of the IRA. But they might also be the (translated) words of a Kashmiri leader, or of Yasser Arafat. But no. These words were written by Thomas Jefferson in 1774. They propelled him to the Congress in Philadelphia as a representative from Virginia. Jefferson was clearly accusing George III of the form of terrorism according to the usage I listed first in this memo. This was before the Jacobins came to power and the word "terrorist" became popular.

Indeed on July 4th every year Americans celebrate the day when terrorists became patriots and rebels became statesmen.

I then go on with my difficult questions.

13. Were the perpetrators of the Boston Tea party "terrorists" as George III might have said, or freedom fighters? They wantonly destroyed private property but they killed no one.

14. Almost everyone in the USA and many others seem to agree that the people who deliberately flew airplanes into the world trade center were terrorists. But the further one gets into the complicated disagreements, the more difficult it is to agree upon a consistent definition.

15. In May 1940, after Dunkuerque, most Englishmen feared a Nazi occupation of England within a few weeks. Teenagers, including myself, learned rules of unarmed combat. While before 1939 we had been taught the "Queensbury Rules" of boxing, we were now told: "always hit below the belt" and "stamp on the instep." I was shown how to creep up on a German sentry and cut off his head with a sharp wire such as used for cutting cheese. Was this education in resisting unwanted occupation a training in terrorism or training in fighting for freedom?

The birth of Bangladesh 30 years ago illustrates how a metamorphosis can come about. Some people in East Pakistan picked up guns to oppose the government of West Pakistan. They were clearly terrorists. As the weeks passed they became freedom fighters. When they succeeded they became the first statesmen of their new country. But the Pakistani Army objected even as they were losing. On December14th, "Martyred intellectuals day", the Pakistani army systematically slaughtered hundreds of intellectuals: judges, lawyers, physicians and professors. Such behavior, disguised to appear as a legitimate and proper response to those trying to destroy law and order can also be assumed to be a deliberate attempt to deprive a new nation of its leadership, is all too common and can be seen today. How does one choose sides?

Opinions of people will differ on each of these cases, and few will come out on the same side on all of them. But we can probably all decline the irregular verb and say literally, "I am a statesman. You are a freedom fighter. He is a terrorist"

A. As Dr Elena Bonner said about the fighting between the Armenians and the Azeris in the early 1990s, both sides did bad things but (in her view) the Azeris were bad first because they massacred ethnic Armenians in Sumgait just north of Baku. But is that enough reason in itself for choosing sides? If not what are the criteria?

Nowadays, in the USA, the distinction tends to be made between individual terrorism and state sponsored terrorism although the President of Pakistan (among others) recently insisted that he opposed both equally. Most Americans seem to think that only the former (individual terrorism) exists even though the word seems to have been first applied to the state terrorism of the French Jacobins, and the much support for the IRA in Ireland against the British came from the USA.!

B. The late Edwin H. Purcell, Nobel Laureate in Physics and for six years a member of the President's Science Advisory Committee, used to describe his view of the US administration's position (which he opposed, particularly as it applied to Vietnam): "A terrorist is a man with a bomb and no airplane to drop it from".

C. This talk was first given in Chatham House where William Pitt (the elder), Earl of Chatham, once lived. After a distinguished period in office, George III replaced him as prime minister. Chatham said in his last speech: "My Lords, if I were an American, as I am an Englishman, while a foreign troop was landed in my country I never would lay down my arms- never, never, never." I would not rest until the last foreign soldier had left my soil". I commend these words to statesmen in any country whose troops are on the soil of another.

The Planners and Financiers of Terrorism

It becomes even more complicated when one discusses the planners, and financiers, of terrorism. President Bush explicitly stated that he would consider them equally. If we take the implicit modern American usage of a terrorist who opposes by illegal force, including attacks on civilian targets, the established government, President Bush must clearly oppose strongly (and even prosecute) the IRA and its financiers, widely believed to reside in Boston and New York. Fortunately the IRA seems to have got the message (although in September 2002, Mr. Trimble and others claim that it is not disarming but should do so).

President Bush has frozen the assets of Hezzebolla because he claims that it is a terrorist organization. The Lebanese government has stated its reluctance to do so. Hezzebolla, in the Lebanese view, are freedom fighters trying to liberate southern Lebanon. Which is correct? Will we have a situation where many organizations have assets frozen in one country but not another? And particularly not in Switzerland or the Bahamas?

Some observers (e.g. Baroness Cox) have noted that financiers with contacts with Al Qaeda, own major blocks of shares in companies in sensitive positions in western countries. These holdings clearly have the potential to cause great trouble. Far worse however, would be secret dealings. Indeed it is hard to see how one can have anything approaching global security with the secrecy of the tax havens so many countries like and economists have been slow to oppose. I believe that strong international agreement to prevent tax havens is very important. In the wake of the Enron, Anderson and Worldcom scandals, maybe the U.S. congress will muster the courage to propose such a step. Civilian or Military Targets?

Many people with whom I have discussed this issue claim that attacks on civilians break the important barrier that distinguishes a real terrorist from a justified freedom fighter. Some would add the adjective "unarmed" before civilians. Some would add: "with intent to kill." According to this view an attack by an individual against an occupying army or police would not be a terrorist attack, but would be justified resistance. But that leads to problems also. The Boston tea party perpetrators and the Palestinian youth who threw stones at soldiers would clearly not be terrorists according to this definition. But would the Palestinians be terrorists if they threw stones against Jewish worshipers in Jerusalem even though there was no intent to kill? What about bullets against armed settlers even though, according to their contention and belief, the settlers had stolen their land? When applied to state actions, such a definition would have to apply to many more actions that are often accepted. Were the air raids, primarily against civilians in Dresden, Hiroshima and Nagasaki in World War II justified or were they unacceptable state terrorism? What about the actions of a country (USA) that anticipates and accepts "collateral damage" in Vietnam and Afghanistan?

Finally, during the cold war, the USA and the USSR could be said to have terrorized each other by the policy of Mutually Assured Destruction (MAD). It was mad indeed. My family and I were scared at the time of the Cuban missile crisis when the USA had about 70 nuclear weapons and the USSR had about 40. If 40 bombs is enough to deter a people (if not their government) why did we make so many thousands of bombs? And what is the merit in reducing from 5,000 to 2,000 as is now being discussed? Even 2,000 is far more than necessary for the stated purpose of terrifying another country.

Much more important is the question: are not both the USA and Russia terrorizing the world by keeping even 10 bombs on dangerous "trigger alert?" Dismantling the bombs so that their use would require 3 days notice would avoid destroying the world accidentally by mistakes such as that of 1995. Why are not Bush and Putin both evil for refusing to follow the duty under article VI of the non-proliferation treaty and dismantling the nuclear bomb arsenal completely?

Indeed I blame both Mr. Putin and Mr. Bush for signing the recent agreement on nuclear arms. It is a step back from the SALT2 treaty we signed but never ratified. It allows nuclear weapons to be decommissioned rather than just destroyed. It reverses the 30 year old ban on weapons defense. Perhaps the saving grace of the last is that most scientists agree that the "Strategic Defense Initiative" will never work. However it can be a "cover" for other weapons activities and give a very dangerous false sense that there is a technical solution to a problem that is a permanent political problem; one to which we must pay attention until the end of the human race. Cowardly acts.

I emphasized the importance of definitions and in particular the importance of using words so that they may be understood. Sometimes, of course, politicians deliberately use words in ways to confuse. A professional should not accept this. The complications also enter when the adjective cowardly is carelessly used, particularly when attached to the noun terrorist. It has become all too usual to describe "suicide bombers" as "cowardly." I first heard this word when General Haig described the man who drove a truck full of explosives into the U.S. Army barracks in Lebanon as a coward. Although Humpty Dumpty said "I pay the words extra and make them mean what I like," I believe that this is NOT a useful use of the word coward. By its pejorative meaning, it tends to prevent the listener from thinking about the root cause of the action being discussed. But it has been used again and again recently.

But were the Japanese Kamikaze pilots in World War II cowards, or misguided patriots? I believe that Colonel Claus von Stauffenburg was a brave man as he carried his briefcase bomb into the conference room with Hitler. He is reported to have said after gaining access to Hitler's briefings: "Fate has offered us this opportunity, and I would not refuse it for anything in the world. I have examined myself before God and my conscience. It must be done because this man [Hitler] is evil personified." But Colonel von Stauffenberg became a coward when, and only when, he refused to stay with the bomb to ensure its success. He was also careless. He was outside when the bomb blew up and left. When Hitler came staggering out he could easily have been killed right then.

Who were the greater cowards: the Israeli pilots who dropped bombs on the UN refugee camp in Lebanon from a safe height, or the Palestinians who chose certain death to ensure the killing of people, including a dozen unarmed civilians, in Israel? Does it make a difference that the Israeli government apologized for the mistake (but without paying compensation) in the first case, whereas a number of Palestinians were jubilant in the second?

Historically countries have romanticized war. The bravery of the soldiers was extolled: one who refused to go into battle was labeled a coward. The bravery of one's adversary was acknowledged even as he was being killed. In my boyhood I saw several films and read books about World War I, and how the British Air Force in particular, honored the bravery of the German pilots. This romanticization of war has, I am glad to say, gone out of style and the demonization of an individual adversary, particularly a weaker one who fights in a different way, has replaced it. The replacement sentiment is, I believe no better, and is perhaps worse because it is a negation of thought. An ABC talk show host was roundly criticized for making some of the above distinctions in late September 2001. That makes the situation even sadder and even more dangerous.

DEFENSE IN DEPTH

This was a long time in preliminaries. But the preliminaries are essential to be sure that we are talking about the same subject. I now come, at last, to the three independent steps that I believe to be essential if we wish to combat terrorism. As is usual in discussions of series of events, it is easier and more important to address the first step in the chain.

Step 1: The root causes of Terrorism

Terrorism has been with us for centuries and seems to be a permanent facet of our existence. I therefore think it is very important to attempt to find, and eliminate or reduce, the root causes of terrorism. Among these root causes are clearly frustration and despair caused by poverty, hunger, ignorance, injustice and intolerance. In the various long run disputes that plague the world, most people are not armed; and believe in peaceful solution to problems. But when oppression becomes, or is perceived to become, intolerable, these peaceful people will refrain from denouncing those that take up arms in their cause. Those that are killed while fighting become martyrs and are honored. It is not hard to see that these "freedom fighters" can go over the edge. Terrorism then becomes an end in itself independent of the cause.

Terrorism has been described as a cancer in our society. If we develop the analogy further, I note that cancers can be controlled and even cured until they metastasize to another location. When IRA terrorists, now seemingly, and most of us hope permanently, unemployed as terrorists at home, started training terrorists in Columbia, such metastasis occurred. Many of us fear a metastasis of the Palestinian/Israeli conflict. Indeed one Israeli foreign Ministry representative, talking in February 2002 on National Public Radio, implied that metastasis had already occurred by blaming the Palestinians for setting a bad example to other Arabs. Most of us agree that these long running disagreements can be a breeding ground for terrorism. Edward Rothstein, writing in the New York Times of November 17th 2001, seems to dispute this but that may merely be his interest in a particular case. When disagreements are also seen, or perceived, to exist side by side with wealth, extravagance and aggression of another group, particularly an oppressing group, there is likely to be trouble. In my view the solutions must lie in charity, tolerance, and humility in understanding and helping other peoples.

To this end I have circulated the following statement and encourage others to support it:

"We at (state your group), a diverse community of many races, religions, cultures and nations, commit ourselves to work for peace and justice everywhere in the world. We invite others to join in this commitment. We must and will fight ignorance, poverty, hunger, intolerance and injustice wherever and whenever they show their ugly faces.

We must succeed so that no one state, no one group or even one individual will ever again have the desperation to perform such an abominable act as the attack on September 11th 2001 or shelter one of the perpetrators."

I have no patent on this idea, and indeed it is very similar to one the citizens of the city of Hamburg in Germany adopted in 1998. I would be grateful if any group who decides to say the same would let me know.

It is, however, difficult to put the aims of the perpetrators of 9/11 in the categories above. The perpetrators were Egyptians and Saudis—surely not countries being (directly) oppressed by another country. But many analysts have noted that these two countries have governments that are responsive to the needs of the rich but not of the poor. They also leave little room for the poor to express themselves politically. There is no opposition party in the western sense. The poor, and the middle class people who support the poor seem to have no option but to turn to organizations such as the Moslem Brotherhood (in Egypt) who seem to have people dedicated to help the poor. Both the people of the USA and their governments prefer to deal with a stable, even though undemocratic, government than one in political turmoil. The U.S. government supports the governments both of Egypt and Saudi Arabia; providing aid in the former case and protection in the latter. This automatically makes the U.S. complicit in the government's actions and a target for those (the suicide hijackers and Bin Laden) who object. There is no easy way out. The USA gave strong support for President Syngman Rhee of South Korea, and we were fortunate that the Koreans eventually made their own internal reforms. The recent attacks were clearly against symbols of America's domination: the Pentagon with its military domination and the World Trade Center with its financial domination. I think that it is important to note that they were not against other targets in America which, as I will discuss later, could do much more damage to U.S. civilian life.

There is an interesting cheerful corollary to the above thought. The population of Iran has more than doubled since the Shah was overthrown and the clerical government took over. A majority of the population is under 30 and never knew the Shah. These are the young people who might engage in violence. Yet their frustration with lack of progress of the country seems to be aimed at their government, not at us. For the USA can hardly be blamed for supporting the existing, clerical, government. To the very limited extent that President Bush is correct in calling the government of Iran as evil, this does not seem to apply to the young people.

Step 2: Keeping Terrorists at Arm's Length

I believe it would be stupid to believe that one can correct all the root causes of terrorism, and perhaps not even many of them. The consequence then, is that there will be terrorists who must be contained, isolated or eliminated (killed). In the immediate aftermath of the World Trade Center destruction, President Bush assembled a truly remarkable coalition of world leaders to denounce terrorism. One must not belittle the importance of this achievement by comments that many of them are not leaders of democracies, or are in some way oppressing other people. Some of the most emotional support for America has come from people from other countries who are trying to build American values in their 3rd world countries. Yet there is a perception that American actions do not always follow the stated ideals. Palestinians and nearby Arab states, for example, complain that the U.S. government continues to subsidize, and provide arms to Israel, regardless of what Israel does. Indians complain that we fail to denounce the failure of Pakistan to halt terrorism in the Kashmir.

There is general agreement with Jefferson's concept that "no society can survive without a decent respect for the opinion of mankind." (quotation from memory). This unanimity in the world is probably greater than at any time since 1945 when several unlikely major countries were allies against the scourge of Hitler. We must capitalize on it. In this context, I commend and support a fine op-ed piece in the NY Times by Mikhail Gorbachev who argued that we had set up an organization in 1945 to cope with matters such as these and we should use the UN. But of course we should not hesitate to modify it if necessary. Indeed, I believe that modification is appropriate. In the General Assembly the voting power of populous countries like USA, Russia, China and India is no greater than the voting power of the many small countries, and this has led both USA and USSR to avoid taking to the UN issues of importance to Russia or the USA. Something must be done to avoid this international impotence.

While almost all of us believe that religions have played a major part in making the world a better place for its citizens, there is no doubt that wars fought in the name of religion, particularly in the crusades and the wars of the 17th century, have created major havoc. Thus has been built the concept of religious freedom and the vital importance of tolerance for the religion and opinion of another. But there are limits to tolerance. Society cannot survive if it allows the extremists of any religion to attack others. Most Moslems might insist that "jihad" means an inner struggle. The capturing or restriction of the word to mean armed struggle against another person is already a sign of trouble and western society has become wary of groups such as "Islamic Jihad." The defining and enforcement of these limits is one of the most important problems of this second step in combating terrorism.

More recently we learn (e.g. interview with Kuwaitis on "60 minutes" on November 18th 2001) that the world is not unanimous and that support for the U.S. may not be as firm and strong as desired. In my view that is partially because the U.S. has not faced up to the difficulty of defining terrorism, and modifying its own thoughts on the contentious issues mentioned earlier to more nearly accord with international views. It is urgent for all people of good will to discuss these issues.

Finally I believe that although the UN has been wise in restricting its actions to internal rather than domestic problems, (because otherwise it would be overwhelmed), I believe it must intervene and act and act firmly, with justice and generosity, in any conflict that has existed for more than 50 years. These include Ireland, Sri Lanka, Kashmir, and of course the Holy Land. If the world waits, the wound to society will fester.

Step 3: Making Society Safer

America is an extraordinarily safe place – although there is a higher murder rate in America than in England. My father's house in London was robbed 3 times in 25 years. My house in America has never been robbed in 46 years, although we accidentally left the doors unlocked for a month during one vacation. That is, in fact, one reason why the 2,800 people killed in the World Trade Center attack was so troubling. It is here that President Bush has paid most attention, and created the Office of Homeland Security. It is here that Risk Analysts such as those who go to PSAM6 meetings can and should provide the most help. The problem must be considered carefully.

Postmortem on the World Trade Center
Worrying about the World Trade Center is somewhat like fighting the previous war – with all the strategic mistakes that trying to fight the last war encourages. Nonetheless I start with my own postmortem on the World Trade Center collapse. I have read, and recommend the report in May 2002 of the Federal Emergency Management Agency (FEMA), and also an important factual paper, "The World Trade Center Catastrophe: Was the Type of Spray Fire Proofing a Factor in the Collapse of the Twin Towers?" by Dr. Arthur M. Langer and Dr. R.G. Morse which appeared in the July 2002 issue of the Journal of the Indoor and Built Environment. As I read the FEMA report I believe it missed the major conclusion. Although the building was a strong building, and built according to code, no one in the building industry, had considered what Norman Rasmussen emphasized. This is what safety analysts such as the participants in PSAM6, consider every day: the low probability high consequence accident. A terrorist will consider a high consequence event and convert it from low probability to high probability. We must consider such accidents in advance of the terrorist and make our society as secure as we can. In that we have available the tool of the event tree. In this connection I note one paper that was presented to the 2002 PSAM6 conference, Dr Christie and collaborators. If a full risk analysis is made, including full attention to the non-safety related procedures, a nuclear power plant has a fatality risk that is 30 times smaller than if the plant designers and operators merely meet codes and NRC regulations. That probably applies all over society. My major conclusion is that the building industry, as all other industries, MUST do a full event tree analysis and pay particular attention to high consequence events.

There are smaller problems with the FEMA report. Steel buildings, and in particular steel supports are more vulnerable to fire that concrete or even wood. U.S. builders may not have understood this, but the captured tape that was released on December 14th 2001 showed that Osama bin Laden understood it well. Steel conducts heat more readily, and can bend and melt at fire temperatures. At the World Trade Center, the steel uprights and horizontal floor supports were originally planned to be insulated with asbestos to retard fire. Langer and Morse suggest that the inferior properties of the fiberglass insulation as compared to asbestos was an important issue in the collapse. Certainly the insulation did not stick to the beams at the time of collapse. These authors suggest that the material was sprayed on steel beams that were rusty and the material may well have peeled off again. Electricians and members of other crafts often scrape off insulation to install their own devices. Some photographs of the fallen beams suggest that, indeed, many of the beams were denuded of insulation. It appears that no one checked that the insulation was secure after the other construction trades had done their worst. There were no enforced regulations at the time. It is possible that if the original asbestos had been used, or the building redesigned, it would be standing today. It is irrelevant whether Langer and Morse are right. What IS relevant is that no one seems to be able to disprove their suggestions. This suggests that any and all tall buildings built at that time be checked in detail to see whether the insulation is still present.

My colleague, Dr. Pompei, suggested a simple method. Test the insulation by a reverse process. Apply heat to a steel beam at one location, measure the temperature at all nearby locations and compare with a calculation assuming that all insulation is in place. This might cost $50 million per building. But that is cheap compared with bombing Afghanistan.

It is also not correct that no one raised a warning. The man who was most responsible for the use of sprayed on asbestos, the late Mr. Herbert Levine, founder of Asbestospray, was concerned. He told anyone who would listen (including me in 1991) that "if a fire breaks out above the 64th floor (where asbestos stopped) the building will fall down." This raises another question. Should one pay attention to every warning? I suggest that this warning was a warning of a vulnerability that should have been examined.

Again nothing is perfect, and we should have had defense in depth. Evacuation of people in the anticipated 4 hours time available in which the fire resistant material would last was foreseen and indeed evacuation occurred to a remarkable extent, but not everyone would get out, and there was major property damage as the buildings fell. Many disaster movies have shown helicopters picking people off the roof of a burning skyscraper, and spraying foam into the fire below. Where were the helicopters on September 11th? Were there any disaster plans? Clearly any new tall building should have had, and must now have, plans to cope with such disasters and must take account of events of low probability and high consequence.

Buildings can be protected from airplane attacks. In World War II, cables were hung from barrage balloons to cut off the wings of any aircraft willing to fly into them. Sensitive facilities at Los Alamos are protected by cables hanging from tower – no more conspicuous than cell phone towers. These would not completely protect against air attack, but the probability of serious consequences would be diminished.

Although most of the public discussion is about preventing an accident of the same type as occurred on September 11th I believe it is unlikely that it will be attempted again soon. For the last 10, years airplane hijackings have been handled peacefully by the pilot following instructions of the hijacker and arguing (negotiating) when the plane has landed. Pilots basically "gave in." After September 11th, that has clearly changed. Pilots will obviously resist even though the probability of a terrorist being a suicide bomber is probably small. As we saw, the consequences of a successful suicide hijacking are large. But there are a number of technical steps that can be taken. They have even been suggested and put aside. Barring the cockpit door is obvious. The pilot could have a special button that a pilot can press to alert FAA of a hijacking just as bank tellers alert police by a button when a bank robbery is in progress. It is also possible to set by such a button, or by command from the ground, a present flight and landing pattern. These have their own possibilities for sabotage, but there seems to have been no study and discussion.

THE GENERAL VULNERABILITY OF SOCIETY

Fuel storage

It takes very little thought to realize that society is very vulnerable to sabotage and terrorism. But it can be made more secure. We could start by taking basic safety precautions. There is clearly potential for a terrorist to cause great harm by making sure that we do not store a lot of fuel in one place nearby a lot of people in one place. Oil tanks and Liquefied Natural Gas (LNG) facilities should be in remote areas. In my opinion it is more important to locate such sensitive facilities in remote areas than it is to locate nuclear power plants in remote areas. I commend the citizens of London who, a century and a half ago in 1848, decreed that petroleum products not come up the river Thames closer than 30 miles east of London bridge. The accumulation of over one hundred 17 million gallon tanks (LNG, oil, ammonia) in Canvey island (30 miles east of Tower Bridge) was not good. That planners allowed seaside vacation bungalows to be built at the east end of the same island, with two bridges to the mainland converging on one traffic circle (roundabout) was NOT good. It prevented evacuation if trouble occurred whether caused by the IRA, Okaeda or the Tamil Tigers. But the decision of the UK government to ask the Atomic Energy Authority experts in Risley to carry out a safety analysis was excellent. Their (1978?) report, CANVEY, to the UK Health and Safety Executive is an excellent example of clarity of thinking and exposition. One can doubt their numerical assessment of safety, particularly because they did not address international terrorism although they addressed sabotage; but it is hard to doubt the improvement that addressing their simple improvements achieved. But few localities have been as cautious as the good citizens of London 150 years ago. I give here a number of examples in my personal experience and knowledge of how this simple rule is frequently violated.

Co-location of long unprotected rail, gas pipe and water pipe lines is a recipe for disaster. I am well aware of the financial and social advantages that using a common, already paid for both politically and financially, right of way can afford, whether in a capitalist country or one with a "centrally planned economy." But we only have to look at the Soviet LPG accident in the late 1980s, when a gas pipe line leaked and was set alight by a couple of electric trains on the co-located railroad to see the problem. In this little publicized accident 800 people were burned to death – far more than Chernobyl, yet with less international publicity and consequent domestic concern. In the USA, an overloaded freight train derailed in Cajun Pass and broke the accompanying gas pipeline which later exploded – killing 2 people. This has always seemed to me fruitful ground for a terrorist – and terrorists like Osama Bin Laden are now more intelligent than many politicians.

In 1972 or 1973 I had a phone call from a distraught resident of a suburb of Providence, Rhode Island. The local gas company was planning to put a big multi-million gallon LNG storage tank 500 feet from a local school. There were other sites. One obvious one was ruled out because it was 500 feet from a power line (surely less important than a school). I gave testimony suggesting that there was inadequate caution and was on the witness stand for 6 hours. But the local residents won. In 1975 I reviewed a risk assessment for an LNG tanker terminal on the west coast near a major city. The calculated risk was small (10^{-35}). But the study had had left out sabotage or terrorism where the risk is unfortunately much bigger. I pointed this out to a director of the gas company who had paid $1,500,000 for the study. I suggested that he rethink the conclusions. If he used the study to justify building the terminal, it could (and might well) destroy him.

The methane in an LNG tank only has to be mixed with easily available oxygen to be highly inflammable and in some circumstances explosive. In contrast neither the fuel itself nor the stored fuel in a nuclear power plant is easy to sabotage in the same way. In Boston there are two 17 million gallon tanks within 2 miles of the center. If mixed stochiometrically with air each would have the energy content of 3 Hiroshima bombs. 25 years ago I participated in a study for the General Accounting Office (GAO) and in a session deliberately unrecorded, we found many ways to wreak a lot of havoc. These scenarios were deliberately not written down and will not be here. Suffice to say that a week or so later, I stopped for coffee along the Massachusetts turnpike and found three trucks side by side at the rest stop. One was a gasoline truck. Another a liquid Oxygen truck. A third was an LNG truck. I went on to the next rest stop. We must now pay close attention to these events of low calculated probability but high consequence. The terrorists will.

Hydroelectric Dams

Hydroelectric dams are necessarily upstream of an estuary. For reasons of easy communication by sea, society has usually built a town at the estuary. Hydroelectric dams have sometimes given way naturally, and at one time the "natural" failures made hydropower one of the more dangerous energy sources. Natural failures have been reduced, but few analysts have considered sabotage. In 1944 an Englishman destroyed a hydroelectric dam in Germany under very unfavorable circumstances. He had to do so from the air (with a 7,000 pound bomb) while being shot at from the ground by merciless anti-aircraft fire. This was documented in the film: "the dambusters." With more modern explosives, this could be done with a 1000 pound bomb from the ground. To test the possibility of this route of sabotage I deliberately drove out onto an unguarded dam in the upper Connecticut River, stopped long enough to take such a heavy object from my car and drove away. No one said anything. The late Professor Arthur Casagrande, one of North America's major dam designers, told me 30 years ago that if a dam in the upper Missouri were to fail naturally or be destroyed deliberately in time of flood, then all the dams downstream would fail until near St Louis, where he had deliberately designed a dam to cope with such a contingency. At the Connecticut River, we both had little doubt that if I had blown up this dam on the upper Connecticut in time of flood, all dams would fail in turn down to the sea. After I related this story at the PSAM6 meeting, a risk analyst in the audience told me that he had studied the risks of all of these dams for an insurance company but had failed to consider that these failures might be correlated (common mode failure).

Anthrax and Smallpox

The anthrax scare was technically easily avoidable. Surgical equipment in hospitals is sterilized at modest expense by gamma irradiation. It would not be unduly expensive to pass ALL mail in a sorting office past a cobalt 60 (or Cesium 137) unit that sterilizes everything within. Society might decide that this would be undesirable as a general rule. It **would** stop my wife sending flower seeds to our children through the mail. But the equipment needs to be ready to be used immediately on the first outbreak. Indeed this seems to be happening. A smallpox scare could be worse since it is airborne. Vaccinating everyone might be a solution, but this would subject everyone to a risk, about one in a million lifetime risk. Experts now recommend that vaccine be made and stored but used only after an initial outbreak is detected. This is an interesting recommendation because it is a clear risk-risk comparison of the type we at PSAM6 always recommend.

Agricultural Chemicals

We did not learn as much as we should have from the Bhopal accident in India where a lot of isocyanate, used as an intermediate in fertilizer manufacture, was stored in one place and housing was allowed to be built nearby. I tend to believe the claim by analysts at Arthur D. Little that the release was deliberate sabotage by a disgruntled employee. But the designers and operators of the plant were delinquent in many ways. They designed a plant which was easy to sabotage; they stored more isocyanate in one place than they needed; they allowed people to live nearby, and they failed to train the employees and community in the simple precautions (put a wet handkerchief over your face).

Ammonia is used as an agricultural chemical intermediate and used to be stored in large tanks – 17 million gallons – often close to a community. If released over a residential area there would be a large loss of life. The day after Iraq invaded Kuwait, both my friend Dr. Adnan Shihab Eldin, former director of the Kuwait Institute of Scientific Research, and myself remembered that there was a large ammonia tank in the port of Shuwaikh, only 1/4 mile upwind from a population area. I don't doubt that this would have been released, when the wind blew in the right direction, to add to the mess created by the oil fires. We discussed how to get someone to empty the tank. We later found out that a Kuwaiti who was in the country at the time had had the same thought and emptied the tank into the sea while telling no one.

Timothy McVeigh took advantage of easily available fertilizer, ammonium-nitrate, to fashion an explosive that destroyed a building in Oklahoma city. This fertilizer is still easily available. After the Oklahoma bombing, Russell Seitz suggested at a Congressional hearing that all agricultural fertilizer be mixed with urea – to make it impossible to detonate. But farmers object because it makes the fertilizer stink. Maybe this should be reconsidered.

Drinking Water

Drinking water supplies can be easily contaminated and even the threat of contamination can upset a community. As a beginning graduate student I had to do some silver plating with silver cyanide solution. When I got a headache I looked up the poisonous properties and realized that I had enough cyanide in the cupboard to poison the whole city of Oxford. Of course this last remark is about as useful as the oft repeated remark that a kilogram of plutonium could poison the world. The poison would have to be spread uniformly. But I went on and found out exactly where to drop the material (from a small footbridge) to do the most harm. The Oxford water supply system has been upgraded but similar problems remain. Most water systems can be easily sabotaged. But the solution is simple. A state can make available a portable system that could be rushed to any threatened system to provide emergency water. Such systems exist: they could provide 10,000 gallons a day at a cost (including paying off the loan) of 1.5 cents a gallon – somewhat cheaper than the bottled water many people store for such emergencies.

Nuclear Power Plants

There has been recently a lot of public attention paid to possible accidents in nuclear power plants, plant safety, including accidental aircraft hits. Now they must be specifically applied to possible terrorist attacks. Yet few other facilities are studied with the same thoroughness. In this, we can thank once again those who made the decision 40 years ago to build strong containments. The record shows that these are among the few facilities where sabotage has been considered, and even direct hits from large aircraft. Those close to airfields (such as Seabrook NH) are designed to withstand a crash of a Boeing 747 at 500 mph. Others will withstand a large aircraft at landing speed (200 mph) but even if parts of a faster plane penetrate the containment, there is no reason to believe that such a release could be large. A direct hit from a large aircraft could put such a power plant out of action – maybe forever. The most important issue for public confidence is the possibility of radiation release. The probability of release is hard to calculate, and the Nuclear Regulatory Commission is rightly reexamining the issue as a matter of urgency. One matter is clear: hitting the containment vessel will not cause the worst accident. 20 years ago I discussed sabotage with Norman Rasmussen. "It is hard for a saboteur to do more than the clowns at Three Mile Island did on their own." But the probability can be increased. Many in this audience know better than I that there are some places an airplane could hit that might cause real trouble. But do not ask me – except in general terms. I might tell a terrorist by mistake. Fortunately hitting some spent fuel in its storage casks will not do as much as many people fear. The casks are hard to break open; almost impossible to burn. There is no radioactive iodine left, and it is hard to vaporize the fuel.

Blackouts

The above examples focused on actions that can cause death. But even actions that cause no casualties can be serious, as I reminded NAE, a simple relay failure started the sequence of events that led to the blackout of the northeastern United States in 1966 (or maybe it was 1965). A saboteur could do this – but he would have to know what relay! But a terrorist group may well be diligent enough to find the weak link. A single substation failure at Naperville, Illinois shut down the landing control system for O'Hare airport (AND, more important to me personally, shut down the e-mails from my son at FERMILAB).

WHAT SHOULD WE DO?

In all the above examples most elements of society have not even begun to think about the societal vulnerabilities that exist. Firstly society needs to consider the most elementary precautions using the defense in depth philosophy. Then we can use the full panoply of techniques to assess the relative vulnerabilities of different parts of society. We can, and should, study sabotage and terrorism with the imagination (perhaps the imagination of a physicist) which we apply to other potential accidents. We should imagine what a terrorist might do and then devise a system to make it hard for him to do it. This is the "defense in depth" and the "Event Tree Analysis" that are already successfully applied to nuclear power as nuclear power plants. We must imagine what a terrorist might do, make it unattractive, and also make the consequences low. This should be done in a comparative way so that excessive resources are not spent on one vulnerable point in society to the exclusion of all others. The actual risk that a terrorist poses is hard to calculate. We may therefore need an intermediate goal, in the same way that NRC has an intermediate safety goal for U.S. light water reactors; the reduction of core melt frequency to less than 1 in 10,000 per year. I suggest that assessed vulnerability could be the basis for such a goal. The Department of Homeland Security has been created and is being funded. It is our job to influence that department and to make sure that they use the best techniques that we can offer. In that direction, why has the head of that department not come to this meeting? Was he invited?

But we should be a little careful about doing too much. I understand that New York State has taken a lot of map directions off its web sites to avoid giving easy instructions to a terrorist. This is reminiscent of May 1940 when all the (road) signposts in England were cut down in anticipation of an imminent German invasion and the state controlled terror that we all anticipated. Such actions will make a terrorist's life more difficult, but may not reduce the probability of his success by much. In performing them we should be aware of Edward Teller's most frequent recent utterance; unnecessary secrecy harms society more than it harms the would-be enemy, whether state, saboteur or terrorist.

Until recently America only experienced random, uneducated, terrorists. Until 1970 few experts thought further. But in 1970 it became clear that there could be educated terrorists with a "cause." These educated terrorists might take a reactor safety course at MIT to learn the weak points of a reactor, or my "Risk Analysis" course to learn all sorts of risky technologies that could be disturbed. But I thought that 19 terrorists acting in concert was very unlikely. I was wrong, and all of society must now recognize that the probability is, alas, quite large.

Those who have been unable to get public attention properly latch on to any seemingly related event or idea to raise their unheeded concerns. I am among them. I am, therefore, in delighted agreement with the general idea that there is now MORE emphasis among the U.S. public on considering the dangerous proliferation of nuclear weapons. In that sense 9/11 may have been a blessing in disguise. 9/11 was a "wake up call" to America. Just as Chernobyl may have been a "wake up call" to the USSR and a blessing in disguise. Marshal Yazov, defense minister of the Soviet Union, at a small meeting in his office in May 1991 stated to a small group of us that the Chernobyl accident persuaded hard line Soviet generals that a nuclear war could not be won." If a reactor that was not supposed to explode made this much mess, a nuclear war would destroy the planet". I have worried about nuclear weapons proliferation for 50 years. I have worried about biological weapons for 40 years. I have worried about chemical weapons for 60 years since I was trained to cope with them in World War II. However, although very nasty, chemical weapons are not really weapons of mass destruction in the same sense. But on issues of weapons of mass destruction it is not enough to raise concern in the State Department. Concern about proliferation of weapons of mass destruction must be raised in every citizen by instruction in every school, not only in the USA but all over the world. Mankind has a capability, which since 1945 has become very clear, of destroying itself completely. Indeed, from a technical point of view, destruction of the human race by these weapons of mass destruction seems far easier than planning for the continuation of the human race. A terrorist may prefer to destroy the human race. Most of us prefer to plan for its continuation. But it is not enough to prefer it. We must think and act. As scientists said loudly in 1945 – everything (technically) has changed but our ideas have not.

Sabotage and terrorism are unfortunate facts of life. They will be with us until the end of the human race. Indeed, if we do not pay attention to them, there may well be a premature end to the human race. The countries of the world must get together and pay attention to the three facets above. We must resolve conflicts and situations that breed terrorism, isolate the terrorists, and make modern large-scale technologies ever more difficult to attack.

COMPARISON OF RISKS

I frequently urge that everyone would gain perspective by comparing the risks of the activity one is considering with other risks, which may be more familiar. I believe that it is useful to do this for terrorist activities.

2,800 people were killed at the World Trade Center. This was indeed terrible. But over 40,000 people are killed every year on U.S. highways by automobile and truck accidents. Is this not more terrible? Yet somehow it does not seem so. I can identify two aspects, which account for the difference. Firstly, a large number of people killed at the same time is psychologically more disturbing than the same number of people killed over a period of time. This seems to be true of other accident situations. Secondly, terrorism and the fear of more, even worse, terrorism seems to be even more disturbing than an accident of equivalent magnitude. Analytically, in a decision theoretic framework, one can take account of this by assigning a higher amount of money to avert a terrorist risk than other risks – perhaps $50,000,000 per life rather than the $6,100,000 per life now being used by U.S. EPA and its equivalent in NRC.

It is hard to quantify the importance of living in a free society with our human rights that are so important to us. We must beware of giving up these rights for too small a benefit. I do not believe I am alone in thinking that it is these rights as a free man that makes life worth living.

Much more important is a comparison with the narcotics industry. Although the deliberate destruction of life and property on 9/11 was an evil act, its consequences were far less than the yearly evil of drug traffic. Drugs kill or destroy many more people and are far more destructive of U.S. society. Drug addiction can create despair. Desperation is, I believe, one of the motives that drives people to terrorism. We also must not forget the drug that society has accepted and society is intermittently trying to eradicate – nicotine. The New

Yorker caught this idea well with Gregory's cartoon (available as <u>Cartoon bank</u> ID 47397) in February 2002. One Afghan was talking to another. "If you still want to join an organization dedicated to killing Americans there is always the tobacco lobby."

6. CONFRONTATIONS AND COUNTERMEASURES: PRESENT AND FUTURE CONFRONTATIONS

TOWARDS AN UNGUIDED WORLD?

ANATOLY ADAMISHIN
Moscow, Russia

I always liked the famous sentence by Albert Einstein "The most unconceivable thing about this World is that it is conceivable".

A lot of predictions of the great scientist, even some of those that he himself later renounced, proved to be true.

But it is probably more difficult to deal with the human world than with the physical one. At least those who, in their vanity, tried to foresee the future of mankind were not especially lucky.

The events of September 11th 2001 took us back to sinful Earth. In a brutal way they showed that our understanding of the world is again lagging far behind the world itself. Conciousness proved to lag behind existence. It is marxist but nevertheless it is true.

The political class' inadequate thinking, even in most advanced states, became evident.

Stepping into a new stage of development, the world today definitely entered the turbulence zone. Usually such periods are accompanied by a sharp decrease in controllability. And usually this is perceived as an approach to the end of civilization in general. At least we heard about the end of the story.

The fact that our civilization is still alive does not automatically guarantee that it will successfully cope with the present crisis. A lot will depend on the conscious activity of the political leaders of the states that can still influence the world's evolution. And on those who are capable of giving them the right recommendations.

The 21st century has begun with a considerable gap between the world affairs that have undergone colossal changes, on the one hand, and the behavioral rules in this world, on the other.

In the days of the Cold War there were two poles of force, each of whom wanted to rule the world in its own way. While they were both tugging on the rope, the world was a rather dangerous place to live (remember the Caribbean crisis).

Later on some sort of behavioral rules emerged between them. These rules were considerably influenced by the Third World. Naturally, the non-aligned states tried to benefit from the contradictions between the two superpowers. But in general the non-alignment movement played a great positive role in setting new and common game rules.

They are not only fixed by the UN charter which – although not instantly – became a sort of an international legal code. The rules of behavior are the sum of the inter-state agreements and their implementation practice. And I am not talking here about rules fixed only after WWII. International law has been based on two principles: namely national sovereignty and legal equality of nations – since the 17th Century. It is easy to see how both of these principles have been transformed.

In today's world, states and peoples coexist without a set of defined and generally acceptable behavior rules which makes their life even more complex.

The present monstrous metastasis of international terrorism is a vivid sign of the world's uncontrollability. The effectiveness of the terrorist strikes is, no doubt, fueled by our civilization's high vulnerability and even more so as it acquires global and hence interdependent character.

Internationalization of economic ties has always existed. For example, it had reached a rather high level before WWI. According to the economists' calculations, the same level was hit again only in mid 70s. Then another dash forward followed. The main novelty here is that the roots of this last dash are in the industrial revolution, mainly in the IT area. Definitely, such derivative factors as an increase in the flow of goods and people, growth of foreign trade's share in GDP, an enormous world-wide inter-flow of finance (up to 1,5 trillion dollars per day) which is now mainly out of national governments' control, and many others, play their role as well.

By the way, the weakened state function of control is one of the reasons for the recent U.S. corporate problems. But does the explosion in information and technology exchange explain everything?

Nobody has proved yet that technological, informational and other revolutions, being epochal for civilisation, should necessarily cause such response as international terrorism. Certainly, we know about the Luddites, but they used to smash machines.

Over and over again it has been proved that the most crucial factors (socially) are not the fruits of the civilisation, but how these fruits are used.

The process of globalisation goes hand in hand with the decrease in the number of information and innovation centres of the modern world. Actually, all of them are in the countries usually called "Western." And those who control technologies control the world - this formula has been known since the times of Ancient Rome.

The newly acquired technological superiority sharply increases opportunities for the West to influence all other states. In various forms the principle, "Take as much as you can and leave as little as possible to others" is carried out. One fifth of the world obtains 80% of the global wealth. To make the standard of living of the rest population equal to that of the elite club, resources equal to four planets similar to Earth would be needed. By the end of 19th Century the income per capita in the richest country of the world was approximately 9 times higher than in the poorest one. Today this ratio is 100:1.

The poor received only some remnants from the terrific economic growth of the '90s when the revenue of the rich countries increased by some $10 trillion.

So, what? Is poverty the reason for international terrorism? Certainly it is, but not the only one.

Otherwise it would be difficult to explain, why in some regions poverty results in such extreme forms of social protest as terror, and in others it doesn't. Africa, for example, is one of the poorest continents, but has anybody heard of African terrorism?

I was deeply impressed by the results of an opinion poll in India that showing that a large number of Indians live in awful conditions without considering themselves unhappy.

But still, in my opinion, we shall not find answers to the numerous questions arising today if we stay away from the unsteady ground of various outlooks, moral principles, faith, religion and the use of all this for selfish ends.

Terror nearly always used to explode in places where weakness, humiliation, despair and ignorance reigned. Ignorance of some special sort that is based on intolerance and fanaticism.

This ignorance has been cultivated deliberately for several decades. The ruling circles of some Arab regimes, like Saudi Arabia, tried to avoid the threat of social discontent by several means including the method of stimulating the darkest sides of fanatic Islam and channelling it against the external enemy.

It is hard to get rid of the impression that it was exactly this combination of economics-related factors and cultivated religious fanaticism that gave birth to the explosive mixture of international terrorism, of which Bin Laden has become a symbol. The latter, by the way, is Saudi Arabian by origin.

The United States had their eyes shut to all this for a long time, carrying out the "barter" which Americans themselves now qualify as cynical: constant supply of oil to the U.S. and multibillion arms deliveries to the Arab regimes in exchange for immortalising feudalism and security for the ruling families there.

Add to this the most destructive weapons and instruments that can be used by terrorist organizations, and the perspective becomes gloomy.

The international relations managing system is in crisis. Certainly one can sound the alarm when the UN charter is violated, but one cannot avoid realizing that a number of its important provisions no longer meet today's requirements.

As a result a sort of vacuum has been created in the international legal structure of the world.

Often this vacuum is filled by decisions made by some group of countries. See the bombing of Yugoslavia – or by unilateral actions of a single power. There are a lot of examples.

But it is still beyond their capacity to rule the world in a way that will make everybody happy. To make the world safe enough for all, including the rulers.

With all their power the United States will hardly be able to establish order in this chaotic world, though I would not mind if they succeeded in this. Further still, some American actions destroy the former system of international agreements and treaties and offer nothing in exchange. Hence they themselves are a factor of instability.

The degradation of the multiple arms race limitations have links to mass destruction weapons proliferation which is exactly what Americans consider to be the number 1 problem.

But the Americans have to make their choice since it is not very logical to rely on themselves and ignore the international community to solve a number of problems and then insist on unanimous efforts when and where the U.S. needs them.

As Sweden's and Finland's ministers of foreign affairs have successfully put it in their recent article (IHT, August 3, 2002), "Only a multilateral approach can counter the new threats, those of nuclear, chemical and biological weapons".

The United States are extremely powerful. Sensible use of this power is a great responsibility of the American ruling class. Might and brain have to go hand in hand as Prof. Shea showed yesterday in a convincing example of the Roman Empire.

International cooperation can contribute to America's own interests provided the latter are correctly interpreted.

The world is becoming less governable not only because of globalisation. There is another historical process - disintegration of the international relations system as it was shaped after WWII, disappearance of the Soviet Union from international scene.

Though overstraining itself and spending its potential (which could be used with much better benefit to its own advantage) the USSR was a sort of counterbalance to Western dominance and constrained the extremes of its pressure.

The end of the Cold War led to the end of the ideological confrontation and demolished the stable military balance that had existed for many years.

Ethnic and religious differences between peoples occupied the stage while the breach of balance contributed to their further growth into conflicts.

One can agree or disagree with the civilisations collision theory, but it is difficult to ignore that modern threats and challenges often originate from inter-civilisation fractures.

The exhaustion of natural resources, first of all energetic, the threats, greater than ever, to forests, fish, clean water and air, catastrophic environmental pollution, prompt population increase and constantly increasing rupture in standards of living between rich and poor countries - all these factors expand the basis for wars and conflicts.

I do not believe that we could successfully confront these global problems, the famous 53 planetary emergencies of Professor Zichichi, without substantial improvement of interstate relations. Moreover, we have a window of opportunity for that.

I can refer here to the international diplomacy guru Henry Kissinger. He considers that, "the war against terrorism is not only the prosecution of terrorists. It is, first of all, the protection of a newly emerged, extraordinary opportunity to rebuild the international system."

We should start from that which may be the most difficult: the psychological transformation. Former opponents in the Cold war should really understand that their own survival depends on whether they are able to switch their attention to new challenges.

It is high time to put a final end to the feud that we have been engaged in for the last 40 years within our one civilised family, though it was split ideologically. It is during this period of time that the new threats have appeared and gained strength.

Providing we reach new wisdom, what is the next stage? Here science comes out ahead in trying to unite all creative forces in order to intellectually pave the road towards the changes in world order that are so badly needed.

On this basis we may try to achieve a very important goal: elaborating new rules of international behaviour. Or, better yet, modernise those already existing, accelerating the work that is always in process in the UN.

A new balance between national interests and moral principles will play an enormous role. And the key issue here is: who will decide to use force, and how, in inter-state relations and ethnic conflicts.

A systematic and purposeful search of what can serve as a common denominator in relations between different civilisations and cultures is also needed.

The improvement of the world situation is hardly possible without serious internal changes. First of all comes the building of civil society in countries of different political, religious and cultural orientation. There is a very close connection between mature civil society on the one hand, and normal inter-civilisation relations and the democratisation of international life on the other.

Again and again, the only acceptable perspective is to elaborate a code of international conduct rules that will be accepted by the overwhelming majority of states.

Why could Erice, our organisation, not make its own draft and send it to the governments?

Another big question: who will be the moderator and who will take the decisions? Surely not all the 190 or so states that now exist. They will have to give up some of their powers in favour of an international body. I think it will be the UN. But the renewed UN. And inside it?

I have already mentioned the limitations of the United States in this respect. At the same time only the USA is capable of opposing new crises.

The leading role of the United States is indisputable. It should be exactly that: the leading, not hegemonic role. Ideally, the USA should play a leader's role in a coalition of states including – it sounds natural on my lips – Russia. I do not mean that they have to rule the world. But they have to ensure that the generally accepted rules of behaviour are respected.

It would not be world government, but something approaching it.

TERRORISM – DEFINING THE PROBLEM, ASSESSING THE RISK

CHRISTOPHER DAASE
University of Kent at Canterbury, Brussels School of International Studies, Brussels, Belgium

Terrorism is a contested concept. By disagreeing about the definition of terrorism and the methods of assessing its risk, political cooperation to combat this menace is severely hampered. Discussions in international fora are often stalled due to deeper ideological controversies. The international community of natural and social scientists can help to tackle this problem by engaging in an open, cross-cultural discourse on how to define terrorism and how to assess its risks. The World Federation of Scientists is in a unique position to lead such an effort in order to facilitate a less biased and more successful international strategy towards this "cultural emergency."

To develop this argument, I will, first, stress that the definition of terrorism is not only an academic problem, but that it has implications for political cooperation; secondly, I will show why the risk assessment of terrorism is controversial; and finally, I will point to the virtues of epistemic communities to overcome these problems and to facilitate international political cooperation.

DEFINING TERRORISM

For some, terrorism is like pornography: They know it, if they see it. This famous approach towards tricky conceptual issues, first taken by a U.S. judge, is not without problems, however. It may be pragmatic and individually satisfying, but it may also cause disagreement and prevent collective action. The judge may know what pornography is, but even his wife may disagree with his judgement disapproving of his evening readings. Cooperation it seems, is very difficult without a common notion of the matter on that cooperation is sought.

The same is true with regard to terrorism. There are a vast number of definitions, political and academic, that try to capture the essential features of terrorism. But so far, no single definition has been universally accepted. Even Alex Schmid's attempt to synthesize a comprehensive notion of terrorism out of one-hundred and nine different scientific definitions in order to find the hard conceptual core that distinguishes terrorism from conventional violence has not been very successful.[1]

All these failed attempts have led some experts to become sceptical, if not cynical, about the conceptual debate. Walter Laqueur stated (as early as 1977) that a universal definition of terrorism does not exist and is unlikely to emerge in the near future. But, he maintained, it would be absurd to believe, that without such a definition research on terrorism is impossible.[2] All research, however, relies on some kind of definition, explicitly or implicitly. What Laqueur proposed and upheld throughout his many books on this subject is a pragmatic approach to the definitional problem and a loose notion of terrorism as the illegitimate use of force to achieve political aims through attacking innocent people.[3]

Practitioners in national governments and international organizations have taken a similar attitude, avoiding the hard conceptual work. Sometimes, they acknowledge the inherent problem of defining terrorism, but more often they simply provide their personal definition according to their own interests and values. This pragmatic, but at the same time sloppy attitude towards the definitional problem, I would argue, is one of the main obstacles for a more successful cooperation in the fight against terrorism. By avoiding disputes over words, practitioners (just like academics) have prevented progress in substance. Let me give you some examples.

International Organizations have historically been unable to agree on a definition of terrorism. Since the time of the League of Nations, numerous concepts and opinions of terrorism have been proposed. The 1937 *Convention for the Prevention and Repression of Terrorism* defined terrorism in very general terms as "criminal acts against a State intended to provoke a state of terror in particular persons, groups of persons or the general public." The convention was ratified by a single state only and never entered into force.[4]

When the issue of terrorism was first brought up in the UN General Assembly, a bitter controversy arose about how to distinguish illegitimate terrorism and the legitimate struggle for freedom and self-determination against colonialism or foreign occupation. Since no common ground could be established, the General Assembly adopted a "piecemeal approach." Instead of developing a comprehensive strategy to deal with terrorism, it agreed on twelve international conventions between 1963 and 1999 that address very specific issues and outlaw precise categories of acts such as high jacking aircrafts, assassinating diplomats, and taking hostages.[5] These conventions typically avoid a general definition of terrorism, but

- specify certain acts that are considered offences,
- indicate Member States' obligations regarding the prohibition of these acts under national law,
- and establish the legal basis according to which Member States can prosecute the alleged perpetrators as terrorists.[6]

Some experts hold that this "piecemeal approach" has been relatively successful by outlawing terrorist acts bit by bit and gradually building an international consensus about what constitutes terrorism.[7] On the other hand it must be acknowledged that the international legal framework to combat terrorism is far from being perfect. Although it covers by now most kinds of terrorism, its incremental development has left significant gaps, especially in the area of nuclear, chemical and biological terrorism. Moreover, it is doubtful that the twelve UN Conventions add up to a comprehensive understanding on what terrorism is and why it should be resisted.

Most UN Member States have condemned terrorism in strong terms after the September attacks. But this unanimity has not brought any progress to the negotiations of the remaining two Draft Conventions on the Elimination of Terrorism (introduced by India) and for the Suppression of Acts of Nuclear Terrorism (introduced by Russia). The definitional disagreement of what constitutes illegitimate terrorism and what legitimate political violence still frustrates international cooperation.

In the European Union, too, cooperation on terrorism has been delayed by conceptual disagreement. Only after September 11th, the EU has decided on a more active strategy adopting a common definition and an Action Plan to combat terrorism. This was not easy, since only 6 out of 15 EU Member States (namely France, Great Britain, Portugal, Spain, Germany and Italy) had a national legislation on terrorism, and those who had such legislation had very different definitions of terrorism depending on their own history and experience of political violence in their countries.

Yet on September 21st 2001, the European Council decided that it was necessary to introduce new measures to promote intra- and interregional cooperation in order to eradicate terrorism. These measures included "joint investigation teams of police and magistrates from throughout the EU; a common list of terrorist organizations; routine exchange of information about terrorism between the Member States and Europol; a specialist anti-terrorist team within Europol and the relevant U.S. authorities; and Eurojust, a co-ordination body composed of magistrates, prosecutors and police officers, to be launched on 1 January 2002."

For all these measures, a common definition of terrorism was deemed essential. After lengthy discussions behind closed doors, the EU Framework Decision on Combating Terrorism came finally into force on June 23rd 2002.[8] It defines terrorist offences as "intentionally committed by an individual or a group against one or more countries, their institutions or people with the aim of intimidating them and seriously altering or destroying the political, economic, or social structure of a country." In addition, the Framework Decision specifies criminal offences that should be punished as terrorist acts under Member States's national law if they are carried out by terrorist groups.

Although the EU definition of terrorism increases the chances for cooperation among European states and between the EU and the U.S., it has also received criticism from civil society groups who argue that it is ambiguous and could cover protest.

A final example how conceptual imprecision might hinder cooperation is the U.S. itself. Prior to September 11th, more than thirty different government agencies were engaged in antiterrorist activities, most of them operating on the basis of their own understanding of terrorism, terrorist acts, and terrorist groups. In conjunction with overlapping responsibilities, this conceptual inconsistency has contributed to the inter-organizational confusion that is said to be responsible for the failure to prevent the attacks of New York and Washington.

Although a clear system of hierarchy was in place designating the State Department as the lead agency for countering terrorism overseas, the Justice Department's Federal Bureau of Investigation (FBI) as the lead agency for domestic terrorism and the Federal Emergency Management Agency (FEMA) as the lead agency for consequence management, congressional investigations found numerous instances in which inter-institutional cooperation failed, thus rendering the U.S. antiterrorism apparatus impotent.[9]

Reducing the number of responsible agencies by creating the Department of Homeland Security, streamlining the chain of command, and harmonizing the antiterrorist programs of different government agencies[10] seems to be the logical path to reorganize the institutional base for countering the terrorist threat.[11] Primary responsibility for dealing with international terrorism, however, will rest with the Department of State and the Pentagon, as well as with parts of the law enforcement and intelligence communities.[12] In this situation, the need for conceptual clarity in order to determine a common strategy on the one hand and to delineate areas of responsibility on the other remains a top priority.

But I do not want to overstate my point. A common definition on terrorism is not a substitute for a sound anti-terrorism policy. But it is a first step in this direction, be it on the national, supranational, or international level. Where conceptual difficulties are ignored and competing, or even contradictory definitions of the problem prevail, cooperation in the fight against terrorism will severely be restricted.

True, debates on the meaning of contested concepts can be tedious and frustrating. But there is no alternative. Even if political consensus is unlikely and full agreement on a common definition is not possible, the conceptual debate is of great value. It points to the fact that there are different interests and values behind conceptual disagreements that have to be accommodated[13] if a common strategy is the goal; and nothing less will be successful in the fight against terrorism.

ASSESSING THE RISK OF TERRORISM

Even more tricky than defining terrorism is to assess its danger. Since the surprise attacks of September 11, government agencies and independent experts keep warning the public that new assaults are imminent, maybe of even greater magnitude and with graver consequences. But specific warnings are rare and the intelligence situation is unclear. Vice President Dick Cheney maintains that "the prospects of a future attack against the United States are almost certain", but he admits that "we don't know if it's going to be tomorrow or next week or next year."[14] In the meantime, not only liberals, but also conservatives fear that constant warnings and the permanent state of alert may in the long run actually weaken public vigilance and distract government attention from other important business.

Terrorism shares the difficulty to determine its danger with other new security problems that are felt more urgently since the end of the Cold War: the proliferation of weapons of mass destruction, cyber attacks, environmental degradation, ethnic conflict, fundamentalism etc. What is more, in combination with one or more of these challenges, terrorism might become the mega threat of the 21st century. But still, the magnitude of the threat is hard to determine. The reason is that so many uncertainties are involved, many more than during the Cold War. To make this difference clear, it is helpful to distinguish between threat and risk – a distinction that was first introduced by the NATO Council during its London meeting in 1990.[15]

If we define – for the purpose of this argument – threat as a "bad intention of an actor with the capacity of doing harm,"[16] then it becomes clear that a threat requires three elements, a threatening *actor*, an *intention* to hurt or damage, and a military or other *capability* to do so. During the Cold War, East and West perceived such a threat and made their policy choices accordingly. Risk by comparison, is less easily identified. It can be defined as "the probability of a future yet manipulable harm or damage."[17] It is obvious that risks might exist without identifiable political actors, without the availability of military capabilities, and without malign intentions. Risks are imperfect threats if you will, or "emerging threats" as the Rumsfeld Commission used to term them in its 1998 report.[18]

But again, the emergence of these threats is uncertain. It is the undeniable merit of the Rumsfeld Commission to have highlighted the fact, that new threats are not easily measured with old methods. But it has failed to spell out an alternative methodology and to caution against the possible danger of a politicised risk assessment. Indeed, some experts have criticized the Report for being partisan and unscientific with regard to the "emerging missile threat". Just by changing the parameters of the assessment process, they argue, the Commission has increased the perceived threat tremendously without there being any change in real world conditions.[19] Whether this was intentionally done in order to improve the prospect for a National Missile Defense is a controversial issue and does not interest here.[20] For the problem runs deeper. It concerns the difficulties of a threat assessment under uncertainty.

In this sense, terrorism is a risk rather then a threat, since too many variables of its assessment are uncertain. First, it is unclear who "the terrorists" are. Usually, terrorist groups operate in the dark; they are only weakly institutionalised and able to reorganize if one of its cells or even the leadership has been destroyed. Although governments often "solve" this problem by personalizing terrorism or blaming state sponsors, the elusiveness of "the terrorist" or "terrorism" is a major problem for risk assessments. Secondly, the capabilities are indefinite. While the danger of nuclear, chemical or biological terrorism remains the prime concern, September 11 has demonstrated that low tech terrorism can be just as damaging as high tech terrorism. But what the means of choice of terrorists are, is nearly impossible to detect. Finally, the intentions are dubious. Recent attacks – especially suicide attacks – are difficult to comprehend in terms of Western political rationality; yet it would be unwise to call them irrational thus depriving ourselves of the means to understand terrorist behaviour.

So far, two different methodologies have dominated the risk assessment of terrorism.[21] The first is advocated by terrorism experts and regional specialist. They analyse social conditions, organizational structures and political motivations of regional terrorist groups and try to predict potential actions by extrapolating past behaviour into the future. The trouble with this approach is that it cannot predict spontaneous change, the creation of a new, more aggressive group or the acquisition of new, more damaging capabilities. The effect is that this approach is inherently conservative and tends to downplay the likelihood of dramatic events.

The second approach is favoured by security experts and political planners. It calculates the risk of terrorism in terms of the well-known formula according to which the risk is the product of the probability of a terrorist attack and the magnitude of its consequences. The problem with this approach is, as Brian Jenkins said in a Congressional hearing, that it does not provide useful data if the consequences are deemed catastrophic, which is the case if one considers terrorist actions with nuclear, chemical or biological weapons. In such cases, the possible averse effects would "overwhelm" even a very low probability. The effect is, that this approach tends to overstate the actual threat and to dramatize the situation.[22]

This, it seems, is not only a problem of the risk assessment of terrorism, but also of anti-terrorist policy.[23] For if one element of the risk equation tends toward infinity, there is no rational measure to determine the extent of counter-terrorist action. Mary Douglas is right in pointing out that if risk is not only the probability of an event but also the probable magnitude of its outcome, "everything depends on the value that is set on the outcome."[24] And it is interesting to note that this approach, taken to its extreme, does no longer respond to real world phenomena, but increasingly only to its own anxiety.

It is important, therefore, to reconnect the risk analysis of terrorism with terrorism analysis, i.e. to integrate the two approaches previously mentioned. For as long as no balanced methodology for the risk assessment of terrorism exists, threat perception and anti-terrorist policy will continue to waver between neglect and overreaction.

THE VIRTUES OF EPISTEMIC COMMUNITIES

But who is going to do this? I argue that scientists, natural and social, have the duty to be involved in the fight against terrorism by keeping the scientific standards of terrorism research and risk assessment. I am not so naïve as to believe that scientific discussions can solve all problems; and I am also not so naïve as to think that scientists are the better politicians. But I believe in the ability of scientists to further an open and cross-cultural discourse on difficult and politically controversial issues.

This after all is what happened during the Cold War among nuclear physicists, political scientists and military strategists. An "epistemic community" emerged in which concepts, theories and strategies about deterrence, stability, arms-control and disarmament have been developed, first in order to manage and then to overcome the East-West confrontation.[25]

With regard to terrorism, we are just beginning to build such a community. Its purpose is not so much to teach anybody what terrorism is and how it should be assessed or be treated. In short: its purpose is not hegemonic risk communication; but rather to understand different approaches and to engage in an scientific discourse on what terrorism is and how it can best be overcome. The World Federation of Scientists and the International Seminars on Planetary Emergencies are in an exceptional position to lead such an effort. They draw on a global membership and on multidisciplinary expertise. If their efforts are focused on these issues, they can make an important difference in the public discourse on terrorism.

REFERENCES

1. See *Schmid, Alex P./Jongman, Albert J.* 1988: Political Terrorism. A New Guide to Actors, Authors, Concepts, Data Bases, Theories and Literature, Amsterdam, 20.
2. *Laqueur, Walter* 1977: Terrorism, London, 5.
3. See *Laqueur, Walter* 1987: The Age of Terrorism, Boston, MA; *Laqueur, Walter* 1998: Dawn of Armageddorn, New York.
4. See *Fernandesz, Silvia/Nohl, Beatrix* 2001: The Legal Framework to Combat Terrorism, MS.
5. See *United Nations* 2001: International Instruments related to the Prevention and Suppression of International Terrorism, New York.
6. See *Fernandesz/Nohl*, op. cit., 2.
7. *Jenkins, Michael* 2001: Terrorism and Beyond: A 21st Century Perspective, in: Studies in Conflict and Terrorism.
8. COM(2001)521 final. Under Article 11.1 all EU Member States shall take the necessary measure to comply with this Framework Decision by December 31st 2002.
9. *New York Times*, May 30, 2002, Self-Criticism and Risk: may Interests to Please; *New York Times*, June 2, 2002, Wary of Risk, Slow to Adapt, F.B.I. Stumbles in Terror War.
10. SSee Statement by Governor Tom Ridge On the Department of Homeland Security Submitted to the House Select Committee on Homeland Security, July 15, 2002 (http://www.uspolicy.be/Issues/Terrorism/ridge.071502.htm 17/07/2002)
11. See *Carter, Ashton B.* 2001/02: The Architecture of Government in the Face of Terrorism, in: International Security 26: 3, 5-23.
12. See *Perl, Raphael F.* 2001 (updated June 21, 2002): Terrorism, the Future, and U.S. Foreign Policy, Washington, DC.
13. On the nature of "essentially contested concepts" see *Gallie, William B.* 1956: Essentially Contested Concepts, in: Proceedings of the Aristotelian Society, London 56: 167-198; *Connolly, William E.* 1981: The Terms of Political Discourse, Oxford.
14. *New York Times*, May 20, 2002, Cheney Expects More Terror for U.S.
15. See *Communique* 1990: North Atlantic Council Ministerial Communique in: NATO Review 38: 6, 22-24.
16. See *Daase, Christopher* 2002 (forthcoming): Internationale Risikopolitik. Ein Forschungsprogramm für den sicherheitspolitischen Paradigmenwechsel, in:

Daase, Christopher/Feske, Susanne/Peters, Ingo (eds.): Internationale Risikopolitik, Baden-Baden.

17. ibid.
18. Executive Summary of the Report of the Commission to Assess the Ballistic Missile Threat to the United States, July 15, 1998, (http://www.fas.org/irp/threat/bm-threat.htm).
19. *Cirincione, Joseph* 2000: Assessing the Assessment: The 1999 National Intelligence Estimate of the Ballistic Missile Threat, in: The Nonproliferation Review 7: 1.
20. *New York Times*, January 14, 2002, How Politics Helped Redefine Threat (second of two articles by Michael Dobbs).
21. See *Falkenrath, Richard* 2001: Analytic Models and Policy Prescription: Understanding Recent Innovation in U.S. Counterterrorism, in: Studies in Conflict and Terrorism 24: 3, 159-181.
22. *Jenkins, Brian* 1999: Testimony before the Subcomittee on National Security, Veteran Affairs, and International Relations, House Committee on Government Reform, 106th Session of Congress, 20 October 1999.
23. See *Christopher Daase* 2002 (forthcoming), Terrorismus – Der Wandel von einer reaktiven zu einer proaktiven Risikopolitik nach dem 11. September 2001, in: Daase, Christopher/Feske, Susanne/Peters, Ingo (eds.): Internationale Risikopolitik, Baden-Baden.
24. *Douglas, Mary* 1990: Risk as a Forensic Resource, in: Daedalus 119: 4, 1-16, 10.
25. See *Haas, Peter* 1992: Epistemic Communities and International Policy Coordination, in: International Organization 46: 1, 1-35.

EUROPEAN SECURITY: NEW CHALLENGES AND PERSPECTIVES

TATYANA PARKHALINA
Institute of Scientific Information for Social Sciences; Centre for European Security Studies, Moscow, Russia

The terrorist attack against the USA on September the 11th of 2001 had serious consequences for the whole system of international relations, global and European security. Terrorism – as a qualitatively new challenge for global and national security – reveals the necessity to re-estimate numerous categories, criteria and models on which relations among subjects of international system were traditionally based.

While analysing the consequences of the above-mentioned tragedy for the world one should have in mind at least three factors:

First: this challenge in not so new for a number of states, in this connotation what was absolutely new was the scale of the catastrophe and its PR character.

Second: the necessity of revising the whole system of international relations is conditioned not only by the new character of this challenge, but also by the tendencies which developed in the world community during the last decade. Among them: integration and globalisation processes, democratisation (internal and external), dissolving of state frontiers, national self identification, increasing gap (material) between poor and rich societies and states.

Third: the attack was directed not only against the United States, but against the lead of the West which typifies its system of values, power, international influence, level of prosperity – achieved on the basis of those values.

On the whole, the existing system of international relations has survived, but as a result we are witnessing a regrouping of forces, a new configuration: former adversaries became allies and friends (the USA and Russia), former partners became adversaries (Taliban and Pakistan).

What are the consequences of the terrorist attack against the USA for Europe and European security system?

It is worthwhile focusing attention on the fact that terrorism is not a new phenomenon for Europe. Such European states and regions as Great Britain, Spain, Italy, the Balkans, the Northern Caucasus, met this challenge long before 2001 and tried to find responses. The results were different and contradictory. One could come to the conclusion that up to now international and European communities have not managed to find adequate answers to this security risk. Neither individual states, nor the international organisations in Europe were prepared for this type of development, as they were founded at the time of Cold War and the confrontation between the two blocks.

A CHALLENGE FOR NATO

After the end of the Cold War this Euro-Atlantic Organisation tried to find its new identity. The first wave of NATO enlargement or opening to the East as well as crisis-management in the Balkans gave the impression that NATO has found this new role – the role of "peace-maker" and "peace-keeper" in Europe. But the Kosovo crisis proved that the process of decision-making inside the Atlantic Alliance could not give immediate and necessary results in the case of military conflict. NATO acted but at the same time demonstrated its slow character.

After September 11th, NATO for the first time in its history applied Article 5 concerning solidarity and mutual assistance not for the defence of Europe as it was planned at the beginning of 1950s, but for the defence of the United States. But instead of using the armed forces of the NATO states and NATO plans, the USA tried to avoid all those. When the American deputy-defence-minister came to Brussels he declared that the U.S. administration was not interested in the formation of the "coalition of those who are ready to act." He demonstrated that the USA welcomed NATO's initiative of solidarity, but they would like to do this job themselves with a group of their assistants. In the process of homeland defence the USA did not want to be dependent upon the opinion of their allies. Washington only asked them to share secret information, as well as the right to use their air space and military bases.

At the same time, to achieve the goals of anti-terror campaign the USA needed partners. They were chosen in conformity with American national interests: Great Britain – a unique NATO state with compatible (to the USA) military capabilities; Russia whose political support was important for a campaign in Asia; Tadjikistan, Uzbekistan and Turkmenistan, who then gave the U.S. the right to use their air-space and military bases; Pakistan whose territory was absolutely necessary for the transportation of military forces and equipment. It was only a certain time later that the USA accepted limited support from their NATO allies.

There are a number of reasons explaining the relatively small role of NATO in the anti-terror campaign: the most polite interpretation is that after the attack the USA wanted to create the preconditions for the "anti-terror war" as soon as possible. But this is only one part of the truth; another could be explained by the long process of decision-making inside NATO. Having in mind the limited military capabilities of their European allies, the lack of corresponding plans (for the fight against terrorism), eventual "war among NATO committees," the USA decided not to rely on the North-Atlantic Alliance.

The fight against the terrorists of "Al-Qaida" as well as the Kosovo crisis demonstrated one extremely important fact – the nature of military conflicts has changed. In the age of the Cold War military blocks did deter one another by the threat of MAD (mutual assured destruction). Today the challenge to the West is coming from a network of terrorist groupings, the main arms of which are not military, but psychological. Their principle moving force – religious ideology; their nourishing space – failing states of the so-called "third world." The instruments of military deterrence are ineffective against terrorists, who are confirmed in their exclusive mission and ready to die.

After the Kosovo crisis and campaign in Afghanistan, the American estimates of NATO functions have changed: the U.S. political and military establishment does not perceive NATO as a collective defence alliance any more. They see its importance in the political stabilisation of Europe: they perceive it as a certain institution (framework) which could integrate Central and Eastern European states, that is why they support "large" enlargement; a good basis to transform relations with Russia (format –20). One of the main problems of NATO is that the Europeans need it much more than the Americans. The Europeans need it as a collective defence organisation and at the same time as an instrument for the common co-ordination of the transatlantic policy of the member-states.

While analysing the present-day NATO situation, I reached the conclusion that little by little it is being transformed from an organisation for collective defence into an organisation for collective security, a regional organisation that could accomplish crisis-management missions in the future. Another challenge for NATO comes from the second wave of enlargement. If the process of decision-making is not changed, 26 national delegations inside the Alliance could block this process. If NATO does not realise, in the very near future, the necessity of the specialisation of its members' armed forces, it will create a lot of problems (different levels of decision-making, financing, operability etc.).

ALTERNATIVES

The existing situation could spoil transatlantic relations. There are three schools of thought (three concepts) on how to overcome it. The proponents of the first support the europeanisation of the Alliance. They hope that one day the USA will withdraw its military forces from the European continent. In this case NATO could transform into something comparable to the OSCE, and the USA will no longer interfere with the situation in the Balkans. Instead, the Europeans will be responsible for the region within the framework of the European Security and Defence Policy (ESDP). At the same time such a division of labour could entail great risk of further differentiation of security policy on both sides of the Atlantic. One version of this model presupposes more active efforts by the Europeans in the field of security and defence policy based on the prior role of NATO (NATO first). But it is the Atlantic Alliance that should elaborate methods of crisis management in the regions beyond Europe.

Here the basic principle is equal risks and not division of labour between NATO and the EU, as well as integration of the ESDP into internal structures and processes of the Alliance. Common structures for planning and management are absolutely necessary to avoid competition between the two organisations, as well as the compatibility of armed forces and armaments.

From the point of view of those who belong to the second school of thought, the ESDP subordinated to NATO, will not have military instruments that could be used independently from the USA or without special instructions from Washington. If the Europeans have independent military instruments, they could lead discussions with the Americans on an equal basis. Only in this case they will be taken seriously by the USA in military terms. Those who defend this concept are ready to co-ordinate certain positions with NATO, but not ready to refuse a certain level of autonomy.

According to the third approach, NATO has a future only if the Europeans are ready to make more serious efforts – first of all to increase defence expenditure. The proponents of this concept consider it as the most effective instrument to adapt the Alliance to the new developments in the field of security, to make it an effective military body of the transatlantic community capable of responding adequately to new challenges (among them international terrorism and non-proliferation). But the question is: are the European governments and parliaments ready to increase military expenditure?

The Europeans are not interested in distancing themselves from the USA nor in playing the role of "junior partner." Decreasing transatlantic links does not correspond to the political and economic interests of the European states in the world. Bearing in mind the processes of globalisation, it does not correspond to the interests of the USA as they could lose their privileged position in European security system.

To become a respected partner of the United States, the Europeans should reform their socio-economic structures: the economy should again become competitive; the systems of health services and social insurance must be effective and not too expensive; the systems of education should catch up on what they have missed. The Europeans should speed up the reconstruction of their armed forces.

RUSSIA AND THE WEST

Here I would like to share my views on Russian foreign policy since V. Putin came into the Kremlin, as without this connotation it is difficult to understand what really happened after September 11th 2001.

Russia tried to reassert its international profile in several directions:

- undertaking bilateral dialogue with the European States and the EU;
- reviving relations with former Soviet allies;
- promoting Russian arms export;
- abandoning the idea of integration within the CIS in favour of bilateral relations with CIS countries.

Key foreign policy principles determined at that period were:

- pragmatic orientation through its emphasis on economic relations;
- not to define any priorities;
- Russia continued to view itself as a global power with world-wide interests;
- Russia tried to use Russia/West-European relations to influence Russia/U.S. dialogue.

In general, before September 11th, Russia's foreign policy under Putin was characterised by ambivalence:

1. by the desire to reshape relations with the West through engaging in and working within core Western institutions and to divide the USA and Western Europe;
2. by the attempts to ensure foreign policy and foreign economy activities through its participation in international institutions such as WTO, G-7, the OSCE, and at the same time by revising relations with so-called problematic regimes which deny those institutions;
3. inspired by the fact that Russia adapted a number of official concepts concerning foreign policy, there was no clear vision what Russia's place in the world and Europe could be, no clear understanding of who the Russian partners are and who the possible adversaries are. This resulted in reactive answers to certain events and not in shaping a strategy of behaviour on the international arena.

The events of September 11th created fresh opportunities for co-operation between Russia and the West as they provided graphic evidence of common threats and challenges.

Now it is an open secret that just after the tragedy in New York and Washington V. Putin invited 21 politicians to discuss the question of how Russia should behave. One of them recommended supporting Taliban; 18 suggested remaining neutral; only two recommended demonstrating solidarity with the United States and the West. Two hours later V. Putin pronounced his famous speech on Russia TV where he explained why Russia would proclaim its support of the USA and the anti-terrorist coalition.

In this connotation I'd like to focus your attention on two facts: 1) inside Russia there is opposition to the new foreign policy line of President V. Putin. 2) Putin's foreign policy has not yet become Russian foreign policy.

There are three serious gaps:

1. between Putin's foreign policy and Russian bureaucracy
2. between new foreign policy and Russian mentality
3. between new foreign policy and domestic policy.

As a pragmatic political leader V. Putin does realise that relations with Western Europe and with the EU could give Russia guaranties of economic security, relations with the USA – guaranties of military security.

NATO was chosen by V. Putin as a dimension in which he tried to divide the so-called "anti-Russian front" at the beginning of the year 2000 when all the European international institutions (the OSCE, the EU, Council of Europe) were extremely critical of Russia due to the second Chechen war. Then in January 2000 he invited the new

NATO Secretary General, Lord Robertson, to visit Moscow. What was the real reason for this initiative?

- to give an impression in the West that the so-called "new" Kremlin team is ready to reopen the dialogue;
- to try to "substitute" the developments in Chechnya for the situation in Kosovo during the crisis and NATO bombings; it is cynical, but in a sense the second Chechen war helped to restore relations with NATO;
- the Kremlin tried to use NATO in their attempts to change the attitude of the West aiming at future support of Russian policy after the presidential elections.

In November 2001 the initiative of British Prime Minister, Tony Blair, on a new Russia-NATO council (format-20), and its realisation in May 2002 in Rome, when the mechanism of 20 was adapted, opened a "window of opportunity" for Russia and the West to establish a new quality of relations

Positive developments will depend on several factors: on the capacities of both sides to learn how to behave in a new situation, on the political will of top authorities in Russia and in the NATO states to establish real partner relations, on the perspectives of USA-Russia and the EU-Russia dialogues.

SMALL WARS—A CHALLENGE FOR FUTURE SECURITY

WOLFGANG MÜLLER-SEEDORF
Commander German Navy, German Armed Forces Centre for Analyses and Studies, Schaumburgweg 3, 51545 Waldbröl, Germany

INTRODUCTION

I would like to thank the World Federation of Scientists for the invitation to come to Erice. I am delighted to have the opportunity to talk to you. I will speak about "Small Wars – A Challenge for Future Security."

But before I start please allow me to introduce myself because it is the first time that I have come to Erice. I am a German Navy Officer and spent 11 years of my career in submarines. During these 11 years my interest in contemporary history, especially in security policy, increased continuously so that I was very happy to have the opportunity to study security and defence in the UK. After graduation I was appointed to the Center for Analyses and Studies, the German Armed Forces think tank, where I am a member of a research team working on a comprehensive research paper about future global challenges and their consequences.

THE CHANGING NATURE OF WAR

The changing nature of war is one of the manifestations of security trends with significant implications for future politics. Until the end of the Cold War, countries were considered to have the monopoly on war, but since then there has been an increased tendency toward the privatization of war, as we heard from Peter Lock yesterday.

The economic, political, and social developments shown will continue to involve significant displacements in many parts of the world. Hence, the future will see more and more non-state actors such as warlords and terrorists, who want to ensure a share in the satisfaction of material and immaterial needs by force of arms for themselves and their people, and who are not interested in ceasing war. This specific means of satisfying needs will take the place of economic life, which, during conflicts between states, is clearly delimited from war. A large number of future conflicts will no longer see a clear separation between the use of force and business, and the violence specialists' independence from civilized society will disappear.

The features of a new form of using force may be characterized as unconventional, or as 'small wars.' Since the new powers in a future world order will no longer permit wars between states, state and non-state actors will increasingly resort to this new type of violence that threatens international security.

This process is enhanced primarily by scientific-technical advances and their potential for asymmetric warfare. Asymmetric wars will thus become more and more attractive as they can be waged more economically and are characterized by a reduced vulnerability on the part of the aggressor. Exchanging violence for money is becoming increasingly popular and is being encouraged by the formation of networks.

The danger that these networks pose to modern societies, as well as their perceived vulnerability, are of great significance when looking at how borders of countries and empires have changed.

According to Herfried Münkler, a German political scientist, the majority of domestic wars that took place over the past decades were waged along the 'soft' borders of large empires. Today, as a result of globalization and its symptoms, e.g. migration, formerly 'hard' national borders are becoming softer and softer.[1]

It is most likely that – as a result of this process – countries will be increasingly confronted with these new forms of conflict settlement within their national borders. On the one hand, this is due to the fact that these forms of conflict may affect countries across their borders from anywhere in the world, thus influencing national security, and, on the other hand, to the fact that the 'soft' borders will only to a limited extent be able to prevent non-state actors from settling the new forms of conflict even within the countries concerned.

As a result, the boundary line between external and internal security will become blurred.

With no clear boundary line between the use of force and business, the use of force will begin to evolve into a matter of routine. Wherever political structures and local economies decline, or are caused to decline through preceding violent conflicts, war will become the way of life pursued or suffered by people.

For generations, the use of force will become an integral part of social life, and it will be difficult for the fragmented warrior societies to return to an organized civilized society (look at Palestine, Afghanistan or Northern Ireland).

The fact that these societies will be built around a war system *and* a war mentality results in the unification of social space and the battlefield, as well as in the denationalization of war and its consequences for international security.

In the final analysis it can be determined that, in terms of security policy, we now find ourselves in a phase of transformation which is characterized by interdependent security risks. They cannot be managed by military means alone, but only at multinational and inter-ministerial/inter-departmental levels.

A further increase in the democratization of the use of force can be expected, as well as the achievement of technological breakthroughs (new sources of energy, voyages into the solar system and the microcosm) and the worldwide increase in the production of knowledge.

Given these global developments and the increasing networking of all spheres of life, the number of actors who are relevant to security policy and who resort to violence will rise.

THE "SMALL WARS" PHENOMENON

Let us now have a closer look at some aspects of what I today refer to as "small wars."

From recent history we know that the number of wars between states tends to decrease. Domestic wars, i.e. civil wars, account for two thirds of all wars that have been waged since 1945.[2] As I move on with my presentation I will – for the sake of simplicity – now use the term *'small wars'*[3] when talking about those wars that are not waged between states.

I am aware of the fact that the term 'small wars' does not fully take into account the nature of that phenomenon, since 'small wars' are not necessarily smaller than wars on a larger scale – neither in terms of intensity and duration nor in terms of their destructive power nor – referring to our colleague Christopher Daase – in their effects.

Thus, 'small wars' encompasses large-scale violent conflicts lasting for a prolonged period of time and taking place not only between state and non-state actors, but between non-state actors as well.

Waging a war by complying with conventions is a phenomenon typical between states. The 'small war' constitutes the prototype of war, where there are no rules and which inherently attempts to violate existing conventions.

States with unstable structures and with weak, disintegrating, and criminal regimes, as well as the globalization process, have contributed to the fact that more and more non-state actors resorting to organized force are emerging in international relationships. This is what clearly threatens the process of civilizing and pacifying international politics.

Peter Lock in his presentation already emphasized the privatization and economization[4] of war. But this is only the one side of the coin. The other side is the ideologization of war. It is the ideological motives in particular which lend political conflicts an extreme fierceness.

Religion, no matter whether it is the own or an adapted religion, in many cases fulfils a collective identity-building function[5] and manifests in increased self-confidence combined with the urge to either expand to other cultural circles or to clearly dissociate from these. Within the own environment, ideologized religion may appear as the solution to political and social problems in order to push through the own spiritual tendencies in a militant-fundamentalist manner. This will often be effected in conjunction with religion or by the abuse of religion within the framework of power and pressure politics. Recent example was the employment of ideologically disguised 'Warriors of God' of a terror network against the Western World, abusing Islam for their aims.

THE CONSEQUENCES FOR SECURITY POLICY

The consequences of "small wars" change international politics!

The privatization of the use of force because of the eroding governmental exclusive right to use force and the destruction of the peace economy, the fact that the dividing line between war and peace becomes increasingly blurred, the merging of the use of force and business as well as the growing congruence of social space and battlefield are tending to make a clear distinction between combatants and non-combatants impossible.

Regular forces lose their importance; instead, almost all parts of society participate in the use of force, which will penetrate deeper and deeper into the entire societies whereby warfare will become an economic source of income. War will be totalized, war will become a way of life!

Having heard my speech so far, what are now the consequences for security policy? Or, toward what direction do we – we as scientists – have to stimulate the politicians to change their policy?

Precondition for a stable peace economy is a clear separation of war and peace and thus the separation of use of force and business. In view of the denationalization and economization of war the traditional dividing line between external and internal security becomes blurred. It is therefore difficult, for example, to tell whether a breakdown of the information system is caused by a planned attack or only by failure.

While multinationality is nothing new in the field of external security, it certainly is in the field of internal security. National differences in the legislation relevant to internal security as well as different standards, among other things in protection of data privacy, preliminary police investigation, surveillance of suspects and criminal prosecution, impede the fight against criminal organizations and terrorists operating at international level. For this reason, the balanced international cooperation of police, intelligence and secret services is of utmost importance for future preventive security measures.

In future, security cannot be looked at in isolation from the point of view of one ministry only because political, economical and social developments can result in a threat to security. Therefore, security problems should rather be resolved through a holistic approach. This holds true at national level as well as within international bodies.

Today, the responsibility for the resolution of these problems lies with bodies and institutions which for the most part act independently of each other and whose activities have to be coordinated in a new manner. They compete for resources (manpower and funds), but depend on each other during operations.

Against the background of limited resources this means that the maximization of the effect of preventive security systems not only requires unified control during their employment, but ultimately also common planning. In future greater emphasis should be placed on unified coordination and control of the activities of different bodies dependent on each other.

Prevention is generally difficult to calculate since local leaders in conflict areas will not keep quiet, if only because of the fact that otherwise western funds in favor of needy parts of the population and the stabilization of the region would cease to flow. A comprehensive prevention policy at national level is also impossible, as it would always require the consensus of the international community.

To what extent preventive measures of all kinds will be taken depends on the one hand on the own interest in becoming active at all, and on the other hand on whether politicians are able to legitimate their action toward their own public. In doing so, it is certainly not only more promising but also easier to 'sell' a structure-oriented approach with different political measures than to intervene in a purely event-oriented manner mainly with military means.

For the prevention itself, especially for the structure-oriented prevention, much time is necessary, time, which politics often does not have.

Prevention by deterrence can be useful in preventing the creation sanctuaries for terrorists; military intervention for the purpose of preventing or ending severe violations of human rights (for example genocide) is also legitimate in certain cases, but ultimately the approach based on the motto 'Getting into the minds and winning the hearts of the people' appears to be most promising approach in the long term.

This must include, however, the ability to take rapid decisions supported by the international community – an indication of the creative political task waiting to be tackled by the international community in future.

We can conclude that the following consequences *as to security policy* can be drawn:

1. Security risks are interdependent.
2. The dividing line between war and peace will become blurred.
3. Preventive security measures can no longer be accomplished at national level.
4. Preventive security measures require an inter-ministerial approach.
5. Vulnerability of post-modern industrialized states, especially with regard to asymmetric forms of violence, is increasing.

From these changes in the security environment the following consequences can be derived *for the states' executive instruments.*

The executive instruments of the civilized nations will have to contribute, as part of a comprehensive political strategy, to the maintenance and stabilization of an economically, socially and politically dynamic world order. The questions as to whether and how this contribution will be made must principally be reviewed anew. This contribution includes:

- first, and that should have priority, the ability to maintain a world order which allows the development of civilization and
- second, the ability to intervene against developments if they pose a threat to international security.

REFERENCES

1.   Münkler, Herfried. *Krieg und Politik am Beginn des 21. Jahrhunderts.* Opening lecture at the 'Philosophicum Lech'. Berlin, Lech/Germany, 2000 (http://www.philosophicum.com/archiv/Band4.pdf, p. 10.

2.   Imbusch, Peter, *op.cit.*

3.   The term 'small wars' goes back to Carl von Clausewitz. He used this term to distinguish this kind of warfare from the "Great (interstate) Wars". - Synonyms for 'small wars' are 'low-intensity conflicts' (LIC), 'asymmetric warfare,' 'partisan warfare,' 'neo-Hobbes' warfare," 'guerilla warfare,' 'new wars,' 'postmodern wars' and 'degenerated wars.' Christoph Daase. *Kleine Kriege – Große Wirkung. Wie unkonventionelle Kriegführung die internationale Politik verändert (Small Wars – Big Effect. How Unconventional Warfare will Change International Politics).* Baden-Baden/Germany: Nomos-Verlagsgesellschaft, 2000. (Book review by Martin Hoch. Hamburg Institute for Social Research. Insert in Mittelweg 36, Hamburg/Germany: Verlag Hamburger Edition, 1/2001, p. 45) and Kaldor, Mary. *Neue und alte Kriege. Organisierte Gewalt im Zeitalter der Globalisierung.* Frankfurt am Main/Germany: Suhrkamp Verlag, 2000, p. 8f. (English Edition: Kaldor, Mary. *New and Old Wars: Organized Violence in a Global Era.* Cambridge / United Kingdom: Polity, 1999).

4.   Lock, Peter. *Ökonomien des Krieges(Economies of Wars).* Lecture at the Workshop "'Small Wars' – a Challenge for Security Policy." Waldbröl/Germany, 14/15 January 2002.

5.   Mey, Holger. *Deutsche Sicherheitspolitik 2030 (German Security Policy 2030).* Frankfurt am Main, Bonn /Germany: Report-Verlag, 2001, p. 71.

WAR FOR WATER? TRANSBOUNDARY FRESHWATERS: CRISIS AND CONFLICTS IN THE SHORT FUTURE

ANDRÉ BEAUCHAMP
Commission on the Ethics of Science and Technology, Government of Quebec, Quebec, Canada

This communication will be on the present and predictable conflicts related to Fresh Water at the international level. I must apologise, as I am not an expert either in water or in international politics. My main fields are public consultation and participation, conflict resolution mostly relating for environment and environmental ethics.

THE CASE OF THE PROVINCE OF QUEBEC (CANADA)

During the year 1999-2000, I was the President of the Province of Quebec Commission on Water Management. Even if Quebec doesn't have any water shortage, the major public issues of the hearings were:

- Exportation of fresh water and marketing of it on a free market like any other natural resource;
- Privatisation or at least an opening to the private interests in the public services of water;
- Intensification of the use of groundwater by big businesses already controlling international market;
- Water management at the watershed level;
- Trust and mistrust of the population, especially regarding surface waters and health issues;
- Desire for better information and public participation in water management.

The public awareness is very high on themes like "blue gold," free access to the water for the poor and charter of the water. Because water is essential to life for which there is no available substitute, people insist on *precautionary principle* and are very aware of climate change, desertification and aquifer depletion. Because water is so essential to life, they see any possibility of water shortage as a possible source of conflict. Many observers use the term water war, in a metaphoric sense.[1] It is interesting to note that, in French, riverain (riparian) and rival (rival) have the same linguistic root: the Latin word *riva*, shore of a river. A rival, an enemy, is the person who lives on the other side of the river. It can also be the one who lives upstream or downstream. But, in history, we also know that, in quasi desert lands, the wells are the meeting places where people discuss, negotiate and make agreements.

The water crisis can be a source of conflicts and wars, or a source of new international agreements.

WHAT IS THE QUESTION?

First, let us talk about fresh water. Most of the water of the earth is saltwater. Fresh water represents only 2,5% of all the water of the earth, and we think that 99% of this soft water are in the glaciers and in the subsurface waters.[2] On a global scale, there is enough fresh water for human and natural life. But on local scales, it is quite different because water is diversely distributed, due to climate, temperature, rain, drainage and so on.

Jean Margat, a French expert, suggests the notion of 1000^{m3} per person per year with 50 % of the exploitation of the resource to qualify the poverty in water availability. Falkenmark suggests 1700^{m3} per person per year to draw the line between the frontier between stress and comfort.[3] Margat calls scarcity a situation where the availability of water is less than 500^{m3} per person per year, with an exploitation of the resource near to 100%. With these numbers, Margat estimates the future of the humanity as follows:[4]

	1995		2025	
	Number of states	Population 10^6	Number of states	Population 10^6
Poverty	8	72	9	800
Scarcity	15	53	26	345
Total	23	125	35	1145

In less than 25 years, over one billion persons will be in a situation of poverty or of scarcity of water. And what about the quality of the water! These numbers seem to be quite conservative.[5] The situation is the result of different factors. Among those, let us look at: use, pollution and population's growth.

Intensification of the use of the water for different purposes: irrigation for agriculture takes about 70% of the resource with a dramatic expansion since the green revolution; industrial use 22%; municipalities and domestic use 8%. The issue of agriculture is very important because irrigation induces over exploitation of groundwater (including fossil water) resulting in increasing salinity;

Intensification of pollution: in agriculture with pesticides, chemical fertilisers and excess of manure; in cities, because of the lack of municipal waste water management both for domestic and industrial pollution;

The growth of population, mostly in the third world and in developing countries. For instance, there are a million new Egyptians every nine months.[6] The growth of cities in the third world represents a terrific challenge in many countries, as the criteria of modern life for health and comfort require more and more water.

Speaking of a water crisis is not an exaggeration. The presence of the water is not by itself a warranty of prosperity; but absence of it is often an important restraint to development. There is no evidence between water's availability and GNP. But the importance of the symbolic dimension transforms the technical issue in a politic and ethic issue.

WHAT ARE THE SOLUTIONS?

There is not only one solution, but rather a mix of different means in a global approach, including public involvement. The activist environmental movement tries first to fight the commercial trade of water, while the pro-technical party understands the problem more as one of supply.

An in depth analysis is impossible at this time. But we can indicate briefly, a few paths:

1. As for energy, we must develop demand side management, including progressive prices for industrial and agricultural uses. In many cities of the world, progressive prices are also in place for domestic water: in those cases, there is a special problem with the poor, for those who cannot pay, because water is essential to life.

   In agriculture, the hypothesis of drip-irrigation,[7] and the development of new biotechnologies to face dryness and salt seem to bring new hope. In the driest countries, a change of the import-export of crops is also interesting but raises the question of food-security and international confidence.

2. Development of new and cheaper technologies to prevent pollution and to treat waste water; a few breakthroughs are also predictable in municipal sectors to reduce consumption and prevent losses;

3. New management experiences including private and public sectors, with a better involvement of the public;

4. Research of new sources of water including desalinisation of sea water, new exploitation of groundwater including fossil water, transfer of water by containers, balloons, diversion, and so on. In each case, we need a very strict assessment, both economic and ecological. Water is not only a resource. It's a part of life itself. The keyword here is sustainability.

But, there will always be countries unable to satisfy their developing needs because of their insufficiency of water resources. For them, the only solution seems to keep water upstream in another country or to use entirely and intensively the waters flowing on their land, allowing nothing to flow downstream. This is a source of numerous conflicts.

CONFLICTS IN THE USE OF WATERS

There is a possible source of conflict when a watershed or a river basin (river, lake or aquifer) is shared by two or more countries. There are more than 200 international rivers in the world, covering more than one-half of the total land surface.[8] A recent survey indicates that there exist 145 treaties on water, of which 124 concern only two countries and 21 include three or more parties.[9] These treaties focus mostly on hydropower and water supplies, but also industrial uses, navigation, pollution and flood control.

The most difficult conflicts are those with multiple partners and multiple issues, including water quantity and quality and many other issues (politics, history, ideological debates, and strategic considerations). We currently speak about *hot spots* all over the world. The more important of them are surely:

- The Jordan watershed including West Bank Aquifer, concerning Israel, Jordan, Lebanon, Palestine and Syria;
- Euphrates, concerning Turkey upstream, and Iraq and Syria downstream.
- Nile, concerning 10 countries, mostly Egypt but also Sudan, Kenya, Ethiopia and six others.
- Ganges Brahmaputra, affecting especially China, India, and Nepal.
- Indus, affecting Afghanistan, China, India, Pakistan.
- Mekong, affecting six countries, among which China, Thailand and Vietnam.
- Danube affecting 16 countries.[10]

With all these treaties and conventions, with the involvement in Dispute resolution on water related conflicts, a new ethos emerges concerning the rights and the duties of each partner in this type of conflict. The doctrine of absolute sovereignty, which is called Harmon Doctrine, no longer makes sense. Seemingly, the doctrine of historic rights or prior appropriations is not sufficient. We must speak of shared responsibility upstream and downstream, which can mean responsibility to share water, always keeping in mind the risk for the resource itself since water, rivers and watersheds are fragile and related to the equilibrium of all the ecosystem. The idea of a right to the water is vague and general. If you live in a dry country, do you have the right to the same amount of water than those who live in a country with abundant water? There is room for discussion.

It's not surprising that many observers are suggesting a World Chart of Water and a World Court to arbitrate water disputes. Many experiences are emerging, like GWP (Global Water Partnership), Water Supply and Sanitation Collaborative Council, World Water Council, Secrétariat mondial de l'eau, and so on. Military power cannot be sufficient. Will we have time and wisdom enough to find our way without violence? Nothing is sure.

REFERENCES

1.   Cans, Roger, *La bataille de l'eau*, Paris, Le Monde Editions, (1994) 1997. The book descrives mostly the competition between big companies for the taker-over of the market.

2.   Delisle, André, in Institut national de la recherche scientifique, *Symposium sur la gestion de l'eau au Québec*, Québec, 1999, vol. 1, p. 20. See also *National Geographic*, Sept. 2002.

3.   Quoted by de Villiers, Mark, *Water*, Toronto, Stoddart, 2000, p. 54.

4.   Margat, Jean, in Institut national de la recherche scientifique, *Symposium sur la gestion de l'eau au Québec,* Quebec, 1999, vol. 1, p. 35.

5.   The theme of scarcity is already use in the Johannesburg Earth Summit, called Rio + 10.

6.   de Villiers, Mark, 2000, p. 17 and 238-240.

7.   Postel, Sandra, *Pillar of sand*, New-York, London, WW Norton & Co, 1999, p. 171-179.

8.   Beach, H.L. Hammer J., Hewitt , J.J. and alii, *Transboundary Freshwater Dispute Resolution,* Tokyo, New-York, Paris, United Nations University Press, 2000, p. 39.

9.   Beach and Alii, 2000, p. 49.

10. Beach and Alii, 2000, p. 79-130. See also Sironneau, Jacques, *L'eau nouvel enjeu stratégique mondial*, Paris, Économica, 1996.

LIMITATIONS OF INTERNATIONAL TREATIES ON WEAPONS OF MASS DESTRUCTION—ESCAPING THE PRISON OF THE PAST

TERENCE TAYLOR[1]

International Institute for Strategic Studies – U.S., Washington DC, USA

INTRODUCTION

In examining a future arms control and non-proliferation policy agenda an analysis cannot escape the domination of the existing treaties and their regimes. However, the treaties themselves are prisoners, in important respects, of the time in which they were negotiated. A clear understanding of the constraints of this factor is essential for their successful implementation and enhancing international security. Not only will such an understanding help with existing treaties but also with the negotiation of new ones. A failure to appreciate the limits of treaties – in their political, economic, scientific and technical dimensions – can result in less security rather than more. At its extreme the most dangerous aspect is an almost ideological drive to enforce the implementation or negotiation of a treaty without taking full account of these limits. For example, the possibilities for effective verification of compliance with a treaty depend on the scientific and technical nature of the subject of the treaty. It is easier to verify the presence or absence of a missile with clearly defined characteristics, than to monitor a wide range of activities in, for example, the chemical or biotechnology industry.

SECURITY FIRST

At the end of the Cold War it seemed that arms control became an unfashionable phrase. In the perception of some it even acquired pejorative overtones. Books and articles appeared with such titles as "House of Cards – Why Arms Control Must Fail;"[2] or, perhaps with a title more apt for this conference "Arms Control – What Next?"[3] These authors were rightly challenging the conventional wisdom, but unfortunately some of the Cold War era attitude to treaties still prevails. This is particularly true in the sense of seeing treaties as global instruments at the leading edge of arms reduction or elimination detached from the deep-rooted regional security concerns such as those in the Middle East, South Asia and the Korean peninsula. However, seen overall, the second half of the 1990s, despite setbacks, has seen a revival of arms control in some important respects. This is illustrated by such developments as the indefinite extension of the Nuclear Non-Proliferation Treaty (NPT) IN 1995 along with its increase in membership and the entry into force of the Chemical Weapons Convention and its increased number of adherents. There are now 187 States Parties to the NPT; a greater number than any other security treaty. Also, with the nuclear tests in South Asia and the difficulties with North Korea, it is easy to overlook the fact that there are now fewer states with active nuclear weapon programmes than at the start of the decade. South Africa dismantled its nuclear weapons in 1993; Argentina and Brazil ended their nuclear weapons and missile programmes by 1992. Russian nuclear weapons, along with their delivery systems, have been removed from Belarus, Kazakstan and Ukraine. These actions were a direct result of cathartic change in their domestic politics and the international security environment. All these countries are now members of the NPT. When arms control regimes are perceived to have failed it can be the result of a failure to appreciate the limits of treaties and their place in international security policy. Some would see the opening for signature of the Comprehensive Test Ban Treaty (CTB) and the treaty banning anti-personnel land mines as successes – others would point to failure of certain important states not joining these treaties as serious setbacks which undermine the norms set out in these accords.

ARMS CONTROL AND SECURITY POLICY

In analysing future security policy agenda there is a danger of falling into compartmentalised thinking about the treaties. This is particularly true of the nuclear treaties. A sound analysis must encompass legally and politically binding arrangements, non-proliferation and confidence-building measures. These arrangements might be multilateral, bilateral or unilateral. Limits must be set somewhere thus, for the purpose of this analysis. Excluded are policy and plans for war fighting and the destruction of weapons and their production facilities by military action. As always the real world undermines attempts to draw conceptual boundaries in thinking about arms control and security policy. In addition to disarmament or arms limitation by military action and negotiation, there is a third means, which is by imposition. The 1919 Versailles treaty is an early 20th century example. A more recent one is the UN Security Council's mandate for the UN Special Commission (UNSCOM), and its successor organization, the UN Monitoring and Inspection Commission (UNMOVIC), and the International Atomic Energy Agency (IAEA) to dismantle Iraq's weapons of mass destruction and missile programmes. This task is astride the boundary described above. On the one hand the mandate derives from a cease-fire arrangement imposed on a losing side after a war; on the other hand it deals with breaches of arms control treaty obligations to which Iraq is party. However, this does not undermine the utility of a conceptual boundary. On the contrary, it can enhance understanding by making clear the limits of arms control treaties and agreements. It also helps make clear which lessons from Iraq are relevant for arms control and which are not. It is important to take into account activities outside but related to the treaties. For example, the 1994 Framework Agreement involving South Korea, Japan, the European Union and the U.S. is an important part of the process by which North Korea may be brought back into compliance with the NPT. Also, legitimately part of the arms control agenda, is the bilateral leverage exercised by the

U.S. in stemming North Korea's long-range missile programme[4] – which, while its relationship to weapons of mass destruction are obvious, is not an activity directly related to a legally-binding treaty regime. In dealing with these difficult cases, extra-treaty arrangements, perhaps associated with a regional or bilateral agreement, may be more successful than attempting to modify treaties or working solely through the treaty organisations.

THE WEAPONS OF MASS DESTRUCTION TREATIES

To expand on the thought that treaties are prisoners of their time, a brief examination of the three principal weapons of mass destruction treaties (the Biological Weapons Convention (BWC), CWC and the NPT) will serve to illustrate this perspective. The discussion is confined to three aspects: political, economic and technical (or scientific). Before doing so a cautionary reminder is necessary that these weapons treaties deal almost entirely with the supply side of the weapons proliferation problem. They take second place to the resolution of the political, ethnic and social conflicts that give rise to weapons of all kinds.

Nuclear Non-Proliferation Treaty
The implementation of the NPT has a particular political and historical difficulty to overcome in that the treaty recognizes five nuclear weapon states, while all other parties undertake not to develop or acquire nuclear weapons. Many non-nuclear weapon states view this as an inequity and seek to redress this through the NPT provisions and the Statute of the International Atomic Energy Agency (IAEA). The compliance monitoring provisions of the NPT are conducted on behalf of the treaty parties by the IAEA through separate bilateral agreements. At least two-thirds of the IAEA's resources are taken up by activities other than compliance monitoring. There are legitimate reasons for this, which flow from its primary purpose in the original mandate to promote the peaceful uses of nuclear energy through technical cooperation and assistance and advice on safety. The safeguards system focuses on materials accounting and does not have a state-to-state challenge inspection provision. The Director-General initiates all types of inspection activity. This contrasts sharply with the Chemical Weapons Convention (CWC), in which the implementation organization, the Organisation for the Prohibition of Chemical Weapons (OPCW) is devoted solely to the treaty and is under the direct control of the member states. Nearly three-quarters of the personnel of the CWC organization, and two-thirds of its financial resources, are devoted to verification of compliance. While the routine inspection system under the CWC is the most costly element, and has some of the drawbacks of the IAEA system, there is a state-to-state challenge inspection provision, which is a valuable deterrent to would-be violators. These stronger compliance provisions could only be negotiated in the immediate post-Cold War political and security environment. With regard to the economic incentives, these do not lie so much within the NPT but more in the IAEA, which acts an agent for the treaty members in operating the safeguards system, and provides technical cooperation and assistance.

Chemical Weapons Convention

In the case of the CWC negotiated some twenty years after the NPT, it was possible to incorporate an economic element more directly into the treaty. Members of the CWC are precluded from trading with non-members in certain widely traded chemicals listed in schedules that are an integral part of the treaty. There is a strong economic incentive for states to join the CWC in order not to suffer trading disadvantages by being on the outside of the treaty regime. Unlike the nuclear industry the chemical industry is largely in the private sector and in dollar terms vastly greater and, particularly at the low technology end, involves production in a much greater number of countries.

While this factor is an incentive for joining the treaty it also represents a verification challenge. The routine inspection system under the CWC can look at only a small fraction of this industry and unless these inspections are targeted to places of particular concern it does not represent a strong deterrent. The targeted part of the verification system, the short notice inspection provisions, which can be initiated by any member state. Also these inspection provisions are an integral part of the treaty and do not require each member state to sign a separate protocol with the treaty organisation, the Organisation for the Prohibition of Chemical Weapons (OPCW).

Biological Weapons Convention

The Biological Weapons Convention (BWC) is a stark example of a treaty that sets a global norm banning a weapon as a legal arrangement without any verification provisions. After the treaty came into force (in 1975) one of the three depositary powers, the Soviet Union, continued an illegal offensive biological weapons programme, even expanding it in the 1980s with the investment of substantial additional resources. The Soviets exploited developments in biotechnology to gain a technical military advantage that they could not achieve in other strategic military capabilities. The United States and the United Kingdom are engaged with Russia, under a trilateral agreement,[5] in what has become a protracted confidence-building process to gain assurance that this program has ended. This process involved intrusive visits to biological facilities in Russia and, as part of the bargain, reciprocal visits in the United States and the United Kingdom. While the trilateral process is stalled for the time being it represents a method by which investigations can take place using national resources as opposed to an international organisation.

Concerns about non-compliance in Russia and elsewhere have led to efforts to negotiate a verification protocol for the BWC, which has been under consideration by parties to the treaty for the past six years. These efforts were stalled in December 2001 when the U.S. rejected the draft protocol saying that it was not possible to devise a verification system that could be truly effective.[6] There are particular technical challenges in going beyond a confidence-building measure regime to enhance compliance with the BWC. To stand a chance of being an effective deterrent to cheating, a verification regime would have to be even more demanding than that of the CWC, which is generally recognized to represent the limits of what was politically possible in the political and security environment of the early 1990s. A determined violator could hide an offensive programme in a small clandestine facility, or in an otherwise legitimate commercial or academic activity. A routine inspection system would stand little chance of being effective. A challenge inspection system would work only if it were conducted with a strong state-to-state element enabling the use of intelligence resources available from national sources.

The use of intelligence from national sources, as the UNSCOM experience shows, is understandably a particularly sensitive issue in multilateral compliance monitoring activities. Nevertheless, it is an aspect that needs to be dealt with directly and does not apply only in the BWC context. It is hard to see how in the difficult cases where states are determined to avoid their obligations, particularly in areas such as biotechnology that are relatively easy to hide, how multilateral inspection activities can be successful without this kind of assistance. The use of intelligence in multinational verification processes needs to be maintained and careful study is required into how this may be achieved. A dilution of the contribution of intelligence will limit further the role these organisations can play in assuring compliance with treaties. In scientific and economic terms the biotechnology industry has experienced phenomenal growth in the past decade. This rapid growth seems set to continue both in terms of its scientific and technical advances and its diffusion to a larger number of countries around the world. The verification protocol under negotiation in Geneva is in danger of being overtaken by events. The industry has spread well beyond the traditional pharmaceutical industry into agriculture, the food industry and may even enter the information technology sector. Billions of dollars and substantial proprietary stakes are involved. A global verification system, even with very intrusive rights and a very large inspection organization, would face a daunting task.

ENHANCING SECURITY—REGIONAL APPROACHES

It is a much easier task to point to the difficulties in the effective implementation of multinational treaties than propose solutions. Beyond the important role of establishing international legal norms there is a limit to what the treaties and their organisations can do. The parties to a treaty are "bound only by ropes of paper" as a distinguished ambassador to the Conference on Disarmament once said.[7] Treaties depend on a confluence of interest between the member states for their implementation and evolution. It is easier, but still often difficult, to achieve such a confluence at the bilateral or regional levels. The major advantage of a regional approach is that it can take place in the context of a security discussion that deals directly with the security concerns of the states involved. It can also help free the treaties from the political and security constraints of the past. This approach can draw on the existing treaties and establish regional compliance and verification systems that could have more intrusive rights and obligations than a global regime. In particular, regional approaches can more easily accommodate national inspectors as do the U.S.–Russia bilateral nuclear agreements such as the Strategic Arms Reduction Treaty (START) I, the Conventional Armed Forces in Europe (CFE) Treaty and a number of confidence-building measure regimes around the world. Regional arrangements can and should be supported by the appropriate treaty organisation if one exists, as is the case with the NPT and CWC. Technological developments will increasingly favour states playing a role with national surveillance means on a more equal basis than in the past at the regional level. In particular, the enhanced capabilities of remotely piloted vehicles are likely to be more generally available within the next decade. They will provide an overhead surveillance capability on a par (or perhaps better in terms of response time and in certain weather conditions) with that enjoyed by major powers with satellite capabilities.

Regional arrangements can be an integral part of either a regional or sub-regional security agreement or a peace settlement, and are not a new idea. Examples include the Multilateral Force Organisation in the Sinai and, more recently, the arms control arrangements under the 1995 Dayton Agreement for Bosnia. The dismantling of weapons of mass destruction programmes and reductions and limits on deployment of conventional weapons are likely to form part of security agreements for the Middle East (a distant prospect at the moment) and the Korean peninsula, in the event of the unification of the two Koreas. In these situations what would be needed is an oversight organisation or commission that integrates all the disarmament and arms limitation activities. The single-issue organisations (such as the IAEA, OPCW and other bodies that in future may be operating under the BWC and Comprehensive Test Ban Treaty Organisation) should be called upon to support an organisation of this kind as appropriate. Such an organisation could be set up as part of a regional agreement or by the UN Security Council.

In this regard there are a number of valuable lessons, both political and technical, which should not be lost sight of in the fog of current events. One of the many political lessons is that the task of disarming Iraq of all three weapons of mass destruction, and its missile programmes, was dogged by divided responsibilities between the IAEA and UNSCOM. The recent difficulties with Iraq should not obscure the remarkable achievements by UNSCOM and the IAEA in finding and dismantling major portions of Iraq's nuclear, biological and chemical weapons and missile programmes by non-military means – although from time to time being backed by the threat, or use of force. The technical lessons from the experience are many and some have already been taken on board, for example, the improved IAEA safeguards (93+2 agreement) have incorporated environmental monitoring procedures. One of the more challenging lessons for standing organisations to deal with is the wide range of up-to-date scientific and technical capabilities required of inspectors in order to uncover a clandestine programme. Some of UNSCOM's more successful biological weapons inspections, included inspectors with a wide range of disciplines such as civil engineering, veterinary science, chemical engineering, medicine and an explosives expertise. This spread of expertise within a single inspection team was not uncommon. It would be too much for an international organisation to be able to keep such a range of expertise, and for it to be up to date, within its permanent staff. At least arrangements should be made to call on such people when needed. They would have to be designated and declared to the inspecting organisation in advance to make such a system work.

ESCAPING THE PAST

No treaty can escape the prison of the past entirely. Greater empowerment of and investment in treaty organisations will not necessarily improve the implementation of the treaty regimes and enhance the security interests of their members. There are dangers in expecting too much of the global treaties in trying to deal with the more difficult cases at the expense of their vital role in reinforcing global norms. To deal more directly with the interests of member states, and to overcome some of the anachronisms in them, support should be given to processes that deal with the total regional security environment. The existing treaty organisations can have an important role in this regard provided they have sufficient flexibility to inter-operate with the regional arrangements in a coordinated way, particularly if a range of different weapons is involved. An important issue that should not be ducked because of the recent difficulties over UNSCOM and the creation of its successor organisation is the use of information from a variety of sources to support verification and monitoring activities.

Another factor that complicates confidence in the implementation of treaties that are required to monitor the activities of private industry is the nature of transnational research, development, production and trading. This is particularly true of the chemical and biotechnology industry. In the case of the latter, for example, governments are lagging far behind in their regulatory efforts in keeping pace with the rapid scientific advances and their industrial application. It is the advances in the private sector, motivated for sound commercial and medical reasons, which have led to the possibility of improved biological weapons for those whose objectives lead them to misuse these advances for such a purpose. Both the Soviet and the Iraqi biological weapons programmes exploited advances in the private sector to develop their weapons capabilities. The private biotechnology and pharmaceutical industry, which has traditionally resisted international regulation with regard to their activities, needs to be encouraged to take responsibility in helping to manage the risks arising from their activities. A more constructive relationship needs to be developed between government, academia and private business to safeguard the enormous benefits the advances in biotechnology will continue to bring. The traditional pre-globalisation era way of doing business will not advance the cause of enhancing global security.

More attention, however, must be paid to the demand side of the equation than the supply side in the form the availability of the technologies. In analysing the arms control agenda for the future the leading edge of arms elimination and reduction is the resolution of the major political differences in the various regions of the world. The arms are not necessarily the problem but the deadly symptom of the failure to resolve these differences. In policy terms this means that investment in processes that reduce the demand for weapons of mass destruction is likely to bring a higher return than reinforcing global monitoring regimes that deal only with the supply side. Given the nature of the developments in global trading, and the speed at which technology diffuses, the latter investment can bring only a very modest return at best; at worst single minded devotion to this approach can undermine security. The two approaches are complementary and one does not exclude the other. However, pragmatic policies that support the dismantling of weapons of mass destruction, such as the U.S. Cooperative Threat Reduction (CTR) programme with Russia under which many hundreds of nuclear weapons are being dismantled,[8] is a substantial activity that enhances international security. The UK and its European partners have contributed to similar activities in Russia in a modest way with similar activities but substantially more resources could be devoted to this kind of activity by the Europeans to good effect in reducing a major source of proliferation. As far as other parts of the world are concerned, policies that support conflict resolution in the Middle East, the Gulf region, South and East Asia will bring greater dividends in stemming proliferation than modest enhancements to global weapons of mass destruction treaties. The limits of these treaties need to be fully recognised to avoid raising unjustified expectations and creating what could be in effect false security. The idea of living with risk, engaging all the stakeholders, must be inculcated into policy-making instead of the traditional government-centred simplistic risk elimination. The scientific community could make a valuable contribution to more effective policy-making conducting multi-disciplinary research into new methods of risk assessment.

REFERENCES

1. Terence Taylor is President and Executive Director of the International Institute for Strategic Studies – U.S. and Assistant Director of the International Institute for Strategic Studies, London. The views in this paper are entirely his own and do not represent those of the Institute or any other organisation. This paper is based on written testimony given to the Foreign Affairs Committee of the House of Commons, London

2. Colin S. Gray, Cornell University Press, 1992.

3. Lewis A. Dunn, Westview Press, 1993.

4. The U.S. struck a bargain with North Korea by easing sanctions in return for the latter suspending its missile-testing programme.

5. The Trilateral Agreement between Russia, UK and U.S. was signed on 19 September 1992.

6. On 7 December 2001, at the closing session of the 2001 Biological Weapons Convention Review Conference the U.S. rejected the conference chairman's text for a verification protocol and stated that it did not wish to pursue further negotiations with the expert group set up for this purpose.

7. Ambassador Paul O'Sullivan, Australia, at the 1992 session of the Conference on Disarmament, Geneva.

8. The CTR programme was extended for four years by a protocol signed between Russia and the U.S. in June 1999. It also covers the dismantling of chemical weapons.

7. CONFRONTATIONS AND COUNTERMEASURES: PSYCHOLOGY OF TERRORISM

THE PSYCHOLOGY OF TERRORISM: FANATICAL IDENTITIES

GRETTY M. MIRDAL
Department of Psychology, University of Copenhagen, Copenhagen, Denmark

BACKGROUND AND DEFINITIONS

In Hanif Kureishi's novel, *My Son the Fanatic*, one of the main characters is a middle-aged man, Parvez, who was born in Lahore but lived in London all his adult life. Well aware of the problems which the sons of other Muslims encountered in England, Parvez did not want to make the same errors with his own son. He therefore brought his son up as an English child, bought him fashionable suits, good books, computer discs, video tapes, a guitar... only to find out one day that they were no longer father and son:

> In a low and monotonous voice the boy explained that Parvez had not, in fact lived a good life. He had broken countless rules of the Koran, eaten crispy bacon, ordered his wife to cook pork sausages, drank alcohol, gone with women.
>
> The problem is, the boy said, "You are too implicated in Western civilisation."
>
> "Implicated!" Parvez said. "But we live here!"
>
> "The Western materialists hate us," Ali said. "Papa, how can you love something which hates you? My people have taken enough. If the persecution doesn't stop there will be *jihad*. I, and millions of others, will gladly give our lives for the cause."
>
> "What has made you like this?" Parvez asked him, afraid that somehow he was to blame for all this. "Is there a particular event which has influenced you?" (Kureishi 1997: pp. 119-131)

This paper deals with some of the same questions that Parvez asked his son. How and why do people become fanatics and terrorists, and what characterizes those who do? Are they influenced by particular events? Do they have common personality-traits or sociological attributes? Are they mentally unbalanced? Are there typical trajectories leading to membership of a terror organization?

The Psychology of Terrorism (at the Individual Level) Deals with Questions Regarding the Making of a "Terrorist":

- How and why do people become terrorists, and what characterises those who do?
- Do they e.g. have common personality-traits or sociological attributes?
- Are they mentally unbalanced?
- Are there typical trajectories leading to membership of a terror organisation?

"While nothing is easier than to denounce the evildoer, nothing is more difficult than to understand him." (Dostoevsky)

METHODOLOGICAL PROBLEMS IN ANSWERING QUESTIONS ON THE ANTECEDENTS OF TERRORISM

1) Since September 11, a large number of articles and books have been published on the psychology of terrorism, which might give the impression that there is a fair amount of information and knowledge on the topic. Few of these publications are however scientifically based. Until the 11th of September there were very few **databases** on terrorism (e.g., Edward F. Mickolus's and the Rand-St. Andrews University Chronology of International Terrorism) and these were largely incident-oriented. Biographical databases on large numbers of terrorists were not and are still not available, and the small number of profiles that are available are hardly sufficient to qualify as representative for the different types of terrorists in different parts of the world at different historical periods, (see Hudson's report for the Federal Research Division of the Library of Congress, 1999).

2) The second reason for the paucity of scientifically valid answers on the making of a terrorist has to do with the difficulties in defining who is a terrorist. No one is a terrorist in his own eyes. During the Second World War, the men of the Danish Resistance who we now call heroes, were then seen as terrorists by the Germans as well as by the Danish Police forces. They were caught and jailed by their own countrymen. In their own understanding however, they were fighting for their nation. Throughout history groups of people have killed other groups to protect their freedom, or assert a cause, a religion or an ideology. The fact of the matter is that we do not have satisfactory guidelines for classifying persons as terrorists or combatants. Whether they are seen as freedom-fighters or terrorists depends on the eyes of the beholder.

I am not putting this as a political or philosophical question but as a scientific and methodological question. If we want to study the possible personality traits of patients with e.g. asthma, it is obvious that we have to specify our selection criteria in order to differentiate them from a control-group of patients without asthma. It is absurd to postulate that we are studying the psychology of asthma, if our group consists of heterogeneous patients whose illness ranges from a regular cold to lung cancer. What I am saying here is a banality, and yet it is the situation in the literature on terrorist.

Most of the people who have been killed in recent wars have been non-combatants, who were killed by a smaller group of soldiers in uniforms. The armies of the so-called decent, law abiding citizens have thrown toys to children from airplanes, toys that exploded in their hands while they were enthusiastically picking them up from the ground. The rhetorics and metaphors of military powers are surprisingly similar to the ones used by terrorist organizations. We do not have controlled studies. And finally we know from the classical studies on authoritarianism that over 80% of us are willing to carry out appalling things when we are given orders to do so. Who then is a terrorist?

3) It is more feasible to grasp the complexities of these questions in art and literature than it is to investigate them in science. What we are able to study in scientifically acceptable terms is not always emotionally meaningful, and what is psychologically and existentially meaningful is extremely complicated and hard to investigate systematically. The questions go beyond intellectual curiosity and general interest in the acquisition of knowledge. They deserve care and precision because they constitute the basis of prevention programmes and countermeasures to be taken against terrorism.

For all these reasons, I would feel much more comfortable if the title of my talk were: "What we do not know about the psychology of terrorism." It might not be the most glamorous and exciting title, but if our purpose here is to collect information in order to take measures of prevention such as the construction of profiles for identifying terrorists, it seems rather important to start by defining our terms and to get a feeling of what we do not know.

What we do not know about the psychology of terrorism

- The questions which are interesting are inaccessible to scientific investigation
- The "answers" are not scientifically founded
- In any other domain, the present results would not be regarded as valid and reliable

---

PSYCHOLOGICAL THEORIES

Let me rapidly summarize the main lines of psychological theorizing about the antecedents of terrorism. I have grouped these into the following four categories:

The psychological hypotheses on the antecedents of terrorism:

a. frustrating psycho-social conditions
b. severe psychopathology
c. personality disorders: identity problems and self-hatred
d. fanaticism

FRUSTRATION DUE TO MARGINALISATION, POVERTY, UNEMPLOYMENT, AND SOCIAL ALIENATION

One of the oldest and most widespread **sociological** theories on the causes of terrorism is that terrorists come from groups that experience marginalisation, poverty, unemployment, and social alienation. People with such social disadvantages are thought to be at a higher risk for getting generally involved in acts of violence, and by inference in terrorism. Several paths have been thought to lead from social affliction to violence, I will here mention two of them: the **frustration-aggression hypothesis** and **the hypothesis on vulnerability to fanaticism.**

It is fairly well-established that frustration in both humans and animals generally leads to aggression, although it is too simplistic to postulate that frustration always leads to aggression (frustration can for example also provoke stress and depression). And all aggression does obviously not spring from frustration. For a long time, however, the frustration-aggression hypothesis played the most important role in the literature on terrorism and still figures as a major causal factor.

According to Joseph Margolin's (1977:273-4) often cited work, "much terrorist behavior is a response to the frustration of various political, economic, and personal needs or objectives." Others (e.g., Knutson 1981) have also suggested that some people engage in terrorism as a result of feelings of rage and helplessness over the lack of alternatives, e.g. regarding education or social mobility. There is little doubt that young poeple with little education, such as Palestinian youths in the Middle East, or second generation immigrants in the underpriviledged areas of big European cities live in constant frustration at being excluded from the higher status majority groups that surround them, from the realization that they do not share the same opportunities, and from lack of hope of ever improving their living conditions. The higher rates of aggressivity and criminality found among such minority groups compared to the same age groups of the majority could lend support to the frustration-aggression hypothesis.

However many of the persons who have committed acts of violence against civilians in the recent times do not show this kind of profile. Many are well-educated, goal-directed, and not particularly necessarily underpriviledged.

Bin Laden, for example, is definitely not a prototype of an economically disadvantaged person. This of course, does not mean that there have not been other types of frustration in his life, which have led him on the path of terrorism, frustrations of a more psychological rather than sociological character, which leads us to the next category of explanation which is more related to individual characteristics than to social conditions.

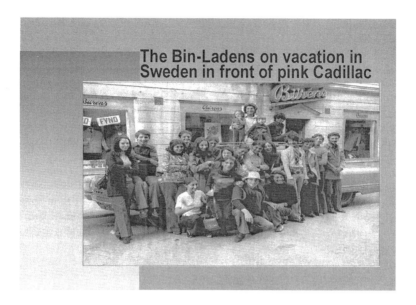

The Bin-Ladens on vacation in Sweden in front of pink Cadillac

PSYCHOPATHOLOGY AND SEVERE MENTAL DISORDERS

It is very understandable that persons who commit acts of extreme abuse and destruction, killings and massacres have been regarded as inhuman, crazy and abnormal. In the early 1970's the American psychologist Berkowitz (1972) described six psychological types who would be most likely to threaten or try to use WMD: paranoids, paranoid schizophrenics, borderline mental defectives, schizophrenic types, passive-aggressive personality types, and sociopath personalities. He considered sociopaths the most likely to use WMD (weapons of mass destruction).

Thirty years later, there is however very little evidence that terrorists are more likely to be psychiatric diagnosis or a personality disorder than non-terrorists from the same background. For example, comparisons of terrorists with non-terrorists brought up in the same neighborhoods show psychopathogy-rates similar and low in both groups, (McCauley, xxxx) Crenshaw (1981) found that "the outstanding common characteristic of terrorists is their normality." C.R. McCauley and M.E. Segal (1987) wrote in a review of the social psychology of terrorist groups that "the best documented generalization is negative; terrorists do not show any striking psychopathology." Maxwell Taylor (1984) found that the notion of mental illness has little utility with respect to most terrorist actions. He pointed out several differences that separate the psychopath from the political terrorist, although the two may not be mutually exclusive. And Heskin (1984) did not find members of the IRA to be emotionally disturbed. It seems clear that terrorists are extremely alienated from society, but alienation does not necessarily mean being mentally ill.

Post's conclusion was likewise (1990) that "most terrorists do not demonstrate serious psychopathology" (Post 1990, p. 31). Taylor and Ethel Quayle (1994:197) concluded similarly that "the active terrorist is not discernibly different in psychological terms from the non-terrorist." In other words, terrorists are recruited from a population that describes most of us. Taylor and Quayle also assert that "in psychological terms, there are no special qualities that characterize the terrorist." Just as there is no necessary reason why people sharing the same career in normal life necessarily have psychological characteristics in common, the fact that terrorists have the same career does not necessarily mean that they have anything in common psychologically." (Hudson 1999).

Finally Nuclear terrorism expert Jessica Stern (1999:77) is of the same opinion. She believes that schizophrenics and sociopaths, for example, may *want* to commit acts of mass destruction, but that they are less likely than others to succeed. Furthermore terrorist organizations will probably be rather reluctant to enroll mentally ill persons in their groups, and it is probable that a certain informal screening already takes place where serious psychopathology is discarded from organized terrorism. Lone bombers or lone gunmen who kill for political causes may indeed suffer from some form of psychopathology. But terrorists in groups, especially groups that can organize successful attacks, are also, according to McCauley (2000?), likely to be within the range of normality.

More recent positions:

- "the outstanding common characteristic of terrorists is their normality." Crenshaw (1981)

- "the best documented generalization is negative; terrorists do not show any striking psychopathology." (McCauley and Segal (1987)

- "most terrorists do not demonstrate serious psychopathology (Post, 1990)"

- "it seems clear that terrorists are extremely alienated from society, but alienation does not necessarily mean being mentally ill." (Hudson,1999)

PERSONALITY DISORDERS: NARCISSISTIC AND BORDERLINE DISORDERS[1]

People drawn to terrorism may, however, have milder forms of psychopathology such as personality disorders or troubles of identity. The problem here is that they are generally identified as terrorists after a longer period of affiliation to a segregated group, and one does not know if the so-called narcissistic traits that can be observed in some terrorists, (for example extreme sensitivity to criticism, lack of solid relations with other people, inability to form intimate bonds, tendency to split the world into black and white, lack of nuance, extreme fluctions of mood, lack of sensitivity to other's needs and feelings, unrealistic self-evaluation and poor reality testing) are the cause or the result of belonging to a fundamentalistic, fanatical or otherwise terroristic organisations.

Characteristics of the borderline/ narcissitic personality:

- instability of mood and self image
- emotional lability
- law frustration tolerance
- feelings of emptiness
- fear of being abandoned, of being alone
- pronounced self-centeredness
- need for constant attention and admiration
- unrealistic evaluation of own abilities

We can again turn to yet another brilliant writer, Dorris Lessing for a description of *A Good Terrorist*. This is in fact the title of her book from 1985. It is a sensitive portrait of a terrorist, where one does not know at the end, whether the main character was drawn into terrorism because of an initial personality disorder, or if she becomes that way because of what happens to her. In the beginning of the story, Alice Mellings is in her mid-thirties, she is an excellent organiser, who knows how to cope with almost

---

1 The term "borderline" derives from older psychoanalytic theory which held that these patients' problems stood on the border between neurosis and psychosis. Borderline and narcissistic personalities are overlapping categories, and will, for practical purposes be used synonymously in this presentation.

anything, except the vacuum in her own life. She lives in a squatters' commune fixing, replacing, cooking, always reliable, giving her time and effort to running the house so that the others are free to take part in the demonstrations that are the motivating force of their lives.

Suddenly, some people in the group appear to have ties to insurgents in Northern Ireland and the Soviets. Alice finds herself at the center of a circle on the verge of collapse, and it falls to her to make decisions that entail a kind of terrorism - political and personal - that she has never really meant to involve herself in, but which, finally, she may be helpless to avoid.

We have living examples of trajectories, where people end up getting involved in terrorist organisations little by little, at times by coincidence, and often without having taken a decision to do so. After September 11th, for example, there were interviews with the mother of one of the apprehended terrorists, Zacharias Moussai on the French television and in the press. Aicha Moussai, originally from Morocco, speaks French fluently and gives the impression of being quite well-integrated in French society. On the wall behind her there was a picture of Zacharias in cape and gown taken at his graduation from a British University with a degree in international economics. "In my son's eyes, I am an infidel, a non-believer," she said.

She was born in Morocco, got married when she was 14, and divorced after 10 years and four children. Zacarias was the youngest and brightest of the four. As a child, he was not remarkable in any way. After elementary school, he wanted to go to highschool, but was directed toward a professional school instead. His mother overheard his teacher say: "That's good enough for an Arab." Later he changed schools, came into contact with a group of juvenile delinquents, dropped out of school. His criminality became more and more serious. He was also impossible at home, and his mother ended up throwing him out of the house. Finally an Islamic organisation took hold of him and redressed him. He went back to school, contacted the family, presenting excuses and asking for his mother's forgiveness. Everyone was elated. This in turn rewarded and reinforced his affiliation to the Islamic brotherhood. But then he became more and more involved, more and more fanatic, which led to new problems between mother and son.

The key words here are "vacuum," lack of purpose, and negative identities. Particularly for people who have few reasons to feel proud and worthwhile, affiliation to a group can feel like a redemption. When people therefore mention narcissistic or borderline personalities (I will use the two terms as synonyms for the present purposes) it is therefore not because these character traits predispose to violence or terrorism, but because they make the person extremely vulnerable to group influences, and what Stephan Zweig has called, "fanatic devotion to a group." This can be a religious, a political or any other type of group. If its leader is fanatic and prone to terroristic activities, narcissistic personalities can then engage in a terroristic carreer.

REFLECTIONS ON FANATICISM

This leads us to the last of the psychological hypotheses on the antecedents on the paths of terrorism. In the original sense of the word a fanatic (from *fanum* meaning a holy site in Latin) is a person who is passionately engaged in a religious cause. His belief dominates all other aspects of life, and signs that contradict it are ignored. Earlier alliances are deserted and feelings of compassion blunted. Individuality is replaced by allegiance to a group of co-believers, and by obedience to its leaders. To a fanatic the world is divided into two categories, those that are with him and those that are against. There are either allies or enemies.

Similarities between Narcissistic and Fanatical

- a common tendency to see the world as black and white
- a common tendency toward narcissistic rage
- "an excess capacity for fanatical devotion" (S. Zweig)

In Freud's words:

"...a religion, even if it calls itself the religion of love, must be hard and unloving to those who do not belong to it. Fundamentally indeed every religion is in this same way a religion of love for all those whom it embraces; while cruelty and intolerance towards those who do not belong to it are natural to every religion." (p. 98)

The most important thing is belonging to a group and togetherness with its members. One seeks affirmation of one's existence in the group:

> ■ *Group narcissism...is extremely important as an element giving satisfaction to the members of the group and particularly to those who have few other reasons to feel proud and worthwhile. Even if one is the most miserable, the poorest, the least respected member of a group, there is compensation for one's miserable condition in feeling "I am a part of the most wonderful group in the world. I, who in reality am a worm, become a giant through belonging to the group." Consequently, the degree of group narcissism is commensurate with the lack of real satisfaction in life. Those social classes which enjoy life more are less fanatical (fanaticism is a characteristic quality of group narcissism) than those which, like the lower middle classes, suffer from scarcity in all material and cultural areas and lead a life of unmitigated boredom. (Erich Fromm)*

For the fanatic, *Cogito ergo sum* ("I think, therefore I am"), is replaced by *Sumus ergo sum* ("We are therefore I am").

From Several Identities to a Single Identity:

* reducing contact with persons of different opinion;
* excluding earlier identifications and identities;
* inability to switch between different identities

It is in this allegiance to the group, also described by the Lebanese-French writer Amin Maalouf in "Identités meurtrières" that we find the spring from fanaticism to terrorism.

CONCLUDING UNSCIENTIFIC POSTSCRIPT

Considering the fact that I started by deploring the fact that we do not have reliable knowledge on the psychology of the making of a terrorist, it would be inappropriate to draw definite conclusions at this point. I shall however, take the liberty of presenting an "unscientific postscript" in guise of a conclusion:

* Terrorists are neither insane, inhuman or abnormal
* Anyone can, under circumstances of extreme fear, stress, and pressure commit acts of terror and violence against defenseless persons

- It is easier to commit acts of terror when one "dehumanizes" the Other
- Humiliation leads to hate and to loss of identity and self-respect
- Humiliation increases thereby the risk for fanaticism and terrorism
- Every time we humiliate another human being, we get closer to becoming a terrorist and to begetting one

THE LIST OF REFERENCES IS AVAILABLE FROM THE AUTHOR

THE PSYCHOLOGY OF TERRORISM

AHMAD KAMAL
Senior Fellow, United Nations Institute of Training and Research, New York, NY, USA

While nothing is easier than to denounce the evil-doer, nothing is more difficult than to understand him. – Dosteyevsky

The events of 11 September 2001 in the United States have focused our minds acutely on terrorism, far more than ever in the past. In a way, this is surprising, as terrorism has been around for hundreds of years, and there are perhaps many other countries and societies that have suffered substantively more from it during the course of their respective histories.

With all the spotlight on the Al Qaeda these days, one has the tendency to ignore the exceptionally long list of organizations that have practiced terrorism over the years. The Zealots go back to the 1st Century, the Hashashin to the 12th Century. In modern times alone there is an extraordinary list, ranging from the FLN in Algeria, the FARC in Colombia, the Aum Shinrikyo in Japan, the Bader Meinhof in Germany, the IRA in Ireland, the Irgun and Stern in Israel, the Mao-Mao in Kenya, the Sandinistas in Nicaragua, the Hizballah and the Hamas in Palestine, the Shining Path in Peru, the ETA in Spain, the LTTE in Sri Lanka, the PKK in Turkey, the Symbionese Liberation Army in the USA, to name just a few from an endless list.

So who are all these "terrorists" and why do they expend so much effort in the implementation of their objectives?

THE DEFINITION

The United Nations has struggled for almost forty years now to agree on some sort of definition of terrorism, and has still not succeeded. The reason is deceptively simple – one man's terrorist is another man's freedom fighter. History is replete with the story of those who were successful in their national liberation struggles, and became heroes in their independence movements. History is equally replete with the story of those who failed, and were labeled as terrorists. It is tempting to see the dividing line not in their actions, but rather in their successes or failures. It would be interesting to see how the "other side" would have labeled George Washington or Charles de Gaulle, had they failed in their respective endeavours.

The State Department of the United States has its own definition, which reads as, "premeditated, politically motivated violence perpetrated against non-combatant targets by sub-national groups or clandestine agents, usually intended to influence an audience." This is obviously a loaded definition. The emphasis on "sub-national groups" is meant to eliminate any application of this definition to excesses by agents of state, whether in uniform or otherwise. This fits in with the current official position under which actions by defense or occupation forces against civilian targets become understandable, but actions by resistance groups against occupation forces are reprehensible.

A third definition is simpler, namely, actions which endanger or kill innocent civilians. However, this immediately becomes applicable to agents of state. Ever so many innocent civilians have been killed in wars in so many countries, either deliberately, or due to the use of indiscriminate tactical weapons like carpet bombs or butterfly mines, etc. In most cases these civilian deaths are euphemistically described afterwards as "collateral damage."

The Non-Aligned Movement examined this issue some years ago, and agreed that terrorist actions by agents of state, or state sponsored terrorism, constituted "the worst form of terrorism." That voice was lost in the wilderness.

THE MOTIVATION

Much thought has been given to the psychology of the terrorist, and to his profile. On the one hand, there was the classification into sick forms of behaviour, that of the psychopath, or the fanatic. Then there was the physiological examination into terrorist behaviour by identifying the absence of chemicals like norepinephrine or acetocholine or some endorphins in their bodies. Then there was the theory that all terrorists were brain-washed ideologically into abnormal and suicidal behaviour, like that of the LTTE, which still holds statistical pride of place among suicide bombers.

Only recently have some explanations gone deeper into motivations. A recent State Department study on the mind-set of terrorists, commissioned after the events of last year, mentions rather casually that terrorists are, (a) unable to achieve goals by conventional means, (b) try to send an ideological message by terrorizing the general public, and (c) target symbolic or representative items in the achievement of that objective.

That is something that Margolin and Knutson had discovered years ago, namely, that much terrorist behavior is a response to the frustration of various political, economic, and personal needs and objectives. This was then amplified further as "rage and helplessness over the lack of alternatives."

What are the reasons for this intensity of rage and helplessness? It is after all highly abnormal for relatively well brought up, well educated, and technically qualified individuals to embark on actions which they know will inevitably culminate in suicide or certain death. What then is the idealism or nationalism that moves them so deeply.

There are peoples who have endured brutal occupation now for three generations or more. There are peoples whose fundamental beliefs are anchored in social democracy, but who are condemned to live in absolute monarchies, frequently bolstered and sustained from abroad. There are peoples whose inherent search for liberty and freedom and self-determination has been stymied by the foreign policy interests of others. There are peoples whose deep desire to participate in their local political processes is drowned by their own petty dictators.

THE RESPONSE

Perhaps we should not be examining the psychology of terrorism at all, but rather the psychology of our own response to this situation. The frustrations of the down-trodden and wretched of this earth are perhaps understandable, but our inability to see the obvious and to empathise with them is not. We have after all turned our face away from some of the most festering denials of human rights for years, if not for centuries. Even the magnificent social revolutions of the 18th Century, with all their brave declarations about the equality of man and the inalienability of their fundamental rights did not prevent the very formulators of these impressive principles from indulging in slavery or colonialism or racism in subsequent decades and centuries.

We have gone even further. Dictatorial regimes have been propped up in many parts of the world against the desires of their own populations, not because of any abiding commitment to these countries, but rather in the advancement of our own foreign policy objectives. We have had the intellectual arrogance to choose and impose leaders on others, and to justify this on the grounds of freedom and security, not their security, but our own. How do we possibly imagine that history will just forget such excesses that are committed in the name of liberty and freedom.

It is absolutely essential for us to realise that most of our policies are perceived elsewhere, either as a mere prolongation of the status-quo in areas where change is necessary, or as a mere prolongation of injustices in different regions, in both cases in the interests of our own security concerns and our foreign policy and economic objectives. The two tectonic forces that have shaped our world over the past thousand years, namely, the progressive spread of democratic thought, and the expansion of economic opportunity as a result of the shrinkage of space, have both created an atmosphere of earnest anticipation, about justice, about opportunity, about development, about social balance. Alas, we have then been found lacking in the implementation of our standards. Our practices fall so short of our precepts. This just cannot endure. Unless we understand that the principles that we have identified and enunciated must be truly and impartially implemented in a global village, the frustrations that we have seen in recent times will only increase. Our feeble attempt to analyse the psychology of others will not help. This is not a North-South divide, or a Clash of Civilisations, or a simple differentiation between "us" and "them." It is basically a divide between "us" and "us," between our own moral principles and our own amoral actions. We have to resolve that dilemma ourselves without pointing fingers at others.

No, it is not the psychology of the terrorist that needs to be examined, but the psychology of our own response to a situation of our own creation. *Honi soit qui mal y pense.*

8. CONFRONTATIONS AND COUNTERMEASURES: DEFENSIVE COUNTERMEASURES

NUCLEAR AND BIOLOGICAL MEGATERRORISM[1]

RICHARD L. GARWIN
Senior Fellow for Science and Technology, Council on Foreign Relations, New York, NY, USA

The loss of 3000 Americans to Al Qaeda terrorism September 11, 2001 brought to many the sudden recognition that America was no longer leading a charmed life. Since then, a great deal of hand wringing and discussion has ensued, but the problem is a serious one and won't go away. Not that it was unrecognized and unpublicized. For instance, in 1999 the Commission chaired by former U.S. senators Gary Hart and Warren Rudman reported:

> "There will...be a greater probability of (catastrophic terrorism) in the next millennium...Future terrorists will probably be even more hierarchically organized, and even better networked than they are today. This diffuse nature will make them more anonymous, yet their ability to coordinate mass effects on a global basis will increase...Terrorism will appeal to many weak states as an attractive option to blunt the influence of major powers...(but) there will be a greater incidence of ad hoc cells and individuals, often moved by religious zeal, seemingly irrational cultist beliefs, or seething resentment...The growing resentment against Western culture and values...is breeding a backlash...Therefore, the United States should assume that it will be a target of terrorist attacks against its homeland using weapons of mass destruction. The United States will be vulnerable to such strikes." — U.S. Commission on National Security/21st Century, *New World Coming: American Security in the 21st Century*, September 1999, p. 48.

The concept of megaterrorism was well known: the warning was there; only the date, place, and nature of the deed were in question to those who had looked at the prospects.

---

[1] This paper is an expanded version of an article to appear in the September 2002 issue of MIT Technology Review, titled *"The Technology of Megaterror."*

NOT TERRORISM, BUT GENOCIDE

It is important to recognize that some of the most important threats do not have the object to instill terror in the population, but simply to destroy vast numbers of people and even their accomplishments. The Nazi campaign of extermination of gypsies, homosexuals, and Jews was not oriented toward terror and publicity, but only on the goal of genocide. As will be seen, the empowerment of the individual by modern technology (which increases lethality and which has increased vulnerability), together with the willingness or the desire to die in the act of destruction, can greatly reduce the effectiveness of some of the most important tools of counter terrorism: post-attack attribution and punishment— e.g., by the promise of reward. Nevertheless, such tools are vitally important in other cases and can serve as an important deterrent to terrorist organizations and acts.

This paper is focused largely on the threat and only secondarily on the potential remedies. And it concentrates on vulnerabilities of U.S. society. But this is only by example; other societies are at least as vulnerable, and may find themselves also the target of terrorism and megaterrorism. Furthermore, the solution to terrorism does not lie in actions by the United States alone. The talents and efforts of many throughout the world can reduce the threat of terrorism. In particular, the World Laboratory may provide a mechanism for initiating such contributions to the good of humanity.

Before concentrating on analysis of terrorism and potential solutions, it is a good idea to introduce and define terrorism and its nature. There are many types of terrorists, many types of victims and targets, and several categories of actions against those targets. Thus we consider *actors, targets,* and *actions.*

First, the actors - humans. A robot, an emplaced explosive, or a trained animal can conduct terrorism, but for the near term we count those as mechanisms and the terrorists themselves as human beings. There can be state-sponsored terrorism, individual terrorists with their own agendas, and a whole range between. State-sponsored terrorism might use individuals of the sponsoring state; it is as likely to depend upon other individuals who act for hire, or who are motivated by similar causes as those that impel the state sponsoring the terrorism.

The individual terrorist, such as Ted Kaczynski, can have a range of grudges ranging from strong feelings against abortion to equally strong feelings against the use of animals in research or commerce, to the preservation of trees, to race hatred, to a grudge against a movie star or a president. Such groups or individuals can be loosely affiliated, or isolated. "Copycat" terrorism can spread from one group to another without direct communication between the groups.

Then there can be terrorist organizations, either sponsored by a state or not, more or less closely organized to carry out a campaign which, if not dictated, is at least outlined from the top.

There are distinctions among actors—emphasized most recently to the American consciousness by the fact that some individuals don't mind or even prize losing their lives in carrying our terrorist acts. This should be no surprise, since suicide bombers in Israel have been doing this for many years. The professional anti-terrorism community for decades observed that not only did terrorists not wish to die, but also they really did not wish to kill very many people. Their purpose was to bring their cause to world attention in a favorable light, and that does not occur by victimizing and killing large numbers of innocent civilians. The terrorists and their cause must appear to be the victims. The professionals were largely correct: for that era.

A hired killer will take a risk of death, but it is a rare one who will commit himself or herself to death for the cause—and then only if the fee for hire goes to the family, for instance. But the Kamikaze pilots of the Zeros in WWII, and suicide bombers in Israel, and the 19 who died (or at least the four who were in charge of the aircraft hijackings on 9/11) show that there is no shortage of people who fit this mold. This is important not only because it shows increased dedication to the cause, but also because it enables means of action that are otherwise outside the capability of many individuals or groups.

Thus, to bring ten kilograms of explosives into a crowded mall and to detonate them at the desired moment where the crowd is most dense while remaining safe, oneself, is more difficult technically than pressing a button to detonate explosives on one's own body.

Now, the targets. If they were governments and government activities, the deed might not be so much terrorism, but, for instance, revolution. An act of one government against another government constitutes an act of war, declared or undeclared. In any case, governments in general have the resources to protect their personnel and facilities better than do corporations and citizens. Attacks on families of government workers, including families of personnel in the armed services are not a direct attack on government facilities or powers. However, they are little different from attacks on the population, selected groups, or on facilities not belonging to the government, so this paper does not discriminate between government facilities and those belonging more generally to the population and infrastructure.

Terrorists may attack infrastructure, such as transportation nodes, water supply facilities, sewage facilities, electrical transmission, and the information or the financial infrastructure. Such would not have large immediate death tolls, but could bring a society to its knees and focus the attention of the population on the immediate problem rather than on economic activity, health, and the survival of the society.

Some terrorist attacks would deny substantial areas to occupancy or even to transit. Among such are the widespread scattering of antipersonnel mines; the dissemination of intense radioactivity; the spreading of anthrax spores or of other durable BW agent. In part, the denial may be self-denial, because the risk of re-occupancy may not be very great. Yet in a society which has felt at peace for a long time, it is difficult to feed into the calculus of everyday life even a small probability of being blown up in the marketplace, or a tiny enhancement in the probability of dying of cancer.

Some terrorist acts, on first thought, would get a substantial amount of moral support from the population attacked. The Internal Revenue Service appears to be a focus of domestic terrorist resentment. But the IRS impacts economic activity a year ahead. An attack on the system by which the government pays its bills would affect commerce and government within days.

At this point, I give my judgments, which are that the world should fear first megaterrorism by biologic agents—smallpox, anthrax, and the like; and next in line is nuclear megaterrorism—either from the clandestine transport of a nuclear weapon stolen in Russia, or from the assembly in the United States of an improvised nuclear device (IND) based on high-enriched uranium. More about this when we get to the "actions."

Not all agree on the importance of megaterrorism, BW or nuclear, or even chemical agents, as compared with small-scale terrorism using explosives, for instance.

One pole of this debate is represented by a particularly well-informed participant:

"The main trend (in international terrorism) is the trend away from state involvement and state sponsorship (compared to) 15 years ago...I believe that the specter of terrorists, especially international terrorists, using chemical, biological, radiological, or nuclear means has...diverted our attention from what...will continue to be the main threat, which is the infliction of loss of life through conventional means...(There were) two attacks on the United States. The one that used box cutters and aircraft hijacking is the one that killed almost 4,000 people; the one that used anthrax spores has so far killed five. We ought to reflect on that; I can assure you the terrorists will reflect on that." — Paul Pillar, National Intelligence Officer for the Near East and South Asia and former Deputy Director for Counter-Terrorism, CIA, *National Journal*, January 28, 2002.

Whatever the purpose of terrorism, terrorists have limited resources. Such limits were clearly not financial in the case of the damage inflicted by the hijacked aircraft 9/11/2001; there are estimates that the overall direct cost of this activity was $65,000. Be that as it may, if terrorists are limited in lives to be expended, the 9/11/01 events provided the grand benefit-cost ratio of 3000/19. This derives from 3000 dead in the terrorist collisions with the two World Trade Towers and the Pentagon, and 19 terrorists who sacrificed themselves in the process, including those on the aircraft which went down in Pennsylvania because of the heroic actions of the passengers and crew. Although these attacks succeeded—according to Bin Laden beyond his wildest expectations—the result is still a benefit-cost ratio of 3000/19, or about 150:1.

From a cold-blooded reckoning of lives taken against terrorist lives lost, this is "only" 150 to 1. However, the impact on American society, economy, and the world was very much larger than would have been the death by accident of 3000 on an ocean liner, which shows that lives lost are far from the only metric on either side.

And so Pillar is right, in part. It is a lot easier to cause deaths of this magnitude by conventional means than by the display of imagination and organization required for the events of 9/11/01. In particular, if terrorists are satisfied with such an exchange ratio, the tried and true means of obtaining it is to bring down aircraft by the use of explosives on board. And if explosives in luggage unaccompanied by the passenger will not do, then an explosive charge secreted on the body (in the shoes!) or in the carry-on luggage of a willing passenger is available. Such passengers would be more likely to fly on heavily laden flights than on the lightly loaded flights of 9/11/01. And the simultaneous destruction of about a dozen U.S. aircraft, planned by Ramsi Ahmed Yousef in 1995, was designed to obtain just this impact. The chill would begin with the air transport system, and have a substantial impact on the economy. But it would not have the impact of the highly visible destruction of the World Trade Center in New York City.

AGENTS

We have already discussed the agent of a hijacked large aircraft, crashing into a building of symbolic significance and/or which houses many people. This is self-induced vulnerability, but one which can hardly be eliminated at this stage of our society, and in any case not without some years of action. But it can be ameliorated: by strengthened and locked cockpit doors on large passenger aircraft, and by greater control over freight aircraft and private aviation.

My fears—megaterrorism by means of BW agents or nuclear weapons—deserve a bit more description.

Biological warfare agents perfected by the major powers in the immediate post-war period include diseases of plants, animals, and humans. They are further divided into diseases that are only *infectious*, and those that are also *communicable*, or *contagious*. A disease such as anthrax will cause disease in its target by infection with the bacterium or virus which is disseminated in the attack. But there will not be significant spread from one victim to another target in the population.

This does not mean, of course, that there is zero probability of contracting anthrax by contact with a person who has the disease. The difference between a contagious disease and one which is infectious, really lies in the magnitude of probability of cross-infection, rather in its existence. If the magnitude is substantially less than one—say, 10% probability of a secondary case—the impact of a BW attack with that agent is little increased by the possibility of transfection.

On the other hand, if each primary victim infects (by contagion) three secondary victims, then each secondary victim might be expected to infect another three, so that after about 14 days the number of primary victims is multiplied by three, then again by three after the next 14 days, and so on.

Depending upon the state of immunity in the society, and the planning and organization for countering such an infection or for public health in general, the initial infection of 100,000 people might lead to infection of many tens of millions, and (with a smallpox fatality rate of 30%) the death of 30 million Americans within four months.

Anthrax was weaponized by the United States and a number of other countries in the years before President Nixon's 1969 Executive Order banned offensive work on biological warfare agents, forbidding the development, stockpiling, and of course the use of such agents. The Biological Weapons Convention of 1972 has been signed by 145 states and ratified by almost all of these. It is, of course, far from perfect protection against the use of BW by a state in violation of its pledge, or by terrorists who have no standing.

Anthrax has, for the weaponeer, the desirable feature that the bacterium forms a *spore*, which is extremely durable not only in storage, but even in the ground for decades. Under appropriate conditions, the spores revert to the *vegetative* state, and the bacteria then multiply rapidly in the host, as is the nature of bacteria.

The five deaths caused by anthrax-bearing letters—probably from a single domestic terrorist incited by 9/11—and a number of illnesses have taught us a lot about inhalation anthrax which we did not know before. Quite apparent, and not surprising, is the fact that the spores may reside for weeks and months in the host, before vegetating—even in the presence of effective antibiotics, which have no effect on spores—and if antibiotics are withdrawn from the healthy person, an ensuing infection is then largely lethal within days, unless promptly treated. The likelihood of prompt treatment has, of course, increased greatly, since a disease almost unknown to the ordinary medical practitioner is now at the top of everybody's alert list.

A U.S. Army publication shows a number of the agents weaponized by the United States or other countries, with their LD-50, and their division between morbidity and mortality-- the causing of illness on the one hand, or death on the other.[2]

Of course, there is some immunity to some of these diseases, but widespread immunity due to smallpox has largely disappeared (especially in the United States) since vaccination stopped in 1972, in the expectation that smallpox would be eliminated in its natural state worldwide by 1980, as was the case. And immunity to smallpox in a well-vaccinated individual is expected to decay after 10 years.

Clearly, if the United States and the world considered it a priority to develop vaccines against all potential BW agents, this would be a useful contribution to the reduction of terrorism.

Some Candidate Remedies

One might counter terrorism by intervening at any point in the chain, Actors-Actions-Targets. Nothing the U.S. government says or does outside the narrow counter-terrorism field will dissuade *all* terrorists; but such government behavior may well reduce the number of *candidate* terrorists by a large factor.

A similar factor is available if access to terrorist targets or to the mechanisms of terrorism is limited to "trusted persons." Such measures have worked effectively (but not perfectly) in the granting of security clearances. More particularly, they have provably worked to secure El Al aircraft against an intense terrorist threat. In 1989, the author had a stressful two-hour interview at Tel Aviv airport with airport security, in part because a sudden change in schedule forced him to buy a one-way ticket to London and to leave his wife in Israel to return separately to New York.

---

[2] Appendix C: BW Agent Characteristics, of USAMRIID's Medical Management of Biological Casualties Handbook, available at http://www.vnh.org/BIOCASU/26.html

The cost of such interviews would be much reduced, and effectiveness increased if they formed part of a database of information on trusted individuals, together with personal history. A person would be trusted for some months or a year after a satisfactory interview, and access (to aircraft, vulnerable and hazardous facilities, working as a truck driver, etc.) would be possible only if the person passed a biometric test (iris scan, fingerprints, or the like) to verify that the person's identity was as claimed, and matches that of a trusted person.

Beyond that, of course, is the necessity to ensure that a trusted person is not acting under coercion, as was the case in some of the truck-bomb attacks in Northern Ireland-- where an ordinary citizen was blackmailed into cooperating by the threat that his family would be murdered if he did not comply.

What to do about Hijacked Passenger Aircraft as Weapons

The instigators of the 9/11 attack knew better than to imagine that they could break into the cockpit and depend upon a threatened commercial pilot to drive the aircraft into its target. Evidently no pilot would do that at the certain cost of his life and those of the entire crew and passengers. To prevent a repetition, all that is necessary is to strengthen the cockpit door. That and the informed determination of cabin crew and passengers using improvised weapons will sufficiently lower the chance of success that such an attempt will rarely succeed. Thus, it will not even be attempted.

But there are other scenarios of aircraft as manned missile. A commercial pilot might kill the co-pilot within the locked cockpit, and this could be done within 30 minutes of a scheduled landing in the area of the desired target. A partial solution is in the trusted person approach, including its extension to foreign pilots entering the United States as well.

Fighter aircraft are unlikely to be able to respond in such a short time to destroy an airliner-become-missile, although one could envisage almost instant warning as an aircraft diverted from its computer-monitored declared flight path-- a system which is long overdue and which would help to improve the capacity of the airways and safety and reliability as well[3].

Freight Aircraft and Private Aviation as Manned Missile

Hundreds of very large aircraft are used in the United States and elsewhere in freight service, where there would be no cabin crew or passengers (or on-board hijackers). With better piloting skills than were shown by the 9/11 hijackers, such an aircraft, fully fueled, could be stolen from an airfield and flown to its target. Evidently there are many opportunities for countering this action. They range from improved "ignition key" locks to an additional device recognizing a secure token carried by the intended pilot, if the device is removed or not satisfied, it would disable a portion of the aircraft essential to takeoff.

---

[3] Boeing "free-flight" approach. Also Air Traffic Control Panel Report of the President's Science Advisory Committee, R.L. Garwin, Chairman (1971).

How to Counter Private Aviation as a Flying Bomb

Light aircraft and their fuel load cannot do damage comparable with that from a half-million pound gross weight airliner. But a large fraction of the light aircraft are capable of carrying half ton of explosives – either dynamite or military explosives or, more likely, the ammonium nitrate used in the Oklahoma City bombing. Many light aircraft take off from fields where there is no full-time human presence. It would be helpful for every takeoff to be registered by telephone or computer first, and then confirmed by radio, including the flight plan and the identity of the pilot. Biometrics in the form of a thumbprint reader in the aircraft would be helpful together with the trusted-person interview of all with a pilot's license in the United States. Such a device and its interface with the radio might sell for $200, including the appropriate encryption/validation mechanism.

Half a ton of explosives detonated against the side of a building might initiate progressive collapse, or it might not. Government buildings of great prestige such as the White House or the Capitol could be protected with very short-range antiaircraft missiles. Nuclear reactors might also be in this category; France has deployed such missiles for the protection of the reprocessing plant at La Hague, in Normandy.

Countering Hijacked 18-Wheelers as Weapons

Bill Wattenburg has proposed and tested a means of preventing the use of a hijacked 18-wheeler as a weapon. The scenario is that a truck driver is accosted and killed as he or she is about to reenter the truck after a rest stop. The hijacker then drives the hazardous cargo (possibly gasoline, but there are much worse) at high speed toward a pre-arranged target. Large trucks are extremely difficult to stop at a road block; Wattenburg's idea instead is to fit each truck with an exposed air-brake hose at the rear, equipped with a cutter than can be activated by a push-bumper now found at the front of many highway patrol cars. Within a minute or so after the act, the truck brakes set, and the truck becomes immobile.

Truck Bombs or Hazardous Cargo Piloted by Terrorist Drivers

In this case, no hijacking is required, since the driver has spent years in training and getting assigned by a transport company to driving a truck. It could be loaded with many tons of explosives by accomplices, or the normal cargo could be explosives, chlorine, or the like. A solution is the trusted-person approach, whereby not only the driving skills but also the background would be determined in an interview and investigation, before the driver's license (biometric-enabled) would be issued. In addition, as will be discussed under "securing targets," only approved combinations of driver, truck, and cargo might be admitted to sensitive areas such as Manhattan. Such an extension of EZ-Pass might be called a SafeTpass and would not slow vehicles so equipped.

What to do about Radiological Terrorism

At a hearing of the Senate Foreign Relations Committee March 6, 2002 Henry Kelly, President of the Federation of the American Scientists, presented extensive testimony on the impact of radiological dispersal devices (RDD). Kelly's testimony was based on a paper by physicists Michael Levi and Rob Nelson, and is available on the Web.[4] RDDs might be used to disperse radioactive material most hazardous if inhaled and deposited in the lung. For this purpose, the particles should be in the range of one to five microns in diameter. In our book we report a hypothetical attack on Munich with one kilogram of plutonium dispersed by high explosives.[5] Assuming a very pessimistic low wind speed so that the cloud remains over the city for 12 hours, the net result is that 120 people would die of cancer after 40 years or so.

Radioactivity is easily detectable in the most minute amounts. The average person every second is host to some 8000 disintegrations of potassium-40, created in the supernovae which produced all of the heavy elements of which we are formed. And this is only 5% of the background to which we are normally subject – from the rocks around us, cosmic rays, and from naturally occurring radon.

The effect of radiation on people is to add to the death rate from cancer. Some 20% of us die of cancer, but only about 0.5% of us from cancers presumably induced by the normal background radiation.

Yet the deposit of radioactive materials sufficient to triple the annual average exposure to an individual, as the result of the Chernobyl disaster of 1986, was sufficient to provoke general evacuation of the population by the Soviet authorities. For a lifetime of exposure in the contaminated area, an additional 1% of the population would die from cancer.

Kelly's testimony included the example of the radioactivity of a single cobalt-60 pencil (or "rod") from a food irradiator, explosively dispersed in lower Manhattan with a wind aligned with the axis of the island. There are many uncertainties in the calculation, including the rate of deposition (fallout) of the finely dispersed material, the depth of penetration into the soil, and the like. The point is that except in the immediate vicinity of the explosion, the populace need take no early action, since a week of exposure would be 250 times less dangerous than the lifetime of exposure (here the lifetime of Cobalt-60: about 5 years) that would lead to the cancer toll indicated. .

A single Co-60 rod or "pencil" contains typically 10,000 curies of radioactivity. The pencil could be stolen, transported in a shield cask of lead or iron, and removed from the shield only shortly before it is to be dispersed. Hundreds of millions of curies (a curie is 37 billion disintegrations per second) of Co-60 have been shipped for use in clinical sterilization machines and food irradiators. The spices in our kitchen cupboards are irradiated before shipment from their origin in India or elsewhere. The actor for many RDDs can be following a script, rather than have thought out the plot himself. The

---

[4] At http://www.fas.org/ssp/docs/kelly_testimony_030602.pdf
[5] "Megawatts and Megatons: A Turning Point in the Nuclear Age?" by R.L. Garwin and G. Charpak (Alfred A. Knopf, October 2001), pp. 341-342.

radioactive material might have been stolen within the country by other members of the cell, or even imported by aircraft or shipping container.

Opportunities for Countering Co-60 Rdds

Of course, protection at the source is highly desirable, and that includes not only food irradiators and the like the world over, but medical radiotherapy devices such as that which in 1987, taken from scrap metal, contaminated much of the town of Goiania, Brazil. The villagers used their fingers to spread the glowing powder on their skin and some ingested it with their food. Fifty-four people were hospitalized; four died; and the cleanup of the town by the International Atomic Energy Authority (IAEA) required the disposition of 4000 tons of contaminated buildings and soil.

There is also the opportunity of interdiction of the material on the way to its dispersal target. Co-60 is widely used also as a high-energy x-ray source for radiographic industrial castings, structures, and the like. The penetrating radiation can be shielded in increasing amounts by increasing thickness of shield, but highly sensitive detectors can detect the specific gamma-ray lines of Co-60 or the other common industrial and medical sources. Such detectors are being deployed in various areas, and are increasingly linked in a network, so that a moving source that does not spend enough time near a single detector can still be reliably detected and identified as it moves through the system. But an effective system of this kind depends upon larger and more widely deployed detectors that are commonly present.

Improved security over intense sources of radioactivity in the health and industrial sector is evidently necessary to counter the threat of terrorism, since the existing measures were directed largely towards safety and not security. Increased costs associated with such protection will in some cases drive the process to replace the radioactive source with a compact electron accelerator, which can pose no threat of use as a radioactive dispersal device.

Bioterrorism

My chief concern is not with 10,000 anthrax letters, or even the equivalent of 100,000 distributed in a fashion conducive to inhalation anthrax: 80% fatal if untreated. I am concerned about the use of biological agents that are contagious as well as infectious.

Smallpox will make the point. The world has a lot of experience with smallpox, which by foresight and aggressive action on the part of the World Health Organization was rendered extinct in 1980, since it has no host other than human. Two stocks of smallpox virus were officially maintained—one in the United States and one now in Russia—but testimony from one of the workers in the Russian BW program attests to the fact that the Soviet Union had weaponized smallpox. Numerous ballistic missile warheads filled with BW agents were reportedly deployed, as was discovered in 1991 to have been the case with Iraq. But here we are concerned not with these BW agents in wartime, but its use by terrorists.

Some of the Soviet military BW agents may have been stolen or diverted; the U.S. has never had access to these former military BW installations in Russia. It is also likely that some individual researchers whether in military or civil programs did not destroy their stocks of smallpox virus when their nation signed the Biological Warfare Convention of 1972, but kept some for a rainy day: perhaps without any malevolent intent. Some of these stocks may have fallen into the hands of terrorist groups; stored, they could be multiplied by the same techniques used to grow viruses for human or animal vaccines, and could be available for widespread dispersion by nebulizer from a moving car or truck. The BW agent is difficult to detect in a sealed container, even in amounts of 100 lbs. or so.

At the time vaccination was abandoned in the United States in 1972, I argued strongly in the President's Science Advisory Committee that because of the coming extinction of smallpox, society would be too vulnerable to intentional attack, and that vaccination should be continued, despite the two or three people per year who might die from the continued vaccination program. The U.S. now has 15 million standard doses of smallpox vaccine, but recent experiments have shown that the vaccine is effective in doses five times as dilute. And a further economy may be achieved by a bifurcated needle, which holds the liquid, rather than relying on liquid which has been applied to the skin. If exposure is known to have taken place, the vaccine is apparently still effective if given within the next four days. In late March, 2002, it was revealed that some 85 million additional doses of smallpox vaccine exist in the United States; these also can be extended by dilution, so that there is now more than enough for every U.S. resident, even without the new-production vaccine planned for availability in 2003.

But there are many potential BW agents, such as that of glanders (Burkholderia mallei), for which there is no vaccine. They might be disseminated within a large building, and distributed by the circulating air in the HVAC (heating, ventilating, and air conditioning) system, or outdoors, to expose a whole city. It is of interest that a person within a building without filters will receive the same dose of BW or CW agent as a person outside directly exposed to the passing cloud. If the windows are open, this is not surprising, but even if the windows are closed so that there is a typical exchange of air only every 30 minutes, the slow influx of BW or CW agent is matched by the slow efflux, so that the integrated dose is the same. This is strictly true only if the deposition time of the BW or CW agent is very long.

The situation is different if there are in place effective filters against BW. High efficiency particulate air filters (HEPA) are available with face velocities (air flow per unit area) identical with that of normal air filters used in circulating systems (500 ft—170 meters—per minute) and a pressure drop which is the same as that of a normal filter partially loaded with dirt. HEPA filters trap 99.97% of particles larger than 0.3 microns in diameter—compared with an anthrax bacillus of perhaps one micron diameter by three microns in length.

Although the smallpox virus is much smaller (as is the toxin of botulinum), such tiny particles agglomerate, attach to dust or droplets, and may also be effectively filtered by HEPA. More research is necessary to determine the practical effectiveness of these widely available filters. An example is a normal home with a blower circulating air at 2000 cfm (cubic feet per minute) and occupied by several people, each breathing at a resting ventilation rate of 8 liters per minute or 0.3 cfm. A particle infiltrating the home through a crack in the door is 6000 times more likely to be caught in the filter than in a particular person's lungs. But the person's exposure is not reduced by a factor 6000 because of the circulating system. In a normal home of 2000 sq ft and volume of 16,000 cubic ft, the circulating air changes every eight minutes, while air exchange with the outside occurs on the average every 30 minutes. Thus particles which infiltrate are in the air for about 8/30 as long as if there were no circulation or filtering. The improvement in indoor air quality due to filtering circulating air in this case is a modest factor four, and that is the factor by which exposure to the BW agent will be reduced.

Positive Pressure Collective Protection
But if the living space is maintained at positive pressure so that any leakage of air through the cracks of the enclosure is out instead of in, HEPA-filtration of this "makeup air"—that required to maintain the necessary pressure against infiltration—can reduce the exposure by a factor thousand or more. The required pressure is just the "stagnation pressure" at the wind speed V—$0.5\rho V^2$. For a brisk wind of 20 miles per hour, this amounts to about to a pressure of 0.2 iwg in practical units (inches of water–gauge), or about 0.5 millibar. It is also relevant that this is about 1.1 lbs per sq ft (psf), so that the force on an exterior door is about 20 lbs.

Such positive pressure with filtered makeup air can be readily applied under certain circumstances to office suites. It is more complicated with a centralized building HVAC system and implementing it would require professional advice.

In a home, special attention must be paid to vents from furnaces and water heaters, although such appliances can experience similar circumstances if a door is left open on the upwind side of the house in a strong breeze.

In any case, I strongly advocate positive-pressure collective protection. Of course, this does nothing for people who are outside during the typical 20 minutes or so of cloud passage, but most people are inside. And it is entirely possible to provide collective protection with positive-pressure filtered air in public transport or even private automobiles.

BW agents act as individual microbes, despite the widespread confusion about a "5000-spore lethal dose" for anthrax. This simply means that a single anthrax spore residing in the lung has about 1/5000 probability of causing death, if untreated.

So if air filtration reduces the dose to the average person by a factor 100, and if the BW agent was efficiently distributed so that unprotected people received no more than the average lethal dose, the number of people dying would be reduced by a factor 100.

A citizen (or especially a politician) might say that 1/300 chance of dying in a BW attack is too great a risk, but from the point of view of protecting people, 0.3% instead of 30% is a tremendous factor. If instead of one million deaths one has ten thousand—99% protection—this is the difference between life and death for 990,000 people.

The search for perfection often stands in the way of tremendous benefit.

Vaccines against BW

Before the AIDS epidemic and the resurgence of tuberculosis, it was a common expectation that humanity was well on the way to vanquishing infectious diseases. In reality, microbes readily acquire resistance to antibiotics and in this sense do learn to fight back.

Vaccines can be very effective against infection, although to prevent epidemics and in favorable cases to bring about extinction of the microbe, it is only required to reduce the transfectivity below one on the average. If it were taken as three for smallpox, as in the previous example, then a vaccine that was 80% effective would do the job. Greater effectiveness is sought against BW agents, but in reality modest effectiveness can make all the difference.

But vaccines may not be effective against different strains of the same microbe, as is universally recognized with influenza. Each year brings the need for a different vaccine, because of the rapid mutation of the influenza virus, and the peculiarities of its transfection and modification in passing from bird to pig to human.

In addition to vaccines, there is the prospect of antibiotics to interfere with the growth of pathogenic organisms, or even antitoxins to counter the specific mechanism by which anthrax, for instance, or botulinum toxin claims its victims. Apparently anthrax produces three proteins which, together account for the virulence of the disease. These proteins are very specific, and with modern techniques it may be possible to block their action and thus convert anthrax to a nuisance rather than a highly dangerous infectious agent.

Terrorist Nuclear Explosives

A terrorist nuclear explosive would devastate a city, whether detonated in the hold of a ship in harbor, in a cargo container, in a cellar, or in an apartment. The essential ingredient for a nuclear explosive is fissile material: highly enriched uranium (HEU) or plutonium. Although the yield of the uranium bomb that devastated Hiroshima was 13 kilotons (13,000 tons of TNT equivalent), and the plutonium bomb which destroyed Nagasaki yielded 20 kilotons, nominal U.S. and Russian strategic weapons now are in the range of 150 kt. A recent report details the damage of what we expected from explosions of 1, 10, and 100 kt at ground level in a city. The Table taken from NCRP shows the approximate radii to which the quality or destruction extends, for the 1 kt and 10 kt yields.[6]

Consider a 1-kt explosion. This might occur from a gun-type device with less material than was used at Hiroshima, or a plutonium implosion-type device made from reactor-grade plutonium and yielding only a "fizzle" because of a large neutron background from the reactor-grade plutonium. On the other hand, the plutonium device might yield 10 kt, so both are shown in Table 1.

---

[6] Extracted from "Management of Terrorist Events Involving Radioactive Material," Table 3.7 on p. 23 of NCRP Report no. 138 of 10/24/01, Recommendations of the National Council on Radiation Protection and Measurements, 7910 Woodmont Avenue, Bethesda, MD 20814-3095.

Table 1. Summary of ranges for significant effects (in meters).

Yield (kt)	(a)*	(b)*	(c)*	(d)*
1	275	610	790	5500
10	590	1800	1200	9600

a* Range for 50% mortality from air blast (m)
b* Range for 50% mortality from thermal burns (m)
c* Range for 4 Gy initial nuclear radiation (m)
d* Range for 4 Gy fallout in first hour after blast (m)

Considering the numbers for 1 kt, we see that people out to 275 m (900 feet) are likely to die from the blast. We can transform the first three columns into the number of Manhattan city blocks which would be destroyed, simply by equating the area within the circle of 50% effect to a number of city blocks.[7]

The conversion was made by noting that Central Park is 836 acres, and there are 247 acres in a sq km. Thus Central Park is 3.38 sq km. Extending from 59th St. to 110th St., it is 51 blocks north-south and three large blocks east-west. Thus it has 153 large Manhattan blocks. There are thus 45 Manhattan blocks per sq km.

The city blocks destroyed by air blast (50% mortality in the "cookie cutter" approximation - 100% lethality out to the 50% line, and 0% mortality beyond that): 11.

City blocks in which almost everyone would die from thermal burns: 53.

City blocks in which people would get a lethal dose of prompt nuclear radiation: 88.

For the 10 kt explosive, the results are 49, 457, and 203 city blocks.

To convert these areal measures into fatalities, we might take a particularly high local daytime Manhattan population density of 125,000 per sq km or an average of about 2360 people per Manhattan block. So for the 1-kt explosion, some 210,000 people would die-- mostly from prompt radiation within a week or so. Of these, 30,000 would have died from blast earlier, and about 100,000 from burns.

For the 10-kt explosion, about a million people will die from burns. Less than half of these would have died from radiation exposure.

As for fallout, the Table is to some extent misleading, since this provides the distance at which lethal fallout within one hour might be deposited, but it is not a circle of that radius. From the 1977 "Effects of Nuclear Weapons," Table 9.93 (p. 4.30) we see that for a reference dose rate (i.e., for a 1 kiloton explosion) of 3 Sv per hour (300 rads/hr), the downwind distance would be 4.5 miles, and the width about 0.15 miles, for a region affected on the order of 0.7 square miles or 1.5 square kilometers, or 80 Manhattan blocks. So the fallout, although lethal, would not totally dominate the casualties from a nuclear explosion.

Compared with an air burst of a large nuclear weapon at an altitude designed to maximize the blast damage, the prompt radiation and the fallout are far worse with a terrorist explosion. This comes about because the bomb detonated at or near surface of

---

[7] In the "cookie cutter" approximation, assuming that damage beyond the 50% damage expectation contour is equal to the less than total damage within that contour.

the Earth throws up an enormous amount of earth and vaporized structure, which descends in the immediate neighborhood, providing lethal fallout, which is essentially absent when the fireball does not touch the ground.

If it were known that a nuclear explosion was to take place, evacuation would be highly desirable. And as in the case of potential reactor accidents (with or without terrorist involvement) it would be very useful to have distributed and ready for use potassium iodide (KI) tablets or capsules. A 130-mg dose would block the uptake of radioactive iodine to a young thyroid (or to a nursing mother), and avoid many thyroid cancers which would destroy the thyroid and might be lethal.

Of course, hospitals would be overwhelmed with the number of people actually injured by flying glass, suffering from radiation exposure, and the like. Furthermore, transit in the city would be disorganized in the regions effected. With buildings down over a square kilometer or so, as was evident in the case of the World Trade Center collapse covering 1% of that area, severe damage to the communications and transportation infrastructure would be expected.

Organized medicine would be unable to cope. A volunteer emergency medical corps, with adequate planning and practice, could save some people who would otherwise die.

Nevertheless, a terrorist nuclear explosion would explode in one place, or a very few, compared with the nuclear attack which we feared for many years and decades from the Soviet Union. So other localities could send personnel and supplies and be a destination for evacuation from contaminated areas.

Public safety personnel would need to use radiation detectors to determine places which posed no continuing radiological problem; regions in which people could not stay for even an hour or five hours without a high likelihood of dying within weeks from radiation damage; and regions in which radioactivity was clearly evident, but which would add perhaps only 1% to the 20% of American citizens who ultimately die of cancer instead of from some other disease.

The effects of a nuclear detonation in a city are so horrendous that it is clear that most effort should be placed on preventing access by terrorists to nuclear materials or weapons; to interdicting the transportation of weapons or the building of improvised nuclear devices; and to keeping them out of areas of large population density.[8]

Unlike the case of large-scale nuclear war, a single terrorist nuclear explosion would not eliminate the resources of the rest of the country, so healthy survivors could be accommodated elsewhere. Those in the regions subject to substantial fallout could receive expedient medical care, but little can be done for those exposed above the levels shown in the table. Unlike BW attack, a nuclear explosion is evidently far better prevented than treated.

Stolen or diverted military nuclear weapons are rugged, but they are usually provided with substantial protection against unauthorized detonation, so considerable

---

[8] A set of pages portraying the course of a terrorist nuclear explosion in New York: http://www.atomicarchive.com/Example/ExampleStart.shtml

skill might be required to employ one. On the other hand, an improvised nuclear device (IND) would not have this problem, but can be difficult to carry off. The fissile material is not an article of commerce and itself would have to be stolen or diverted. The first plutonium bomb incorporated 6 kg of weapon-grade plutonium, of which more than 250 tons has now been made worldwide—enough for 40,000 such crude weapons. Almost all were produced by the United States and the Soviet Union.

In addition, every large nuclear power reactor produces annually on the order of 200 kg of plutonium, which is not and need not be weapon grade to make an improvised nuclear device. In January 1997, the U.S. Department of Energy stated of reactor-grade plutonium, "Proliferating states using designs of intermediate sophistication could produce weapons with assured yields substantially higher than the kiloton-range possible with a simple, first-generation nuclear device."

At the March 6, 2002 hearing of the Senate Foreign Relations Committee, Senator Joseph Biden quoted former Los Alamos National Laboratory Director Harold M. Agnew to the effect that "If somebody tells you that making a plutonium implosion weapon is easy, he is wrong. And if somebody tells you that making an improved nuclear device with highly enriched uranium is difficult, he is even more wrong." Plutonium metal can be safely accumulated in spherical form up to the so-called "critical mass" of 10 kg for weapon-grade plutonium or 13 kg for reactor-grade plutonium. The analogous critical mass for 94% U-235 is 52 kg, and these numbers set the scale for the amount of fissile material required for a nuclear weapon.

Instead of being assembled by high explosive as in the plutonium bomb (which can also be used for assembly of a uranium core) the Hiroshima bomb was two solid masses of highly enriched uranium metal, one of which was propelled in a shortened, converted naval gun to form more than a critical mass with the stationary uranium metal. Although less efficient, this is far simpler than is the plutonium IND.

With the enriched-uranium gun-type weapon, there is an additional means of preventing significant nuclear energy release. Guns are exquisitely sensitive to the presence of neutrons—a relatively few neutrons will guarantee that only a very small amount of fission energy is released. This is evident from the prompt criticality accidents at Los Alamos, which killed people in the room by acute radiation sickness over a period of weeks, but did not even disrupt the fissile assembly. It is possible with a neutron source of one kind or another to flood the uranium remotely with neutrons at such a rate that, even if the smokeless powder is fired to assemble the uranium, no significant yield will result.

The best single protection against the terrorist use of such weapons is to deny the acquisition of the necessary plutonium or enriched uranium. The low-enriched uranium used in U.S. nuclear reactors (typically 4.4% U-235) can in no way be used directly to make a nuclear explosive. That is true up to about 20%, for which the critical mass is 800 kg. HEU is used not only in nuclear weaponry, but in some research reactors and in fuel for naval reactors, such as propel our aircraft carriers and many of our submarines. Likewise, Russian nuclear-propelled ships use HEU. And in Russia particularly, stocks of HEU and plutonium (even weapon plutonium) do not have nearly the security provided to their nuclear weaponry.

After some months of denigrating U.S. programs which have existed since 1994 to help Russia protect weapon-usable materials, the Bush Administration in December 2001 recognized the seriousness of this problem and that something can be done to solve it, and has increased the budget for such Cooperative Threat Reduction activities.

The U.S. is buying 500 tons of HEU (diluted in Russia to LEU to fuel U.S. reactors) over 20 years, at a cost of about $12 billion. Here is a threat which will persist for mush longer than necessary. It would be a simple matter for the United States and/or the international community to advance Russia the much smaller amount of money required to blend down the remaining 370 tons (and perhaps another 700 tons of HEU not included in this deal) to 19.9% U-235, thus essentially unusable for nuclear weaponry. This could be done quite readily in about two years, and the money would be repaid by Russia with or without interest at the same time this 19.9% materials (remaining in Russia) was later further blended to the 4% range for transfer to the United States. These funds should come from the G-7.

Weapon-usable materials might be detected in transit. Normal uranium metal is detectable primarily because of gamma rays of near 1 MeV energy, although relatively few are emitted, since the half-life of U-238 is 4.5 billion years. U-235 has a shorter half-life (700 million years) but its decay scheme is far more difficult to detect.

The intense radioactivity of plutonium is largely alpha-particle emission in its decay to U-235. The half-life of 24,000 years means that 6 kg of Pu is about 500 curies. Pu is a serious hazard if inhaled, but has very little external radiation. Nevertheless, appropriate counters detect it at a considerable distance, although it is easier to shield than is U-238.

Weapon uranium is only very weakly radioactive, with U-235 having a half-life 30,000 times that of plutonium.

There have been many hoaxes in the United States, mostly extortionists demanding money in order not to detonate a nuclear weapon they say is ready to explode someplace in Boston, New York, or elsewhere.[9] To find such emplaced explosives and to disable them, the government created the Nuclear Emergency Search Team (NEST) which now has the ability to deploy about 600 people with appropriate detection and disabling devices.

But a terrorist with a mission actually to kill people would certainly not alert the authorities to the existence of a nuclear explosive. It would need to be detected either following intelligence tips, or by generalized search, or in transit to its emplacement.

This is a tall order for NEST, even granting substantial improvement in their capabilities.

---

[9] "Defusing Nuclear Terror," Bulletin of the Atomic Scientists, March/April 2002, pp. 39-43.

SUMMARY

In looking at a particular terrorist act as involving an actor, an action, and a target, we find that different acts may be impeded in a variety of ways. But there is some generality to the solutions that will reduce terrorism, even though it will not be possible to eliminate it. The U.S. and other states should act to:

1. Directly and indirectly minimize the number of people who wish to become terrorists against us.
2. Move against the actions and to harden targets so that the actor needs more training to carry out the deed.
3. Introduce trusted-person databases and a biometric-based personal identification to reduce the access of un-vetted persons to hazardous areas or hazardous tools.
4. Modify aircraft standards (strengthen cockpit doors) against hijacking; harden freight and private aircraft against unauthorized use.
5. In the bioterrorism area, urgently expand development and production of vaccines, not only in the most highly industrialized states but also in India, for example.
6. Develop and implement in the government and civil economy, collective protection by positive-pressure filtered air and filtered circulating air (and masks where desired). Reduction by a factor hundred or even 20 of deaths due to bioterrorism is a worthy goal.
7. Improve security over radioactive sources to reduce the threat of radiological dispersal devices (terrorism by contamination with radioactivity). The cost of adequate security will encourage the substitution of radioactive sources by electron-beam accelerators.
8. Have contingency plans and public education so that people will not move precipitously and dangerously when there would be no significant hazard in remaining in place and living a normal life for a week or more.
9. Replace absolute limits for radiation protection by a market-based approach, in which, for instance, full disclosure and inspection would quantify the increased cancer hazard for a particular home in a contaminated area, and it could be transferred at a market price to people who would on the average be older and have fewer children. Recall that 20% of us will die from cancer. Life is too short for the individual to worry about an additional 1% probability in the remote case of terrorist attack, although it is an important topic in public health.

These partial remedies are not now available, and they will not exist unless the United States creates a technical organization responsible for evaluating the terrorist threat, identifying potential remedies, and evaluating capabilities at any time. This needs to be done with wartime urgency, the same urgency that drove the creation during World War II of the radar lab at MIT and the Manhattan Project for the development of the nuclear weapon. Sections of a small number of existing government or national laboratories might initially be put under the firm control of a homeland-defense analogue of J. Robert Oppenheimer—a person with technical leadership and total dedication to the cause of reducing the vulnerability of society.

A homeland security institute is one of the major recommendations of a recent report.[10] I was a member of the authoring committee and of its panel on nuclear and radiological issues. The United States is creating a Department of Homeland Security; if headed by a 21st century counterpart to General Leslie R. Groves of Manhattan Project fame, it could in principle realize some of the near-term remedies advocated here. It could also mount a longer-term program of research and development to reduce the likelihood of catastrophic terrorism and—in the case of bioweapons and radiological dispersal devices—to reduce the economic and human costs in the event of actual attack. The solution is not in more organization but in ensuring that competent people can do their jobs.

The peril is global; and so should be the response. Vaccine development can proceed in India as well as in the United States. Advances in techniques for cleanup of radioactive contamination can proceed worldwide. Intense sources of radioactivity are present in many countries; an effort led by the IAEA could improve their security against theft. If the resources of the world are to be marshalled for the benefit of humanity, they should not be diverted unnecessarily to countering terrorism. Hence the need for collaboration and efficiency in solving this new and urgent problem.

---

[10] "Making the Nation Safer: The Role of Science and Technology in Countering Terrorism" The National Academies Press, Washington, DC, June 25, 2002. (Available at http://www.nap.edu).

HAS AIR POWER COME OF AGE?

DONALD A. YERXA
The Historical Society, Boston, Massachusetts, USA

Precision weapons, stealth technology, sophisticated sensors, and global positioning, we are told, have ushered in a revolution in military affairs.[1] In this new era of information-age hyperwarfare, air power – more specifically, American air power[2] – has finally come of age. Not surprisingly, for those enamored with this line of thinking, the Gulf War is paradigmatic. Ever since that lopsided conflict, a chorus of American voices has been singing the praises of air power.[3] For example, in 1992 Richard Hallion, now the U.S. Air Force's chief historian, proclaimed that "simply stated, air power won the Gulf war."[4] Colonel John Warden, one of the principal architects of the air campaign against Iraq and a prominent air power theorist, has gone further to assert that the Gulf War was "the first conflict in the first true military technological revolution in history."[5] As one might expect, however, more cautious voices have entered into what has become an important debate about the nature and future of air power.

The American air power debate, as Benjamin Lambeth has noted, is really a cluster of debates. One centers on the relevance of classic air power theory, particularly "whether 'strategic bombardment' ...can compel an adversary to capitulate." Another revolves around the relationship between air and surface forces in joint warfare: more to the point, whether air power has displaced heavily armed ground forces as "the dominant form of military might."[6] Yet another relates to whether air power can effectively exert coercive diplomatic pressure. My focus – a broad one to be sure – will be on the evolution of classic air power theory and its relevance to current debates; my perspective will be, in the main historical.

A BRIEF HISTORICAL SURVEY OF THE CONCEPT OF AIR POWER

Despite the undisputed importance of air superiority in modern warfare, efforts to develop a clearly defined theory of air power have been less than satisfactory.[7] Since the 1920s, there has been no dearth of air power enthusiasts; nevertheless, retired airman and military historian David Mac Isaac confessed in 1986 that "air power, the twentieth century's peculiar contribution to warfare, continues to defy our attempts at analysis."[8] In order to assess the current air power debates and address the question of whether air power has indeed come of age, it is necessary to examine briefly the history of the concept of air power. At the very least, such a historical excursion will demonstrate that in many important respects the issues raised in current debates are not new, though the technology certainly is.

Much like their contemporary counterparts, military analysts in the years following World War I believed they were in the throes of a revolutionary situation. New weapons on land, sea, and air – not to mention the horrible stalemate of the war in Europe – provided ample evidence that the character of warfare had changed fundamentally. As a result, the inter-war years witnessed bold schemes utilizing the new technologies to reintroduce mobility to land warfare, develop a modern doctrine of amphibious warfare, and exploit the potential of military and naval aviation. None of these developments was more celebrated or more controversial than the claims General Giulio Douhet (1869-1930) and Brigadier General William "Billy" Mitchell (1879-1936) made on behalf of air power .

These early air power advocates were not philosophers of war on a par with Antoine-Henri Jomini, Carl von Clausewitz, or even Alfred Thayer Mahan; rather, they were polemicists arguing that the airplane had become the predominant instrument of war.[9] Essentially, Douhet and Mitchell preached a doctrine – not dissimilar from that of today's air power advocates – "that the airplane possesses such ubiquity, and such advantages of speed and elevation, as to possess the power of destroying all surface installations and instruments, ashore or afloat, while itself remaining comparatively safe from effective reprisal from the ground."[10]

For Douhet, who began his military career as an Italian artillery officer, air power was the use of the third dimension to decide war on the surface. Borrowing, whether intentionally or not, from the concept of sea power put forth by Alfred Thayer Mahan and refined by Sir Julian Corbett, Douhet argued that the first order of business in war was securing command of the air.

By no means was this a function of one-on-one romantic dogfights. Command of the air would result from huge fleets of "battle planes" bombing enemy ground installations and factories supplying materiel. Once command of the air was achieved – and he believed this could happen rapidly – air power would be exercised decisively, not against an enemy's armed forces, but against his cities and infrastructure, thereby shattering civilian morale and will to resist.[11] Douhet accepted the harsh consequence that "victory by swift obliteration" came at the high price of obliterating the distinction between soldier and civilian: "all citizens...will become combatants."[12] The air war Douhet envisioned would be "vicious and terrifying," but as one historian has put it: "war decided in the air would be a merciful substitute for the hell of the trenches."[13] While Mitchell agreed with Douhet about the importance of attacking cities and the infrastructure of an enemy in order to break morale, he believed that enemy surface forces, both ground and naval, remained important targets for air power. Mitchell's main concern, however, was establishing an autonomous air command to co-ordinate all of the nation's air assets.[14]

No commonly accepted theory of air power emerged during the inter-war years. MacIsaac contends that despite the efforts of Douhet and Mitchell, neither proved to be a Mahan or a Jomini from whom the air power enthusiasts could draw the secrets of the third dimension in warfare. Rather, the airplane's application was the product of separate choice within each major nation, reflecting an effort to integrate the unique capabilities of aircraft in support of land and sea forces, or in independent operations, in a manner that was both affordable and attuned to the achievement of national objectives.[15]

While a strong theory of air power was absent, several air power doctrines, with distinct national flavors, emerged during the interwar years.[16] In the American context, in fact, this occurred at the think tank of air power,[17] the U.S. Army Air Corps Tactical School at Maxwell Field, Alabama, where officers studied the possibility of identifying, bombing, and destroying the key industrial and infrastructure targets that constituted an enemy's strategic center of gravity. Creating massive air fleets with the capabilities that the prophets of air power envisioned in the 1920s was not feasible, neither technologically nor budgetarily in the 1930s. But a new bomber with improved range, speed, altitude, and bomb load capacity, the B-17, was in the works, as was a more precise bombsight. The American air doctrine of "daylight, high altitude, precision bombing of selected targets" emerged from the interplay of budgetary constraints, existing and new technology, and air doctrine.[18]

Strategic bombardment was not the only air doctrine developed at the Air Corps Tactical School in the inter-war years. American airmen also studied the use of air power in support of ground operations. "Attack aviation" or tactical air was assigned three missions in descending order of priority: (1) achieving air superiority in the theater of operations, (2) isolating the battlefield by attacking military and logistical targets beyond the range of artillery, and (3) engaging in close air support on the actual battlefield.[19] But tactical air never attained the status of strategic bombardment. In August 1941, Lt. Col. Harold L. George and a group of officers in the U.S. Air War Plans Division drafted A WPD-l, a plan for "winning the war with air power." Reliance on strategic bombardment was at the core of this war plan. After Pearl Harbor, George's group drafted a more extreme plan, A WPD-4, for winning the war possibly by air power alone. This plan put even more emphasis on strategic bombardment and called for aircraft production to be given "overriding priority." Predictably, the Allied Combined Chiefs of Staff rejected A WPD-4 in favor of a modified version of A WPD-l.[20]

The United States, then, entered World War II without a comprehensive theory of air power, though it did have a variety of air doctrines. The Navy forged its own doctrine of carrier-based naval aviation, while the Marine Corp specialized in close support of ground forces. The Army Air Corps, for its part, developed separate tactical and strategic air doctrines.

Without question, military aviation was crucial to the outcome of World War II. Achieving air superiority was essential for the success of most ground and sea operations; losing it almost always led to failure. But while tactical and naval air power proved to be of enormous importance, the effectiveness of the strategic air campaign has been in dispute. This brief historical survey is not the place to rehearse these debates in any detail. A simple listing of the variety of concerns raised by the strategic bombing campaign will have to suffice: (1) the effectiveness and morality of the RAF's policy of "area bombing directed against German civilian morale" and the "precision bombing" of the United States, (2) the shift in 1945 of American bombing toward area bombing, especially the devastating attacks on Japanese cities, (3) the question of whether racial prejudice led to a more callous disregard for the Japanese civilian population, (4) the question of whether the enormous resources of the strategic air campaign could have been more effectively employed in other ways, and (5) the necessity and morality of dropping atomic bombs on Japan.[21]

One final point about air power and World War II. Quietly in July 1943, the American military took an important step toward developing a comprehensive view of air power. Following the ineffective performance of American air-ground operations at Kasserine Pass in February 1943, the decision was made to reorganize all theater air forces under a single air commander, rather than assigning air assets piecemeal to subordinate commanders. This decision was codified in the U.S. War Department's slim, fourteen-page *Field Manual* 100-20: *Command and Employment of Air Power,* arguably the most important volume in the history of air power since Douhet's *Command of the Air. FM100-20* presented an outline for a comprehensive view of air power (except naval) based upon the premise, printed in capital letters in the opening sentence: "Land power and air power are co-equal and independent forces: neither is auxiliary of the other." Asserting that air power should be directed both at strategic targets and in support of ground operations, *FM* 100-20 represented a compromise between the two dominant schools of American air power, strategic bombardment and ground support-a compromise that, despite its fragility and frequent imbalance, has been in effect ever since.[22]

After World War II, theorizing about air power became entangled with strategies of nuclear war and deterrence through massive retaliation. Delivery of nuclear weapons, it was thought, had finally provided air power with the decisive capability prophesized by the early air power enthusiasts.[23] Once the USAF became independent in 1947, it considered its primary mission to be conducting of strategic operations against an enemy's vital center to destroy his ability to fight. In a military culture dominated by the Strategic Air Command, tactical air doctrine languished. Despite the importance of conventional air power in the Korean War, that conflict was viewed as an aberration. Consequently, the United States entered the air war in Southeast Asia relying on overwhelming firepower to attain political goals well beyond the reach of air power. The details of the Vietnam War need not detain us here. It will be enough to conclude that Vietnam exposed the consequences of the priority American airmen placed on nuclear strategy at the expense of conventional air power and especially the error of committing air power in piecemeal fashion.[24]

Vietnam was a "defining experience for American air power."[25] As a result of the soul-searching that occurred after the war, the air force went about improving "the sharp end" of air power: achieving air superiority and the ground-attack mission. Training and tactics improved greatly, as did the capabilities of new aircraft, munitions, and other hardware. Air planners had three opportunities during the 1980s to evaluate their investment in air power vicariously in 1982 when the Israeli Air Force used the latest American equipment in the Bekaa Valley against Syrian forces, in 1983 when the navy conducted air strikes against Syrian proxy forces in Lebanon, and in the 1986 El Dorado Canyon operation against Libya. The results, particularly in the 1983 Lebanon operation, were not always spectacular, but valuable lessons were learned as American air power underwent transformation.[26] Nevertheless, despite the attempts to forge an effective air instrument after the debacle of Vietnam, there was a sense in 1990 that the U.S. Air Force was conceptually adrift. According to one officer, it was "a conglomerate of specialists with greater loyalty to machines and sleeve patches than to any single unifying theme or to the Air Force itself."[27]

The impressive military results[28] of the Gulf War seemingly changed all this. With minimal combat losses (17 coalition airplanes and 148 American combat fatalities out of more than 500,000 military personnel assigned to the theater versus an estimated 100,000 Iraqi lives), coalition forces overwhelmed the Iraqi military in one of the most lopsided victories in modern military history. The plan for the Gulf War air campaign, however, was actually the result of a set of very contingent events, dubbed "the 'airpower compromise' of 1990-91."[29]

Shortly after Iraq's invasion of Kuwait on 2 August 1990, Army General Norman Schwartzkopf was given operational responsibility for the war. Early on he asked the Air Staff to put together an air campaign for him to consider. Ordinarily, responsibility for this should have fallen on Lt. Gen. Jimmie Adams, who believed ground support was air power's primary mission. But since Adams was on leave, Col. John A. Warden, III drew the assignment. Warden held a very different view of air power. He and his group of planners drafted a bold plan for a six-day campaign of intensive simultaneous attacks against a relatively small number of strategic targets – "the nerve centers of Iraqi national power" – with the intention of incapacitating Iraqi leadership and destroying key military capabilities. The plan, named Instant Thunder in obvious contrast to the failed gradualism of the ineffectual Rolling Thunder campaign against North Vietnam, was designed to showcase the war-winning potential of the new air power. This would be a truly strategic campaign where air power – if not by itself, then almost so – would win the war.[30] Following an initially enthusiastic reception, Instant Thunder ran into opposition from the more tactically oriented staff of the U.S. Air Forces Central Command (CENTAF) led by Lt. Gen. Charles Homer. Homer commanded the theater air assets, and his inclination was to direct coalition air power against the Iraqi military. Eventually a compromise was reached, and a composite campaign plan emerged. After a first phase that looked much like Instant Thunder, air operations would focus on gaining air superiority and then be directed against Iraqi ground forces.[31]

The performance of air power in the war was nothing short of spectacular for the victors and devastating for the vanquished. Coalition air forces achieved air superiority from the opening moments of the campaign, and in the first 24 hours of operations, virtually every major strategic target was hit in the largest single air offensive since World War II. Having gained strategic control in the first days of the war (depriving Iraq of effective air defense or "situational awareness"), coalition commanders had the luxury of allowing air power to beat down enemy ground forces before launching the ground assault. Some argue that engaging an enemy's army wholesale with virtual impunity may well be the real legacy of air power in the Gulf War.[32]

Since the Gulf War, there have been three major tests of American air power. The first two were attempts at conducting coercive air diplomacy. Operation Deliberate Force was a brief, eleven-day U.S.-led NATO air campaign in 1995 against Bosnia Serb targets, and Operation Allied Force was the 1999 U.S.-led NATO air campaign against Yugoslavia designed to get Serbian strongman Slobodan Milosevic to stop human rights abuses. The third test is, of course, the ongoing war in Afghanistan prompted by the attacks against the World Trade Center and the Pentagon on 11 September 2001. Whereas most analysts agree that Deliberate Force was a reasonably successful example of coercive air diplomacy, the efficacy of Allied Force is much debated. Despite its obvious operational shortcomings, some see this 78-day campaign; which witnessed the operational debut of the B-2 stealth bomber, the first ever downing of a F-117 stealth aircraft, the mistaken bombing of the Chinese embassy in Belgrade, and eventually Milosevic's yielding to NATO's demands; as a demonstration of the capabilities of air power as a tool of policy.[33] Others, most notably Andrew Bacevich, warn that while the results of such operations may be acceptable in the short run – especially since America's risk of casualties is considerably reduced – these episodes of coercive air diplomacy may seduce Americans into thinking the United States can become a global policeman "on the cheap" and that air power can be effective in all situations, including those where restraint would be the best counsel.[34]

The jury is still out of course, but all indications are that the "new American way of war" is here to stay. According to a current blueprint for military transformation, Joint Vision 2020, the United States seeks "full-spectrum dominance...to defeat any adversary and control any situation across the range of military operations." Just weeks ago in California, the U.S. Joint Forces Command conducted Millennium Challenge 2002, a combination of live field exercises and computer simulations to test the some of the principles outlined in Joint Vision 2020 in a "small-scale contingency that has the potential to escalate to a major theater war."[35] Specifically, Millennium Challenge 2002 examined the concept of rapid decisive operations (RDO), the current American expression of the revolution in military affairs.[36] As one would expect, air power plays a major, but certainly not exclusive, role in these efforts to transform the American military into an effective instrument in the information-age.

THREE VIEWS ON THE CURRENT AIR POWER DEBATES

While no one seriously contests the importance of air power, nevertheless, a debate is underway in the United States on its very nature and proper function in 21st century warfare. A brief summary of three prominent analysts' views will provide the reader with a flavor of these discussions. They are selected not because they represent the full spectrum of positions in the air power debate. They don't. Rather, the following perspectives have particular bearing on the question posed at the outset: Has American air power indeed come of age?

THE SYSTEMS APPROACH OF JOHN WARDEN

John Warden has been hailed as one of the most important air power theorists since Douhet and Mitchell. We have already seen that he is an unabashed advocate of strategic air power, but unlike Douhet et al., his focus is on the enemy's leadership, not its civilian morale. Warden adopts a systems approach to analyzing an opponent's strategic centers of gravity. "The enemy," he asserts, "is a system, not an independent mass of tanks, aircraft, or dope pushers."[37] Consequently, military operations should seek to paralyze at a strategic level by preventing the "system's" leadership from gathering, processing, and using information. Given its enhanced capabilities, this can best be done by air power adopting a strategy of parallel attack, subjecting the "enemy system" to many near-simultaneous attacks that overwhelm his ability to react, defend, or repair the damage. According to Warden, the number of truly significant strategic targets is surprisingly small; they are very expensive, have few backups, and are difficult to repair. If a significant percentage of these targets can be appropriately identified and hit in parallel, "the damage becomes insuperable." Based on this line of thinking, vindicated by the Gulf War, Warden proclaims that air power is now truly dominant in warfare.[38]

COLIN GRAY'S STRATEGIC ORIENTATION

Colin Gray, one of the most respected contemporary American strategic thinkers, does not fully agree with Warden. Of course, Gray acknowledges the spectacular success of air power in the Gulf War. Indeed, the lethality of air warfare is unprecedented. But he believes that it is essential to anchor discussions of air power in the larger context of America's geo-strategic position and its national strategic culture. According to Gray, inflated claims of air power's utter dominance betray muddled and potentially dangerous strategic thinking. For one thing, there is danger in making generalizations about air power based upon the optimal conditions coalition air forces experienced in the Gulf War. More importantly, Gray objects to the hyperbolic assertion - harking back to Douhet and AWPD-4 - that air power has developed to the point where it can win wars by itself. Over the years, this notion has retarded the development of a mature air power theory and needlessly polarizes the current air power debates. Moreover, ever since Douhet, Gray argues, air power enthusiasts have confused air power theory with a theory of war. Air power can still be recognized as "an essential player in conflict" without the distracting and exaggerated claims that air power is so dominant that it can win wars alone and thereby exercise a decisive influence on the course of history.[39]

Has air power finally come of age? Has Douhet been vindicated? Gray believes that it is time to move past these unhelpful questions and ask what does it mean for the United States to be the leading air power?[40] Answering this question, however, requires an assessment of America's overall geo-strategic position. Gray contends that the United States is a dominant great power with a continental outlook, maritime situation, and an air power preference. While the strategic heritage of the U.S. is a mixture of continental and maritime elements, the American way of war has been essentially continentalist.[41] Consequently, Americans have favored military approaches that promise swift victory usually as the result of decisive battle. American national and strategic cultures tend to embrace new technologies, while manifesting an indifference to history and careful strategic analysis. Moreover, Americans consider the resort to force as the last alternative, but once engaged, they "expect a thumping triumph." They are impatient with subtle applications of military force and favor tactical approaches that feature overwhelming firepower and conservation of American lives.[42] America's geo-strategic position and its national and strategic culture, Gray maintains, uniquely favor air power. Indeed, the U.S. is "more truly an air power than it is a maritime or continental power."[43]

BENJAMIN LAMBETH AND THE TRANSFORMATION OF AMERICAN AIR POWER

RAND Corporation senior staff member Benjamin Lambeth offers a third perspective on the air power debates. Lambeth believes that the new capabilities of air and space technologies have transformed American air power to a point where "it has become truly strategic in its potential effects.[44] The effectiveness of American air power has improved to such an extent that, in principle, it offers American theater commanders the promise of engaging and neutralizing opposing military forces "from standoff ranges with virtual impunity, thus reducing the threat to U.S. troops." The same capabilities offer the potential for "achieving strategic effects" at the outset of a joint campaign with attacks on "an enemy's core vulnerabilities with both shock and simultaneity." This transformation in capabilities, Lambeth argues, "is the essence of American air power's recent coming of age.[45]

The debates about the role of air power, Lambeth argues, have paid far too much attention to the question of strategic bombardment. For one thing, research reveals the repeated failure of strategic bombing to break civilian morale and the questionable military impact of air attacks against enemy infrastructure. Moreover, refinements in technology and concepts of air operations have rendered the question of strategic bombardment passé. There are much better ways to think about air power than "by seeking guidance from the now-antiquarian writings of the early-20th-century air power classicists."[46] The sooner we recognize that Douhet's concept of air power has been rendered obsolete, the better.

For Lambeth, the truly significant development is that air power has become so lethal it can proceed directly to strategic goals that "bypass any compelling need to attack an opponent's urban-industrial assets." To be sure, some infrastructure targets (electric power stations and transportation grids) will still be bombed, but not in order to erode the enemy's civilian morale. Rather, the purpose of such attacks is "to deprive an enemy directly of his ability to continue fighting." Far too many air power professionals mistakenly portray strategic air warfare in terms of vital target *types* (key manufacturing systems, sources of raw materials, strategic stockpiles, power and transportation systems, telecommunications networks, etc.) not operational and combat *outcomes.*[47]

Beyond the important task of removing some conceptual shoals, Lambeth assesses the "changed essence" of American air power. In doing so, he strikes a balance between those, like Warden, who argue that air power can come close to winning wars by itself and those who question that the revolution in military affairs is really all that revolutionary. With due recognition of its limitations, Lambeth concludes that the ability of air power to place constant pressure on an enemy from a safe distance, to increase the number of "kills per sortie," to target selectively with a minimum of unintended damage, and to deeply compromise an enemy's ability to control his forces - all suggest that "the relative combat potential of air power in comparison to other force elements" has dramatically increased.[48] Additionally, he argues that the transformation of American air power will save lives: the enemy's by reducing noncombatant death, and American military lives by substituting technology for manpower.

CONCLUSIONS AND OBSERVATIONS

Despite Gray's objections, the question of whether air power has come of age is still relevant, at least for the immediate future. And after so much in the way of preamble, the reader is entitled to some authorial comment. So I conclude with a resounding "yes and no!"

Warden is absolutely correct in wanting to exploit the dramatically enhanced capabilities of air power. And it is obvious that air power will play a major – probably leading – role in the military transformation now underway. But while it would be foolish to ignore the potential for air power to create strategic paralysis in some situations or exert coercive pressure in others, it would be shortsighted to downplay the importance of the joint nature of most military operations. Millennium Challenge 2002 suggests the United States military has not bought the argument that air power alone is the dominant tool of war and coercive diplomacy. Air power can truly come of age only when it is fully integrated with the other forms of warfare.

Gray's conclusions about the compatibility of air power to American national and strategic culture are intriguing. He would surely agree, however, that cultural affinity and even geo-strategic warrant might be a recipe for over-reliance. Bacevich and others are right to question whether air power can be a flexible and convincing instrument of coercive diplomacy. In fact, many analysts worry that reliance on air power could signal that the United States is so reluctant to risk its soldiers' lives, that it lacks the commitment to back up its extensive global commitments. Air power can come of age only when its limits, not just its advantages, are soberly assessed.[49]

Gray's discussion of the American strategic culture also points to another concern. A good case could be made that the American military, in general, and air theorists, in particular, are overly enamored with technological fixes – what military historians have called the "gee whiz" or materialist approach to strategy. As Richard Szafranski has noted, American planners may be so fixated on the tools of war that they risk forgetting that "warfare is about human beings, human aspirations, and human passions." Air power, Szafranski fears, "seems to have become no more nor less than the power of detached, dispassionate technology."[50] In many of the strategic debates of the past century, those impressed with the revolutionary potential of new technology have been pitted against those whose strategic instincts are rooted in historical analysis. The current air power debates are no exception; "technicists" engage in verbal jousts with "historicists."[51] The resulting tension is healthy. Air power can come of age only when technology is subjected to sustained and sober historically informed strategic assessment.

A sign of maturity in the air power debates is the erosion of support for the doctrine of strategic morale bombardment, surely "one of the most repugnant forms of 20th-century warfare."[52] To be sure, a robust debate continues around Warden's systems approach and whether so-called "center of gravity targets" or strategic outcomes ought to be the focus of air power, but strategic bombing directed against civilian populations in order to break a society's will to resist has been soundly discredited. Precision bombing does not remove all risk of non-combatant casualties. Even with the advantages of satellite technology, mistakes will be made. But hopefully, gone are the days of airmen advocating the bombing of people in order to change their minds. Lambeth is wise to note that air power could never come of age as long as it was so closely identified to strategic bombing.

After almost a century, air power remains an operational reality in search of a theory. In 1986, MacIsaac observed: "One might conclude, with some distress, that technology itself may be today's primary air power theorist; that invention may, for the moment, be the mother of application."[53] In 1994, the late Carl Builder bemoaned the fact that air power still lacked a theory.[54] For most of the 20th century, air power lacked sufficient conceptual heft; it was essentially an efficient means of delivering ordnance, an extension of artillery. Air power theory amounted to little more than general notions of air superiority coupled with the suspect concept of strategic bombardment. As the preceding survey has demonstrated, operational and technological factors have generally been more important than theorizing in the development of air power. The current debates confirm the need for a theory of air power appropriate to the new realities and especially applicable, as Lambeth argues, to theater warfare. Perhaps air power's fit within the "rapid decisive operations" strategy will give impetus to a new theory of air power. But until a more mature theory is developed – one that, for example, honestly assesses air power's potential in missions of "air-suasion" and coercive diplomacy – air power will not fully have come of age.

Admittedly, this essay has thrived on the ambiguity of the phrase "come of age." From an operational standpoint, air power, despite its mixed historical record, has clearly matured. The fact that modern warfare is unthinkable without taking the third dimension into account certainly suggests that air power has come of age; indeed, it did so over a half-century ago. But viewed from a conceptual perspective, air power may still be in its adolescence. To be fair, Britain's naval mastery had been established for a century before Mahan and Corbett gave analytical precision to the strategic and operational instincts of generations of Royal Navy officers and a few perceptive Prime Ministers. That being said, however, would-be theorists of air power may not have the luxury of leisurely reflection. If some futurists are correct, then cyberspace, not aerospace, may be *the* operational dimension of the 21st century.[55] If so, will the question of air power's coming of age even matter?

QUESTIONS FOR DISCUSSION

The preceding survey and commentary suggest a number of questions for discussion at these seminars.

1. What would a mature theory of air power look like? And how much does it really matter?
2. Is air power, for all its razzle-dazzle, still essentially an extension of artillery? And if so, will blowing things up eventually give way to disabling systems and infrastructure in more subtle ways? Will the *atmospheric* indeed give way to the *infospheric?*
3. How helpful is it to adopt the essentialism of strategic cultural analysis?
   a. Is there an American "way of war"?
   b. Is there a Western "way of war"?
   c. Is the former a "frightful incarnation" of the latter?
4. Assuming that strategic cultural analysis is legitimate and helpful, is air power indeed a distinctively American way of war?
5. What are the implications for the United States to be so enamored with air power?
   a. in the light of the absence of a comprehensive theory of air power?
   b. in the light of American hegemony?
   c. can air power adequately support America's military and diplomatic responsibilities?
6. What of the need for air bases?
7. Do the enhanced air technologies encourage "interventions on the cheap?"
8. Does the reluctance to risk American lives cause friend and foe to question American resolve?
9. In the light of the increasing military power differentials with other nations?
   a. "is partnership possible?"[56]
   b. will joint operations with allies be diplomatic covers for essentially American-run affairs?
   c. are truly joint operations with allies possible?
10. Does the high-tech America way of war encourage terrorism of either the low-tech suicide bombing variety or high-tech cyber-terrorism?

REFERENCES

1. In the current jargon of the American military, the notion is simply expressed as *transformation.*

2. Clearly, air power is not the exclusive preserve of the United States, but for obvious reasons this examination will focus on the American context.

3. See, for example, Michael Kelly, "The American Way of War," The *Atlantic Monthly,* 289:6 (June, 2002), 16-18; Donald B. Rice [Secretary of the U.S. Air Force], "Air Power in the New Security Environment," in The *Future of Air Power in the Aftermath of the Gulf War,* Richard H. Schultz, Jr. and Robert L. Pfaltzgraff, Jr., eds. (Maxwell Air Force Base, AL: Air University Press, 1992), 9-16.

4. Hallion quoted in Benjamin S. Lambeth, The *Transformation of American Air Power* (Ithaca, NY: Comell University Press, 2000), 261.

5. John A. Warden, III [Col., USAF], The *Air Campaign,* rev. ed. (San Jose, CA: to Excel Press, 2000), 160; "Air Theory for the Twenty-First Century," in *Battlefields of the Future: 21st Century Warfare Issues,* Barry R. Schneider and Lawrence E. Grinter, eds. (Maxwell Air Force Base, AL: Air University Press, 1998), 121.

6. Lambeth, *Transformation of American Air Power,* 262-63; Rice, "Air Power in the New Security Environment," 11.

7. Writing in 1941, Edward Warner noted that it was "only in a limited sense that one can speak with literal accuracy of theories of air power." Forty-five years later David MacIsaac concluded that air power, while used widely as a generic term, had "yet to find a clearly defined or unchallenged place in the history of military or strategic theory." Edward Warner, "Douhet, Mitchell, Seversky: Theories of Air Warfare," in *Makers of Modern Strategy: Military Thought from Machiavelli to Hitler,* Edward Mead Earle, ed. (Princeton, NJ: Princeton University Press, 1941),485; David MacIsaac, "Voices from the Central Blue: The Air Power Theorists," in *Makers of Modern Strategy : Military Thought from Machiavelli to the Nuclear Age,* Peter Paret, ed. (Princeton, NJ: Princeton University Press, 1986), 624.

8. MacIsaac, "Voices from the Central Blue," 625.

9. MacIsaac, "Voices from the Central Blue," 626; Colin S. Gray, *Explorations in Strategy* (Westport, CT: Praeger, 1996), 55.

10. Warner, "Douhet, Mitchell, Seversky," 485.

11. Richard H. Kohn and Joseph P. Harahan, "Editor's Introduction," to Giulio Douhet, *The Command of the Air,* translated by Dino Ferrari (Washington, DC: Office of Air Force History, 1983), viii; Warner, "Douhet, Mitchell, Seversky," 489-92. While Douhet is generally credited with developing the doctrine of strategic bombardment, the Germans in World War I were the first to conceive and execute a truly strategic air campaign (against London in the summer and fall of 1917). See Lee Kennett, *A History of Strategic Bombing* (New York: Charles Scribner's Sons, 1982), 23-26. A little known event off the coast of New England at the outset of the War for American Independence suggests that the concept of bombing a civilian population in order to break its will to resist substantially pre-dates aviation technology. In October 1775, a small Royal Navy squadron, with

orders "to lay Waste" virtually every port between Boston and Canada, bombed Falmouth (now Portland, Maine). While the town was almost completely destroyed, the coastal population's morale was not. Moreover, news of the bombardment served to enhance revolutionary zeal throughout the colonies. See Donald A. Yerxa, *The Burning of Falmouth, October 18, 1775* (Portland, ME: Maine Historical Society, 1975).

12. Douhet, *Command of the Air,* 10. The phrase "victory by swift obliteration" is from Warner, "Douhet, Mitchell, Seversky," 492.

13. Kennett, *History of Strategic Bombing,* 55-56, 179.

14. Lambeth, *Transformation of American Air Power,* 264; MacIsaac, "Voices from the Central Blue," 631.

15. MacIsaac, "Voices from the Central Blue," 635.

16. See, Kennett, *History of Strategic Bombing,* 72-88.

17. See the comments of O.P. Weyland [Gen. USAF (Ret)] in "The Perceptions of Three Makers of Air Power History," in *Air Power and Warfare,* Alfred F. Hurley and Robert C. Ehrhart, eds. (Washington, DC: Office of Air Force History, 1979), 190-191.

18. MacIsaac, "Voices from the Central Blue," 633-35; Michael S. Sherry, *The Rise of American Air Power: The Creation of Armageddon* (New Haven, CT: Yale University Press, 1987), 51-53. Its application was, of course, also a function of the politics of service and joint Allied war planning.

19. MacIsaac, "Voices from the Central Blue," 638.

20. There are interesting parallels between this episode and the decision-making that went into the American air campaign against Iraq. See Edward C. Manu, III [Col. USAF], *Thunder and Lightning: Desert Storm and the Airpower Debates* (Maxwell Air Force Base, AL: Air University Press, 1995), 4-46.

21. Mac Isaac, "Voices from the Central Blue," 636-37; Sherry, *Rise of American Air Power,* 60, 244-45; john W. Dower, *War without Mercy: Race and Power in the Pacific War* (New York: Pantheon Books, 1987).

22. Manu, *Thunder and Lightning,* 51-54. Naval aviation, though not immune from similar dynamics, really was a separate matter.

23. Williamson Murray, " Air Power since World War II: Consistent with Doctrine?" in *Future of Air Power,* 97.

24. Mac Isaac, "Voices from the Central Blue," 643-45; Lambeth, *Transformation of American Air Power,* 12,48-53,314; Murray, "Air Power since World War II," 97-110.

25. Lambeth, *Transformation of American Air Power,* 48.

26. Lambeth, *Transformation of American Air Power,* 54-102.

27. Manu, *Thunder and Lightning,* 163-65.

28. The political results, however, were far from clear cut.

29. Manu, *Thunder and Lightning,* 185.

30. Lambeth, *Transformation of American Air Power,* 104-05; Manu, *Thunder and Lightning,* 27-47; Warden, *Air Campaign,* 144-61.

31. Lambeth, *Transformation of American Air Power,* 105-07; Manu, *Thunder and Lightning,* 60- 63.

32. See Lambeth, *Transformation of American Air Power,* 103-117.

33. Lambeth, *Transformation of American Air Power,"* 216-32.

34. Andrew j. Bacevich, "The Bombing: Over-the-Top Statecraft," *Washington Post,* 28 March 1999, Bl. See Stephen Biddle, "The New Way of War?" *Foreign Affairs,* 81:3 (May/june, 2002), 138-44; jeffrey Record, "Collapsed Countries, Casualty Dread, and the New American Way of War," *Parameters,* 32 (Summer, 2002),4-23. Eliot A. Cohen's comment bears repeating: " Air power is an unusually seductive form of military strength, in part because, like modem courtship, it appears to offer gratification without commitment." Cohen, "The Mystique of U.S. Air Power," *Foreign Affairs,* 73:1 (Jan/Feb, 1994),109.

35. American Forces Information Service, "Joint Vision 2020 Emphasizes Full-Spectrum Dominance," 2 June 2000, www.defenselink.mil/news/Jun2000/n06022000 20006025 .html; U.S. Joint Forces Command, "Millennium Challenge 2002," www .jfcom.mil/about/experiments/mc02.htm.

36. In preparing for and conducting a *rapid decisive operation,* the U .S. and its allies "asymmetrically assault the adversary from directions and against which he has no counter, dictating the terms and tempo of the operation. The adversary, suffering from the loss of coherence and unable to achieve his objectives, chooses [either] to cease actions that are against U.S. interests or has his capabilities defeated." Although RDO is a joint force doctrine, the influence of Warden's Instant Thunder air campaign is clearly evident. See U.S. Joint Forces Command, "M i l l e n n i u m   C h a l l e n g e   2 0 0 2   G l o s s a r y , " www.jfcom.mi1/about/glossary.htm#RDO.

37. Warden, "Air Theory for the Twenty-First Century," 111.

38. Warden, "Air Theory for the Twenty-First Century," 114-21. See also Warden, *Air Campaign,* 144-61.

39. Gray, *Explorations in Strategy,* 56-59.

40. Gray, *Explorations in Strategy,* 60.

41. Gray appreciates that the U.S. is also a maritime power - indeed, for the last half-century the world's leading naval power. Cf., Richard Hallion's notion that "[a]s dominant land power characterized a *Pa.x Romana,* and dominant sea power a *Pa.x Britannica,* dominant air power is the characteristic of modern America." Hallion quoted in Gray, *Explorations in Strategy,* 55. For a different - and, to my thinking, more persuasive - analysis of America's strategic heritage, see Clark G. Reynolds, "Reconsidering American Strategic History and Doctrines," in *History and the Sea~. Essays on Maritime Strategies* (Columbia, SC: University of South Carolina Press, 1989), 108-36.

42. Gray, *Explorations in Strategy,* 85-98. In these respects, the American way of war represents a "frightful incarnation" of the so-called "Western way of war" thesis. See Geoffrey Parker, "The Western War of War," in The *Cambridge Illustrated History of Warfare,* Geoffrey Parker, ed. (Cambridge: Cambridge University

Press, 1995), 2-9. According to military historian Victor Davis Hanson, "the idea of annihilation, of head-to-head battle that destroys the enemy, seems a particularly Western concept largely unfamiliar to the ritualistic fighting and emphasis on deception and attrition found outside Europe." See Hanson's *Carnage and Culture: Landmark Battles in the Rise of Western Power* (New York: Doubleday, 2001), 21-26, 444-55. The phrase "frightful incarnation" is from Hanson's "America and the Western Way of War," *Historically Speaking,* 3:2 (November, 2001), 7.

43.   Gray, *Explorations in Strategy,* 85. Eliot Cohen is even more emphatic: "Reliance on air power has set the American way of war apart from all others for well over half a century. ...Air warfare remains distinctively American-high-tech, cheap in lives and (at least in theory) quick. To America's enemies - past, current and potential - it is the distinctively American form of military intimidation." Cohen, "Mystique of U.S. Air Power," 120.

44.   Lambeth, *Transformation of American Air Power,* 298.

45.   Lambeth, *Transformation of American Air Power,* 11.

46.   Lambeth, *Transformation of American Air Power,* 264-265, 268-271. For a similar perspective, see Air Vice Marshal Tony Mason [RAP (Ret.)], *Air Power: A Centennial Appraisal* (London: Brassey's), xvi, 273-274. See also Kennett, *History of Strategic Bombing,* 185.

47.   Lambeth, *Transformation of American Air Power,* 269-270.

48.   Lambeth, *Transformation of American Air Power,* 297-303.

49.   Something, by the way, Gray takes pains to do.

50.   Richard Szafranski [Col. USAF], "Parallel War and Hyperwar: Is Every Want a Weakness?" in *Battlefield of the Future,* 143.

51.   See Ignatieff, "New American Way of War," 46. For example, novelist and Israeli veteran Mark Helprin, a historian, asserted in 1998 that "in regard to the present revolution in military affairs, nothing yet described in the public record is entirely novel or without a fairly long history." Helprin, "Revolution or Dissolution?" *Forbes ASAP,* 161:4 (23 February 1998), 98.

52.   Eliot A. Cohen, "The Meaning and Future of Air Power," *Orbis,* 39:2 (Spring, 1995), 198. 53 MacIsaac, "Voices from the Central Blue," 647.

54.   Builder cited in Szafranski, "Parallel War and Hyperwar," 143.

55.   See Richard Szafranski [Col. USAF] and Martin Libicki, "...Or Go Down In Flame? An Airpower Manifesto for the 21st-Century Air Force," in 2025: *Executive Summary* (Maxwell Air Force Base: Air University, August 1996, http://www.au.af.mil/au/2025/. Szafranski and Libicki contemplate an "infospheric" rather than atmospheric air force, charged with "information dominance" missions that have little directly to do with "the human mastery of flight."

56.   The phrase is from William Wallace, "Living with the Hegemon: European Dilemmas," in Social Science Research Council, Essays after September 11, http://www.ssrc.org/sept11/essays/wallace.htm.

ENGAGING THE SCIENCE COMMUNITY FOR HOMELAND DEFENSE

WILLIAM A. BARLETTA[1]
E. O. Lawrence Berkeley National Laboratory, University of California, Berkeley
California

ABSTRACT

Science without secrecy and without borders can and does provide direct and indirect benefits vital to the domestic security of all nations. After the terrorist attacks of last September in New York and Washington, many members of the university research community in the U.S. have eagerly sought to find ways in which they could respond to the emerging threat to security at home. Enthusiasm was followed by the debates addressing practical realities of performing security-related research on university campuses and in other open research institutions. From a University-of-California-centered perspective this paper presents a view of how the scientific community can assist in increasing homeland security.

SUPPORTING HOMELAND SECURITY IN A UNIVERSITY ENVIRONMENT

Last September's terrorist attacks have prompted many members of the University of California research community to consider how we as scientists and technologists could assist our nation in combating terrorism and in restoring a feeling of security among our population. In addition to numerous informal discussions among researchers, many deliberations took place at all levels of institutional management. As the shock of the attacks subsided, we gradually reached consensus concerning an approach.

As an aside, we should observe that from an operational point of view the definition terrorism is irrelevant to our enterprise. We need only understand that a threat to domestic security exists and then we need to identify how to increase our security and the perception thereof in the face of that threat. In the meanwhile social scientists can debate and conceptualize the political and ideological frameworks that engender disruptive attacks on civilian society. Even in our considerations of how to work to increase the nation's security, most of us have opted to limit our attentions to how to stabilize and minimize the effects of asymmetrical attacks upon civilian society.

The greatest strength of our universities and of our non-defense scientific and technical communities is open and free inquiry combined with the ability to engage the very best minds regardless of their country of origin. The campuses of the University of

California and our Berkeley Lab are embodiments of open science, without secrecy and without borders. To ensure that this essential environmental characteristic is not violated by our efforts related to homeland security, the leadership of the Berkeley Laboratory has settled on the following guiding principles to regulate our activities:

- Do not compromise the open research environment
- Base participation on special scientific/technical expertise and experience
- Addresses a clear national need
- Be a proactive resource to the local community.

As we have put together a program appropriate to our institution over the past year, we have observed that especially in the areas of our competence, open science has been and will likely continue to outstrip defense science in many of the areas that have been identified as being most vital to assuring infrastructure security. For example, applied genomics and proteomics are vital to future bio-defense; rapid sequencing of bacterial DNA is already available. Information technology is crucial to rapid use of developing science and technology. Nanoscience will permit novel imaging, spectroscopic techniques for inspection and forensics. Furthermore, we find have found that the most fruitful avenues of contribution are in applying the research in which we are already actively engaged.

The remainder of this paper describes some of the ways in which the Berkeley Laboratory is contributing to homeland security. The general areas can be broken into 1) protecting our critical infrastructure, 2) protecting our people against physical threats, 3) protecting our people against biological threats.

PROTECTING CRITICAL INFRASTRUCTURE

The first critical infrastructure is the air we breathe, in particular, the air in our public and critical governmental buildings. For the past few years a consortium of DOE laboratories has modeled airflow and the transport of airborne contaminants in buildings, subways and other confined spaces. Berkeley's contribution builds on its long history of seeking to understand how to improve the air quality in commercial and residential buildings to make the indoors a healthier environment. Our research activities related to homeland security include simulating indoor dispersion of chemical and biological agents, validating computer simulations through controlled experiments, and providing design tools for first responders. The anthrax scare following September 11th has heightened the importance of this work.

The second critical infrastructure is the network of waterways that provide drinking and irrigation water as well as transportation. To address concerns of potential dispersal of chemical and biological agents in aquifers, our Berkeley's Center for Environmental Biotechnology is seeking to apply its expertise in hydro-meteorology, bio-geo-chemistry and large-scale modeling and its research on the biology and ecology of microbes in realistic environments. The goal is to provide sensitive, real-time monitors of water quality. A promising approach is to apply a fundamental understanding of bacterial chemotaxis (the "bacterial nose") to develop a simple, easily engineered receptor-actuator system to detect water-borne agents.

The third critical infrastructure is the electricity grid. Homeland security requires assuring electric reliability[2] and energy security in the face of malicious action. Berkeley is home of the project office of the Consortium for Electric Reliability Technology Solutions (CERTS). The aim of CERTS is to develop and disseminate new methods, tools, and technologies to protect and enhance the reliability of the U.S. electric power system in the face of both natural and man-made disturbances. Some members of the consortium have the defensive task of assessing the vulnerability of critical nodes in the grid. The proactive goal of Berkeley's contribution is to enhance energy security through distributed power by transforming the electricity grid into an intelligent network that senses and responds automatically to changing flows of power.

A fourth critical infrastructure is the information "superhighway" network and its node points. This network is especially sensitive in that it connected in an intimate way to very high value assets (both civilian and military) such as the electricity grid. Precisely as we aim at increasing the security of physical infrastructures via the use of "intelligent" information networks, we create a new source of potential single-point vulnerability that must be analyzed and controlled. We expect that the tools for enhancing information security will be driven by commercial and other civilian requirements of protecting the ever-more pervasive role of information technology in the commercial and academic sectors.

PROTECTING OUR PEOPLE AGAINST PHYSICAL THREATS

In the U.S., the September 11th terrorist attack has dramatically increased the perceived need for the rapid and reliable detection of explosives and fissile materials in containers, be they luggage or large shipping containers. In many scenarios, the detection must be performed without direct access to the enclosure/container in which the material is being transported. Screening must be rapid; the false alarm rate must be low, and the miss rate must be exceedingly low.

A versatile approach to such analysis is the active interrogation[3] of luggage and containers using a controlled neutron flux. The underlying scientific principles for active neutron interrogation are well understood and documented.[4] In contrast with X-ray scanners, neutrons can penetrate significant distances through packaging materials to produce a variety of penetrating diagnostic signatures (gamma rays and secondary neutrons) from enclosed objects. The energies of the gamma rays are specific to elemental make-up of the target. Analysis of the observed elemental profile can be used to distinguish among a variety of materials including explosives, nuclear materials, and shielding materials. The presence of prompt and delayed neutrons is diagnostic for the presence of fissionable materials. If multiple neutron energies are used in the probe beam, isotopic ratios can be measured.

Rapid neutron interrogation of luggage and cargo requires new sources with fluxes and lifetimes 100 to 1000 times greater than provided by commercially available neutron tubes. Choosing among the radiation detector options involves trading off detector efficiency against energy resolution, counting rates, and position encoding that impact analytical sensitivity, specificity, elemental range, and exposure times. To measure the of neutron-induced radiation from the target, these new sources must be combined with field deployable, high performance sensors that are outgrowths of detector development for high-energy physics research. Gamma-ray detector may range from simple NaI or CsI scintillators (high detection efficiency with poor energy discrimination) to more complex germanium or CZT detectors[5] with lower efficiency but good energy discrimination. Measuring prompt and delayed neutron emission involves similar tradeoffs in the design of the detection system. Given the detailed spectral data from the sensors, automated software analysis of detected events combined with expert system or trained neural nets can rapidly select anomalies from the primary screening data. Additional software, including image reconstruction algorithms, would provide the more complete characterization. The underlying technology can also be adapted to the humanitarian mission of detecting unexploded ordinance such as land mines.

Another technique for screening the contents of cargo is being investigated at LBNL. This technique will take magnetic resonance methods, NMR and MRI, into exciting new territory by implementing the novel, seemingly impossible, methods and devices of "ex-situ" and "remote" detection. Such a tool, NMR and MRI–outside the magnet[6]–will benefit materials and life sciences, nano-technology, earth sciences, biomedicine and counter-terrorism. While NMR and MRI have extraordinary advantages as non-invasive modalities of imaging and spectroscopic analysis, they typically require that samples be immersed in huge, immobile, expensive and often hazardous magnets designed for high homogeneity, in order to provide the greatest resolution. In the case of cargo screening it is impractical to insert the luggage of container into the gap or bore of a high-field magnet. To address such cases, Pines and his co-workers propose to use an "inside-out magnet with" a tunable, dynamic "sweet spot" that can be scanned over the intact object or subject, in order to acquire magnetic resonance information with compact, portable spectrometers.

Once terrorist attacks have occurred, domestic security forces are often faced with the daunting task of sorting through pulverized, burned and dispersed materials to search for tiny clues revealing the identify and the methods of the perpetrators. In such circumstances the materials are often too small to be analyzed using standard forensic instruments, even at infrared wavelengths. Here the many synchrotron light sources in the open scientific community offer a new and powerful forensic tool, "infrared spectro-microscopy."[7] Infrared spectroscopy is an extremely powerful analytical tool because infrared photons can couple directly to the vibrational modes of molecules in the sample so as to provide a unique signature for many molecules. The frequency spectrum of such modes forms an infrared molecular fingerprint of the compounds in a sample. The challenge of employing this tool in an open environment is related to maintaining the "chain of custody" of evidence without undue intrusion in the research environment.

PROTECTING OUR PEOPLE AGAINST BIOLOGICAL THREATS

The anthrax-filled letters that were mailed to the press and members of the U.S. Congress only a few weeks after September 11th indicate both the vulnerability of the public to bio-terrorism, but also the extreme fear that even limited bio-attacks can generate. Among the problems facing responders to bio-attacks are the detection of pathogens, the characterization of the nature of the bio-agent and the determination of whether potentially exposed individuals have been infected. At Berkeley one possibility for symptomatic diagnosis of anthrax infection relies on the fact that in infected individuals the anthrax endospore-macrophage system becomes a bioamplifier enabling detection long before onset of anthrax-specific symptoms. The IR-active vibrational modes of these biomolecules are dynamic multispectral IR signatures. Therefore broad-band synchrotron IR spectra can identify markers for the endospore-macrophage system. For field application, laser diodes tuned to the biomarker frequencies replace the synchrotron leading to a hand-held detection system for rapid, positive identification of infection.

An extremely difficult challenge is the combination of high selectivity and high sensitivity in detecting pathogens. The Superconducting Quantum Interference Devices (SQUID) Based Pathogen Detection[8] being developed by Clark and his co-workers at U. C. Berkeley and LBNL offers an approach that is selective, easy to use, rapid (seconds), and extraordinarily sensitive. Their technique relies on a microscope with a high-Tc SQUID that detects the binding of magnetic nanoparticles (such as antigens) to the target. A sample containing target agents is added to the magnetic particles in the well of the magnetic microscope and a two second measurement is made. In contrast with other techniques, such as fluorescence, unbound particles do not give a signal, thus no "wash" step to remove them is required. The prototype device at UC Berkeley detects the presence of fewer than 2000 magnetic particles. This number could translate to fewer than 100 bacteria or viruses.

Protein crystallography beamlines and associated robotics and processing software allow for rapid determination of protein structure relevant to design of protein-based assays for pathogens.[9] Such facilities exist at the LBNL's ALS,[10] Stanford's SSRL, and Argonne's APS and as well as at other synchrotron light sources worldwide. As the biotechnology industry develops the approach to rapid drug design based on crystallographic data, medical science will have a powerful tool to control and mitigate the effects of biological attacks.

Another aspect of biological characterization is genomics:[11] The Production Genomics Facility (PGF) of DOE's Joint Genome Institute (JGI) is one of the most rapid and cost effective sequencing facilities in the world. The JGI was established as a partnership of Lawrence Berkeley, Lawrence Livermore, and Los Alamos, National Laboratories to complete DOE's portion of the Human Genome Project. The PGF is essential to that effort because it combines advanced sequencing machines, robotic instrumentation, and computational resources in a high throughput production setting. While not uniquely dedicated to microbial sequencing, a portion of this established capability has been directed toward sequencing microbial pathogens considered to be potential biothreat agents and related but non-pathogenic microbial species. These sequence data on pathogens are needed for (1) identifying pathogen-specific genomic regions for DNA-based detection and diagnostic technologies, (2) deciphering the molecular mechanisms responsible for an organism's virulence, and (3) identifying genetic variations to differentiate among strains of a given pathogen. The understanding gained will be extremely valuable to researchers and agencies developing medical prophylaxis and treatment for biothreat agents and better forensics to determine genetic signatures.

CONCLUDING COMMENTS

In light of the dramatic and rapid developments in electronics, biotechnology, robotics and information technology for research and commerce, it is unlikely that defence science will keep pace with open science in the areas that are most vital to assuring infrastructure security. Applied genomics and proteomics, biotechnologies that are vital to future biodefence are developing at a rapid pace; rapid sequencing of bacteria is already available in open, government-supported and commercial laboratories. Information technology is crucial to the rapid application of developing science and technology. Data mining will be crucial in providing law enforcement and intelligence agencies early warnings dangerous groups and to provide supporting forensic information. Nanoscience and the associated technology of designer materials will permit novel imaging and spectroscopic techniques for cargo inspection, forensics, and material tagging. The bottom line is that law enforcement, intelligence and defense agencies must engage the academic and commercial worlds, if they are to be at their most effective in combating international crime and terrorism. The mode of that engagement must respect the open environment at heart of scientific creativity.

ACKNOWLEDGMENTS

I would like to acknowledge the efforts of all my colleagues who are working on the areas described in the text and especially to Prof. Ka-ngo Leung and his group in my division at LBNL for their remarkable developments in plasma-based neutron generators. I thank Jody Westby for many long discussions concerning information security in the context of the terrorist threat. I am deeply grateful to Prof. Antonino Zichichi and the staff of the Ettore Majorana Center for Scientific Culture for their hospitality during this International Seminar. This work was supported by the Office of Science of the U.S. Department of Energy under Contract No. DEAC03-76SF00098.

REFERENCES

1. The author is Director, Accelerator and Fusion Research Division and Director, Homeland Security and Non-proliferation.
2. http://eetd.lbl.gov/ea/certs/CERTS_Pubs.html#RTTools
3. http://www.lbl.gov/Tech-Transfer/collaboration/techs/lbnl1814.html and http://www.lbl.gov/nsd/annual/2001/preview/isotopes/firestone4_PGAA.pd
4 . http://accelconf.web.cern.ch/AccelConf/p95/ARTICLES/FAG/FAG14.PDF and http://www.fas.org/irp/ops/le/docs/gcip/appd.html and http://www-hoover.stanford.edu/research/ conferences/nsf02/gozani.pdf
5. http://www-phys.llnl.gov/Organization/NDivision/pdf/Detector_Summary.pdf
6. A. Pines et al., *Science*, July 6, 2001.
7. T.J Wilkinson, Dale Perry, Wayne McKinney and Michael Martin, *Physics World*, March, 2002 pp. 43.
8. Y.R. Chemla, H.L. Grossman, Y. Poon, R. McDermott, R. Stevens, M.D. Alper, and J. Clarke, *Proc. Nat. Acad. Sci.* 97(26), 14268 (2000).
9. http://www.llnl.gov/str/June02/Balhorn.html
10. http://www-als.lbl.gov/als/science/sci_archive/superbend.html
11. http://www.lbl.gov/Science-Articles/Archive/JGI-homeland-security.html

9. CONFRONTATIONS AND COUNTERMEASURES: PREVENTIVE COUNTERMEASURES

LITERATURE IS LANGUAGE STRUGGLING FOR MORE MEANING (WORDS TO HURT AND WORDS TO HEAL)

JOSEF JARAB

Palacky University, Olomouc, Czech Senate, Prague, Czech Republic

Just a biased reminder that language and literature may still essentially be one, and that poetry still matters today. At the same time, a few doubts (sneaking in) that this need not be necessarily so any more.

In her Nobel Prize acceptance speech in 1993 the African-American writer, Toni Morrison, reminded us of the fact that we people are mortals: "We die," she said, and "that may be the meaning of life." Yet then she went on saying: "But we do language. That may be the measure of our lives."

Such observation need not be considered a discovery or a revelation pertaining to the modern times; already Shakespeare's contemporary, Ben Jonson, believed that "language most shows a man," and wanting to know a person he demanded: "Speak that I may see thee!" Later, as history saw literacy grow among the populations over the centuries, simultaneously conditioning the process of democratization of societies within our civilization, the wish and desire to identify and assess individual people or individual communities would most likely include as well an inquiry after their reading which amounted to a precept, "tell me what you read and I will tell you who you are." A number of wise persons are being quoted for having said something to that effect and we may remember our teachers reminding us of this maxim in our own young years when exposed to a process called formal education.

Indeed, we have been taught, and have ourselves empirically learned a great deal about that complex phenomenon called LANGUAGE: as an instrument of communication, as a social agency, as a system, and also as a living thing. It grew with us as we grew, and it behaved and performed as a challenge when we faced the challenges of the courses of events in our personal, communal or national histories.

Personally, I found it puzzling, to say the least, that the tongue I used at home when communicating with my mother and friends was, so were we told, not good enough as a language of instruction at school, when, at the beginning of World War II, German was to replace my Silesian-Moravian Slavic dialect which I had been happy with until school-attendance age. After the war ended and we were liberated from the alien power and language, I had to first learn Czech as a system and norm before I could accept and employ it as a mother tongue, as "the blood of the soul, into which our thoughts run, and out of which they grow" to use one poet's adequate and beautiful description of language as an environment and tool of intellectual activity. (Cf., Oliver Wendell Holmes.)

During the time of adolescence, when, after the communist putch in 1948, the educational system was rigidly controlled by the authorities and free thought was straitjacketed by dogmatism, a shock of recognition was to dawn upon me and my schoolmates that language can also be exploited as a severe violator of knowledge and truth. Instead of offering a path to further learning, my own language, as officially imposed on us then at school and through media, was obviously intended to limit if not close access to "undesirable" information, to new knowledge.

It took us a while to grasp and evaluate the situation of language abuse before we started learning to read between the words and between the lines, and went on inventing our own ways of communication. Our learning about the world beyond the "iron curtain," especially through other languages, in my case English, also contributed to the enlargement of our knowledge of our own world, and of at least theoretically possible alternatives of organizing life. And after I got involved in the exciting business of translating from English, a new stage of intensive learning about my language (and world) as much as about the other language (and world) began, and I assume that it will never end.

"That everything we do and think creates, changes, destroys, or otherwise influences language is self-evident," Mario Pei, author of a skillfully and enjoyably written book *The Story of Language*, declared half a century ago. And the eminent linguist, born in Italy, educated and later settled in the United States, continued with a meaningful warning: "What is not so obvious, perhaps, is that language in return affects all our actions and thoughts." I am convinced that my own personal experience, even as sketched above, would not be an isolated confirmation of professor Pei's thoughtful words.

Here and now, however, I wonder how the language of the contemporary powerful mass media and globalizing advertisement mechanisms can and will affect the population's "actions and thoughts" in our consumer democracies. But then again, when I come across a letter that reads, "this generation is given over to the making and spending of money, and is losing the capacity of thought. It wants to be amused, and the magazines amuse it," and realize that this was written as a complaint of an American critic to an English one in 1873 I may get less skeptical. (Charles Eliot Norton to Thomas Carlyle.) Another cause for some optimism I find in my literary seminars at the university where I see the students growing very much aware of the superficiality characteristic of so much of the present "popular" and "official", i.e. populist language; and I am happily surprised that they are not just willing but truly anxious to turn to more meaningful texts, to turn to the riches of literature which "is news that STAYS news," literature which is considered classic not because someone decided so but "because of a certain eternal and irrepressible freshness," as Ezra Pound maintained.

Now I would dare join those philologists of the old days who believed that language and literature are essentially one. What both language and literature share is the permanent, or rather continued, unending, openness to new experience. "Language can never live up to life once and for all. Nor should it... Its force, its felicity is in the reach toward the ineffable," wrote Toni Morrison, and a similar statement could be offered about literature, including Ms. Morrison's own fiction, which was praised by the Swedish Academy for its "visionary force and poetic import." (One American critic and poet, Donald Hall, characterized poetry as "The Unsayable Said".)

According to Ezra Pound and many others, it is the good writers who keep the language efficient, who keep it alive and responsive. Even more it is believed they often see something the rest of the population does not immediately see and, therefore, they may serve as cthe antennae of the race." (In the recent times of darkness that ruled the Soviet-dominated world, our sensitive and brave artists were often referred to as "the conscience of the nation". What seems at present rather sad, a mere decade after the unexpected, though not unwanted, fall of communism and arrival of freedom, is the short and failing national memory of exactly this role that the writers fulfilled and performed so well. Is it uncomfortable to look into the mirror they kept offering? Do we not need any public conscience any more? One wonders. When some of the writers, then dissidents, now critically point their fingers at something disturbing them, some of our politicians are ready to call them self-appointed moralists and preachers, an accusation from which not even Václav Havel, the onetime playright and contemporary President of the country, is entirely safe.)

And it was, indeed, the words of the writers, such as Václav Havel, Czeslaw Milosz, or Anna Achmatova that was liberating people, encouraging them to the bravery of choosing "life in truth." The Czech poet Jaroslav Seifert's Nobel Prize became a political act not because of the poet's political "provocations" but because of the lyrical force of his verse which was so much at odds with the blank official language of the times. And the Czech people learned affectionately so many of his poems by heart, and thus wandered out of the prison taking a step towards liberation of their minds and souls.

The power of poetry can hardly be supported with a weightier argument than was to be found in the Soviet gulag-camp environment. Zoja Marchenko, Yelena Vladimirova and many more of the prisoners turned to writing and reciting poetry for themselves and others at the risk of being severely punished. And why? "To save our humanity, and to escape into a depth where we could not be reached by our tormentors and by the regime," as one of the luckier survivors testified.

After his heroic life-long effort to create more space for poetry in the modern world, the American beat poet and activist, Allen Ginsberg, came in his final years to the simple conclusion that "poetry's task is to reduce human suffering."

It should not be surprising if the poets themselves remind us that the Greek word *poietes* stood for "maker" or "creator," and the Latin *auctor* for someone who produces, increases, or adds to something already available. The American philosopher and poet Ralph Waldo Emerson believed that "every word was once a poem," and "language is fossil poetry." Ezra Pound, a century later, still insisted that "your language is in the care of your writers." And his friend and co-founder of the very influential "imagist" movement, the English philosopher and poet, T.E. Hulme, stated that language is born in poetry, used in prose, and dies of abuse in journalism.

If we ever shared such belief in the role of the writer, and above all the poet, do we think it still holds today? What influence do poets have at present over the users of language? Does a critical mass of those users still pay attention to what the poets do with words and what they say? "Literature, the literary work, remains incomplete until it has passed from the desk to the marketplace," wrote the ever-provocative critic Leslie Fiedler in his boook *What Was Literature?* And the very popular historian Barbara Tuchman brought up another point for our deliberations when she said that "to be a bestseller is not necessarily a measure of quality, but it *is* a measure of communication." Can and should literature classes at school pick up the task of making literature a more central topic of the learning discourse? Will posters with short poems in the Prague metro cars have some impact on the language and thought of the passengers? Etc., etc., – endless questions and queries with many more answers needed. But the very fact of asking those questions is undoubtedly relevant. Also for the health of our language, of our languages. When last year, after September 11, we heard again and again that the tragic event was "beyond words" and "beyond human imagination" were we admitting a failure of language as a means of conveying the unbelievable sight or something even more essential?

As a mere coda to my remarks – here is some verse, some poetry for specific consideration. What the three poems I have chosen have in commom is the theme of war, of fighting, of killing and/or being killed for something or nothing relevant, depending on the angle from which the reality and the poems are read. Certainly, Walt Whitman was aware that it was nothing but wishful thinking, and an attempt at magic incantation, when he recited "Away with themes of war!" suggesting that it would also mean "Away with war itself!" On the contrary, in wars, language has always been an important instrument - whatever the goal. Words are being used to arouse the killing spirit, the bravery or brutality, the justified revenge or motivated fight for some kind of interests; words are also being used to ask the reflective "why," to express one´s doubts, to seek understanding, tolerance, peace, even affection, to try to heal afflicted wounds with human empathy and compassion, with evocation of beauty.

The first poem, "If We Must Die," is a "revolutionary sonnet" by a Jamaican poet, Claude McKay – it was written in 1919 to boost the rebelling and defying spirit of the New Negro in the aftermath of World War I in Harlem. At the time of its publication, Senator Henry Cabot Lodge had its text entered into the Congressional Records as a sample of the threat coming from contemporary black America.

If we must die, let it not be like hogs
Hunted and penned in an inglorious spot,
While round us bark the mad and hungry dogs,
Making their mock at our accursed lot.

If we must die, O let us nobly die,
So that our precious blood may not be shed
In vain; then even the monsters we defy
Shall be constrained to honor us though dead!

O kinsmen! We must meet the common foe!
Though far outnumbered let us show us brave,
And for their thousand blows deal one deathblow!

What though before us lies the open grave?
Like men we'll face the murderous, cowardly pack,
Pressed to the wall, dying, but fighting back!

But the author never agreed that his poem be read as a Negro poem. He wanted it to be seen as a universal poem for all those who were "abused, outraged and murdered, whether they are minorities or nations, black or brown or yellow or white." The irony is that it worked that way. Winston Churchill used it in the British Parliament to bolster the morale of his nation during the moment of deep crisis in World War II, not mentioning, and perhaps not even knowing, the race of the author. A number of American soldiers had the text copied and carried it on them in combat on both fronts, as later records proved. All this may be rather surprising as the poem is not just universal it is also quite abstract using very general and not quite original language and imagery. And it is hardly rendered in moving personal terms. Yet, it seemed to have had a general appeal because it is universal through abstraction, and because it is built on the constantly repeated conflict of *we* against *they*, because it is a powerful battle-cry... – I can imagine that it could be appropriated by some freedom fighter or terrorist even today.

The other two poems come from Yusef Komunyakaa, another African-American and one of the most impressive poets of contemporary America. Unlike Claude McKay, he had a personal experience with war – having been a correspondent and later a soldier in Vietnam. For Komunyakaa his involvement in this war conflict is a cause for deep reflection on what the whole affair really did mean to individuals involved; above all to himself. What is grasped is the movement from innocence to experience and disillusionment. The result is not a complaint, however, but rather a lesson to be learned, and an invitation to sharing in that lesson through telling laguage, images, functional use of cliches, even "foreign" words, such as the pun-like title "Tu Do Street" (also to be read as Two Door Street). It is musical in a very spontaneous, jazzy way – and, like jazz, it really works across racial, national or other possible borders.

To Do Street

Music divides the evening.
I close my eyes & can see
men drawing lines in the dust.
America pushes through the membrane
of mist & smoke, & I'm a small boy
again in Bogalusa. White Only
signs & Hank Snow. But tonight

I walk into a place where bar girls
fade like tropical birds. When
I order a beer, the mama-san
behind the counter acts as if she
can't understand, while her eyes
skirt each white face, as Hank Williams
calls from the psychedelic jukebox.
We have played Judas where
only machine-gun fire brings us
together. Down the street
black GIs hold to their turf also.
An off-limits sign pulls me
deeper into alleys, as I look
for a softness behind these voices
wounded by their beauty & war.
Back in the bush at Dak To
& Khe Sang, we fought
the brothers of these women
we now run to hold in our arms.
There's more than a nation
inside us, as black & white
soldiers touch the same lovers
minutes apart, tasting
each other's breath,
without knowing these rooms
run into each other like tunnels
leading to the underworld.

The poem "Facing It" presents as a site and symbol the Vietnam Veterans Memorial in Washington and makes the place a painful reminder of the casualties whose names are enumerated in the stone. Like the shiny stone, the poem itself, reflects on the historical event in very complex, intimate and yet universally accessible and comprehensible human terms. And it suggests the possibility of reconciliation and redemption, namely through the uncompromising, and most likely unparalleled, effort to challenge the painful experience with words exploiting the poet´s art and ethics of the poetic creation.

Facing It

My black face fades,
hiding inside the black granite.
I said I wouldn't,
dammit: No tears.

I'm stone. I'm flesh.
My clouded reflection eyes me
like a bird of prey, the profile of night
slanted against morning. I turn
this way – the stone lets me go.
I turn that way – I'm inside
The Vietnam Veterans Memorial
again, depending on the light
to make a difference.
I go down the 58,022 names,
half-expecting to find
my own like letters like smoke.
I touch the name Andrew Johnson;
I see the booby trap's white flash.
Names shimmer on a woman's blouse
but when she walks away
the names stay on the wall.
Brushstrokes flash, a red bird's
wings cutting across my stare.
The sky. A plane in the sky.
A white vet's image floats
closer to me, then his pale eyes
look through mine. I'm a window.
He's lost his right arm
inside the stone. In the black mirror
a woman's trying to erase names:
No, she's brushing a boy's hair.

It is a very private poem, like the process of healing. It is no more *us* against *them* but a WE composed of a number of selves – that is where it all begins and ends.

PREVENTING TERRORISM – FROM REACTIVE TO PROACTIVE STRATEGIES

CHRISTOPHER DAASE
University of Kent at Canterbury, Brussels School of International Studies,
Brussels, Belgium

I have been asked to make a second presentation today in form of a short intervention, and I would like to use this privilege to talk briefly about the shift in policy that has occurred after September 11th in addressing international terrorism. In particular, I will argue that the U.S. is increasingly relying on a proactive strategy. While this is a logical consequence of the September attacks, it also implies some serious problems especially as far as prevention with military means is concerned. But let me first clarify what proactive security policy is, and, secondly, show how U.S. anti-terrorism policy has changed over time.

PROACTIVE SECURITY POLICY

During the Cold War, security policy was relatively simple. It had to react towards a known threat and to counter it either by building a credible counter-threat (through conventional weaponry or nuclear deterrence), or to reduce that threat cooperatively (through arms-control and political détente). Security policy *after* the Cold War, however, can no longer be *reactive* in this sense, but has to be more *proactive*, because the threats and challenges are manifold and uncertain. In such a situation, the goal is to reduce security risks by diminishing the probability of a loss or damage and by reducing the possible impact *before* an event can happen. Thus, a policy is proactive if decisions are taken in anticipation of future problems, needs and changes.

Proactive policy can address either the causes or the consequences of security risks, i.e. it can be preventive or precautionary. This distinction is important, because it is often mixed up. The purpose of prevention is that an averse effect does not occur; the intention of precaution is to mitigate the consequences if such an effect does occur nevertheless.

Preventive and precautionary security policy can both be either cooperative or repressive, i.e. they can rely either on political collaboration or on political and military coercion. Hence, there are four ideal-type policies how international risks and challenges can proactively be addressed (preventively by cooperation or intervention and precautionary by compensation or preparation).

The point I want to make here is that proactive security policy can have different forms. They all have their merits, but they all have also their specific problems and shortcomings. I cannot address them all here, but I will concentrate on the coercive measures to prevent averse effects, namely terrorism, since this is the direction the United States develops its foreign and security policy. In the words of President Bush: "The war on terror will not be won on the defensive. We must take the battle to the enemy, disrupt his plans, and confront the worst threats before they emerge... [O]ur security will require all Americans to be forward-looking and resolute, to be ready for pre-emptive action when necessary to defend our liberty and defend our lives."

THE TRANSFORMATION OF U.S. ANTI-TERRORISM POLICY

This is indeed a major shift in the policy to address international terrorism and in the U.S. foreign and security policy more generally. For I would argue that U.S. counter-terrorism remained by and large reactive until the September events, although at times military attacks have been employed against terrorism, notably by the Reagan and Clinton administrations.

When the Nixon administration first had to deal with international terrorism in the early seventies, it adopted a political strategy that stressed international cooperation to reduce the likelihood of future attacks. President Carter went one step further by announcing a program to address the root causes of terrorism—poverty, injustice and suppression—linking this effort to the promotion of human rights. The Islamic revolution in Iran, however, brought an end to this program compelling Carter to take a tougher stance on the terrorism issue.

Ronald Reagan then took up the antiterrorist policy where Carter had left it, but increased the rhetoric. On the ideological assumption that behind all terrorist action was a communist state sponsor, he finally ordered the first military attacks in retaliation to terrorist acts in Berlin and other places against Libya. But although the *Task Force on Combating Terrorism*, chaired by then Vice President Bush sen., proposed a proactive approach and Secretary of State George Shultz argued for a much more aggressive policy, the use of force against states sponsoring terrorism during the Cold War remained rather limited and reactive.

The same is true for the Clinton administration. Even under domestic pressure and in the face of mounting attacks, the Clinton administration remained committed to its four maxims of counterterrorism: 1.) to reduce vulnerability overseas and at home, 2.) to increase deterrence through a clear no-concessions policy, 3.) to respond to terrorist acts with all appropriate means, and 4.) to prevent the proliferation of weapons of mass destruction. Proactive was this policy only in the sense that it increased the precautionary measures, mainly by hardening soft targets like U.S. embassies abroad. The military attacks, first ordered against Iraq in 1993, then against Sudan and Afghanistan 1996 were clearly reactive and had mainly a punitive purpose. Until September 11th, then, U.S. counterterrorism, although military measures were employed from time to time, remained largely reactive.

All this has changed. The main lesson the Bush administration has drawn from the attacks of New York and Washington is that "a nation that has experienced the horrors and costs of September 11th, a nation that has experienced a taste to what catastrophic terrorism may bring in the future (...) can no longer afford the luxury of relying on strategies and tactics that allow potentially catastrophic attacks to happen and after they are over, to react to them."[1] In front of the German Bundestag, President Bush said, "If we wait for threats to fully materialize, we will have waited too long."[2]

The argument is compelling and several proactive elements will be included in the Bush Administration's first National Security Strategy later this year. What we can see so far are three things: First a new reliance on covert operations, including assassinations; secondly a new doctrine of pre-emptive action against states and terrorist groups trying to develop weapons of mass destruction; and thirdly a new tactic of "defense in depth" that stops terrorists and terrorist activities before they infiltrate into the United States.

Earlier this year, President Bush has authorized American Special Operations forces and the CIA to kill Saddam Hussein, but "only in self defense." Although Administration Officials have stressed that this order "would not waive the prohibition on assassinating a foreign leader," it is important to note that only two words, "self-defense only," separate this policy form terrorist attacks, as Hussein himself once had planned against President Bush sen., and that the meaning of those words is rather opaque.

This is not the place to go into the details of the new Department of Homeland Security and how it will not only change the government structure but also the American society. Enough is to say that it will run into international conflicts when the interception of alleged terrorists infringe on the sovereignty of foreign countries. Port inspections are here a case in point.

The most dramatic shift, however, is the emerging doctrine of pre-emptive strikes. Especially in combination with the recent Nuclear Posture Review it marks one of the biggest changes in the history of the U.S. armed forces. Bush hinted first at the new doctrine in his State of the Union address in January 2002 when he labelled Iraq, Iran and North Korea an "axis of evil" and warned that he would not tolerate them to threaten the United States with weapons of mass destruction.

But let me here point to the inherent problems of that strategy. The main problem, I have already mentioned in my previous talk. If the intention is to prevent terrorism, i.e. to stop a terrorist event, before it happens, where is the right point in the causal chain of terrorism to counteract? The logic of prevention provides not guidance, no rational limits how far back from a possible attack action should be taken.

A similar problem is the evidence that legitimises pre-emptive action. As President Bush has made clear, the U.S. does not know whether Iraq has acquired nuclear or biological weapons, but he suggests that the only prudent course is to assume it has.

The legal problem is simple by comparison. In international law there simply is no right of defensive intervention. As you know, even the notion of humanitarian intervention is controversial, but pre-emptive strikes are plainly unlawful without UN mandate. I know, international law is not a very hard currency these days. But if we want to keep a minimal international order, I suggest to think about pre-emptive strikes very

very carefully. For nothing can and will keep other nations from immediately follow the American lead and use a policy of pre-emption to their own advantage. Israel, India and China, but also North Korea and other risky states come to mind.

I am not saying, though, that states should wait until they are hit by terrorist attacks before they act. But I have pointed to other, more cooperative proactive measures against terrorism that could be employed. But what is most important, is that states and International Organizations should consider the long-term consequences of their decisions. Prevention, after all, may be better than cure; but only if prevention does not cause bigger problems that have to be cured on much higher costs later.

	Cooperative	Coercive
Preventive	Cooperation	Intervention/Preemption
Precautionary	Compensation	Preparation

REFERENCES

1. Perl, Raphael 2002.
2. *New York Times*, June 17, 2002, "Bush to Formalize a Defense Policy of Hitting First."

ROLE AND SIGNIFICANCE OF SCIENTIFIC COMPONENT IN THE STRUGGLE AGAINST TERRORISM

ASHOT A. SARKISOV
Nuclear Safety Institute, Russian Academy of Sciences, Moscow, Russia

In a long-term perspective, the actions responding to terrorism cannot be efficient without a deep involvement of the integrated scientific potential of terrorism-resisting countries. The scientific component in the anti-terrorism activities is very important, and I would like to dwell on this problem in my talk.

We are the witnesses of gradual forming of a new area of scientific knowledge directed to:

- analysis of fundamental roots of terrorism;
- analysis of the technosphere of modern civilization from the point of view of its vulnerability for terrorist actions;
- substantiation and development of measures for preventing and minimizing consequences of terrorist attacks.

This field of knowledge includes a very wide range of different scientific disciplines. Its development requires major consolidation efforts of different specialists. I do not pretend to give a complete review of all specific scientific problems in this field. I will give only some examples to illustrate topicality, scope and complexity of the scientific component in the anti-terrorism activities.

Thus, investigations of fundamental roots and nature of terrorism are of prime importance. From the scientific point of view this problem is not simple at all.

The solution of this problem could help in developing strategic recommendations for prevention or, at least, localization of terrorism at national and international levels.

To analyze safety at industrial facilities, probabilistic methods have been applied in recent years. The methods of probabilistic analysis progressed most when analyzing safety at nuclear industry facilities. The application of probabilistic approach in combination with deterministic analysis proved its high efficiency.

The experience demonstrates that the perception of accidents, catastrophes and terrorist attacks by the population and the whole society is not adequate, especially if radioactivity is involved. As a rule, the estimation of consequences of such events by the population exceeds many times the actual damage.

Well-organized monitoring over hazardous chemical and radioactive substances within territories under the control is an important factor of ensuring collective protection against terrorist attacks. The development of a concept and realization of such monitoring, the selection of territories, the development of technical means and of the whole monitoring system represent another important scientific task. Competent solution of this problem will help in mitigating the consequences of potential terrorist attacks.

Quite often, however, the consequences of terrorist attacks, as well as of technogenic catastrophes and natural disasters, are aggravated many times, because the population and the society as a whole have no relevant knowledge and are not prepared to effective and competent activities in extreme situations.

Presently educational activities among the population in the field of antiterrorism should be systematic and comprehensive.

The development of a concept of educational and information policies in the field of antiterrorism becomes an acute problem.

ADVANCES IN BIOTECHNOLOGY: SAFEGUARDING THE OPPORTUNITIES AND MANAGING THE RISKS

TERENCE TAYLOR
International Institute for Strategic Studies – U.S., Washington DC, USA

RAPIDLY ADVANCING SCIENCE AND TECHNOLOGY

Extraordinary advances in biotechnology over the past decade have brought enormous benefits to medicine, public health, the food industry, and agriculture. At the same time, the risks to public security from the misuse of this technology have increased. Government- sponsored weapons programs and possibly terrorist groups can now, if they perceived that it suited their purposes, exploit the technology to develop more efficient and destructive biological weapons. In addition, as biotechnology diffuses worldwide, the chances increase for industrial accidents through misunderstanding and inadvertent misuse of the technology. In the case of nuclear technology after 1945 it was an industrial accident at a civilian facility in 1986 in Ukraine that caused major loss of life and widespread environmental damage rather than the use the technology as a weapon.

THE PRIVATE SECTOR

Private industry, academia and other private institutions are at the leading edge of the burgeoning biotechnology industry and the dissemination of the science and technology. Any international effort to deal with biological risks to public safety and security that does not engage the private sector directly will be seriously lacking in effectiveness and ultimately unsuccessful. The relatively youthful biotechnology industry is growing rapidly. It is no longer simply the preserve of the medical sector and therapeutic drugs but rapidly extending into the agriculture and food industries and others. Its boundaries are constantly moving and, at its leading edge, biotechnology is penetrating the materials sector and even information technology. The rapid evolution of the biotechnology industry is raising a host of public safety, security, and ethics issues for the industry itself including adverse public reaction and ethical concerns about such issues as genetically modified crops and cloning. Another issue is the contribution of advancing biotechnology to the threat of enhanced biological weapons. These are also key concerns for governments, which are struggling with the need for national and international regulation of the biotechnology industry and the possible regulation of the advances in the life sciences in the face of these developments. However, the speed of advances in the life sciences is outpacing national and international attempts at legal and regulatory action.

INFORMATION TECHNOLOGY AND BIOTECHNOLOGY

The manner of the development and diffusion of the information technology (IT) industry provides some important indicators for the likely trends in the biotechnology sector. There are similar patterns such as:

- The private sector leads and is resistant to government regulation;
- Innovation and major breakthroughs derive from individuals or small groups (primarily originating from academia);
- Large industrial concerns buy in the technology and adapt it to meet their commercial requirements in their domestic operations as well as in subsidiaries in other countries;
- The technology has diffused globally defying government attempts to restrict it (e.g. the easing of controls on cryptographic technologies and computing power);
- Governments have drawn on the advances in IT in the private sector for their armed forces.

This is not an exhaustive list and these developments are not necessarily a bad thing. While there are downsides, many countries and societies have benefited from these advances. Even in the military sector, it could be argued, these advances have reduced (but not eliminated) the potential for misunderstanding and misperception through the development of better communications and surveillance capabilities. Nevertheless, there is an uneven diffusion of the technology that has led to what some describe as a "digital divide." This is mainly due to a number of countries being unable to exploit the technology for economic or political reasons, including in some cases being faced with long-running armed conflicts and other instabilities.

Despite the similarities, including what is effectively a "biological divide," in the pattern of development and diffusion in the two industries the differences are extremely important. Major ones are:

- First, while IT is bringing considerable enhancements to military capabilities, it is not a weapon itself. The misuse of the life sciences and biotechnology has the potential to produce weapons that can kill hundreds of thousands of people and wreak havoc with the environment; a true weapon of mass destruction in the wrong hands;
- Second, while IT has posed certain challenges to societies in the handling of information (such as in the areas of individual rights and privacy), the ethical issues posed by developments in biotechnology are in many ways more far-reaching in human, animal and plant biology.

GOVERNMENT AND PUBLIC CONCERNS

There are growing public and governmental concerns over developments in biotechnology, and government action and public understanding are in danger of being overwhelmed by the accelerating advances. The challenge is how to engage the private sector, including academia, to take full account of legitimate concerns about safety and security without harming innovation and inhibiting efforts to exploit the science technology for its many substantial benefits. The lessons from the failed government attempts to regulate the IT industry should be taken to heart. In many respects it is a good thing the some of the attempts at restricting the industry failed in the interest of economic benefits and individual and collective freedoms in the dissemination of information; this is an important lesson in itself.

ACTION REQUIRED

The Biological Weapons Convention

There are a number of areas in relation to concerns about the developments in biotechnology in which action can be taken that have a genuine prospect of enhancing public safety and security. First, in the government sphere it has to be recognised that efforts at developing a verification protocol for the Biological and Toxin Weapons Convention will at best bring only minor enhancements to improving safety and security. This is not to say that the Convention itself is unimportant. It is of fundamental importance to support the norm, already established in customary international law, that it is prohibited to use, develop, produce or stockpile biological weapons. The treaty is an invaluable instrument in building coalitions against those who breach this international norm.

Private Industry

A second sphere of action is that of engaging private industry. Governments have an important role to play in setting the regulatory framework for safety standards and setting the ethical boundaries. However, this is largely left to national legislation that will be varied and patchy in its nature and implementation. Private industry also has a history of escaping domestic regulation by setting up subsidiaries or engaging sub-contractors in countries where the operating environment is more liberal. This tendency highlights the necessity of engaging the biotechnology industry itself. This may be best achieved from within by exploiting its self-interest. It would be very much in the interests of the biotechnology industry to cooperate in promoting proper, safe, and ethical business practices and facilities around the world. This is a daunting challenge, since like the IT industry, much of its success derives from highly individual research and development and innovation. However, given the inherent enormous potential dangers in the technology through accident or misuse it should not be beyond the bounds of possibility to encourage some stronger form of self-regulation and co-operation with governments.

Given the way the industry is developing it would be important that such an effort should be an international one. In the leading countries in this sector there are already trade associations and, as in other industrial sectors, it is possible to conceive of an international one. The industry is inevitably going to be faced with increasing government regulation and legitimate public concerns. It would benefit greatly from co-operation internationally to gain a proper understanding of the wide variety of national legislation and regulations as well as to make an impact on any international regulation that might be being contemplated or is actively under negotiation. Also, the industry would benefit from an international exchange on safety and security measures in the operation of their facilities so that standards could be raised worldwide. Indeed, in the wake of the Chernobyl nuclear accident referred to earlier the private nuclear industry set up a World Association of Nuclear Facility Operators (WANO) with the express purpose of enhancing safe operation of their facilities. In preparation for the Year 2000 rollover, this organisation played a critical role in assuring safety at that time. There could be great benefits to industry and the public in setting up a WABO, a World Association of Biotechnology Facility Operators. In this context, given the close links between the industry and academia, the latter could play an important role in fostering such a development.

It is an extremely urgent and important matter to engage private industry effectively, and on an international scale in the effort to assure public safety and security in the field of biotechnology. A major part of this effort is best carried out by the industry itself. It is not enough to leave it to government regulation, as patterns in the development of the IT industry make clear.

Other Steps
Also needed is an approach that deals with biological challenge along the complete spectrum of public safety and security from naturally occurring diseases, re-emerging diseases, anti-biotic resistant diseases, accident or misadventure (through industrial activities or academic research) to deliberate use by a state or non-state group. In addition to engaging private (at the leading edge of diffusion of the science and technology) industry, three things need to be done:

- A truly international scientific, technological and political effort is needed to enhance the quality of epidemiological. The World Health Organisation makes an excellent effort with slender resources – but there are serious gaps, particularly in the developing world.
- A body should be created to track scientific and technical developments in the life sciences and biotechnology to help ensure the opportunities are fully and properly exploited – but also that policy makers are alerted and well informed on those areas where national and international regulation might be needed.
- More research on methods of risk analysis needs to be undertaken to assist in the decision-making and allocation of resources to meet the biological challenge.

10. SCIENCE AND TECHNOLOGY: EMERGENCIES

DO WE MAKE OURSELVES?

JÜRGEN MITTELSTRASS
Center for Philosophy of Science, University of Konstanz, Konstanz, Germany

INTRODUCTION

Since antiquity, one has distinguished, in the European tradition, between the biological and the cultural nature of Man, in other words between what is natural to him in a physical and biological sense, and what pertains to him culturally, what is his cultural essence. A question such as "Do we make ourselves?" would have to be answered affirmatively if directed at the cultural essence, and negatively if it is so at his natural one. Perhaps a slight reservation might be required with regard to the art of medicine, which in its theapeutic aims intervenes in the physical nature of Man, as for instance today in the case of a plastic surgeon, who sometimes heals and sometimes deceives, or in that of hygienic measures or fitness sports. The fundamental difference between the cultural and the natural (physical and biological) essence of Man is, however, not thereby called into question. On the contrary, it is rather confirmed, for it is a matter here of dealing with natural givens.

But this state of affairs seems today to have changed dramatically. The question "Do we make ourselves?" no longer stops at the cultural essence, the cultural nature of mankind, but is posed in the future tense, namely as the question "Will we make ourselves?" with regard to physical and biological nature. With the progress of biology and medicine, for instance in genetic technology and reproductive medicine, a new image of Man begins to form, according to which the latter makes himself in his physical and biological nature, and in which the question "Do we make ourselves?" loses its culturally restricted sense. The old question of what makes Man human becomes an open one in the light of biological and medical possibilities of intervention. And it becomes troubling in contemporary debates, in so far as one seems to think that one should answer it in a purely biological context, namely by referring it to biological facts. But whoever thinks that it can be restricted in this way does not realise what he is doing, or at the very least he loses sight of what is or at least was essential to the question of what makes Man human. Biological insights help us to understand what we are as <u>empirical</u> beings, but they do not answer the question concerning the <u>being</u> of humans.

Thus it is no surprise that discussions concerning this question turn into wars of faith instead of rationally conducted debates, above all when they are connected, as is the case today, with the question concerning the beginning of human life. This is connected in part to ideological points of view that people are reluctant to examine, but also with fears concerning scientific developments and, lastly, with simple misunderstandings. Many are apparently convinced that there must be definitive answers here, for otherwise mankind will endanger, or indeed destroy itself. The question is a legitimate one: Is this really so? Do modern biological developments actually threaten that which they seek to explain, namely the human being? And are those who support these developments actually inhumane? Philosophy and the tradition of anthropological thinking inherent to it, which concerns itself with answering the question of what Man is, thought and think otherwise. And this is also true today. Three short remarks on this topic:

1. Man is a natural being, who can live only as a cultural being and can find his purpose only as such. Descriptively, within the context of biological systematics, mankind is a sub-species of the species homo sapiens, namely homo sapiens sapiens, and thus the only recent member of the genus Homo. But this definition includes only the empirico-physical side of Man, not that which makes up the essence of humanity ascriptively, namely its form of self-description and (not conclusively established) self-determination. This latter was described classically as the animal rationale, a being endowed with and determined by reason, or as a being lying between animal and God. Newer anthropologies (after Nietzsche) capture this notion in the concept of a "*nicht festgestellten*" or "unbound" being (both biologically and culturally). One makes a category error, if one interprets our actions and thoughts as the products of natural processes, whereby even the act of interpreting becomes part of nature, a natural fact. But we fall into a new form of naiveté if we oppose to such a view the claim that scientifically discovered facts have no influence, or at least ought to have no influence on the self-determination of Man. Thus it is a matter of adopting a scientifically informed and philosophically reflected position, one which is beyond mere biologism and culturalism, which is in other words beyond an absolute distinction between biological and cultural explanations, and which refers to both the lives and the laws that we live out. Such a position should reduce mankind neither to (pure) nature nor to the (absolute) spirit he wants to be.

2. There is much to suggest that lurking in the background of the fierce debates concerning scientific progress in the context of biology, medicine and ethics (concretely: the ethical problems concerning prenatal and preimplantation diagnostics, research on embryos, and the use of stem-cells in therapeutic or even reproductive cloning), we shall find the false dichotomy between biologism and culturalism. Some see a fundamental threat to human nature in biological progress and its medical and social implications. Others descry in unscientific descriptions of the essence of humanity a new domination by the humanities and theology. What is at stake here is specifically the question of when human life begins. In fact, both positions give one the impression that the fate of the West, and of humanity itself, somehow depended on the answer to this question, and the related one concerning the point at which that which comes into being, the human, acquires human dignity.

Here again one is concerned with a question about the point in the development of the human at which it acquires its being both descriptively, in the sense of a biological systematic, and <u>ascriptively</u>, in the sense of a <u>cultural</u> systematic, which being is then to be protected by means of the concept of human dignity. The actual problem is once again that according to some, both the descriptive and ascriptive aspects coincide, so that it is biologically given when the human life to which the dignity argument refers in fact begins.

But, in a strong sense, there is no unequivocal <u>biological</u> answer to the question of when human life begins, or when exactly in the development from conception to birth we first are dealing with a human being. And because this is so there is (although not only because this is so) no unequivocal <u>ethical</u> answer either. Is a fertilised egg already a human, or does a human first come into being on fertilisation? How should one deal with gametes, that is to say with haploid egg- and sperm-cells, whose genetic fate is, under appropriate conditions, that is on fertilisation and implantation, also predetermined? What should we make of the argument that one can speak of a (developing) human being only once the central nervous system has formed? What here is description, and what is ascription, what is naturally given and what is culturally ascribed? The biologist will justifiably decline to answer, and the answers of laymen will doubtless be varied.

In other words the idea that human life begins with the fusion of the egg and sperm-cell is only one possibility of determining something like a beginning. There is, in truth, no absolute beginning, because this is neither biologically nor ethically determinable. In any case, the developing clump of cells obviously needs the mother, that is to say a symbiosis with the maternal organism, in order to develop on the pattern of a human being, which is why much speaks for regarding implantation, in other words the point at which the fertilised egg becomes implanted in the lining of the uterus, as a critical stage on the road to human development. In general, when we attempt to answer the question concerning the point of origin of a human life with recourse to the concept of <u>human dignity</u>, we do not achieve greater clarity. Doing so only distracts us from the real problems of determining biologically appropriate criteria, or, worse still, it dogmatically breaks off such efforts.

In fact the concept of human dignity is often applied in contexts where one is not yet able or willing to provide well worked-out justifications. Many people apparently take the suggestion that human dignity is at risk as a sufficient ground for ending a debate, to forbid further deliberations and to ban, among other things, research. Put otherwise, the concept of human dignity is supposed to do argumentative work, but it is not in fact able to perform that work, because it is too unspecific and because it is applied to early, at least when it is supposed to be applied to biological facts. It assumes the role of a taboo, and this in a culture that views itself as rational, that understands itself as founded on (reasoned) arguments and (verifiable) justifications. By the way, if it were in fact the case that the fertilised egg was already possessed of human dignity, then we ought really to celebrate our date of conception and not our birthday, and we would have to bury the fertilised cell with all the usual religious rituals.

Following a long anthropological tradition, we may observe that the notions of a <u>person</u> and of <u>reason</u> are central to that of human dignity. By means of the notion of a person, we try to connect ascriptively the autonomy and the identity of the human being.

That is why one speaks of <u>personal</u> <u>identity</u> and <u>personal</u> <u>autonomy</u>. By identity we mean not the empirical identity of the human being with itself, as for instance might be determined by biological traits, but rather a conception unity, namely that of a rational being. Autonomy refers to the capacity to act with self-determination, to set one's own goals and to realise them. Here the notions of person, reason and dignity are connected to one another, for instance in the impressive formulation of the categorical imperative for the determination of what Kant called the "dignity of a rational being." This formula goes: "Act so that you use the humanity either in your own person, or in that of any one else always as an end, and never merely as a means." Only the "rational being" exists as "an end in itself," which is why for Kant only rational beings have "dignity." So it is clear to Kant: Human beings are not given merely by virtue of belonging to the human species, that is to say in the context of biological systematics, but only by virtue of being bearers of reason, that is to say they first acquire dignity in light of their rationality.

So there will necessarily be difficulties in this connection if one extends the protection of the human individual from external determination, still formulated today by means of the argument from human dignity, either to the preliminary stages of a developed rational being, for instance the fertilised egg, or to later interventions in the "genetic identity" of the individual. One runs the risk of confusing yet again descriptive and ascriptive aspects, for example in those cases in which one fails to distinguish between external determination that is directed against self-determination and external determination which, as in the case of the embryo, affects entities which are not yet self-determining.

Evidence for the polemical nature and the carelessness with which the debate concerning the beginning of human life is conducted can be seen in the speed with which it is claimed that merely by considering differentiation within the notion of human dignity one is putting the human dignity of the mentally handicapped, of Alzheimer's sufferers and coma patients up for grabs. As if one could not distinguish between sick people and a fertilised egg before implantation, and as though, in a society and a legal system that successfully protects personal property, the last wishes of the deceased, and the rights of authors and of animals, we were unable to protect developing human life without immediate recourse to a concept of human dignity that brooks no objections. And such protection could be implemented in manifold ways, both at the beginning and the end of human life, in other words before both birth and death.

3. In an unpublished manuscript "On truth and lie in an extra-moral sense", Nietzsche makes the following comment: "What does Man actually know about himself? (...) Doesn't nature conceal almost everything from him, even concerning his body, in order (...) to drive him and enclose him within a proud and magical consciousness! She [nature] threw away the key." Although this remark is hardly up to date from a biological point of view, it remains quite current from the anthropological one. The human condition is still characterised by a need for self-determination, by a search for the self-determining essence of Man. And for this very reason we should not be looking for a lost key. There is no such key. Self-determination is not only the fate of the individual, but it is also the fate of humanity itself, it belongs to humanity's essence. When one overlooks

this, for instance when we search for the biological or the ideological answer, we are threatened on the one hand by biologism (Man is only a biological species) and on the other by ideological dogmatism (Man is lost in his own ideologies). And so, even in the face of a steadily growing body of biological knowledge and a biological nature that is increasingly at the disposal of that knowledge, it is still essential that Man take control, that he take reasonable control, of his own ascriptions, of his self-definition and his designs.

We could also say that it is Man, as opposed to nature or a transcendent authority, who remains the measure of things. This means, however, that he must determine a measure for himself, that he must strive against both the threat of scientisation and that of ideology. For Man has always tried to draw an image of his future perfection—as individual apotheosis or as social utopia—and has repeatedly turned from this icon in horror or in boredom. This shows that the human condition in which we describe our particular essence is in a sense not to be optimised, in that such an optimisation threatens to dissolve our condition, precisely because this condition is the essence of humanity. What would remain would be either gods or machines, and neither of these share in what makes us human - our warmth, our odour, our happiness and our pain.

This does not mean that we ought not work to change our essence, to alter that human condition that defines the space between the available and the unavailable, between happiness and pain, between god and beast. On the contrary, this is precisely our task, and this task is served both by ethics and by science, not on separate worlds, but on a single one. For not only science learns when ethics learns, in that it measures its own actions against ethical standards; but ethics also learns when science does, in that it takes account of scientific states of affairs, as in the biological-empirical essence of humanity.

LANGUAGES AT RISK

ALAIN PEYRAUBE
Directorate of Research, Ministry of Higher Education and Research, Paris, France

INTRODUCTION

There are today between 5000 and 6000 languages spoken in the world. By the end of this century, if the situation does not improve, half of them at least will be dead. More pessimistic evaluations even state that 90% of them will vanish. Some 25 languages are dying every year while new languages are very rarely emerging. Small communities of course speak most of them. 90% of the 5000 to 6000 languages are used by only 5% of the world population, 600 languages only are spoken by more than 100,000 people, and 500 of them are by less than 100 people (Hagège, 2000: 199).

As human languages are the most achieved expression of the history and the diversity of cultures, to save endangered languages is to prevent cultures from sinking into oblivion.

What is a dead language, and first of all, what is a language? No two linguists will agree on a single definition of language. We will adopt the Saussurian one: "a language (*langue*) is both a social product of the faculty of language (*langage*) and a set of necessary conventions, adopted by the society to allow the expression of that faculty by individuals" (Saussure, 1916). A dead language is a language that no longer has any speakers. Some dead languages, although no longer in general use as a means of oral communication among a people, are still used and studied, such as Latin that gave birth to eleven Romance languages (Spanish, Portuguese, Italian, French, Romanian, Galician, Catalan, Occitan, Rhaeto-Romance, Sardinian, Corsican), Classical Chinese that developed into Medieval Chinese and Modern Chinese, or Sanskrit that evolved first into several modern Indo-Aryan languages, before giving birth to several languages spoken today in North India.

However, these are exceptions. The common rule is that dead languages are extinguished, annihilated, with very little hope to be revived.

CLASSIFICATION OF WORLD LANGUAGES

Languages are usually classified into 400 to 500 language families. Some of them group a large number of languages like the Austronesian family (1200 languages), others, known as isolates, count only one language, like Basque (in Spain and France), Burushaski (in Northern Pakistan) or Ainu (in Japan). There are few languages in Europe: 88 according to the *Atlas Linguarum Europae*, divided into six families or *phyla* and 17 branches, Indo-European being one family assembling twelve branches (Contini, 2000).

Twentieth-century linguists, with a few notable exceptions, have been hostile toward all attempts to connect a linguistic family with any other linguistic family. One major counterweight to that general apathy, however, has been the work of Greenberg who, over a period of fifty years (1950-2000), classified the languages of Africa into four macro-families (Greenberg, 1963); the languages of Papua New Guinea into two macro-families (Greenberg, 1971); and the languages of the Americas in three macro-families (Greenberg, 1987). He also proposed a Eurasiatic macro-family (Greenberg, to appear), connecting Indo-European languages with other language families in Eurasia (Uralic, Altaic, etc.), recovering a former hypothesis of a Nostratic macro-family, put forward by the Dane, Pedersen (1903), and developed later by the Soviet scholars Illich-Svitych and Dolgopolsky (see Dolgopolsky 1998).

In the 1980s, Starostin proposed a family including North Caucasian, Sino-Tibetan and Yenissean, which he named Sino-Caucasian (Starostin 1989). Later, Sino-Caucasian was connected with Na-Dene, a family already proposed in the beginning of the 20th century by Sapir. This larger family is now usually called Dene-Caucasian (Ruhlen 1992, 1994).

If we accept the proposals outlined above for Eurasiatic, Amerind, and Dene-Caucasian as well as the hypothesis of an Austric macro-family (grouping Austronesian, Tai-Kadai, Miao-Yao and Austro-Asiatic) that was first proposed by Schmidt (1905), and developed later by Reid (1994) and Blust (1996), we may now classify the world's languages into the following twelve macro-families, as did Ruhlen (1997): Khoisan, Niger-Kordofanian, Nilo-Saharan, Afro-Asiatic, Kartvelian, Dravidian, Eurasiatic, Dene-Caucasian, Austric, Indo-Pacific, Australian, Amerind.

The geographical distribution is given below.

<u>Africa</u>

1. Khoisan (South Africa, Tanzania)
2. Niger-Kordofanian, a family of languages spoken in Sub-Saharan Africa, which is composed of two main branches: Kordofanian (in the South of Sudan) and Niger-Congo, with hundreds of Bantu languages (more than 400 for the sole Nigeria) like Zulu, Swahili, etc.
3. Nilo-Saharan, in the North of Central Africa and in East Africa, with a dozen sub-families such as Nilotic.
4. Afro-Asiatic, grouping Semitic (Arabic, Hebrew), Chadic (more than a hundred languages like Haussa, Bole, Ngamo, etc.), Berber (some thirty languages), Ancient Egyptian, Omotic (Kafa, Mocha, Dime, etc.), Cushitic (about 40 languages, such as Afar, Somali).

Southeast Asia and Pacific

5.   Austric is the only macro-family grouping all the languages spoken in Southeast Asia, traditionally distributed among four families:

    (i) Austro-Asiatic (grouping some 25 Munda languages spoken in Northern India, and a hundred of Mon-Khmer languages like Vietnamese and Cambodian);

    (ii) Miao-Yao or Hmong-Mien (in South China and in Vietnam);

    (iii)Tai-Kadai or Daic (circa fifty languages in Thailand, Laos, Southern China)

    (iv)Austronesian: 1200 languages spoken in Taiwan, Malaysia, Indonesia (670 languages), Philippines, Madagascar, New Zealand, Tahiti, etc. According to Blust (1997), the Austronesian language family is divided into ten branches: nine of them, grouping only 26 languages are in Taiwan, the tenth one counts more than 1100 languages spread out from Madagascar to the East of Polynesia.

Three macro-families are present in Pacific Oceania: Austronesian (belonging to Austric, see above), Indo-Pacific and Australian.

6.   Indo-Pacific: languages spoken in Papua New Guinea (there are about 800 languages in Papua New Guinea, both Indo-Pacific and Austronesian).

7.   Australian: still 200 or so languages spoken in Australia.

Americas

Following Greenberg (1987), the indigenous languages of the Americas are to be classified into just three families: Eskimo-Aleut, Na-Dene, and Amerind. Only one of them, the last one, is a macro-family, and is still quite controversial now. The other two are components of other macro-families: Eurasiatic for the first one, Dene-Caucasian for the second one (see below).

8.   Amerind, a macro-family that can de divided into eleven sub-families and comprises: in North and Central America, Algonquian (c. 35 languages), Salishan (23 languages), Siouan (c. 20 languages), Uto-Aztecan (c. 35 languages), Mayan (31 languages), Otomanguean (c. 40 languages), Penutian, etc.; in South America, Arawakan (c. 65 languages), Cariban (c. 60 languages) Chibchan (c. 20 languages), Tupian (c. 60 languages), Quechua, etc.

More than two hundred indigenous languages are spoken in Mexico, as well as in Brazil.

Eurasia

The four remaining macro-families ate located in Eurasia.

9. Dravidian (in South India): no more than 25 languages like Tamil (the most important one) or Brahoui.
10. Kartvelian or South Caucasian (only four languages in Georgia).
11. Eurasiatic. The Eurasiatic macro-family is also much debated. It includes:

- Indo-European family, with almost twenty different branches, such as Anatolian, Tocharian, Albanian, Hellenic, Armenian, Germanic languages (English, German, Icelandic, Swedish, etc.), Celtic languages (Cornish, Welsh, Irish Gaelic, etc.), Italic (including Romance languages as outlined above), Balto-Slavic (Lithuanian, Polish, Czech, Slovene, Bulgarian, Russian, etc.), Indo-Iranian (Persian, Kurdish, Pashto, Hindi, Bengali, etc.), etc.
- Uralic, with its two branches of Finno-Ugric (some twenty-five languages like Finnish, Estonian, Hungarian, Ostyak, Lapp, etc.), and of Samoyed.
- Altaic family, with its three subfamilies, Turkic, Mongolian, Tungusic-Mandchu.
- Korean, Japanese, and Ainu.
- Gilyak (Nivkh), an isolate spoken in Kamchatka (Russia)
- Chukchi-Kamchatkan, languages spoken in North and East Siberia.
- Eskimo-Aleut, in Alaska, in Greenland.

What are the differences between Nostratic and Eurasiatic? Both groupings include Indo-European, Uralic, Altaic, and Korean, but Eurasiatic adds to these Japanese, Ainu, Gilyak, Chukchi-Kamchatkan, and Eskimo-Aleut, while Nostratic adds Afro-Asiatic, Kartvelian, and Dravidian.

12. Dene-Caucasian, another controversial macro-family, including, according to Starostin (1989), Bengston (1991) and Ruhlen (1992), the following families:

- Basque, an isolate spoken in Northeast Spain and Southwest France,
- Burushaski, an isolate spoken in the mountains of North Pakistan,
- (North) Caucasian: some thirty to thirty-five languages, such as Chechen,
- Yenissean, with only one living language, Ket, spoken in Central Siberia.
- Sino-Tibetan, some 300 languages traditionally grouped in two branches called Tibeto-Burman (more than 200 languages, such as Tibetan, Burmese, Lolo, Jingpo, etc.) and Sinitic languages, divided into seven groups (Northern Chinese, Wu, Min, Hakka, Yue, Xiang, and Gan).
- Na-Dene, a family identified by Sapir (1915), including some 35 Althabaskan languages in North America and other languages spoken in the Southern coast of Alaska).

Those twelve macro-families hypotheses postulating remote relationships such as Amerind, Eurasiatic, Dene-Caucasian and Austric have been rejected by a majority of mainstream historical linguists. However, they have been partially confirmed by human geneticists interested in the classification of populations. Starting in the 1980's, the geneticists found that the biological classification of human species parallels the linguistic classifications in macro-families quite closely as they have been proposed by the American and Russian "unifiers". See Greenberg *et al.* (1986) for New World populations, Excoffier *et al.* (1987) for Sub-Saharan Africa, Sokal *et al.* (1988) and Barbujani *et al.* (1990) for Europe, Poloni *et al.* (1997) for several populations in Africa and Europe, and mostly Cavalli-Sforza *et al.* (1988) who have built a tree of genetic distance for forty-two human populations from different continents.

The question then arises whether the twelve macro-families are really independent, with no visible connections. During the past decade, the question of monogenesis of human language, which has been a linguistic taboo during the most part of the 20th century, has once again arisen in the works of scholars who have gone beyond the myth of well established families (like Indo-European, Austronesian, etc.) independence. Thus, some scholars are now working on even longer "long-range comparisons" and try to connect Eurasiatic and Dene-Caucasian, or Austric and Dene-Caucasian, allowing the question of monogenesis to be broached. All languages of the world could then be affiliated to only one Proto-World-Language, the "mother language" of all humans, descending from TMRC "the most recent common ancestor", dated by Underhill *et al.* (2000) to 140,000-40,000 years ago. But this is another problem outside of the scope of the present paper.

MECHANISMS AND MOTIVATIONS OF LANGUAGE DEATH

The mechanisms of language death are known. Languages die through transformation, substitution, or extinction. This last process is, of course, the most worrying. It is less worrying if a single language, before being extinct, is diversified into several languages, or is replaced by a newly created language.

Single languages may indeed be transformed into several new languages. This has been the case of Vulgate Latin that gave rise to eleven Romance languages, the case of Buddhist Sanskrit and of Pr_kr_t that developed, through various complicated stages, into several languages spoken today in North India.

Creole languages offer many instances of language substitution by the creation of new languages. See below.

The main motivations of language death are also known. They have little to do with linguistics. Languages never perish through decay due to internal processes of change leading to some type of deterioration. The motivations are either physical or political.

Physical causes may be of different kinds: natural disasters, genocide, epidemics, forced migrations. As an instance of natural disaster, one can cite the elimination of the entire Tambora population (and therefore the language they spoke) in 1815, in the Sumbawa island, located in the small Sonde islands in the Indonesian archipelago, between Java and Timor, after a big volcanic eruption.

Genocide of languages, through the genocide of the populations speaking them, is infrequent, but we nonetheless know of several cases, like the annihilation in 1226 of the Xixia or Tangut people – and consequently of their language that was a Tibeto-Burman language – in Western China, by the Mongolians of Genghis Khan.

Smallpox and syphilis decimated several Australian aboriginal' populations and their languages were lost.

Political causes include cases of languages that have been immolated on the altar of States. Well-known examples are the disappearance of hundreds of languages brought by the Spanish colonization to Central and South America, the English colonization in North America (disappearance of Dutch in the states of Delaware and New Jersey, of French in Maine). In some cases, however, the invaders have been linguistically invaded. This is the case of the Franks who did not impose their Celtic language on the Gaulo-Romans they conquered, or of the Mandchus who ruled China between 1644 and 1911 and were completely sinicized.

Another cause, which is of purely linguistic nature, could be the absence of script. Actually, languages that have scripts are more likely to be able to resist than languages without script. But this is not always true. The Xixia and the Mandchus, mentioned above, had scripts, but were nevertheless destroyed by the Mongolians and Chinese.

ASSESSMENT

Languages proliferated until the 16th century. Then the decline began, obviously linked to European expansion and domination. Great concentrations of endangered languages are now - with a few exceptions like the USA, Australia, or Russia - in the less developed regions of the world, especially in the twenty-two countries where a large amount of languages are spoken (Krauss 1992).

Nine of these countries have more than 200 languages: Papua New Guinea (c. 800), Indonesia (670), Nigeria (410), India (380), Cameroon (270), Mexico (240), Congo Democratic Republic (210), Australia (c. 200), and Brazil (c. 200). See below for slight different figures given by international political administrators. Thirteen other countries have each between 100 and 160 languages. They are, by decreasing numbers of languages: The Philippines, Russia, USA, Malaysia, China, Sudan, Tanzania, Ethiopia, Chad, Vanuatu, Central African Republic, Burma, and Nepal.

As a result, 200 languages at least are dying in Africa, and entire families or even macro-families like the Khoisan macro-family are also endangered. In Southeast Asia, languages like Muong, Palaung, Khmu, Bahnar in Vietnam and Laos will probably die soon. Having a very few speakers, these languages are nonetheless very important, as they proved that Vietnamese undoubtedly belongs to the Austro-Asiatic family, in spite of sharing with Chinese (a Sino-Tibetan language) tones, monosyllabicity, and many common lexical items. In Indonesia, 52 languages out of 670 are very endangered, as they have less than 200 speakers. 121 of them having between 200 and 1000 speakers might also be considered as endangered.

The highest risks of extinction of languages are in Papua New Guinea, which is also the region of the world where languages are the most numerous. 130 languages, out of 800, are there spoken by less than 200 people. 290 of them have between 200 and 1000 speakers.

In Australia, the devastation has been rapid and violent. Two hundred years ago, between one and two million aborigines spoke more than 250 languages. Fifty of them died after the arrival of the European colonies, and out of the remaining 200, 150 are in danger today. There are only five to ten languages (according to different, divergent sources) that are spoken by more than 1000 people.

The indigenous languages of Brazil and Mexico are also threatened. In North America (including Alaska), there were only 213 languages forty years ago (Chafe, 1962), out of some 700 that existed in the 16th century. There are less than 200 today; we know of precise instances of languages that died a couple of decades ago, like Cupeño (the last speaker, 94 years old, died in 1987 in Pala, California).

The figures given by the "Program of the United Nations for Environment" at the Nairobi Conference in February 2001, in which seventy Ministers of Environment participated, are about the same or even more pessimistic. There are approximately 5000-7000 languages in the World languages. It is estimated that 90% of them will disappear before the end of the 21st century. 2500 languages are immediately endangered. 32% of these endangered languages are located in Asia, 30% in Africa, 19% in Pacific, 15% in the Americas and 3% in Europe.

The Conference report also provided a list of countries that are especially threatened, with a number of languages spoken in these countries: Papuan New Guinea (847 languages), Indonesia (655), Nigeria (376), India (309), Australia (261), Mexico (230), Cameroon (201), Brazil (185), Congo Democratic Republic (158), and Philippines (153).

One might think that there are language revivals, or newly created languages that could thwart the tendency of language death. Hebrew is actually a well-known case of a language that was revived, by Ben Yehuda, after a lengthy sleep of several centuries. Cornish is another instance of a language revival. Belonging, with Welsh and Breton, to the Brythonic branch of Celtic languages (a subfamily of Indo-European), Cornish was a victim of the Reform in the 16th century and declined considerably before being almost extinguishing about 1800. The Celtic revival in the Romantic and post-Romantic periods in all aspects of culture has been beneficial to the Cornish language.

Esperanto, invented by Zamenhof, a native of North Poland, is a case of a new creation of an artificial language heavily influenced by the properties of existing languages (Latin, Romance and Balto-Slavic languages). Creoles, though transformed from pidgins, are also new creations that replace other indigenous languages. Pidgins usually arise when adult speakers of different languages are brought together and forced to develop a means of communication at least for basic purposes. Canonical examples are the development of pidgins among African slaves and European owners and overseers on

Caribbean plantations. Creoles in the broadest sense are native languages that arise on the basis of a pidgin situation, i.e. where children are exposed to a pidgin in their community and are forced to develop a native language on the basis of that pidgin.

Creoles, as well as pidgins, might indeed be considered as acute solutions found by human communities for maintaining oral communication, which is one of the most vital activities of all societies.

However, revivals are exceptional, and new creations truly marginal. In any case, they cannot match the vanishing of languages, undertaken at such a large scale.

CONCLUSION

A comparison with other living species, either zoological or botanical, might be instructive. The rate of vanishing living species is today one thousand to ten thousand more than it was during the biggest geological periods of extinction. The motivations are also known: intensive agriculture, massive and systematic deforestation, urbanization and globalization. As a result, a large number of the 1,650,000 present species are endangered, either vertebrates (some 45,000), invertebrates (990,000 invertebrates), or plants (360,000).

One should also be aware that out of 4400 mammal species and out of 8600 birds species, respectively 326 (i.e. 7.4%) and 231 (i.e. 2.7%) are endangered (Hagège, 2000: 230). If the extinction rate continues as it is today, 25% of animal species will have vanished before 2025, and 50% before 2100. The proportion is about the same as the one we have given for languages.

There is however a big difference. It is not inconceivable today that the tendency, if not reversed, will decline. The rate might well slow down. The main reason is that powerful international associations, more than forty of them are now sponsored by United Nations, are willing to fight to protect endangered species.

Thus, it might be also be possible to slow down the rate of language death. This could be done through international associations. In fact, when large actions are undertaken, they are generally successful, as exemplified by the revival of Maori in New Zealand in the past few years.

Today it is an urgency, a planetary emergency.

Linguists should also mobilize and urgently explore all unknown languages that are endangered. If this is not done, linguistics will be the only scientific discipline that let 50% to 90% of the material on which it is based vanish.

REFERENCES

1.   Barbujani, G. and R. Sokal (1990). "Zones of Sharp Genetic Change in Europe are also Linguistic Boundaries," *Proceedings of the National Academy of Science* 87:1816-1819.
2.   Bengston, J.D. (1991). "Notes on Sino-caucasian," V. Shevoroshkin ed., *Dene-Sino-Caucasian languages*. Bochum:Studienverlag Brockmeyer.

3. Blust, R. (1996). "Beyond the Austronesian Homeland: The Austric Hypothesis and its Implications for Archaeology," W. Goodenough ed., *Prehistoric Settlement of the Pacific*. Philadelphia: American Philosophical Society. pp. 117-140.

4. Blust, R. (1997). "Subgrouping of the AN Languages: Consensus and Controversies." Paper delivered at the *8th International Conference on Austronesian Linguistics*. Taipei, Taiwan.

5. Cavalli-Sforza, L.L., A. Piazza, P. Menozzi, and J. Mountain (1988). "Reconstruction of Human Evolution: Bringing together Genetic, Archaeological and Linguistic Data," *Proccedings of the National Academy of Sciences* 85:6002-6006.

6. Chafe, W.L. (1962). "Estimates Regarding the Present Speakers of North American Indian Languages," *International Journal of American Linguistics* 28:162-171.

7. Contini, M. (2000). "Vers une nouvelle linguistique historique: l'ouvrage de Mario Alinei, *Origini delle lingue d'Europa*," *Dialectologia et Geolinguistica* 2000-8:13-35.

8. Dolgopolsky, A. (1998). *The Nostratic Macrofamily and Linguistic Paleontology*. Cambridge:McDonald Institute for Archaeological Research.

9. Excoffier, L, B. Pelligrini, A. Sanchez-Mazas, C. Simon, and A. Langaney (1987). "Genetic and History of Sub-Saharan Africa," *Yearbook of Physical Anthropology* 30:151-194.

10. Greenberg, J.H (1963). *Languages of Africa*. Bloomington:Indiana Research Center in Anthropology.

11. Greenberg, J.H. (1971). "The Indo-Pacific Hypothesis," T.A. Sebeok ed., *Current Trends in Linguistics, Vol. 8*. The Hague:Mouton. pp. 807-871.

12. Greenberg, J.H. (1987). *Languages in Americas*. Stanford:Stanford University Press.

13. Greenberg, J.H. (to appear). *Indo-European and Its Closest Relatives: The Eurasiatic Language Family*. Stanford:Stanford University Press.

14. Greenberg, J.H., C. Turner, and S. Zegura (1986). "The Settlement of the Americas: A comparison of the Linguistic, Dental, and Genetic Evidence," *Current Anthropology* 27:477-497.

15. Hagège, C. (2000). *Halte à la mort des langues*. Paris:Odile Jacob.

16. Krauss, M. (1992). "The World's Languages in Crisis," *Language* 68-1:4-10.

17. Pedersen, H.L (1903). "Türkische Lautgesetze," *Zeitschrift der Deutschen Morgenländischen Gessellschaft* 57:533-561.

18. Poloni, E.S., O. Semino, G. Passarino, A. Santachiara-Benerecetti, I. Dupanloup, A. Langaney, and L. Excoffier (1997). "Human Genetic Affinities for Y Chromosome P49a,f/Taql Haplotypes show Strong Correspondance with Linguistics," *American Journal of Human Genetics* 61:1015-1035.

19. Reid, L. (1994). "Morphological evidence for Austric," *Oceanic linguistics* 33-2:323-344.

20. Ruhlen, M. (1992). "An overview of genetic classification," J.A. Hawkins et M. Gell-Mann eds., *The Evolution of human Languages*. Redwood City (CA:Addison-Wesley Publishing Company. pp. 159-189.

21. Ruhlen, M. (1994). *On the Origins of Languages: Studies in Linguistic Taxonomy*. Stanford:Stanford University Press.

22. Ruhlen, M. (1997). *L'origine des langues*. Paris:Belin.

23. Sapir, E. (1915). "The Na-Dene languages. A Preliminary Report," *American Antrhopologist* 17:534-558.

24. Saussure, F. de (1916). *Cours de linguistique générale*. Genève.

25. Schmidt, W. (1905). *Grundzüge einer Lautlehreder der Mon-khmer Sprachen*.

26. Sokal, R.R., N. Oden, and B. Thomson (1988). "Genetic Changes Across Language Boundaries in Europe," *American Journal of Physical Antrhopology* 76:337-361.

27. Starostin, S. (1989). "Nostratic and Sino-Caucasian", V. Shevoroshkin ed., *Explorations in Language Macrofamilies*. Bochum: Studienverlag Dr. Brockmeyer. pp. 42-66.

28. Underhill, P.A., P. Shen, A. Lin, L. Jin, G. Passarino, W. Yang, E. Kauffman, B. Bonné-Tamir, P. Bertrandpetit, P. Francalacci, M. Ibrahim, T. Jenkins, J. Kidd, Q. Mehdi, M. Seielstad, R. Wells, A. Piazza, R. Davis, M. Feldman, L. Cavalli-Sforza and P. Oefner (2000), "Y-chromosome Sequence Variation and the History of Human Populations," *Nature Genetics* 26:358-361.

EUROPEAN SCIENCE IN A KNOWLEDGE-BASED WORLD (RISKS IN A WIDENING EUROPE IN A NARROWING WORLD)

NORBERT KROO
Hungarian Academy of Sciences, Budapest, Hungary

Knowledge has a growing significance worldwide, inclusive of Central and East European (CEE) countries. Scientific and technological knowledge are part of this knowledge base. They are associated with risks and uncertainties of different character. At the same time uncertainties and risks are interrelated.

Public attitudes to risks and the level of their acceptance are critical issues in modern societies and enhance the significance of science-society relations.

Simple simulations of societal behaviour, based on statistical physical calculations, show the significance of external parameters as, for example, the level of information in a crowd of individuals.

The possible solution of existing problems needs multidisciplinary approaches. The importance of precautionary research is also emphasized.

Finally some of the special problems of CEE countries are listed with reference to possible solutions.

The world is narrowing, called by other terms globalization. As a parallel process the significance of knowledge is increasing. From the five main pillars of economies, namely labour, materials, energy, capital and knowledge, the latter has more and more weight. Parallel with the narrowing of the world, Europe is experiencing another process, namely enlargement. It is expected that this process will bring some benefits but not without risks.

Where is the place of science in this general picture? Scientific knowledge is part of the general knowledge pool, playing not only the role of satisfying human curiosity but providing the potential basis of future technologies. The current technologies have a tendency to run out. If we want further development, new technologies are needed which will be based on new ideas, expected mainly from (basic) research. Bio-, nano- and information sciences are perhaps the most important fields which already have a strengthening engineering character and each of them could be the source of at least one revolution, similar to the industrial revolution of the 19th Century. But these revolutions may happen simultaneously.

SCIENCE OF THE 21ST CENTURY

The new science of the 21st Century is different in style than that of the 20th Century as summarised in Table I and has a changing sequence of priorities as shown in Table II.

Where is the place of Europe in this scene? The limited competitiveness of European industry, in spite of a strong (basic) research is often called the European innovation paradox. It is hoped that the European Research Area concept, accompanied by some other measures will lift this paradox. The enlargement process may also contribute to the solution of this problem in spite of the fact that the process has significant costs and bears some risks. But inherently science is a stabilising instrument, it is co-operative and at the same time competitive, with healthy rivalry which is the driving force of development.

As far as Central and East Europe (CEE) is concerned, changes in the scientific structure were introduced earlier than in other fields. There is, unfortunately, a significant gap between the EU and the CEE but there are even larger differences within the CEE countries. These countries had to solve two problems simultaneously, while following global changes as indicated in Tables I. and II. They had to adapt their research structure, financing, etc. to European standards. Changes, however, go together with risks and risks are also correlated with uncertainties.

SCIENCE, RISKS, UNCERTAINTIES

Science and technology have some inherent risks for S and T itself (e.g. radiation hazards, anthrax, etc) and risks for society (e.g. nuclear energy, cloning, genetically modified food, etc.).

But there are also major risks such as the military use of S and T results (nuclear, biological, chemical weapons), terrorism or industrial mismanagement (e.g. cyanide poisoning of sweet water).

How can scientific uncertainties be managed, or uncertainties of general character be managed by scientific methods?

Risk management is nothing else but balancing risks and rewards. For hard sciences risks can be objectively measured, for social sciences they are "culturally constructed". Therefore the treatment is also different in the two cases. Risks may be categorized. Some of them, such as driving a car, are directly perceptible, others are perceived through science (e.g. infectious diseases) while virtual risks are characteristic of issues that scientists do not know, or cannot agree upon (e.g. Creutzfeld-Jacob Disease, suspected carcinogens, etc.)

In the public eye risks are perceived largely on a subjective basis. Significant risks are played down and insignificant ones over-emphasized. Therefore one role of science might be to help by introducing objective measures.

A "Richter Scale" of risks can e.g. be introduced in the R=10+log P form where P is the probability of the event ever occurring at all. For a certain event R=10, for a comet colliding into the Earth R=0,1 and most of human activities with uncertain outcome (gambling, warefare, business) are in the 9<R<10 range. To use radioactive isotopes in medicine is not a serious risk since R~5 for growing a tumour in 20 years on the basis of present practices. On the other hand selling tobacco should be banned since R~7,2 for contracting the same illness within one year, if 10 cigarettes are smoked daily. The sale of alcohol should also be restricted to 1 unit/day in order to keep R<5.

On the basis of quantifying risks science has been effective in reducing uncertainties but less effective in managing them. It has the capacity to render visible dangers which were previously invisible but it will never have all the answers to any issue raised.

Risks and uncertainty

On the frontiers of science we do not always know what will happen. This is often unbelievable for the public since science in schools deals with certainties. But we are surrounded by uncertainties in which only probabilistic statements can be made. The probabilistic statement, however, does not mean that there is a lack of understanding or that it is something beyond the frontiers of present knowledge.

This means that scientific advice to policy-makers can also be only probabilistic. That is, that there is always some risk behind the advice. And people only accept risks easily if they have the illusion of control (e.g. car driving) but reject them (e.g. perceived risks of radiation) even if their probability is vastly lower.

Public attitudes to risks can, however, be influenced (e.g. by the proper wording). "Magnetic resonance imaging" in medicine is accepted but would probably have been rejected if the original "nuclear magnetic resonance" terminology had been used. That is why genetically modified food is rejected although "natural" modification has been a long time praxis.

PHYSICS OF SOCIETY

The statistical (probabilistic) approach in physics stirred debate in spite of the success of the kinetic theory of gases (Maxwell). But the statistical approach started in sociology. Chance and randomness in the world of people and politics seem to have laws of their own. This led to the study of society on a scientific (quantitative) basis as, for example, the use of demographic data or the (Gaussian) distribution of cases.

This experience helped to convince the community of natural scientists (physicists) that statistical mechanics gives an objective description of nature and later the understanding of the statistical nature of quantum mechanics. But in this latter case the unknown has to be replaced by the unknowable.

In recent times the opposite tendency has been observed. Methods of statistical physics are extended to the social sciences. The movement of pedestrians on a crowded street, the crisis of panic situations, etc. can be modelled, but economic processes may also be described by this means.

THE NEED FOR MULTIDISCIPLINARY APPROACHES

Science (but also society, economy, and the environment) is facing complicated problems which can be solved only on the basis of a multidisciplinary approach. Systems contain gradients, which produce the driving forces of development but at the same time produce tensions. Therefore balancing actions are needed. These issues are familiar is natural sciences and contribute to a sort of self-confidence among scientists.

In this situation there is the temptation for science to advocate instead of advise. This should be avoided. Science should not be made more political but rather politics should be made more scientific, (e.g. in connection with nuclear power, genetically modified food, chemicals added to food, etc.). This may imply the need for balance between different interest groups and even between different groups of scientists. And science has the responsibility not for the decision, but for giving several options (possibly with probabilities) together with the consequences for each case to the decision-makers.

Scientific authority should not be put at risk in this process. Science is anyway already feared because of some possible applications and of a new perception of risks involved in research itself. The explanation of this attitude lies in:

- changing context of the production of knowledge;
- declining amount of public money for research and the competition for it;
- the weakening borders between
  - science and technology,
  - research and applications, and
  - knowledge and actions;
- the increasing pressure on scientist's codes of behaviour and scientific ethics, and finally;
- the image of science (as driven by scientific curiosity) is clouded.

The effect of this situation on science is a new scepticism toward science, and a more critical attitude of society toward it.

This phenomenon has to be analysed not only for the sake of science but first of all in the interest of the society. One of the actions to be taken is to carry on precautionary research. This needs permanent questioning of what is done (inclusive ethical, societal, political, i.e. non-scientific considerations). And the responsibility, associated with scientific work, has been born continuously in our mind. And what if scientific opinion is requested in cases when no proof exists yet, but may arise in the future? A trial and error approach may be useful in such cases with corrections whenever possible. But personal judgement, controlled speculation in order to reduce the degree of uncertainty may also be useful.

Positive precaution means that risks should be considered together with potential benefits of S and T advance. And as far as uncertainty is concerned, it begins only when we are unable to attribute numerical values to the elements of risk to allow probability calculations.

Early warning and quick response are also part of this issue. In situations of crisis quick decisions are needed. This puts pressure on science for quick advice. This is not a simple issue since systems are of growing complexity. We have a large quantity of information, which is frequently mixed with uncontrollable rumours and even hysteria.

Critical analysis of recent crises for early warning, the study of correlation between different elements of events, a detailed S and T reference system or an existing network of well informed centres of excellence may ease the fulfilment of the above demand. Training courses and simulations may also be used as special tools.

A FEW SPECIALITIES OF CENTRAL AND EAST EUROPE

In addition to what has been said above, CEE countries face some special problems too. Their recent past can be characterised by the neglect of quality in products and services, of environmental issues and of high tech industry.

They faced distortions of their institutional and social structures and autarchism rooted in isolation from the outside world. People were taught to be successful only at the expense of others and grew up with a permanent enemy image.

The last decade resulted in fast and enormous changes and such processes are characterised by large fluctuations. And large fluctuations result in higher risks.

These negative features are, however, partly compensated by traditional feelings of appreciation for knowledge, first of all scientific excellence, and by a strong societal drive for the solution of existing problems and for integration into the family of the European Union.

SUMMARY

There are two basic problems mankind is facing, namely:

- the fast S and T development with societal attitudes lagging strongly behind and,
- a growing overpopulation with large geographical, economical and social gradients.

Some solutions can be recommended to ease these problems, such as:

- education;
- efforts to decrease economical and societal gaps;
- teaching of modern agricultural and industrial technologies along with the involvement of (basic) research in developing countries;
- protection of the natural environment;
- the practice of effective birth control which can be realized only if the number of citizens is not the source of strength of a particular country (see the USA);
- decreased energy consumption.

Science has to play a significant role in the solution of the above mentioned problems by modelling, risk analysis and management, by decreasing the uncertainties, driving precautionary research, and further by training in research and by education.

Europe with its traditions and strength in research may play a decisive role in coming years in solving these problems for mankind.

Table 1. Changing Character of Research.

20th Century	21st Century
• Problems raised and solved by the scientific community • Disciplinary approach • Knowledge production community homogeneous • Hierarchic and continuous • Quality control based on peer review • Emphasis on individual creativity	• Knowledge production is basically motivated by applications • Inter- and multidisciplinary approach • Knowledge production community heterogeneous • Multiple and intertwined • Societal and economical accountability and related quality control • Increasing role of collective creativity

Table 2. Science of the 21st Century.

1. The 21st Century will be the time for profound changes in research. Instead of being divided and separated it will continue toward cross-disciplinary integration with strengthened problem solving character.
2. The 21st Century will be a Century of global co-operation and competition.
3. The 21st Century will be a Century when science and technology will advance by leaps and bounds leading us into knowledge based societies.
4. The 21st Century will be the age of information, based on highly sophisticated information technologies.
5. The 21st Century will be a Century of life sciences based on molecular, developmental and neuro-biology.
6. The 21st Century will be a Century of new materials and advanced manufacturing techniques.
7. The 21st Century will be the age of extended exploration of space, ocean and deeps inside the Earth.
8. There are chances of an age of broad co-ordination among individuals, society and natural environment. Control of energy and material consumption, protection of the environment, animal and plant diversity, increase of the weight of renewable energy resources will be the basis of the survival of mankind and its cultural and technical achievements.

11. SCIENCE AND TECHNOLOGY: POLLUTION

EXPOSURE TO VERY LOW DOSES OF ENDOCRINE DISRUPTING CHEMICALS (EDCs) DURING FETAL LIFE PERMANENTLY ALTERS BRAIN DEVELOPMENT AND BEHAVIOR IN ANIMALS AND HUMANS

STEFANO PARMIGIANI

Dipartimento di Biologia Evolutiva e Funzionale, Parma University, Parma, Italy

FREDERICK S. VOM SAAL

Division of Biological Sciences, University of Missouri-Columbia, Columbia, MO, USA

PAOLA PALANZA

Dipartimento di Biologia Evolutiva e Funzionale, Parma University, Parma, Italy

THEO COLBORN

Wildlife and Contaminants Program, World Wildlife Fund, Washington, DC, USA

ABSTRACT

Only recently has it been discovered that chemicals in commerce previously thought to be safe have the capacity to disrupt the functioning of the endocrine system at very low doses that are within the range of exposure of humans and wildlife. These chemicals pose the greatest threat when exposure occurs prior to birth or hatching, when irreversible damage to developing organs can occur due to endocrine disruption. Appropriate methods of testing for endocrine disrupting effects are needed in order to have a science-based process of assessing the risk to humans and wildlife posed by these chemicals. New approaches to testing chemicals for endocrine disrupting effects should thus include exposure during critical developmental windows of vulnerability and examination into adulthood or middle age, when the adverse consequences of developmental exposure may become apparent as functional deficits and disease. Of particular concern is the evidence from epidemiological studies of a loss of IQ and changes in social interactions in children exposed to endocrine disrupting chemicals via exposure by their mothers prior to and during pregnancy. These findings have been confirmed in controlled laboratory animal studies. Using an ethological approach to study the long-term effects of fetal exposure to the pesticide, methoxychlor, we have shown that permanent changes in neurobehavioral development, exploratory activity and aggression occurred. Traditional toxicological tests had led to the conclusion that the very low dose of methoxychlor we tested was safe for humans and animals. The widespread use of endocrine disrupting chemicals, as well as atmospheric and oceanic transport of persistent endocrine disrupting chemicals, makes this an issue of concern for the entire world.

INTRODUCTION

Development of the brain and other components of the neuroendocrine system is regulated by genes whose expression is, in turn, regulated by endocrine (hormonal) signaling molecules that are referred to as paracrine compounds (acting within the tissue without being transported by blood) or classical endocrine compounds (produced in one tissue, transported in blood, and acting on cells in another tissue). It is well established that normal brain development in males and females requires the precise amount and timing of release of 3 critical classes of endocrine signaling compounds: the thyroid hormones (primarily triiodothyronine), androgens (primarily testosterone) and estrogens (primarily estradiol) (Ottinger et al., 2002).

It has also now been established that there are chemicals in household products and other industrial products and by-products that can disrupt thyroid hormones, androgens and estrogens, and thus interfere with normal development of the brain and other organ systems (Colborn et al., 1993; Colborn et al., 1998). These environmental chemicals are referred to as endocrine disruptors. Endocrine disrupting chemicals (EDCs) have been defined by a United States Environmental Protection Agency (U.S. EPA) panel as: "An exogenous substance that changes endocrine function and causes adverse effects at the level of the organism, its progeny, and of populations of organisms" (EDSTAC, 1998). A list of some of the chemicals in commerce for which there is evidence of endocrine disruption is presented in Table 1.

The neuroendocrine–gonadal axis regulates the developmental organization and adult expression of behaviors critical for survival and reproduction, such as exploration, competitive aggression, sexual and parental behaviors (Palanza et al., 1999). From an evolutionary viewpoint the "normal" development and subsequent expression of these behaviors determines the reproductive success (i.e. fitness) of the individual.

Neurobehavioral alterations induced by EDCs are especially problematic during fetal development when genes and the intrauterine hormonal milieu orchestrate the ontogeny of male and female traits. Disruption of the normal processes of masculinization of males and feminization of females may undermine the survival and fitness of exposed individuals, and might also destabilize populations (Parmigiani et al., 1998).

Table 1. List of some chemicals for which there is evidence of endocrine disrupting and reproductive effects. From: Colborn et al., 1993.

ENDOCRINE DISRUPTING CHEMICALS

HERBICIDES	INSECTICIDES	INDUSTRIAL CHEMICALS
2,4,-D	Aldicarb	Bisphenol - A
2,4,5,-T	beta-HCH	Polycarbonates
Alachlor	Carbaryl	- dimethacrylate (BPADM)
Amitrole	Chlordane	Butylhydroxyanisole (BHA)
Atrazine	Chlordecone	Cadmium
Metribuzin	DBCP	Chloro- & Bromo-diphenyl ether
Nitrofen	Dicofol	Dioxin (2,3,7,8-TCDD)
Trifluralin	Dieldrin	Furans
	DDT and metabolites	Lead
FUNGICIDES	DDE	Manganese
Benomyl	Endosulfan	Methyl mercury
Ethylene thiourea	Heptachlor / H-epoxide	Nonylphenol
Fenarimol	Lindane (gamma-HCH)	Octylphenol
Hexachlorobenzene	Malathion	PCBs
Mancozeb	Methomyl	Pentachlorophenol
Maneb	Methoxychlor	Penta- to Nonylphenols
Metiram - complex	Oxychlordane	p-tert-Pentylphenol
Tri-butyl-tin	Parathion	Phthalates
Vinclozolin	Synthetic pyrethroids	Styrene
Zineb	Transnonachlor	
Ziram	Toxaphene	

The issue we will discuss, damage to the developing brain due to endocrine disrupting chemicals in the environment, is very important for the future of humans and wildlife. We will review research with wildlife, laboratory animals and humans showing that fetal exposure to EDCs results in a decrease in intelligence and capacity to learn, a decrease in the ability to cope with stress, and alterations in social and exploratory behaviors. In animal studies, these changes are associated with effects of EDCs on brain neurochemistry. The capacity to solve future planetary emergencies could be undermined by exposure to environmental pollutants that result in brain damage, abnormal behavior and a decrease in intellectual potential in our children, grandchildren and future generations. For how ironic would it be if we were to devote all our resources to combating terrorism in an effort to ensure peace and stabilize international relations while, at the same time, ignoring the evidence that environmental chemicals are disrupting brain development.

ASSESSMENT OF SAFETY AND DETECTION OF ENDOCRINE DISRUPTING
CHEMICALS REQUIRES NEW TOXICOLOGICAL TESTS

There is now consensus that prior methods of testing chemicals have been inadequate to
detect adverse effects of the type now known to be caused by chemicals that are
classified as endocrine disruptors (EDSTAC, 1998). Indeed, the recognition of the
inadequacy of current information about health effects of endocrine disrupting chemicals
led the United States congress to mandate in the 1996 reauthorizations of the Food
Quality Protection Act and the Safe Drinking Water Act that the US-EPA establish new
methods of testing chemicals for endocrine disrupting effects. A similar process of trying
to establish a new set of screens and tests for endocrine disrupting chemicals is ongoing in
Europe and Japan through the Organization for Economic Cooperation and Development
(OECD).

One goal of these panels, which have representatives from government agencies,
chemical corporations, non-governmental organizations and academia, is to set priorities
regarding which chemicals to test first. This can only be accomplished once there is
agreement concerning the new screens and tests that will identify which chemicals in
commerce are endocrine disruptors. Of the approximately 87,000 chemicals that are
registered, perhaps 55,000 are actually in use, and of these, approximately 3,000 are listed
as "high volume" chemicals, which are produced at greater than one million pounds per
year.

A major problem associated with human studies of effects of fetal exposure to
endocrine disruptors is the very long period of postnatal development required to reach
maturity. There have thus only been a few longitudinal studies that have tracked cohorts
beginning prior to birth, which will be reviewed below. There is a desperate need for more
information concerning exposure to specific endocrine disruptors during fetal life, and the
relationship between exposure levels and developmental abnormalities and adverse
outcomes not apparent until after adulthood is reached. An estrogenic pharmaceutical,
diethylstilbestrol (DES) provides a human model for specific damage associated with
exposure during fetal life. Millions of women were prescribed this drug beginning in the
1940s through the early 1970s, until its use during pregnancy was restricted. Longitudinal
studies of the offspring of women who took this drug (a prototypical endocrine
disruptor) during pregnancy clearly demonstrated in humans, and subsequently in
laboratory animals that outcomes of developmental exposure to endocrine disrupting
chemicals can be markedly different from the effects of the chemical on adults (Newbold,
1995; Swan et al., 2001). When exposure occurs after organogenesis is completed, the
adverse effects caused by developmental exposure are not seen. For example, all registered
cases of vaginal cancer in women with documented prenatal DES exposure were first
exposed before week twenty of pregnancy, and there is a significant inverse relationship
between the prenatal day of first exposure to DES and risk of genital tract changes in both
humans and rodents. Adults did not show these adverse effects associated with the use of
DES (Johnson et al., 1979; Newbold, 1995; Newbold et al., 1998).

In order to resolve the many questions that have arisen since the phenomenon of endocrine disruption was first introduced, it is necessary to use animal models with much shorter life cycles than humans to predict harm from developmental exposure to endocrine disruptors. Evidence suggests that society cannot wait one or two more generations using long-term epidemiology studies to determine the extent of endocrine disruption on human development and survival. In regard to using animal models, it is important to take into consideration that there has been a high degree of conservation of the genetic and endocrine control systems that regulate developmental processes over the 300-million years of vertebrate evolution (Gilbert, 1999; Baker, 2001; Thornton, 2001). The endocrine systems across genera and species are very similar at the mechanistic level.

For a long time, endocrine disrupting chemicals were overlooked because they do not cause chromosomal damage, and they do not result in mutations, which is what much of traditional toxicology was designed to detect. However, EDCs do interfere with the ability of genes to be activated to engage in transcription, and in so doing, unfortunately, EDCs disrupt development and thus the future functioning of organs.

Of considerable interest is the mechanism(s) by which hormones and chemicals that mimic hormones permanently alter cellular functions when exposure occurs during organogenesis in fetal life. One mechanism that is generating considerable interest is the epigenetic modification of DNA by addition of methyl groups to specific bases located in the promoter region of genes. DNA methylation consists of the covalent addition of methyl groups to the 5-position of cytosines that are 5-prime to guanine nucleotides in the DNA sequence. CpG dinucleotide sequences can occur as clusters in regions known as CpG islands (Gardiner-Garden et al., 1987), which are normally protected from DNA methylation. When methylation occurs at these normally protected sites, there are changes in the chromosome structure and the capacity for the gene controlled by the promoter to be activated.

Methylation of CpG sites occurs in cancer, where the loss of the normal protection against methylation within regions of DNA that control gene expression results in the silencing of critical genes required for the control of the cell cycle (Lyn-Cook et al., 1995; Yan et al., 2000). Thus, a clear adverse outcome of abnormal methylation of genes is the disruption of genes that produce critical factors in cell cycle progression, growth regulation and in tumor suppression. Methylation of such genes acts in a manner analogous to a classical genetic mutation and results in the lack of a functional protein product. The result can be a subsequent breakdown in homeostasis, producing functional changes that could easily be missed in short-term tests for acute toxicity in adults or in vitro tests for classical gene mutations involving changes in base sequences (Jost et al., 1993; Larid et al., 1994). Thus, current toxicological testing methods would not reveal this type of functional damage.

BIOACCUMULATION: PERSISTENT ORGANIC POLLUTANTS THAT ARE ALSO EDCs

In establishing priorities for concern with specific classes of EDCs, the chemicals that persist after release into the environment and that build up in the body and thus can remain in human or animal tissues for years or decades have received the most attention. International concern with these persistent organic pollutants (POPs) led the UN to vote to phase out 12 POPs referred to as "the dirty dozen" (Table 2). There is atmospheric and oceanic current transport, as well as transport through trade and commerce of persistent EDCs, with the result that these chemicals are present in wildlife tissue from the Arctic to the Antarctic, far from the environments into which the chemicals were released. Thus, exposure to these pollutants is a global problem, as opposed to being of concern only to those living in "hot spots:" environments into which these chemicals are directly released (NRC, 1999).

Table 2. The "dirty dozen" persistent organic pollutants (POPs) that were identified by the United Nations as needing to be phased out of production over the next decade.

Pesticides	Industrial Chemicals
DDT	Dioxins
Chlordane	PCBs
Heptachlor	Furans
Hexachlorobenzene	
Aldrin	
Dieldrin	
Endrin	
Mirex	
Toxaphine	

Other EDCs do not bioaccumulate in tissue but are constantly present in the products people have become dependent upon, such as plastic food and beverage containers, building materials, toys and medical equipment (for example, blood storage bags). They range from industrial chemicals to pesticides, plastics, perfumes and cosmetics. Most people do not realize the extent of their exposure to synthetic chemicals in their homes and the workplace.

EVIDENCE FOR NEUROBEHAVIORAL EFFECTS DUE TO FETAL EXPOSURE TO EDCs IN HUMANS

A number of studies has revealed that exposure to EDCs during fetal life via the mother can affect her offspring's future ability to learn, to socially integrate, to fend off disease, and to reproduce. At a prior workshop held in Erice at the E. Majorana Center for Scientific Culture to address this issue, a group of international experts unanimously agreed that chemicals of this nature can change the character of human societies or destabilize wildlife populations without society realizing what is happening. With the following statement they made it clear that future generations are at risk if we do not address the threat caused by EDCs.

We are certain of the following:

Endocrine-disrupting chemicals can undermine neurological and behavioral development and subsequent potential of individuals exposed in the womb or, in fish, amphibians, reptiles, and birds, the egg. This loss of potential in humans and wildlife is expressed as behavioral and physical abnormalities. It may be expressed as reduced intellectual capacity and social adaptability, as impaired responsiveness to environmental demands, or in a variety of other functional guises. Widespread loss of this nature can change the character of human societies or destabilize wildlife populations. Because profound economic and social consequences emerge from small shifts in functional potential at the population level, it is imperative to monitor levels of contaminants in humans, animals, and the environment that are associated with disruption of the nervous and endocrine systems and reduce their production and release (Statement, 1998).

Studies have now confirmed that prenatal exposure to a group of widely dispersed industrial chemicals, such as PCBs, dioxins, and similar chlorinated compounds, can undermine human neuromuscular and neurological development that can be detected at birth (NRC, 1999). Moreover, as the affected children matured, they exhibited short-term memory problems and behavioral problems: they were often difficult to calm down in unpleasant situations. In one study, the more highly exposed children's average reduction in IQ at age 11 was 6 points, with some of the children more than two years behind in reading and school performance. These deficits were significantly related to levels of PCBs detected in maternal and fetal blood (collected from the umbilical cord) at the time of birth, whereas blood levels of PCBs in the offspring after birth did not correlate with these deficits (Jacobson et al., 1996).

In another independent study 10 years later with another cohort of children, researchers found the same problems, but they also found that the affected children cried more, laughed less, expressed more fear, and again, did not habituate well to changes in their environment. Children troubled in this manner have difficulty getting along with their classmates and families (Lonky et al., 1996). It has also been reported that monkeys exposed to PCBs *in utero* and during lactation exhibit impaired ability to perform spatial reversal learning tasks and spatial alternation tasks, and deficits in cognitive function that may last for years (Schantz et al., 1989).

A paper recently published in the American Journal of Public Health raises questions about the possible greater vulnerability of males to neurodevelopmental problems. In this study, approximately 13% of the enrollment in the 4th and 5th grades in a North Carolina, U.S. county were taking prescription drugs for ADHD (attention deficit hyperactivity disorder). When boys and girls were compared, ADHD was reported in 15% of the boys versus 5% of the girls. From the results of this study, the authors feel that the problem of ADHD is generally underreported (Rowland et al., 2002).

Taken together, these findings demonstrate the importance of longitudinal studies where exposure to EDCs is determined during critical periods in organ development and individuals are followed postnatally to determine the consequences of prenatal (in mammals) or pre-hatching (in birds) exposure. This is a critical point, since a number of studies have examined levels of a few chemicals in blood at or close to the time of diagnosis of breast cancer in women (Wolff et al., 1995; vom Saal et al., 1998). Surprisingly, the chemicals chosen for analysis in these studies had already been shown to have anti-hormonal activity (the chemicals would thus be predicted to have a protective rather than an inducing effect on breast cancer). It is thus not unexpected that most of these studies have not shown a relationship between blood levels of these chemicals in the women following their diagnosis of breast cancer. For diseases, such as breast cancer, that may require years or decades between an initiating event and detection, longitudinal studies need to be conducted that address the issue of chemical exposure throughout the lifetime. It is also important to note that only recently have attempts been made to simultaneously measure more than one or two chemicals in epidemiological studies seeking to relate EDCs and adverse outcomes.

EFFECTS OF ENDOCRINE DISRUPTORS ON WILDLIFE

There is a substantial literature documenting effects of EDCs in wildlife populations. One of the best-known study sites is Lake Apopka in the State of Florida in the USA. A chemical spill in 1980 has resulted in long-term effects apparent over many generations. Newborn alligators still show significant damage to reproductive organs even though levels of pollutants in the lake are now very low (Guillette et al., 1996). Effects of EDCs on avian brain, behavior, and reproductive systems have also been reported in wildlife and in follow-up studies in the laboratory (Fox et al., 1978; Fry et al., 1987; Fry et al., 1987; Ottinger et al., 2002). The extensive loss among Forster's terns chicks exposed in the egg to PCBs was in part associated with lack of parental care (Kubiak et al., 1989).

Humans can mate and produce offspring during any season throughout the year, and so the exposure for vulnerable human subpopulations is spread out over 12 months. But many wildlife species, because of their shorter gestation periods and seasonal breeding, limit their critical exposure period to one season, the springtime. And in the case of some avian species that reach sexual maturity within a year, almost all of the females, or half the population, will be producing offspring during a short period of time. If the adult animals are exposed to endocrine disrupting chemicals prior to or on their breeding grounds, this would lead to a clustering of health problems that should be identified in the offspring produced during that breeding season. This is why it was among bird species like terns and gulls nesting in large colonies that the problem of endocrine disruption and the passing of chemicals from one generation to the next was first discovered by wildlife biologists (Colborn et al., 1990; Colborn et al., 1992). These findings then led to epidemiological studies in humans.

In humans, the very long time to sexual maturity plays a role in disguising what happens as a result of contaminant exposure during fetal life (Fig. 1). However, as the second and third generations of humans that were exposed to EDCs during fetal life mature (exposures began in the 1940s after the onset of the post WWII chemical revolution), one could expect to see measurable impacts at the population level of the kind detected in the neurobehavioral study reviewed above conducted by the Jacobsons (Jacobson et al., 1996).

1920s-30s	PCBs and DDT released
1940a-WWII	First wide-scale exposure to man-made chemicals
1940s-50s	First generation exposed post-natally
1950s-70s	First generation born that was exposed in the womb
1970s-90s	First generation born that was exposed in the womb reached reproductive age
1980s-present	Second generation born that was exposed in the womb

Fig. 1. Chronology of Human Exposure.

AN ETHOTOXICOLOGICAL ANALYSIS OF EFFECTS OF THE PESTICIDE METHOXYCHLOR IN MICE

What follows is research that comes from the laboratories of Stefano Parmigiani and Paola Palanza, which provides a bridge between behavioral studies conducted in the ethological tradition and toxicology, with the focus being on administration of endocrine disrupting chemicals (within the range of humans exposure) during critical periods in prenatal development.

Traditionally, behavioral testing in toxicology has consisted of studying animals in laboratory situations that were not relevant to the expression of the behavior being examined in "real-life" situations. In toxicology, the animals were often used as tools to detect perturbations in behavior in response to exposure to a chemical. For example, a monkey might have been strapped into a chair and subjected to some sort of stress while being allowed to bite at a ball as an index of aggression, with the behavior of control (no chemical exposure) and exposed animals being compared. However, in this type of study, it is not appropriate to try and use the animal's behavior to predict whether aggression between monkeys in their natural habitats might be influenced by exposure to the test chemical.

An alternative approach is based on the field of ethology (the evolutionary study of behavior). The ethological approach provides a framework for integrating a functional perspective (i.e. adaptive significance) to toxicological studies. At the Erice meeting in 1995, this type of testing was defined for the effects of toxic chemicals on development and adult expression of behavior as ethotoxicology: *an evolutionary approach to behavioral toxicology* (Parmigiani et al., 1998). Impaired behavioral responsiveness to environmental demands expressed as reduced social adaptation may be a consequence of fetal and/or postnatal exposure to endocrine disrupting chemicals. In the following studies this evolutionary approach was applied to the study of behavior.

The house mouse *(Mus musculus domesticus)* can be used with the ethotoxicological approach to understand more general principles of actions of endocrine disruptors on animals in different taxa (Palanza et al., 1999; Palanza et al., 2001; Palanza et al., 2002). Swiss albino outbred stocks of mice (CD-1) were used in these studies, because they are very similar to wild mice in their social behaviors. The assumption is thus that research findings from laboratory studies can be applied to predict effects of chemicals in other species, including humans, who cannot be subjected to experimental studies. As described above, this is plausible since, at the mechanistic level, with regard to the development of physiological and neurochemical systems, there has been a high degree of conservation throughout vertebrate evolution.

The effects of fetal exposure to the pesticide methoxychlor were investigated using doses previously thought to be safe for both animals and humans, based on toxicological methods now recognized to be inadequate for detecting endocrine disruption (ATSDR, 1994). Methoxychlor is currently used as an insecticide on pets, in home gardens, and on crops and livestock. Methoxychlor is an interesting chemical that has been shown to bind to estrogen receptors and mimic the action of estrogen. In addition, methoxychlor binds to androgen receptors and blocks endogenous androgen (testosterone or dihydrotestosterone) from being able to activate responses; during development this blocks normal masculinization in exposed males. Methoxychlor is thus an estrogen and an anti-androgen (Gray et al., 1999). There is also evidence that methoxychlor acts through other, as yet unidentified, mechanisms (Ghosh et al., 1999).

The effects of exposure to methoxychlor were examined during fetal life on the subsequent neurobehavioral development and socio-sexual behaviors of male and female house mice. Social and nonsocial behaviors sensitive to the action of gonadal hormones were observed. In particular, the key systems under investigation were those behaviors critical for survival and reproduction (for example, maternal behavior, aggression and exploration) whose expression is modulated by the neuroendocrine system and that were shaped by evolutionary processes to maximize fitness.

In social species, such as house mice, an important consequence of aggression between members of the same sex is the regulation of the density of animals, leading to an appropriate spacing of competitive males as well as competitive females. Since sex steroids play a critical role in regulating the development of the neural areas mediating aggression (vom Saal, 1989), as well as the expression of aggression in adulthood (in species that have the genetic predisposition for aggressiveness), environmental chemicals that interfere with the normal actions of sex steroids have the potential to alter levels of aggressiveness and other territorial behaviors, such as urine marking of the environment, in exposed animals (vom Saal et al., 1995). The assumption in these studies is that if environmental chemicals alter aggressiveness or other socio-sexual behaviors, there will be changes in social interactions, which will be reflected by changes in population dynamics (Parmigiani et al., 1989).

The analysis of male aggressive behavior at different ages and in different contexts has shown that prenatal exposure to methoxychlor and another pesticide, DDT, can alter the developmental trajectories of aggression (Palanza et al., 1999; Palanza et al., 2001; Palanza et al., 2002). Specifically, the data show that aggressive behavior of the peri-adolescent male house mouse was altered after prenatal exposure to a 20 µg/kg/day dose of methoxychlor, which was previously thought to be at least 100-times lower than a dose that would cause any harm (ATSDR, 1994). Specifically, around the time of puberty, methoxychlor-exposed male mice showed a decreased frequency of aggressive interactions and a longer latency to attack another male. With increasing age, this effect was attenuated, but was still observed in young adulthood. However, a territorial aggression test conducted in adulthood (Resident–intruder test) did not significantly differ in relation to the prenatal treatment. These findings suggest interference by methoxychlor with the normal masculinization process in males. This is consistent with developmental exposure to a chemical with both estrogenic and anti-androgenic activity (vom Saal, 1989).

EFFECT OF METHOXYCHLOR ON BRAIN RECEPTORS FOR THE NEUROTRANSMITTER DOPAMINE AND EXPLORATORY ACTIVITY

Neurons that use dopamine as a neurotransmitter (the dopaminergic neural system) in the caudate and the putamen regions of the corpus striatum, are involved in the control of locomotor activity, exploration and novelty-induced behavior. This system also influences the expression of social-sexual interactions, such as different types of aggressive interactions and maternal behaviors.

The primary reason for examining methoxychlor in this study is that it can mimic the action of estrogen rather than because of its other modes of actions. The most potent endogenous estrogen, estradiol, can induce permanent effects in specific brain regions in synaptic formation, dendritic length, the distribution patterns of serotonergic and dopaminergic fibers, the density of receptor for these neurotransmitters, and neuronal connectivity (Matsumoto, 1991; McEwen et al., 1999). A first objective was to analyze developmental trajectories (i.e., testing animals at different ages and for different behavioral endpoints). For example, early ontogeny is considered a markedly plastic and crucial stage in the organization and regulation of future behavioral responses. In particular, weaning is an important developmental stage when mice begin to show a marked increase in exploration of the surrounding environment. It has been proposed that hormone levels during fetal life influence novelty seeking and exploratory behavior, with males exposed to elevated levels of estrogen and the lowest levels of androgen having the greatest tendency to leave the home territory and colonize new environments (vom Saal, 1984). Our hypothesis here was that exposure during fetal life to the estrogenic and anti-androgenic activity of methoxychlor would result in animals with an increased tendency to seek novelty and explore new environments.

The corpus striatum region of the brain that integrates neuromuscular and behavioral information was also examined for effects of methoxychlor on dopamine receptors (Morellini et al., in preparation). A loss of dopamine function in the neurons interconnecting the corpus striatum and substantia nigra (in the midbrain) of humans is the cause of Parkinson's disease.

Pregnant mice were administered methoxychlor (20, 200 or 2000 µg/kg/day) or no chemical (controls). The 20 µg/kg/day dose of methoxychlor was included since it is considered to be a "safe" amount for humans to be exposed to per day by the US-EPA. In order to measure the degree to which the offspring engaged in exploration of a new environment, free-exploratory paradigms, where the animals have the opportunity to choose between a novel and a familiar compartment were used (Griebel et al., 1993; Palanza et al., 2002). The behavior of animals exposed to novel situations results from a competition between an exploratory tendency (novelty seeking, curiosity) and a withdrawal tendency (fear). Within a week after weaning, peri-pubertal males and females exposed to the 20 µg/kg/day dose of methoxychlor showed an increase in exploration of a novel environment, with the greatest effect on females' exploratory behavior (Palanza et al., 1999; Palanza et al., 2002).

When examined in adulthood, control mice showed the expected sex differences in locomotor and exploratory behavior, as well as dopamine receptors in the caudate and putamen regions of the corpus striatum (Morellini et al., in preparation). Subsequent to being tested for their behavior, these adult control and methoxychlor-exposed males and females were sacrificed. Through a receptor autoradiography study, different sub-types of dopamine receptors (D1-like, D-2 like and DAT) were analyzed in the caudate and putamen. The number and the affinity of the receptors were calculated from the binding curves.

The control males were more active and had lower D1-like receptors in the caudate-putamen than the control females. Methoxychlor-exposed females (20 µg/kg/day) showed a male-like profile on these measures (Morellini et al., in preparation). There was thus interference with the normal prenatal development of sex differences due to exposure to an environmentally relevant dose of methoxychlor. Prenatal exposure to low doses of methoxychlor previously thought to produce no effects and to be safe for animals and humans produced increased reactivity to novelty, particularly in females, at different developmental stages and in different experimental paradigms. This effect could be due to a non-specific increase of locomotor activity, a decrease in anxiety in response to novelty, or an increase of novelty seeking. Furthermore, an increased reactivity to novel environments could also explain the previously observed increase in urine marking behavior observed in male mice prenatally exposed to low doses of methoxychlor.

CONCLUSIONS

The threat to the health of future generations of wildlife and humans posed by EDCs needs to be addressed immediately. Endocrine disrupting chemicals have the capacity to interfere with brain development, to significantly reduce intellectual potential, and thus to potentially destabilize populations. This is a global threat that can only be solved by fully understanding the complex effects of EDCs and eliminating the use of chemicals at the international level when warranted based on scientific findings.

To address this problem, we need a science-based research agenda ensuring that prior to chemicals being introduced into commerce, adequate health effects studies are conducted. And to achieve this goal there needs to be a set of validated and standardized assays to detect endocrine disrupting chemicals among those chemicals already in commerce as well as new products being developed.

We propose that until currently used "stealth" chemicals (now assumed to be safe) are removed from commerce, it will be impossible to achieve world peace. These endocrine disrupting chemicals have the potential to disrupt the development of the brain of individuals who would otherwise have been the future great thinkers and leaders.

ACKNOWLEDGMENTS

Support was provided to the authors by grants from: the National Institute of Environmental Health Science, NIH (ES11283) to FSvS, The Winslow Foundation to TC, and the Italian Ministry of University and Scientific Research (MURST-COFIN2000), the University of Parma and the National Council for Research (CNR) to SP and PP.

REFERENCES

1.   ATSDR (1994). *Toxicological profile for Methoxychlor*. Atlanta, Agency for Toxic Substances and Disease Registry, U.S. Department of Health and Human Services.

2.   Baker, M. E. (2001). "Adrenal and sex steroid receptor evolution: Environmental implications." *J. Mol. Endo.* 26:119-125.

3.   Colborn, T. and Clement, C. (1992*). Chemically-induced alterations in sexual and functional development: The wildlife/human connection.* Princeton, Princeton Scientific Publishing Inc.

4.   Colborn, T., Davidson, A., Green, S.N., Hodge, R.A., Jackson, C.I. and Liroff, R.A. (1990). *Great Lakes, Great Legacy?* Washington, DC, The Conservation Foundation.

5.   Colborn, T., Smolen, M.J. and Rolland, R. (1998). "Environmental neurotoxic effects: The search for new protocols in functional teratology." *Tox. Ind. Health* 14:9-23.

6.   Colborn, T., vom Saal, F.S. and Soto, A.M. (1993). "Developmental effects of endocrine-disrupting chemicals in wildlife and humans." *Environ. Health Perspect.* 101:378-84.

7.   EDSTAC (1998). *Endocrine Disruptor Screening and Testing Advisory Committee (EDSTAC) Final Report*. Washington, D. C., US Environmental Protection Agency.

8.   Fox, G.A., Gilman, A.P., Peakall, D.B. and Anderka, F.W. (1978). "Behavioral abnormalities of nesting Lake Ontario herring gulls." *J. Wildlife Manag.* 42:477-483.

9.   Fry, D.M. and Toone, C.K. (1987). "DDT-induced feminization of gull embryos." *Science* 213:922-924.

10.   Fry, D.M., Toone, C.K., Speich, S.M. and Peard, R.J. (1987). "Sex ratio skew and breeding patterns of gulls: demographic and toxicological considerations." *Stud.*

Avian Biol. 10:26-43.

11. Gardiner-Garden, M. and Frommer, M. (1987). "CpG Islands in vertebrate genomes." *J. Molec. Biol.* 196:261-282.

12. Ghosh, D., Taylor, J.A., Green, J.A. and Lubahn, D.B. (1999). "Methoxychlor stimulates estrogen-responsive messenger ribonucleic acids in mouse uterus through a non-estrogen receptor (non-ER) alpha and non-ER beta mechanism." *Endocrinol.* 140:3526-3533.

13. Gilbert, S. (1999). *Developmental Biology.* New York, Sinaur Press.

14. Gray, L.E., Ostby, J., Cooper, R.L. and Kelce, W.R. (1999). "The estrogenic and antiandrogenic pesticide methoxychlor alters the reproductive tract and behavior without affecting pituitary size or LH and prolactin secretion in male rats." *Toxicol. Ind. Health* 15:37-47.

15. Griebel, G., Belzung, C., Misslin, R. and Vogel, E. (1993). "The free-exploratory paradigm: an effective method for measuring neophobic behaviour in mice and testing potential neophobia-reducing drugs." *Behav. Pharmacol.* 4:637-644.

16. Guillette, J., Louis J., Pickford, D.B., Crain, D.A., Rooney, A. A. and Percival, H.F. (1996). "Reduction in penis size and plasma testosterone concentrations in juvenile alligators living in a contaminated environment." *Gen. Comp. Endocrinol.* 101:32-42.

17. Jacobson, J.L. and Jacobson, S.W. (1996). "Intellectual impairment in children exposed to polychlorinated biphenyls in utero." *N. Engl. J. Med.* 335:783-789.

18. Johnson, L.D., Driscoll, S.G., Hertig, A.T., Cole, P.T. and Nickerson, R.J. (1979). "Vaginal adenosis in stillborns and neonates exposed to diethylstilbestrol and steroidal estrogens and progestins." *Obstet. Gynecol. Surv.* 34:845-6.

19. Jost, J.P. and Saluz, H.P., Eds. (1993). *DNA Methylation: Molecular Biology and Biological Significance.* Basel, Birkhauser Verlag.

20. Kubiak, T.J., Harris, H.J., Smith, L.M., Schwartz, T.R., Stalling, D.L., Trick, J.A., Sileo, L., Doucherty, D.E. and Erdman, T.C. (1989). "Microcontaminants and reprodcutive impairment of the Forster's tern on Green Bay, Lake Michigan-1983." *Arch. Environ. Contam. Toxicol.* 18:706-727.

21. Larid, P.W. and Jaenisch, R. (1994). "DNA methylation and cancer." *Hum. Mol. Genet.* 3:1487-1495.

22. Lonky, E., Reihman, J., Darvill, T., Mather, J. and Daly, H. (1996). "Neonatal behavioral assessment scale performance in humans influenced by maternal consumption of environmentally contaminated Lake Ontario fish." *J. Great Lakes Res.* 22:198-212.

23. Lyn-Cook, B.D., Blann, E., Payne, P.W., Bo, J., Sheehan, D.M. and Medlock, K.L. (1995). "Methylation profile and amplification of proto-oncogenes in rat pancreas induced with phytoestrogens." *Proc. Soc. Exp. Biol. Med.* 208:116-119.

24. Matsumoto, A. (1991). "Synaptogenic action of sex steroids in developing and adult neuroendocrine brain." *Psychoneuroendocrinol.* 16:25-40.

25. McEwen, B.S. and Alves, S.E. (1999)." Estrogen actions in the central nervous system." *Endocr. Rev.* 20:279-307.

26. Newbold, R. (1995). "Cellular and molecular effects of developmental exposure to diethylstilbestrol: implications for other environmental estrogens." *Environ. Health Perspect.* 103:83-7.

27. Newbold, R.R., Hanson, R., Jefferson, W.N., Bullock, B.C., Haseman, J. and McLachlan, J.A. (1998). "Increased tumors but uncompromised fertility in the female descendants of mice exposed developmentally to diethylstilbestrol." *Carcinogenesis* 19:1655-63.

28. NRC (1999). *Hormonally Active Agents in the Environment.* Washington, D.C., National Academy Press.

29. Ottinger, M.A. and vom Saal, F.S. (2002). "Impact of Environmental Endocrine Disruptors on Sexual Differentiation in Birds and Mammals." *Hormones, Brain and Behavior.* D. Pfaff. New York, Academic Press. 325-383.

30. Palanza, P., Morellini, F., Parmigiani, S. and vom Saal, F. (2002). "Ethological methods to assess the impact of estrogenic endocrine disruptors on behavior: a study with methoxychlor." *Neurotoxicol. Teratol.* 24:56-67.

31. Palanza, P., Morellini, F., Parmigiani, S. and vom Saal, F.S. (1999). "Prenatal exposure to endocrine disrupting chemicals: Effects on behavioral development." *Neurosci. Biobeh.* Rev. 23:1011-1027.

32. Palanza, P., Parmigiani, S., Huifen Liu, H. and vom Saal, F.S. (1999). "Prenatal exposure to low doses of the estrogenic chemicals diethylstilbestrol and o,p' DDT alters aggressive behavior of male and female house mice." *Pharmacol. Biochem. Behav.* 64:665-672.

33. Palanza, P., Parmigiani, S. and vom Saal, F.S. (2001). "Effects of prenatal exposure to the estrogenic chemicals diethystilbestrol, o,p'-DDT and methoxichlor on neuro-behavioral development in the House mouse." *Horm. Behav.* 40:252-265.

34. Parmigiani, S., Brain, P.F. and Palanza, P. (1989). "Ethoexperimental analysis of different forms of intraspecific aggression in the house mouse." *Ethoexperimental Approaches to the Study of Behavior.* R. Blanchard, Brain, P., Blanchard, D. and Parmigiani, S. Dordrecht, Kluwer Academic Pub. 418-431.

35. Parmigiani, S., Palanza, P. and vom Saal, F.S. (1998). "Ethotoxicology: an evolutionary approach to the study of environmental endocrine-disrupting chemicals." *Toxicol. Ind. Health* 14:333-339.

36. Rowland, A.S., Umbach, D.M., Stallone, L., Naftel, A.J., Bahlig, E.M. and Sandler, D.P. (2002). "Prevalence of medication treatment for attention deficit hyperactivity disorder among elementary school children in Johnston County, North Carolina." *J. Amer. Publ. Health Assoc.* 92:231-234.

37. Schantz, S.L., Levin, E.D., Bowman, R.E., Heironimus, M.P. and Laughlin, N.K. (1989). "Effects of perinatal PCB exposure on discrimination-reversal learning in monkeys." *Neurotoxicol. Teratol.* 11:243-250.

38. Statement (1998). Statement from the worksession on environmental endocrine disrupting chemicals: neural endocrine and behavioral effects. 14:1-8.

39. Swan, S.H. and vom Saal, F.S. (2001). "Alterations in male reproductive

development: The role of endocrine disrupting chemicals." *Endocrine Disruptors in the Environment*. M. Metzler. Heidelberg, Springer Verlag. 131-170.

40. Thornton, J.W. (2001). "Evolution of vertebrate steroid receptors from an ancestral estrogen receptor by ligand exploitation and serial genome expansions." *Proc. Nat. Acad. Sci.* 98:5671-5676.

41. vom Saal, F. (1989). "Sexual differentiation in litter bearing mammals: influence of sex of adjacent fetuses in utero." *J. Anim. Sci.* 67:1824-1840.

42. vom Saal, F.S. (1984). "The intrauterine position phenomenon: Effects on physiology, aggressive behavior and population dynamics in house mice." *Prog. Clin. Biol. Res., Vol. 169, Biological Perspectives on Aggression*. K. Flannelly, Blanchard, R. and Blanchard, D. New York, Alan R. Liss. 135-179.

43. vom Saal, F.S., Nagel, S.C., Palanza, P., Boechler, M., Parmigiani, S. and Welshons, W.V. (1995). "Estrogenic pesticides: binding relative to estradiol in MCF-7 cells and effects of exposure during fetal life on subsequent territorial behaviour in male mice." *Tox. Let.* 77:343-50.

44. vom Saal, F.S., Welshons, W.V. and Hansen, L.G. (1998). "Organochlorine residues and breast cancer." *New Engl. J. Med.* 338:988.

45. Wolff, M.S. and Toniolo, P.G. (1995). "Environmental organochlorine exposure as a potential etiologic factor in breast cancer." *Environ. Health Perspect.* 103:141-145.

46. Yan, P.S., Rodriguez, F.J., Laux, D.E., Perry, M.R., Standiford, S.B. and Huang, T.H.-M. (2000). "Hypermethylation of ribosomal DNA in human breast carcinoma." *Br. J. Cancer* 82:514-517.

LONG TERM STEWARDSHIP OF RADIOACTIVE AND CHEMICAL CONTAMINATION

LORNE G. EVERETT, PH.D., D.SC.
Shaw Environmental and Infrastructure, Inc.
3700 State Street, Suite 350, Santa Barbara, CA 93105
lorne.everett@shawgrp.com

STEPHEN KOWALL, PH.D
BBWI
Idaho National Engineering and Environmental Laboratory
P.O. Box 1625, Idaho Falls, ID 83415-2213
kowasj@inel.gov

ABSTRACT

The U.S. DOE is responsible for cleaning up the environmental legacy (estimated cost $300 billion dollars) of the nation's nuclear weapons program and government-sponsored nuclear energy research. The cleanup program is one of the largest and most diverse and technically complex environmental cleanup programs in the world. In February 2002, DOE embarked on an accelerated cleanup and closure program intended to yield more secure protection of our nuclear material inventory, while reducing the cost of storage and protection at multiple sites. Due to the nature and complexity of this approach, as well as the limitations of currently available remediation technologies, much of this radioactive and chemical contamination will constitute a long-term hazard, since significant amounts of it will remain in the ground even after DOE's cleanup goals have been achieved at the 144 DOE sites. Whether contaminants are moved or stabilized in place, the vadose (unsaturated) zone of the earth will host much of the post-cleanup contaminated material, as well as spent nuclear fuel. This approach will require an improved understanding of the processes influencing the subsurface movement of contaminants in the DOE complex in order to support necessary decisions for the short-term management and long-term stewardship of DOE sites. Breakthrough advances in environmental science and technology will be central to that understanding and would have the effect of significantly advancing schedules, and reducing costs, uncertainty and risk.

It is reported that more than one hundred DOE sites will require monitoring for an indefinite length of time at an estimated cost of $100 million per year. More specifically, DOE anticipates that long-term stewardship will be required at various sites to ensure protection from over 75 million m^3 of contaminated soil and 1.8 billion m^3 of contaminated water. Risk-reduction activities will include sampling and analysis of more than 11,000 monitoring wells and maintenance of engineered barriers at hundreds of the over 3,000 existing sites contaminated with hazardous or radioactive materials.

INTRODUCTION

The Top-to-Bottom review of the U.S. DOE Environmental Management (EM) Program (DOE 2002) has noted that the EM cleanup program cost estimate could easily increase to more than $300 billion. Further the report indicated a systemic problem with the way that EM has conducted its activities. The EM program historically has placed major emphasis on managing risk rather than reducing risk on the 2 million acres at 144 DOE cleanup sites. The new proposed approach is designed to reduce risk to public health, workers, and the environment on an accelerated basis. As a result the reorganization of DOE's Environmental Management program has placed greater emphasis on accelerated cleanup/containment and closure of DOE sites.

RADIOACTIVE WASTE HAS BEEN ACCUMULATING IN THE US

The U.S. Navy's nuclear-power vessels, the nation's past production and ongoing dismantlement of nuclear weapons, the commercial generation of 20 percent of the country's electricity, and many research and development activities produce high level radioactive waste. These radioactive materials have accumulated since the mid-1940s and are currently stored in temporary facilities at some 144 sites in 39 states (Fig. 1).

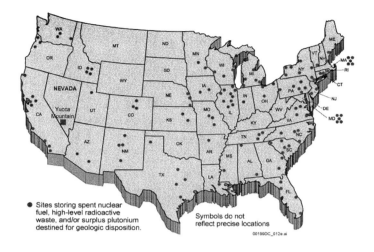

Fig. 1. Location of Radioactive Waste Sites in the USA.

THE LONG-TERM STEWARDSHIP PROGRAM

The mission of DOE's Long-term Stewardship Program is to manage these residual risks and reduce future environmental liabilities associated with the government's continuing operations at many of these sites. As part of its stewardship ethic and vision, DOE is committed to protecting human health and the environment, sustaining natural and cultural resources, and enhancing the use of the Department's land and facilities for the public good. Advances in science and technology will be needed to fulfill this stewardship commitment.

A NATIONAL SCIENCE AND TECHNOLOGY ROADMAP FOR LONG TERM STEWARDSHIP

Federal investments in scientific research and engineering projects are needed to benefit contaminated DOE sites as well as hazardous and solid waste disposal sites across the United States. Rather than leave such investment decisions to individual agencies and independent institutions, a more thoughtful, coordinated approach to research planning is now underway. The Idaho National Engineering and Environmental Laboratory (INEEL) has been directed by DOE to facilitate a national roadmapping process that will provide a scientific consensus for future research investments in the area of long-term stewardship.

The draft roadmap document, scheduled for completion in August 2002, will:

- Reflect a national consensus on near-term (5 year) R&D needs.
- Identify what S&T is needed. It will not identify who will do it, where to do it, or how to do it.
- Provide a strategy to plan and coordinate science and technology investments by interested agencies involved in long-term care of contaminated sites.

The primary focus of the fiscal year 2002 effort is on capability improvements achievable within the next five years. The 4 draft key capabilities are listed in Table 1. For this paper only long term stewardship issues related to monitoring as identified in Table 1 are discussed in detail. The majority of the monitoring ideas have recently been written by the authors for an American audience.

Table 1. Main Long Term Stewardship Needs by Category.

Contamination Containment and Control
- Alternate technologies that detoxify of immobilize contaminants at the source and reduce the volume of groundwater needing to be treated
- Cover and subsurface containment systems that mimic natural processes and accommodate environmental change.
- Models, natural analogues, and indicators that improve design, planning, decision making, monitoring and maintenance.
- Technologies that significantly reduce the need for maintenance of containment systems.
Decision Making and Institutional Performance
- Improved institutional credibility and community interaction to best maintain trust and confidence.
- Continuous improvements of LTS decisions to sustain stakeholder support and reduce life-cycle costs.
- Institutional mechanisms that sustain and improve LTS.
Monitoring and Sensors
- Validation of containment and safety system performance.
- Monitoring systems that can adapt to changes in knowledge of the geologic, hydrologic, chemical and biologic processes at the site.
- Improved multimedia-monitoring capabilities.
- New methods that utilize advances in wireless, miniaturization, non-invasive, and remote interrogation technologies.
- Information management systems that address validity, access, outreach, education, and visualization
Safety Systems and Institutional Controls
- Approaches to select standardized, risk-based safety systems that enhance efficiency of cost and operations.
- Criteria for analyzing data to ensure the integrity of security and access control systems,
- Technology that preserves site information for intergenerational continuity.
- Legal strategies and associates instruments to facilitate handoff of closed sites stewards.

REGULATORY OBSTACLES

The current framework of laws, regulations and cleanup agreements create obstacles to the rapid cleanup and closure of contaminated sites. The Federal mandates, including both RCRA and CERCLA are written by Congress and implemented by the Environmental Protection Agency (EPA). With one exception, Federal regulations do not have an early warning component. The only Federal guidance on vadose zone monitoring (Everett 1986) can be found under RCRA and deals with hazardous waste land treatment Part B permits. This report: *Permit Guidance Manual on Unsaturated Zone Monitoring for Hazardous Waste Land Treatment Units*, 9EPA/530-SW-86-0400 was published in 1986. An interesting component of the EPA Guidance was to recognize that early alert monitoring made sense even in shallow environments (Everett, 2001).

The philosophical position taken by EPA for the vast majority of the regulations however is directed towards regulating contamination after it reaches the saturated zone through the use of groundwater monitoring wells. This approach clearly is flawed if one thinks in terms of long half-life radioisotopes, or in areas of significant depth to the water table, as is commonly found at many of DOE's sites. This is akin to monitoring a patient in a hospital to tell you when the patient is dead.

Most DOE sites will be subject to either RCRA, CERCLA, or both. Both statutes are of recent origin, and both were amended to clarify that they do apply to federal facilities (RCRA in 1992 through the Federal Facilities Compliance Act and CERCLA in 1986 through the Superfund Amendments and Reauthorization Act). The laws are written to provide general control of situations where hazardous substances on a site require some form of management and remediation. Both laws will likely change in the future. The lack of soil cleanup standards has caused great uncertainty in DOE remediation costs and technologies.

The significance of state authority over remediation of DOE facilities within their borders cannot be under-estimated. Many states control corrective action programs through their EPA authorized RCRA programs and environmental restoration through their own CERCLA analogues. Federal facilities not on the National Priorities List (NPL) are subject to state laws on remediation and removal actions (CERCLA Section 120[a][4]). Congress also provided states the opportunity in CERCLA Section 120 (e) to participate in the development of remedial investigations and feasibility studies with DOE and EPA at sites on the NPL. Notice must be given to the affected state within six months of a federal facility being placed on the NPL.

In addition to these environmental remediation laws, DOE sites are subject to other older (~25 years) major federal environmental statutes such as the Clean Water Act, Clean Air Act, Toxic Substance Control Act, Endangered Species Act, and National Environmental Policy Act. Many states will also have laws patterned after these federal laws, and some provisions of the states' laws may be more stringent than the federal laws. Each of these statutes has it own significant regulatory framework and standards that can become site-specific cleanup levels.

Currently there are no set standards for soil decontamination. The National Council on Radiation Protection and Measurements (NCRP) published screening limits for radionuclides in soil that relate an effective dose to a critical group to a corresponding soil contamination level (Everett, 2001). The screening levels are consistent with the NCRP recommendation that the maximally exposed individual should not exceed 0.25 mSv per year (25mrem per year) from any single set of sources. Different screening levels are derived for various land uses from farming to commercial use. However, these limits are stated *not* to be used as cleanup standards on the grounds that they apply to the maximally exposed person and are conservative. A cleanup standard for plutonium in surface soil of 200 pCi/g (7400 Bq/kg) is in use as a de facto standard at NTS. This concentration is estimated to give an exposure of 100 rnrem per year for a full time resident. The U.S. NRC has promulgated cleanup standards for radioactive contamination in soil that are applicable to decommissioning of U.S. NRC-licensed sites. The U.S. NRC ground cleanup standard is based on individual radiation exposures of no more than 25 rnrern/year to an average member of the critical group (10 CFR 20.1402). However, the EPA objects to this standard and recommends a limit of 15 rnrern/year from all pathways, with no more than 4 rnrern/year through the drinking water pathway for decommissioned sites. The appropriate contaminated soil remediation action is determined by the details of the particular situation, both with respect to the degree of health and environmental threats, the availability of practicable remediation technologies, and the financial resources to implement the technologies.

DOE SITE CLOSURE TIMEFRAMES

Over the next 50 years, DOE expects to complete clean up at all of it's sites and transition from a role of providing active remediation to one of insuring stabilization and long term stewardship. Long-term stewardship refers to " all activities required to protect human health and the environment from hazards remaining after cleanup is complete." Figure 2 illustrates the timeline by which DOE anticipates commencing long-term stewardship across 144 sites. While DOE estimates that only about 123 sites will have been cleaned up and put in active or passive stewardship by the year 2006, all 144 sites will be so by 2050 (Fig. 3). Most of these sites, including the most complex ones are located in semi-arid western states with thick vadose zones. The time line driving Doe's cleanup mission, coupled with the prevalence of thick vadose zones at important sites, dictates the need for aggressive, accelerated program to understand vadose zone processes and properties, develop better tools and techniques to characterize and monitor contaminant migration and fate, and develop predictive tools to address and access long term stewardship needs."

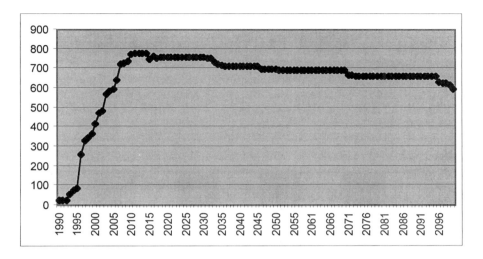

Fig. 2. LTS Activities vs. Time for Implementation.

The National Academy of Sciences based their recommendations on an appendix entitled *Closure Plans for Major DOE Sites.* This excellent appendix represented by example in Table 2 has identified 50 separate sites in 19 different states across America. An evaluation of each of these sites has resulted in a recommendation for long-term monitoring of soil in approximately 21% of the sites. Secondly, a review of the long-term requirements related to groundwater indicates that at least 72% of the sites will have a groundwater-monitoring program. Further, an evaluation of the complete table indicates that in greater than 40% of the sites, a surface cap or barrier will be implemented as a part of the long-term strategy. Although these percentages are hardly exact, they do give an excellent representation of where the emphasis needs to be placed relative to a long term monitoring strategy for DOE sites.

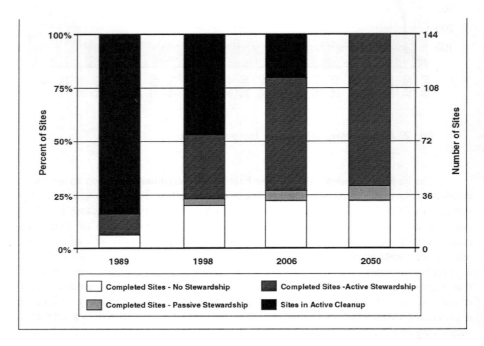

Fig. 3. Stewardship Activities Increase as Cleanup is Completed.

Table 2. Closure Plans for Major DOE Sites (Sources: U.S. Department of Energy [1995, 1996, 1998a, 1999]).

State	Site	Responsibility for Site/End Use(s)	End State	Conditions of Closure	Completion Date
Alaska	Amchitka Island	Release to U.S. Fish and Wildlife Service or U.S. Bureau of Wildlife Mgt.	Greenfield on surface/ institutional control on all sub-surface areas near shot cavities	Sub-surface and groundwater surveillance and monitoring planned for 100 years, but assumed to be in perpetuity; will require controlled access; surface released for uncontrolled use (open space)	2001
California	Energy Technology Engineering Center (ETEC)	Site will be turned over to Boeing/ Rocketdyne	Probably industrial use under surveillance and monitoring and deed restrictions	Remediation of groundwater, soils and decontamination and decommissioning (D&D) of several bldg.; residential inorganic, PCB, semivolotile organic chemicals (SVOC). mercury and dioxin left in soil; contaminated soil over 1×10^{-5} disposed off site; facilities require D&D of radionuclides and sodium under RCRA	2006
California	General Atomics Site (GA)	U.S. Department of Energy (DOE) keeps liability until all waste is off the site then GA assumes site	Greenfield	GA responsible for post remediation monitoring	1999

MONITORING STATE OF THE ART VS. STATE OF THE PRACTICE

It is clear from the preceding discussion related to long-term requirements for groundwater monitoring (72%) and the long-term evaluation of landfill caps (41%) that a significant improvement in the fundamental technologies used in monitoring will be needed. Based upon a review of groundwater monitoring technologies and barrier construction and monitoring designs, the authors are of the opinion that today's state of the art is far superior to the current state of the practice. The implication is that a substantial improvement is needed in applying today's technology. For example, in 1980 the lead author wrote a book entitled *Groundwater Monitoring* (Everett, 1980) which was endorsed by EPA as "establishing the state-of-the-art used by industry today." Remember that state-of-the-art was in 1980. In the book recommendations are made for the use of neutron probes and pressure vacuum lysimeters in landfill barrier designs. If one evaluates the regulatory requirements for landfill cap designs in California (one of the more aggressive environmental states in the union) the monitoring requirements specify neutron probes and pressure vacuum lysimeters. In the 22 years since, this state of the practice has not moved forward, even though there have been substantial improvements in monitoring technology and monitoring strategies. Although several new monitoring technologies have been developed over the past few years, the environmental market has been so weak that manufactures are hesitant to commit to manufacturing new products that may not achieve profitable sales levels. As such, the state of the art continues to move forward while the state of the practice appears to be hung up with 1980's technologies.

CLOSURE BARRIER CONCERNS

The long term prediction and verification of containment barriers at DOE sites is the central theme of an interagency approach to this problem. The DOE, in concert with the EPA and the Dupont Corporation are actively involved in preparing a state-of-the-art document on several issues related to landfill caps, walls and floors. These focus on: the prediction of materials stability and application; the key factors effecting long term performance; matching barrier type and climate; characterizing and quantifying the role of vegetation in long term performance; and, quantifying the influence of erosion, petrogenisis and subsidence on long term performance. Panels deal with the prediction of barrier performance, wherein processes such as the existence of membrane behavior, attenuation, etc. will be evaluated. Groups focus on scale issues such as barrier performance relative to a regional scale. Issues related to the sensitivity of various containment barrier parameters to prediction including their reliability are evaluated. Specific concerns such as predicting the effect of damage on system performance are assessed as well.

Verification of barriers based upon monitoring technologies will consider fundamental questions such as: *What are the current technologies used in verification monitoring of barriers and long term performance monitoring? What are their underlying principals, specific applications and deficiencies?* Further, this group focuses on the actual subsurface-based methods, which are used in verification. Specifically the monitoring methods will focus on barrier physical integrity and validation, contaminant fate and transport, monitoring, surrogate parameters such as water belts, EH, etc. and a comparison surface geophysical techniques and airborne based monitoring technologies. The comprehensive approach to barrier verification and integrity monitoring will be addressed in an expert workshop to be held June 30-July 2, 2002 in Baltimore, MD. Subsequent to the expert workshop an invitation only suite of scientists will prepare a state-of-the-art manual on the subject of long-term prediction and verification of containment and treatment barriers performance. Professor Hillary Inyang from the University of North Carolina and Lorne Everett will edit this document.

BREAKTHROUGH TECHNOLOGIES NEEDED

Initial estimates for the science and technology improvements in vadose zone monitoring alone are estimated to be in the $10's million per year range. These enormous costs anticipate a basic science evaluation with applications through characterization, monitoring and remediation. Examples of the timeframes for monitoring science and technology development are given in Table 3, below. Programs of this magnitude are needed to improve the uncertainty associated with long term monitoring of DOE facilities. However, the prospect of a few breakthrough technologies may have substantial application not only in terms of soil and groundwater monitoring but also in terms of interrogation and verification of barrier and cap designs.

Over 100 years ago, rotary drilling surpassed cable tools as the state-of-the-art in drilling methods. Recently, exciting new laboratory applications of laser drilling techniques have indicated the potential to penetrate hard rock at 100 times faster than conventional boring technologies. Subsurface Laser Applications Incorporated (SLAI) a specialty company set up to capitalize upon laser drilling and laser analytical technologies have been presenting exciting new ideas. Reports by the Gas Technology Institute (Shirley, 2002) have indicated that 50% of drilling time is spent on making hole, 25% on tripping, and 25% on casing and cementing. A conclusion is that major reductions in drilling costs can be achieved by faster drilling techniques and reductions in requirements for drill string removal, bit replacement, and setting casing. SLAI is working on techniques to create casing in unconsolidated sediments, spall rock with specific removal technologies, and to develop down hole and side-wall laser analytical technologies. Clearly, the ability to create micro boreholes in soil, micro groundwater monitoring wells and micro interrogation holes in barriers has huge breakthrough potential. The accuracy of laser drilled holes guided by laser surveying technologies allows the ability to triangulate and to develop exact understanding of rock material and contamination at specific depths.

CASE HISTORY EXAMPLES OF CLOSURE PROBLEMS

During the Vadose Zone Science and Technology Solutions Book (Looney and Falta, 2000) workshop held at Berkeley, CA, representatives from various DOE facilities were quizzed as to why vadose zone data were not collected. The most common response heard was that since there was not a federal regulatory requirement to investigate contamination migration in the vadose zone, therefore early alert monitoring did not receive a high enough priority relative to the dollars available to conduct investigations.

Since vadose zone characterization and monitoring data were not seen as a priority item, the dollars were used for other kinds of activity to satisfy regulatory demands. Further, since there was no regulatory basis for vadose zone investigations, each of the DOE facilities approached the problem in a different manner. This lack of consistency has resulted in a very disjointed DOE early alert monitoring program

Further misuse of the regulatory program can be recognized relative to the UMTRA Program. Several years ago the author (Everett, 2001) had been asked to review the vadose-zone monitoring program associated with the surface capping barriers placed over many UMTRA sites. The evaluation of the vadose zone monitoring concentrated on the use of neutron probes and the use of tensiometers. Everett pointed out that over the years, neutron probes had been lost, damaged, returned to the manufacture for calibration, etc. In addition several new probes had been purchased. In every case, there was no long-term calibration standard set up by UMTRA and as such there was no way to compare any of the data collected against a base-line. As a result, the interpretation of the neutron probe data over time could not be utilized. In the case of the use of tensiometers, an evaluation was done related to the use of Bourdon tubes at high altitudes. The Bourdon tubes, which rely upon a vacuum to operate, exhibit a very narrow range of operation at the high altitude of many of the UMTRA sites including those in the Grand Junction area. Corrections for altitude were not been made with any of the tensiometer data provided and as such this information could not be utilized. Upon making this recommendation to UMTRA, prior to joining Stone & Webster Consultants, the author was told that since vadose zone monitoring was not required at these UMTRA sites, that the ongoing vadose zone program would be canceled rather than corrected.

Table 3. Research Priorities: Sensors and Instrumentation (DOE, 2001).

2004	• Understand the effects of emplacement.
	• Microdrilling and coiled tubing applied as demonstrated minimization of effects at DOE EM sites.
	• Develop new drilling techniques.
	• Deploy prototypes in existing boreholes, to decrease cost and improve spatial resolution (goal; 10 sensors, fit in <2 inch diameter hole).
	• Characterize the geology and hydrology of a contaminated site at the 10m scale throughout the top 50m of the subsurface using methods that have about a one-month turnaround time for processing and interpretation of field measurements.
2010	• Develop minimally invasive methods and begin to correct emplacement effects.
	• Cheaper, smaller, more robust subsurface location devices.
	• Deploy field prototype using alternatives to boreholes (cone petrometers, new emplacements, microdrilling, autonomous devices, penatrators, injectable microdevices) (goal: 50 channels, rice grain size hole).
	• Extend capability to a resolution of 1m and improve the turnaround time to 1 day, for many field sites.

SPACE/TIME MONITORING ISSUES

The ability to extrapolate from small scale monitoring information to field scale problems is one of the most pressing challenges facing soils, groundwater, and barrier design monitoring. Solving these types of scaling problems is central to advancing our monitoring research capabilities. Scaling issues come in a number of forms: 1) the large spatial variability of hydraulic properties in natural geologic systems over a wide range of scales renders estimation of hydraulic parameters and there spatial correlation difficult. 2) The instrument and network scales used to characterize and monitor sites vary among, and even within, the type of geophysical methods being used, thus creating questions about how measurement-related scales effect the obtained values, and how to appropriately incorporate or combine different types of data obtained at different scales and with different methods and instruments. The addition of computer models to this picture makes scaling issues even more difficult. Because many relevant subsurface properties exhibit multiple nested scales of spatial and temporal variability, simulation based on property measurements on one scale may be of little or no use to simulations on other scales effected by different flow and reactive transport processes. In this case standard theory becomes inadequate, because flow and transport at different scales may require the use of completely different mathematical models and/or constitutive relationships.

As noted earlier, the two main soil moisture sampling and indirect measurement techniques for barriers are pressure vacuum lysimeters and neutron moderation probes. The sphere of influence of a model 1920 pressure vacuum lysimeter with a two-micron aluminum oxide ceramic cup is approximately 3-6 feet. The sphere of influence of a 50-milicurry americium beryllium neutron probe is approximately 8 inches in diameter in a wet environment and 3 feet in diameter in a dry environment. Clearly, the measurement radius of these monitoring tools at a landfill tap is extremely small. The question then becomes how does one scale up from these very small precise measurements into a measure of uncertainty relative to the behavior of the rest of the landfill cap? For the most part, the scale up issues from very small-localized precise measurements have not been attempted as yet and consequently, the reliability of the long term performance of these barriers is difficult to monitor.

LONG TERM MONITORING CONCLUSIONS

Many of the research opportunities for monitoring and validation have been covered in the research emphases discussed above. The National Research Council has seen a need for:

- Development of methods for designing monitoring systems to detect both current conditions and changes in system behaviors. These methods may involve the application of conceptual, mathematical, and statistical models to determine the types and locations of observation systems and prediction of the spatial and temporal resolutions at which observations need to be made.

- Development of validation processes. The research questions include (1) understanding what a representation of system behavior means and how to judge when a model provides an accurate representation of a system behavior - the model may give the right answers for the wrong reasons and thus may not be a good predictive tool; and {2) how to validate the future performance of the model or system behavior based on present-day measurements.

- Data for model validation. Determining the key measurements that are required to validate models and system behaviors, the spatial and temporal resolutions at which such measurements must be obtained, and the extent to which surrogate data (e.g., data from lab-.scale testing facilities) can be used in validation efforts.

- Research to support the development of methods to monitor fluid and gaseous fluxes through the unsaturated zone, and for differentiating diurnal and seasonal changes from longer-term secular changes. These methods may involve both direct (e.g. in situ sensors) and indirect (e.g. using plants and animals) measurements over long time periods, particularly for harsh chemical environments characteristic of some DOE sites, This research should support the development of both the physical instrumentation and measurement techniques. The latter includes measurement strategies and data analysis (including statistical) approaches (NRC, 2000).

REFERENCES

1.   Rumer, Ralph R. and James K. Mitchell, 2000. *Assessment of Barrier Containment Technologies*, National Technical Information Service, Springfield Virginia. 437 pp.

2.   Rumer, Ralph R. and Michael E. Ryan, editors. 1995. *Barrier Containment Technologies for Environmental Remediation Applications*,. John Wiley and Sons, Inc. NY. 170 pp.

3.   Everett, L.G., 2001. "Long Term Institutional and Regulatory Policy Issues Relating to the Vadose Zone." *WASTEC, 2001,Tucson Ariz.*, 13 pp.

4.   Everett, L.G., 1986. *Permit Guidance Manual on Unsaturated Zone Monitoring for Hazardous Waste Land Treatment Units*, EPA, Office of Solid Waste, EPA/530-SW-86-040, 111 pp.

5.   Everett, L.G., 1980. *Groundwater Monitoring*, General Electric Company, Schenectady, NY, 12303. 440 pp.

6.   Looney, Brian B. and Ronald W. Falta Editors, 2000. *Vadose Zone–Science and Technology Solutions, Vol. II*, Battelle Press, 1540 pp and I.

7.   National Research Council, 2000. *Long Term Institutional Management of U.S. Department of Energy Legacy Waste Sites*, National Academy Press, Wash. DC 164 pp.

8.   Department of Energy, 2001. *A National Roadmap for Vadose Zone Science & Technology*, DOE/ID-10874, 150 pp.

9.   U.S. Department of Energy, 2002 (February), *A Review of the Environmental Management Program*.

10.   U.S. Department of Energy. 1995 (March) *Estimating the Cold War Mortgage; The 1995 Baseline Environmental Management Report*. Office of Environmental Management, DOE/EM-0232, Washington, D.C.

11.   U.S. Department of Energy. 1996 (June). *The 1996 Baseline Environmental Management Report*. Office of Environmental Management, DOE/EM-0290, Washington, D.C.

12.   U.S. Department of Energy. 1998a (June). *Accelerating Cleanup: Paths to Closure*. Office of Environmental Management, DOE/EM-0362, Washington, D.C.

13.   U.S. Department of Energy. 1999 (October). *From Cleanup to Stewardship: A Companion Report to Accelerating Cleanup: Paths to Closure and Background Information to Support the Scoping Process Required for the 1998 PEIS Settlement Study*. Office of Environmental Management, DOE/EM-0362, Washington, D.C.

12. SCIENCE AND TECHNOLOGY: CLIMATE — GREENHOUSE EFFECT

THE CARBON CYCLE AND ANTHROPOGENIC CLIMATE CHANGE

PIETER P. TANS

Climate Monitoring and Diagnostics Laboratory, National Oceanic and Atmospheric Administration, Boulder, CO, USA

We already have committed our planet to serious climate change that will last for many generations. There are two main reasons for this statement. First, the natural carbon cycle will not be able to absorb the carbon dioxide (CO_2) emitted by the burning of coal, oil, and natural gas in a way to bring the atmospheric CO_2 concentrations back to pre-industrial levels within a few centuries. Second, the warming of the oceans takes about a thousand years before a new steady state is reached at the higher levels of atmospheric CO_2 in which outgoing infrared radiation once again balances the incoming radiation from the sun. Atmospheric emissions of CO_2 will have to be brought close to zero.

THE CARBON CYCLE

Let us first take a look at the carbon cycle. Figure 1 presents direct atmospheric measurements showing the unrelenting increase over the last five decades superimposed upon the seasonal cycle driven by the photosynthesis and respiration of the terrestrial biosphere. The inset puts the increase recorded in the 20th century into the perspective of the last thousand years. Apparently until the last century the earth's carbon cycle was close to a steady state, as CO_2 was remarkably constant. To understand why the sharp increase in the last few decades coincides with the burning of fossil fuels one has to ask what happens to the combustion product, carbon dioxide, once it has been emitted into the atmosphere. There are basically three reservoirs it can go into: it can stay in the atmosphere, where it is not chemically broken down, or dissolve in ocean waters, or it can be turned into wood and other forms of biomass on land through photosynthesis. The global carbon cycle is pictured schematically in Figure 2. By far the largest reservoirs of carbon near the surface of the earth are geological, (Ca, Mg) carbonate rock and kerogen, which is finely dispersed and recalcitrant organic material. However, the natural fluxes of carbon into and out of these reservoirs, erosion and sedimentation, are very slow, and even partially balancing each other. The geological fluxes comprise no more than several percent of the rate of fossil fuel burning. The fossil fuel resources included in Figure 2 only include conventional coal, oil, and natural gas, but not tar sands, shale oils, and methane clathrates. The latter especially are estimated to be extremely large and may double the total resources.

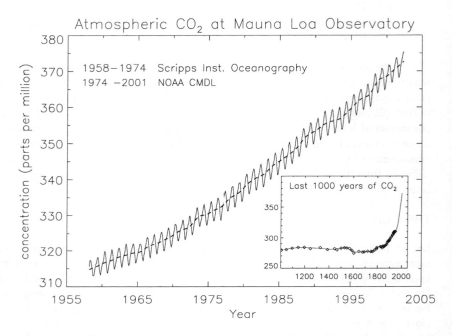

Fig. 1. *Monthly mean atmospheric concentrations of carbon dioxide measured at Mauna Loa Observatory in Hawaii. (C.D. Keeling, Scripps Institution of Oceanography, and Climate Monitoring and Diagnostics Laboratory (CMDL), National Oceanic and Atmospheric Administration). Inset: Atmospheric CO₂ over the last thousand years as recorded in air bubbles trapped in ice in Antarctica. (D. Etheridge, J. Geophys. Res. 101, 4115-4128, 1996).*

The fluxes between the other three reservoirs, the atmosphere, oceans, and terrestrial biosphere, are large. We will therefore call them the mobile reservoirs and they are depicted in red in Figure 2. They were in balance until the 20th century. Today the relatively small imbalance caused by the extra input of fossil fuel-derived CO_2 ($0.55 \ 10^{15}$ mol/yr) is driving the atmospheric increase shown in Figure 1. The oceans and terrestrial ecosystems are not able to take up the additional CO_2 as fast as it is being added to the atmosphere. The ocean reservoir is the largest of the three, but mixing is slow (about a thousand years). Furthermore, the ultimate chemical capacity of the oceans for uptake of the extra CO_2 is not proportional to the total amount of dissolved carbon, but is mostly determined by the total (much smaller) abundance of carbonate ions (CO_3^{2-}) in the global "giant titration" reaction equilibrium:

$$CO_2 + H_2O + CO_3^{2-} \longleftrightarrow 2\ HCO_3^-$$ (Reaction 1)

Once most of the carbonate ions have been converted into bicarbonate ions (HCO_3^-), increasing the acidity of the oceans, the ocean's uptake capacity has been approximately exhausted.

THE CARBON CYCLE

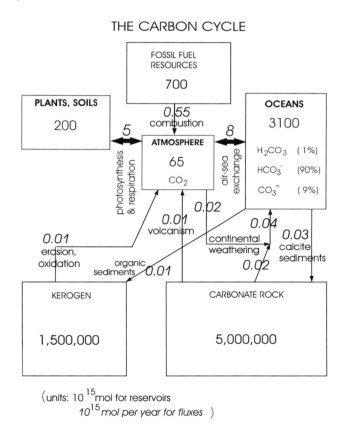

(units: 10^{15} mol for reservoirs
10^{15} mol per year for fluxes)

Fig. 2. The global carbon cycle. One unit of 10^{15} mol corresponds to $12\ 10^{15}$ g C, which, if it had the same density as water, would fill $12\ km^3$.

A fundamental aspect of the carbon cycle is that the erosion-sedimentation processes are very slow. The CO_2 added to the atmosphere, and re-distributed in the mobile reservoirs, is not removed from the mobile reservoirs for many thousands of years by natural processes. The consequence is that, to a first approximation, and neglecting some initial "overshoot" in the atmosphere, the enhanced CO_2 concentration in the atmosphere reflects the sum of all previous emissions rather than the current rate of emissions. If the further rise of atmospheric CO_2 is to be stopped, the emissions have to be brought back to zero. Indeed, all of the stabilization scenarios considered by the Intergovernmental Panel on Climate Change (IPCC) in which the atmospheric CO_2 concentration is to stay below some predetermined level have the CO_2 emissions approach zero. Figure 3 illustrates the point. Let us assume that mankind continues to burn fossil fuels, the majority of which is coal, via two different scenarios. In the first scenario all fuel resources are consumed in a few hundred years, in the second the rate of consumption is held constant at 1990 levels, in which case the resource lasts more than twelve hundred years. A simplified model of the carbon cycle consisting only of the atmosphere and the oceans, with exchange constants calibrated to fit current measurements and the recent past, then predicts future atmospheric CO_2 concentrations for the fast-burning scenario (solid curve, Fig. 3) and the slow-burning scenario (dashed curve). The blue (dot-dash) curve allows for the dissolution of solid calcite sediments on the ocean floor in the fast-burning case, which leads to additional chemical uptake capacity of atmospheric CO_2 by the oceans through the formation of new carbonate ions so that reaction 1 can be repeated:

$$CaCO_3\ (s) \longrightarrow Ca^{2+} + CO_3^{2-} \qquad\qquad \text{(Reaction 2)}$$

Two features stand out in Figure 3. First, the very high levels of atmospheric CO_2 that would be reached if we indeed burn all coal resources, and second, the fact that after the resource has been used it does not make much difference whether that was accomplished in a few hundred years or in 1200 years. The dissolution of calcite is expected to eventually bring the atmospheric CO_2 concentrations back to what they were approximately before the industrial era.

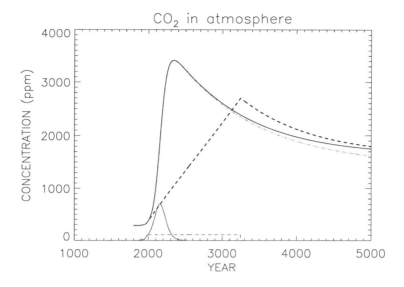

Fig. 3. Potential future concentrations of atmospheric CO_2 if all fossil fuel resources are consumed, either in a fast-burning (solid curve) or a slow-burning (dashed curve) scenario. The two different postulated time histories of burning are depicted along the bottom axis (on an arbitrary scale). The fast-burning case is plotted again with the assumption that calcite dissolution takes place on the ocean floor (blue curve, dot-dash).

The effect on the atmospheric radiation balance if the extra CO_2 were injected suddenly in today's atmosphere (the definition of "climate forcing") would be enormous (Fig. 4), and climate change would almost certainly be enormous as well. The global demand for energy can be expected to increase greatly. It certainly should, to give the people in developing countries a good chance to improve their standard of living. A comparison of per capita CO_2 emissions for three countries is shown in Figure 5. An average citizen in the USA causes 10 times the amount of CO_2 emissions of a citizen of India. It is also striking that the per capita emissions in the USA did not increase during the last three decades despite significant economic growth, and even more striking is that emissions in Sweden were almost cut in half since 1970. The latter is due partially to the increased use of nuclear energy. Such policy choices take decades to reach their full effect. Projections of energy demand for the developed and less-developed economies are presented in Table 1 for certain assumptions. A decrease of 2% per year for the developed countries represents an aggressive schedule of increased energy efficiency, conservation, and alternative energy sources. It is doubtful whether that would be economically feasible, especially if it is to be sustained for more than five decades. It is to be hoped that the less developed countries actually achieve a growth rate in demand of 2% per year. It is clear that better equity among the peoples of the world implies a greatly increased demand for energy. It is also clear that it would be wise to embark upon an aggressive research and development program now to enable the cuts required in fossil fuel consumption in several decades.

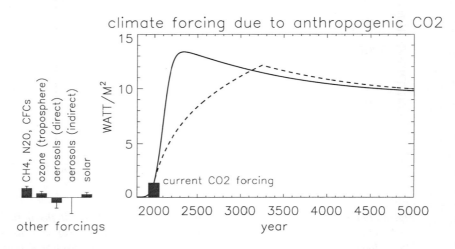

Fig. 4. Climate forcing due to enhanced CO_2 when all fossil fuel resources are consumed. Today's climate forcing is shown for comparison in the bars along the x-axis. For comparison, global average solar radiation absorbed on the ground is about 240 W/m^2.

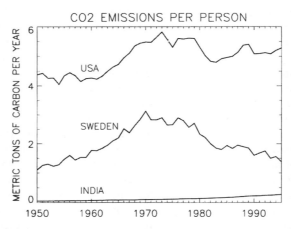

Fig. 5. Per capita CO_2 emissions in the USA, Sweden and India.

Table 1. Global energy demand.

Year	Country	Population (billions)	Per Capita (kilowatt)	Total (terawatt)
1990	Developed	1.2	7.5	9.0
	Less developed	<u>4.1</u>	1.1	<u>4.5</u>
	Total	5.3		13.5
2025	Developed	1.4	3.8 (-2%/yr)	5.3
	Less developed	<u>6.8</u>	2.2 (+2%/yr)	<u>15.0</u>
	Total	8.2		20.3
2060	Global	9.0	3.0	27
		9.0	5.0	45

A BRIEF EXPLANATION OF THE GREENHOUSE EFFECT

Every object in the universe emits what is called thermal radiation, with an intensity and wavelength range that depend strongly on its temperature. The total emitted intensity is proportional to the fourth power of the temperature, implying that an object twice as warm sends out 16 times as much radiation. The sun, with an average surface temperature of 5800 degrees Kelvin, sends out visible radiation in all directions. A very small portion is intercepted by the earth, 70% of which is absorbed, and 30% reflected (Fig. 6, top). The earth also sends out radiation in all directions, but in a different wavelength range, the infrared, which is invisible to our eyes. Over a long period of time the total energy emitted by the earth equals the total amount of solar energy absorbed. This determines the average surface temperature of a hypothetical earth without an atmosphere to be −18°C. If the earth would send out more energy than it received, its temperature would cool, and vice versa.

If we then could surround our hypothetical earth, still with no atmosphere, with a plastic sheet that is completely transparent to visible radiation, but completely opaque (absorbing) for infrared (Fig. 6, bottom), its surface temperature would have to rise. Looking at the earth+sheet system from space, the only radiation leaving would be infrared originating from the plastic sheet, because the infrared coming from the earth's surface cannot get through the sheet. Once the temperatures of the earth and the sheet have stabilized, the sheet radiates into space the same amount as the earth did before, and the sheet's temperature would have be −18°C, in order to balance the total amount of solar radiation absorbed by the earth. The sheet itself absorbs no visible radiation because it is completely transparent at visible wavelengths. The crucial point is that the sheet radiates in all directions, and it sends back to the earth the same amount that it sends into space. Therefore, the earth's surface not only absorbs visible radiation, but also an equal amount of infrared coming from the plastic sheet. Once the earth's surface has stabilized, it will have to send toward the sheet twice the total amount of (infrared) radiation it emitted before. This happens when the average surface temperature has risen to + 30°C.

334

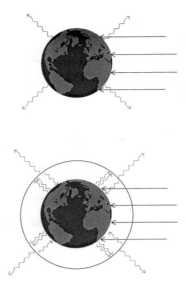

Fig. 6. The principle of the greenhouse effect. Top: earth without an atmosphere. Outgoing infrared radiation is depicted as four wavy lines, symbolizing the same amount of energy as received from the sun, depicted as four straight lines from the right. Bottom: earth surrounded by a plastic sheet, with the earth and the sheet each emitting and receiving equal amounts of energy so that their temperatures are stable.

The atmosphere is much more complicated, but the principle is the same. The atmosphere is opaque only in certain regions of the infrared spectrum and transparent in others (Fig. 7), so that the effect is smaller than in our hypothetical case. Also, energy is transferred by atmospheric motions and by evaporation and condensation of water, not just by radiation. The main gases absorbing infrared radiation in the atmosphere are water vapor, carbon dioxide, methane, nitrous oxide, and ozone. Radiation escaping to space in the spectral regions where the gases absorb has low intensity because the radiation originating at the surface cannot reach space. Instead, that radiation originates at high altitudes where the temperatures are colder. Increases in the greenhouse gas concentrations deepen and widen the regions where the intensity of escaping radiation is low. Since in steady state the total infrared energy lost to space will still have to balance the incoming absorbed solar energy, the radiation in the window region (where no atmospheric absorption takes place) will have to increase. That happens when the earth's surface temperature goes up.

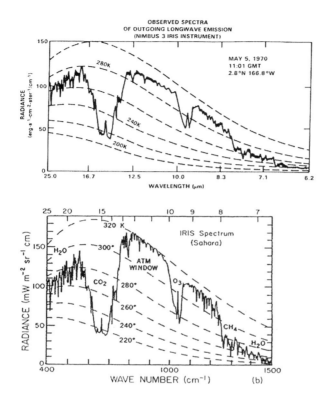

Fig. 7 *Infrared thermal radiation emitted by the earth surface and atmosphere to space from the tropical Pacific Ocean and from the Sahara desert as measured by satellite. Dashed curves indicate the intensity of thermal radiation from a body with a temperature of 280 K (7°C) for example, or 320 K (47°C), etc. In the spectral region where the atmosphere does not absorb ("atmosphere window"), the radiation emitted by the surface reaches space, and one can see that the Sahara is a lot warmer than the Pacific Ocean. In other spectral regions, such as the CO_2 absorption band, the radiation reaching space has low intensity, corresponding to emission from approximately 10 km altitude where the temperature is below 220 K (-53°C).*

THE MAN-MADE CLIMATE CHANGE DILEMMA

An important feature of climate change driven by the current greenhouse gas increases is that the warming of the oceans takes a long time. For the deep waters of the North Pacific

Ocean it has been more than a thousand years since they last saw the surface. Overturning of deep waters is slow, and the heat capacity of the oceans is enormous. Together they dictate a long time for the earth's radiation budget to come back into balance. At this moment the total amount of infrared energy lost to outer space is smaller than the amount of solar energy received because the surplus is going into heating of the oceans. Another slow process is the melting (or growing) of continental ice sheets, which may take thousands of years. Pollution may also be partially masking some of the effects of greenhouse gas emissions because certain aerosols (small particles) scatter solar radiation back to space or impact cloud formation with the same effect. The implication is that with the increase of atmospheric CO_2 that has already taken place we have actually committed the earth to significantly more warming and sea level rise than what we can see today. Decisions on fundamental changes in our energy technology are difficult because of the huge investments involved. The fact that we see far less of the consequences than we would see much later invites skepticism, inaction and delays. Once we decide to make significant changes, continuing emissions at a high rate will continue for several more decades because the energy infrastructure cannot be changed overnight.

A second important aspect of climate change is that the geological record gives us no assurance that the climate is likely to change gradually. Rather the opposite seems to be true. There is evidence in ice cores in Greenland, for example, of temperature changes of up to five degrees taking place in a decade. Ocean bottom sediments indicate that the circulation of the North Atlantic Ocean has undergone massive shifts, and that huge ice-rafting events have taken place during the last tens of thousands of years. The climate forcing by CO_2 and other greenhouse gases increases very gradually, but that does not imply that the climate response will be equally gradual. It thus appears not unlikely that our society will experience some type of major climate shift with serious human and economic costs before we can muster the motivation to take decisive action decreasing our impact on the planet's climate system.

MANAGING THE CARBON CYCLE

One of the approaches to the problem is to create sinks for carbon that can offset the emissions caused by the burning of fossil fuels. Stimulation of forest growth and increasing the organic carbon content of agricultural soils would remove CO_2 from the atmosphere and could have other beneficial effects. There is evidence from atmospheric data that these processes are actually already under way largely unintentionally. Figure 8 shows the global network of regular air measurements maintained by the Climate Monitoring and Diagnostics Laboratory (CMDL). From the data produced by the network we can deduce the average annual mean north-south concentration gradient of CO_2 and other gases in the marine boundary layer (Fig. 9). The concentrations increase going north, mainly because the emissions from fossil fuel burning are strongest at mid-latitudes in the northern hemisphere. Emissions of sulfur hexafluoride (SF_6) have mostly the same pattern in space and time as fossil fuel combustion and SF_6 is chemically very stable in the atmosphere. As a result, it can be used as an atmospheric tracer for fossil fuel CO_2, and allows us to remove the influence of the latter on the interhemispheric gradient (Fig. 9). Sources and sinks of the natural carbon cycle, oceans and terrestrial biosphere, create the pattern in the atmosphere shown as the dashed line. The most striking features are: a very strong sink of CO_2 at mid latitudes in the northern hemisphere, a source in the tropics, and a second large sink at mid latitudes in the southern hemisphere. Additional atmospheric evidence, namely isotopic ratios $^{13}C/^{12}C$ of CO_2 as well as molecular ratios O_2/N_2, indicate that the northern hemisphere sink is mostly terrestrial. To create such a pattern in the atmosphere the northern hemisphere sink has to be very large, at least 2 billion tons C (10^9 tons, or gigatons (GtC) of carbon, or $1.7 \ 10^{14}$ mol) per year. This compares to current global CO_2 emissions from fossil fuels of 6.7 GtC/yr.

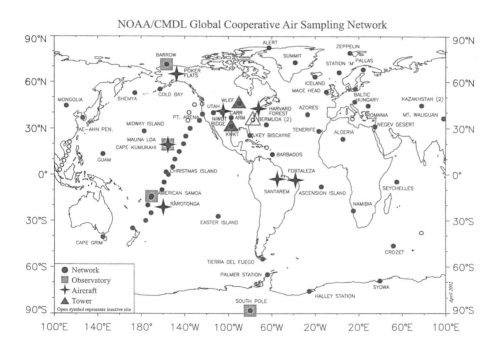

Fig. 8 Surface air sampling network.

338

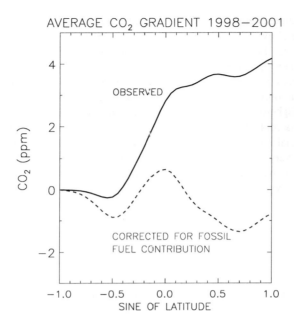

AVERAGE CO₂ GRADIENT 1998–2001

Fig. 9. Average annual mean atmospheric CO_2 gradient from south to north in the marine boundary layer (solid line). The average has been created from measurements performed as part of the NOAA/CMDL Global Cooperative Air Sampling Network. The dashed line presents the same interhemispheric gradient, after the CO_2 data have been corrected for the contribution of fossil fuel burning using the measured gradient of SF_6, the emission pattern of which strongly resembles that of fossil fuel consumption. The corrected pattern reveals the natural carbon cycle underneath the fossil fuel imprint.

The problem is that the atmospheric evidence is not confirmed by what terrestrial ecologists have found when looking for independent evidence on the ground. Their surveys tend to find no more than a relatively small sink. It is imperative that we find out what the true magnitude of the sink is, and what its causes are. If it is mainly due to regrowth of previously cut forests, the sink will probably gradually disappear when those forests become mature. If it is due to fertilization of the entire terrestrial biosphere by enhanced CO_2 and nitrate (also anthropogenic), its future behavior will likely be different. Similarly for agricultural soils, there may be an accumulation of organic carbon due to fertilizer use, reduced tillage, and improved cropping practices. Another potential sink is the replacement of grassland by woody vegetation due to fire suppression and grazing. There are clear management implications because all of these potential causes are directly related to how we use the land. The very fact that there appears to be such a large sink at the same latitudes where humans dominate the land suggests that it has something to do with us. The general drawback of storing organic carbon on land is that it always remains close to the atmosphere, and will likely require continued human management to prevent oxidation. Another drawback is that the amount of carbon to be eventually stored in organic form could become too large. The terrestrial biosphere may have to double or triple in size (compare fossil fuel resources in Fig. 2).

There have been many other proposals for carbon management. One is to fertilize very large ocean surface areas with finely dispersed iron containing particles. There are a few areas where not all of the available major nutrients have been consumed by phytoplankton. It appears that the organisms are starved for iron, an essential micronutrient. Experiments have demonstrated that the addition of iron to the water in such an area stimulates photosynthesis and the production of organic matter. When this can be done in an area of deep water formation, the newly formed organic matter would be carried to the deep ocean. However, this scheme, if it could be carried out at all, represents another huge ecological disturbance caused by us, and may lead to unintended and undesirable side effects. It would not be the first time.

At an electrical power plant CO_2 could be separated from the exhaust gas stream and disposed of in several ways. It could be injected into geological reservoirs, in some cases facilitating the extraction of additional oil or methane from coal beds. It could be injected in liquid form at great depth along the continental slope, and because of its greater density it would tend to flow toward the bottom. The latter approach would bypass the initial atmospheric storage but after a thousand years it would not make much difference, unless the so-called clathrates that are formed (CO_2 molecule bound inside a "cage" of water molecules) turn out to be stable over a very long time. In the case of geological storage we have to make sure that it does not leak out slowly. In my opinion the best proposals have been to chemically react the collected CO_2 into very stable and environmentally benign forms of carbon. One way is to artificially speed up the combination of reactions (1) and (2) above, which would turn the CO_2 into a dissolved salt, namely calcium (or magnesium) bicarbonate. Or it could be reacted with (Ca, Mg) silicates to form stable (Ca, Mg) carbonate, a solid material. The volumes involved are enormous, and the reactions should be fast while not consuming much energy. All of the above represent areas of active research.

If some of the proposed approaches are successful and become part of our strategy to slow down and decrease the "final" magnitude of anthropogenic climate change, they also may give us tools over the very long term to manage the global climate through management of the atmospheric CO_2 concentration.

THE CLIMATE CHANGES IN CHINA RELATED TO GLOBAL WARMING

HUI-JUN WANG, YONG-QIANG YU, REN-JIAN ZHANG, DA-BANG JIANG
Institute of Atmospheric Physics, Chinese Academy of Sciences,
Beijing 100029, China

The global warming issue is widely noted by the scientific world, government, and the public. The Intergovernmental Panel on Climate Change (IPCC) already published three scientific assessment reports in past 12 years. Although scientists are more and more confident of the trend of the global warming as all the climate models simulated, uncertainties still remain in the magnitudes of the changes, the regional details of the changes, and in the capability of the climate model itself.

In this presentation, the author very briefly introduces the climate changes in China related to the global warming.

THE INTERANNUAL AND DECADAL CHANGES OF THE CLIMATE IN CHINA

The El Niño and Southern Oscillation (ENSO) cycle is the largest signal in the interannual climate variability. The interaction between the tropical SST and mid-high latitude atmospheric circulation has been a key topic in meteorology and oceanography since the pioneering works of Bjerknes (1966, 1969). In these works, Bjerknes addressed the teleconnection between the equatorial central Pacific warming and the North Pacific extratropical circulation anomalies.

Some studies (Huang et al., 1989; Wang et al., 2000; Wang, 2001; Ailikun et al., 2001; Wang, 2002) deal with the coupling between the ENSO cycle and the East Asian summer climate. All of them show, to various degrees, the possible linkage between SST anomalies in the tropical Pacific and the East Asian climate. Currently, the ENSO cycle has been an important factor for the extraseasonal short-term climatic forecast in China (Lin, et al., 2000). However, a number of questions remain unresolved. For instance, is the relationship between the EASM and ENSO stable in their long-term march, and what controls the dynamic linkage between them? Torrence et al. (1998) and Webster et al. (1992; 1998) revealed that the relationship between the Niño 3 region SST anomaly and the Indian monsoon is subject to changes over long (i.e., multi-decadal) time scales. Wang (2002) identified that there are periods where the correction between the EASM and ENSO is absent based on the reanalysis data and observed SST data from the National Centers for Environmental Prediction/ National Center for Atmospheric

Research (NCEP/NCAR) reanalysis project (Kalnay et al., 1996). However, observational based data with only 50 years duration are too short for proper analyses of multi-decadal processes.

The East Asian monsoon is shown to be weaker after the end of 1970s, and the correlation of East Asian summer monsoon (EASM)-ENSO relation is proved to be variable in the decadal time scales (Wang, 2001). In addition, a 300 years control integration of a coupled global atmosphere-ocean-sea ice general circulation model (GCM) has been used to study the relationship between the EASM and the ENSO cycle by applying cross wavelet analysis. It follows that the correlation between the EASM and ESNO may break down on interdecadal time scales. Furthermore, the characteristics of summer atmospheric circulation during their high correlation periods (HCP) are quite different from those during the low correlation periods (LCP). Notably, the HCP is characterized by an anomalous low tropospheric cyclone coupled with an anticyclone circulation over the western North Pacific, and a board belt of strong low tropospheric easterly wind anomalies located from the Philippines to the Bay of Bengal. For HCP, large interannual variability is founded in the low tropospheric wind velocity field over Southeast Asia, and the tropospheric temperature and geopotential heights over the tropical western Pacific. In addition, the correlation pattern between summer rainfall in East Asia and simultaneous Niño3 region sea surface temperature (SST) anomalies are significantly different during the HCP and LCP periods.

It is also indicated that in recent 20 years more flood disasters occurs in the Yangtze River valley (for example, the years 1998 and 1999 are flood years for the Yangtze River Valley and they caused serious damages), rather than in the lower reaches of the Yellow River Valley as in the 1950s to 1960s (Wang, personal communication). There is some evidence that the warm winters in North Asia happen very frequently after the end of 1970s. The last winter is the warmest one in past 20 years according to the NCEP/NCAR atmospheric reanalysis, and, interestingly, this extra-strong warm winter event was caused essentially by the interannual scale variability rather than the decadal scale variability.

THE DUST STORMS IN CHINA

In the past 50 years, strong dust storms have occurred more and more frequently. In the 1950s, there were 5 strong dust storms, but in the following four decades such numbers are respectively 8, 13, 14, and 23. In addition, the dust storms tend to be stronger. For example, the dust storm of April 6, 2000 was the strongest one in the past 50 years and it influenced $2/3^{rds}$ of China. It also influenced even the west coastal region of the USA cross the Pacific Ocean.

It is indicated that dust weather in Beijing usually relates with a stable ridge in West Asia and a stable and deep trough in East China Sea region (Zhang et al., 2002). Ye et al. (2000) indicated that La Niña years are usually accompanied with frequent and strong dust weathers in China, and that the temperature and precipitation in spring and the preceding winter are connected to the dust weather as well.

In order to observe the dust storms, a monitoring network has been established in China. The observation stations were set up in Northwest China, Central North China, and East China. In the Institute of Atmospheric Physics Chinese Academy of Sciences in Beijing, a 325m high tower monitors the boundary layer atmospheric meteorology and the air pollution including various chemical components.

THE GLOBAL WARMING SIMULATION IN IAP

The modeling studies in IAP on the global warming related problems started in 1992. After that, in each of the three IPCC scientific assessment reports, IAP model results were cited. The results which were cited in the Third Assessment Report (TAR) of IPCC was done by the coupled atmospheric and oceanic general circulation models. This model also contains a detailed scheme for the land surface processes.

The major conclusions of the model simulations are as follows:

1. The model well reproduced the overall changes of the global mean temperature in 1990-2000. But the model failed to capture the warm period in the 1940s, as many other models did. The model successfully simulated the rapid warming since the end of 1970s as the observation.
2. The model predicts the largest warming in East Asia in spring and largest precipitation increase in winter induced by the CO^2 doubling.
3. The model predicts the larger than average warming over Eurasia, North America, and Australia. While the warming over North Pacific and North Atlantic is the smallest.

As noted by IPCC reports, the regional scale changes are at present highly model dependent. The next generation model in IAP will consider aerosols, chemical processes, and the fresh water input to the ocean.

REFERENCES

1.   Ailikun, B., and T. Yasunari (2001) "ENSO and Asian summer monsoon: Persistence and transitivity in the seasonal march." *J. Meteor. Soc. Japan*, **79**:145-159.

2.   Bjerknes, J. (1966) "A possible response of the atmospheric Hadley circulation to equatorial anomalies of ocean temperature." *Tellus*, **18**: 820-829.

3.   Bjerknes, J., (1969) "Atmospheric teleconnections from the equatorial Pacific." *Mon. Wea. Rev.*, **97**:163-172.

4.   Huang, R. H., and Y. Wu, (1989) "The influence of ENSO on the summer climate change in China and its mechanism." *Adv. Atmos. Sci.*, **6**:21-32.

5.   Kalnay E., M. Kanamitsu, R. Kistler, et al. (1996) "The NCEP/NCAR Reanalysis Project." *Bull. Amer. Meteor. Soc.*, **77**:437-471, 1996.

6.   Li, C., S. Sun, M. Mu (2001) "Origin of the TBO-interaction between anomalous

East-Asian winter monsoon and ENSO cycle." *Adv. Atmos. Sci.*, **18**:554-565, 2001.

7.   Lin, Z., Y. Zhao, G. Zhou, et al. (2000) "Prediction of summer climate anomaly over China for 1999 and its verification." *Climatic and Environmental Research (in Chinese with English abstract)*, **5**: 97-108, 2000.

8.   Lu, R. (2002) "Precursory SST anomalies associated with the convection over the western Pacific warm pool." *Chinese Science Bulletin*, **47**:696-699, 2002.

9.   Ren, B., R. Huang (1999) "Interannual variability of the convective activities associated with the East Asian summer monsoon obtained from TBB variability." *Adv. Atmos. Sci.*, **16**:77-90, 1999.

10.   Tao, S., L. Chen (1987) *A review of recent research on the East Asian monsoon in China*, Monsoon Meteorology, Oxford university Press, 60-92.

11.   Terray, L., S. Valcke, A. Piacentini (1998) *Oasis 2.2 Ocean Atmosphere Sea Ice Soil, User's Guide and Reference Manual*, Technical Report TR/CMGC/98-05, CERFACS, Toulouse, France.

12.   Torrence, C., P.J. Webster (1998) "The annual cycle of persistence in the El Niño/Southern Oscillation," *Q. J. R. Meteorol. Soc.*, **124**:1985-2004, 1998.

13.   Torrence, C., G.P. Compo (1998) "A practical guide to wavelet analysis." *Bull. Am. Meteor. Soc.*, **79**:61-78, 1998.

14.   Wang, B., R. Wu, and X. Fu (2000) "Pacific-East Asian teleconnection: How does ENSO affect East Asian climate?" *J. Climate*, **13**:1517-1536, 2000.

15.   Wang, H.J. (2001) "The weakening of the Asian monsoon circulation after the end of 1970s." *Adv. Atmos. Sci.*, **18**:376-386.

16.   Wang, H.J. (2002) "Instability of the East Asian summer Monsoon-ENSO relations." *Adv. Atmos. Sci.*, **19**:1-11.

17.   Wang, Y., B. Wang, and J.H. Oh (2001) "Impact of the preceding El Niño on the East Asian summer atmosphere circulation." *J. Meteor. Soc. Japan*, **79(1B)**:575-58801.

18.   Webster, P.J., S. Yang (1992) "Monsoon and ENSO: Selectively interactive systems." *Q. J. R. Meteorol. Soc.*, **118**: 877-926, 1992.

19.   Webster, P.J., V.O. Magaña, T.N. Palmer, et al. (1998) "Monsoon: Processes, predictability, and the prospects for prediction." *J. Geophys. Res.*, **103**:14 451-14 510.

20.   Ye, D.Z., J.F. Chou, J.Y. Liu, et al. (2000) "On the dust weather in North China and the countermeasure (in Chinese)." *Chinese J. Geography*, **55**: 513-521, 2000

21.   Zhang, R.J., Z.W. Han, M.X. Wang, et al. (2002) "Some new features of the dust weather in China and the analysis of the causes (in Chinese)." *Quaternary Res.*, **22**:374-380, 2002

FOUR BILLION YEARS OF THE CARBON CYCLE: WHAT'S THE MESSAGE FOR US?

JÁN VEIZER
Institut für Geologie, Mineralogie und Geophysik, Ruhr-Universität Bochum, Bochum, Germany, Department of Earth Sciences, University of Ottawa, Ottawa, Canada

Carbon dioxide, generally believed to be the most important greenhouse gas and climate modifier, is today the centerpiece of a heated political and scientific debate that has polarized scientists, policy makers, and the public. One side maintains that CO_2 is the principal driver of climate, and the sequence of events is this: higher CO_2 equals global warming equals climate change equals disaster. Based on this scenario, the burning of fossil fuels and deforestation will inexorably lead to global warming. The latest models from the International Panel on Climate Change project an average temperature rise from 1.5 to 5.5 degrees Celsius (2.7 to 9.9 degrees Fahrenheit)[1] by the year 2100. Environmental Armageddon is an inevitable consequence of the above equation. The other side claims that the role of anthropogenic CO_2 on climate has not been proved, and that there is therefore no need for emissions quotas such as those mandated by the Kyoto protocol.

As is usually the case with contentious matters, the reality likely lies somewhere in between. So why is this issue so polarizing? First, past, natural variations in the carbon cycle and climate are poorly understood. These variations must be taken into account as a baseline for any superimposed human impact. Second, the climate models are inherently uncertain. Since I am a geologist and not a modeler, I will deal mostly with the first subject, the carbon cycle, contemplating it at time scales ranging from billions of years to the human life span. This perspective is essential, because events on progressively shorter time scales are embedded in, and constrained by, the evolution of the background on longer time scales.

As for the second issue - the uncertainties inherent in the climate models - we must acknowledge the admirable progress in climate modeling. But modeling contains many serious pitfalls, and a number of issues remain to be resolved - for example, the role of clouds and the couplings of climate to the oceanic and particularly the terrestrial biosphere, or land plants.

Consider that, theoretically,[2] cooling by the clouds alone may potentially exceed by up to 5.4 times the warming impact of the greenhouse gases.[3] Such concerns should be given due consideration and resolved before we make any definitive claims based on the climate scenarios. On the issue of modeling, I restrict myself solely to the role of land plants in the carbon cycle because of their potential impact on the "CO_2 sinks" debate, which was the reason for the failure of the 2000 Hague summit, and for the 2001 Bonn compromise.

344

LIFE, WATER, AND THE CARBON CYCLE

The story of the carbon cycle is essentially the story of life. Carbon and water are the fundamental building blocks of living things, and the propagation of life is accomplished via continuous exchange of these two constituents with the atmosphere and hydrosphere – ocean and water bodies on land. Such interactions are termed the water and the carbon cycles. While other cycles, such as those of nitrogen and phosphorus, are also involved, they are of lesser importance for the climate issues discussed here.

To understand the role of atmosphere, water, and life in climate evolution in the geologic past, it is essential to study ancient examples. Yet we have no unequivocal samples of ancient waters, and the oldest samples are bubbles of air that were frozen into Antarctic ice at the time of its formation, only about 420,000 years ago. The situation is somewhat better with the remnants of life, since mineralized shells go back to about 545 million years, and impressions of living things, algae and bacteria, have been found in western Australia in rocks as old as 3.5 billion years.[4] (Fig. 1)

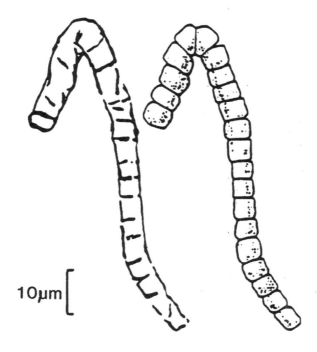

10μm

Fig. 1. Idealized reconstruction of the oldest known fossils, 3.5 billion year-old blue-green algae[4] from Western Australia.

Soft body tissues altered by temperature and pressure referred to as kerogen have been found in still older rocks approaching 4 billion years. This is remarkable, because the oldest rocks ever recovered, found near Yellowknife in northwestern Canada,[5] are of about the same age. The only older things ever found on this planet are a few zircon crystals, such as those used for jewelry, from western Australia, with an age of 4.2 billion years.[6] The core of one of these crystals appears to be only 200 million years younger than the age of the earth itself,[7] which is 4.55 billion years. These remarkable observations tell us that life on this planet goes at least as far back as the oldest rocks. Moreover, some features of that single very old zircon nucleus suggest that liquid water was present on the planet as early as 200 million years after its "birth," implying that conditions conducive to life may go back even further.

HOW MUCH LIFE?

These observations, however, are only qualitative. If we want to understand the operation of the carbon cycle and its role in the climate system, it is necessary to know not only that there was life, but also how much of it there was. In order to establish this, we have to rely on the derivative, or proxy, signals. In our case, such proxies are isotopes, particularly of carbon and oxygen.

Isotopes are atoms of the same chemical element that differ in the number of neutrons and thus in weight. In our example, carbon isotopes of interest have a weight of 13 or 12, and oxygen of 18 or 16 units. These isotopes are present in earth materials in specific proportions which can be altered by processes involving life, such as photosynthesis in the case of carbon, or by the temperature of water at the time of shell secretion, in the case of oxygen. We can collect samples of these shells, minerals, rocks, or organic matter (kerogen) from strata of different ages and measure their isotopic ratios. Employing some assumptions, we can then calculate, for example, the temperature of the ocean at that time, or the proportion of carbon that was sequestered by organisms from the ocean/atmosphere reservoir for generating organic matter. The proportion of carbon is more or less a question of how much biomass was present on the planet at any given time. Note that this "biomass" involves the amount of dead organic matter, or kerogen, and living biomass, the latter always only a minuscule portion of the whole.

From the measurements of isotope ratios of carbon in today's living things and of carbon dissolved in sea water, we can calculate that the rough proportion of oxidized to reduced carbon is about 80:20 percent. The oxidized carbon encompasses sedimentary rocks such as limestones, the bicarbonate dissolved in the hydrosphere, and carbon dioxide in the atmosphere. The reduced carbon includes both the living organisms and the dead organic matter in sediments. Remarkably, when we trace these carbon isotopes back in geologic history, we get exactly the same 80:20 ratio as far back as 3.5, and possibly 4 billion, years ago.[8] Stated rather boldly, not only did we have life as far back as we had rocks, but there was as much life then as today, albeit in its primitive form. Note that even today higher organisms form only a minor portion of the extant biomass. We can conclude, then, that the fundamental features of the carbon cycle were established as early as 4 billion years ago. All subsequent history was merely a series of "boom and bust" oscillations around this 80:20 percent ratio.

YOUNG PLANET: A SUPERGREENHOUSE?

What does this mean for atmospheric carbon dioxide? The simplest assumption would be that it might not have been that different from today. Yet, such a proposition is difficult to reconcile with the so-called "faint young sun" paradox.

Based on our understanding of the evolution of stars in the same category as our sun, the young sun was about 30 percent less luminous than it is today, and became brighter with age. With such low radiative energy from the sun, our planet should have been a frozen iceball until about 1 billion years ago. Yet, from the type of sediments we find from early geologic times, we know that running water shaped the surface of the planet as far back as we can see. In addition, in contrast to the last third of Earth's history, the first two-thirds is remarkable for its general lack of sedimentary rocks laid down by glaciers. The oldest evidence for a relatively localized glaciation is available from South Africa, at 2.9 billion years ago, but the first continental size glaciation, the Huronian of Canada, appears at about 2.2 billion years ago. Subsequently, for 1.5 billion years, there is no evidence to indicate a cold climate until about 0.7 billion years ago, when 2 or more glacial episodes affected all continents. This may have been the coldest period in all of planetary history, with glaciers reaching sea level even at tropical latitudes. Some models, such as the much discussed "snowball earth,"[9] even propose an almost complete freeze-up of all oceans, with ice cover several kilometers thick. Yet, apart from these two intervals, the types of sediments during early planetary history are indicative of a climate that may have been mostly warmer than today. To resolve this paradox, some argue that a massive greenhouse, caused principally by CO_2, must have warmed up the young earth. Theoretical calculations, set up to counteract the lower solar luminosity, yield CO_2 atmospheric concentrations some 1,000 times greater than today's value of 0.035 percent.[10] Yet, if this were the case, not only the chemical equilibria, but also the pH, and potentially the isotopic ratios of carbon in seawater, would have been altered, a prediction not consistent with the observed record. Providing the stellar evolutionary theory is correct, then factors more complex than a massive CO_2 greenhouse would have to be invoked to explain the warming of this planet to temperatures that may have surpassed those of the present day. A plausible alternative is a greenhouse due to water vapor.[11]

Significantly, large numbers of anomalous carbon isotope measurements have been recorded from the two intervals with large-scale glaciations, about 2.2 and 0.7 billion years ago. Unfortunately, our dating of these old sequences is not yet good enough to resolve the timing and correlations of isotopic and climatic events, and this leaves the field open to a plethora of essentially unconstrained scenarios. The correlation capabilities improve considerably with the appearance of shelly fossils, about 545 million years ago, the time interval called the Phanerozoic.

PHANEROZOIC CARBON CYCLE

Once we have framed our understanding of the carbon cycle on billion-year time scales, we can turn to shorter time scales: higher order oscillations on million-year time scales embedded in this baseline.

The previous discussion was based on isotopic proxies measured on rocks, such as limestones. The original sediments deposited on the sea bottom are recrystallized and hardened, eventually to become limestones. This process, called diagenesis, usually preserves the signature of carbon isotopes, but not those of oxygen. This, in addition to dating uncertainties, was the reason we did not discuss paleotemperatures—or temperatures of geologic eras—of the oceans. In the Phanerozoic, some organisms secreted their shells as the mineral calcite ($CaCO_3$), which often survives the vagaries of diagenesis and thus preserves the original oxygen isotope ratio. This ratio reflects two factors, seawater temperature and its oxygen isotopic composition.

As a matter of historical interest, the entire field of stable isotope geochemistry evolved from a post-World War II proposition of American chemist Harold Urey that oxygen isotopes may serve as a potential paleothermometer. To calculate the temperature, we have to know the oxygen isotopic composition of the ambient water from which the organism secreted its shell and the isotopic composition of the shell itself. The composition of the shell is measured directly, but we have no vestiges of the ancient water and so researchers usually operated on the assumption that the isotopic composition of sea water was the same as today. It very quickly became clear, however, that the older the shells, the higher the calculated sea water temperatures, up to 70 degrees Celsius. Considering that some of these were times of glaciation, it was an unrealistic outcome. Consequently, for almost half a century the view prevailed that all older samples had altered oxygen isotope ratios, due to diagenesis. Only the samples younger than a few million years, mostly from drillholes in the world's oceans, were considered well preserved and indeed provided the backbone for the burgeoning field of paleoceanography.

The alternative possibility, however, is that the oxygen isotopic composition of seawater did change over geologic time. Recently, we have generated a very large database[12] based on several thousand well-preserved calcitic shells that cover the entire 545 million year time span of the Phanerozoic eon. These data show that if the results are corrected for such temporal isotopic evolution of seawater, the remaining oscillations correlate well with the climatic history of the planet as deduced from the sedimentary record (Fig. 2).

A semi-quantitative climatic history can be inferred from the type of sediments, such as the distribution of coral reefs, coal measures, salt deposits, soil types, and deposits of glaciers. We therefore proposed that the oxygen isotope trend we observed is a paleotemperature record of seawater for the last 545 million years.[13] Since most of the fossils we studied lived in paleotropical oceans, it is essentially a record of tropical sea surface temperatures, which may have fluctuated by perhaps 5 to 9 degrees Celsius between the apexes of cold and warm intervals, called icehouse and greenhouse times, respectively.

For a geologist, these terms mean extended intervals, of tens of millions of years, of predominantly cold or warm climate. Note that these intervals were not uniformly cold or warm, but were interspersed with shorter intermezzos of opposing climate, called stadials and interstadials. For example, the latest icehouse that commenced with cooling of Antarctica, some 55 million years ago, was in the last 1 million years interspersed by about 10 prolonged cold snaps (stadials) and 10 shorter, warmer, interstadials. We are living in the youngest interstadial of the latest icehouse.

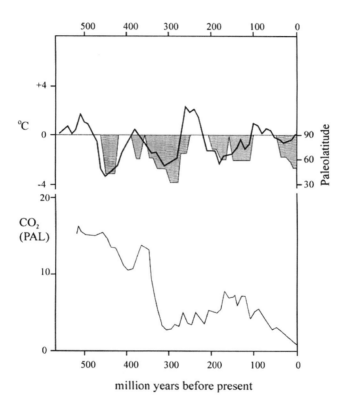

Fig. 2. Reconstructed variations in mean tropical sea surface temperatures during the Phanerozoic eon (545 million years) from oxygen isotopes. Note that at times of cooling, "dropstones" falling to the bottom of the oceans from melting icebergs were found in sediments at almost equatorial (~35∞) paleoaltitudes (shaded).[13] In contrast, the estimated CO_2 atmospheric levels,[14] compared to the present day ones (PAL), do not show any correlation with the temperatures or climate.

If sea surface tropical temperatures have fluctuated by up to 10 degrees Celsius, then cooling and warming modes are global; that is, ocean temperatures during cool modes decline even in tropical areas. This contradicts the widely held belief that during ice ages the tropics contract, but remain more or less at the same temperature, while the cold zones expand. Since the existing climate models generally assume that tropical temperatures are, and were, constant – in clear disagreement with the above experimental data – it may be that the models are calibrated for the modern geography and modern climate mode, a warm period in an icehouse. Therefore, these models are not entirely relevant for climates without polar ice caps, or for strongly glaciated episodes such as the one 15 to 30 thousand years ago.

Another discrepancy arises from the widely held belief that CO_2 is a climate "driver," and therefore that greenhouses are a consequence of the high CO_2 concentrations in the atmosphere, and icehouses of low ones. Comparison of the CO_2 model estimates with the climate record based on sediments or on the oxygen isotope record shows that there is really no correlation (Fig. 2). For example, in the interval from 545 to about 350 million years ago, CO_2 concentrations are estimated to have been high, 10 to15 times present levels,[14] regardless of whether the planet was in a greenhouse or in an icehouse mode. Similarly, for the post-300 million year interval there is almost an opposite relationship between CO_2 and climate, with higher concentrations correlating with cooler climate. This suggests two possibilities; first, that the record for CO_2 in the geologic past is not reliable, or second, that CO_2 is not a climate "driver" and there is no direct causal relationship between CO_2 and climate. In my view, both may apply. The estimates of paleo-CO_2 are based on model calculations that take into account the carbon isotopic compositions of limestones, shells, an iron mineral called goethite, and a type of organic compound called alkenones. A great many model assumptions – parameterizations – are involved before these data can be translated into atmospheric CO_2 concentrations.

If CO_2 is not the culprit, what could the driving force be? The Phanerozoic climate and oxygen isotope record shows that climate undergoes significant warming/ cooling cycles about every 135 million years. No terrestrial or extraterrestrial cycle of such a frequency is known. One may be tempted to speculate that a pulsing solar radiative output may have been the cause, but no theory for such a large pulse exists. Furthermore, if the sun were the culprit, why do we not see any periodicity within the 2.2 to 0.7 billion-year interval? The subsequent regular pulse is perplexing, but remains enigmatic.

THE ICE-CORE RECORD

Drilling in the Antarctic and Greenland has produced a record on millennial to century time scales for the last 420 thousand years. The laminae of ice contain bubbles of frozen air, and there is clear proof that the amount of CO_2 and methane contents in the bubbles increases with temperature.[15] Yet, the cause and effect relationship is a chicken and egg question. New high-resolution studies suggest that at times of transition, temperature changes come first, leading, on average, CO_2 changes by 1,300 years, and preceding changes in the volume of ice by 2,700 years.[16] If so, CO_2 and methane in the past were the products rather than the causes of climate changes, and greenhouse gases yet again served as temperature amplifiers and not as climate drivers.

Moreover, methane, another strong greenhouse gas, is mostly a product of the terrestrial biosphere. This suggests that the climate related oscillations in concentrations of greenhouse gases are strongly influenced by changes in land plant cover and this brings us to the issue of the ill-fated "sinks" that sank agreement at the Hague summit, but were partially reinstated in the Bonn compromise.

THE MISSING SINKS OF CO_2

One of the major unsolved mysteries in the greenhouse scenario is the fate of about one-half of the CO_2 produced by the burning of fossil fuels and deforestation. This CO_2 is not in the atmosphere. Some of it, about one-fourth, has been absorbed by the oceans, but the fate of the remaining one-fourth is unknown. This is the mystery of the missing sink. Some have proposed that this CO_2 was absorbed mostly by northern – boreal forests and their soils, due to enhanced photosynthesis fueled by higher CO_2 concentrations - CO_2 fertilization.[17] The demand of some countries for "green credits" based on such sinks proved to be the major bone of contention at The Hague and Bonn summits.

Our studies of watersheds dominated by northern ecosystems, such as that of the Ottawa River, confirm that the removal of CO_2 from the atmosphere, by photosynthesis, exceeds the export of carbon, by respiration, from the basin,[18] leading to net accumulation of carbon in the ecosystem. If so, the northern forests may indeed be the missing sink. The enhanced photosynthesis may be real, but the chain of events may be entirely different. To fix one molecule of carbon by photosynthesis, a plant has to transpire several hundred to a thousand molecules of water. This is called the Water Utilization Efficiency (WUE). The important point is that the carbon and water cycles are coupled and cannot proceed in isolation. This raises immediately two points.

First, the major factors controlling the rates of photosynthesis are daylight, temperature, and humidity. Considering the 1000:1 WUE, it is likely that the system is water driven and that the carbon cycle is piggybacking on the water cycle, and not vice versa. If so, we are probably dealing not with "CO_2 fertilization" but with "moisture fertilization," and CO_2 becomes a side issue of water balance rather than a driving force. We have shown that if we know the water balance of a watershed, we can make a rough estimate of its ability to absorb carbon.[19]

Second, the air that the plants "inhale" usually contains less than 100 molecules of water for each molecule of CO_2. In order to sustain photosynthesis, the plant has to pump out hundreds of molecules of water from the ground into the atmosphere for each molecule of CO_2 consumed. Yet, water vapor is a potent greenhouse gas, and the net effect of CO_2 lowering may, ironically, be an increase in the greenhouse. I realize that water vapor stays in the atmosphere a shorter time than CO_2, and rains out, to be used again. Nevertheless, before it rains, it acts at first as a greenhouse gas and subsequently as clouds, and the impact on the climate of clouds is large and uncertain.

The important message is that water is important, and that the water and carbon cycles are coupled. This is the case also in short- and long-term time scales. For example, the weathering of rocks is regarded as the most important sink of CO_2 on geological time scales,[14] atmospheric CO_2 being sequestered for chemical reaction with minerals. Yet, in reality it is the water that is the agent of weathering, with dissolved CO_2 accounting for about one-thousandth of the medium. Weathering would proceed without CO_2, albeit with modified chemical reactions, but not without water. In almost any process, and on all time scales, the water and carbon cycles are coupled, and water in orders of magnitude more abundant. Again, it is the carbon cycle that is piggybacking on the water cycle and not the other way around. Depending on whether water vapor warming or cloud cooling prevails, reforestation as a remedial measure for the greenhouse, as opposed to CO_2 abatement, may be an illusory solution. This said, the greening of our planet has its own psychological and environmental merits, and should not be viewed solely from the perspective of an uncertain water vapor greenhouse.

DOES IT MATTER?

Carbon dioxide is a greenhouse gas and, regardless whether it's a climate "driver" or only a temperature amplifier, higher CO_2 concentrations mean higher temperatures. The distinction therefore could be regarded as a moot issue, particularly since the answer to some extent depends on personal perception of what is weather and what is climate. Unfortunately, such a distinction may have an impact on the predicted magnitude of warming.

Most readers do not realize that this planet would be an iceball, at an average temperature of minus 16 degrees Celsius, were it not for a natural greenhouse of 31 to 33 degrees Celsius. Some two-thirds of this temperature enhancement is due to water vapor in the atmosphere and not to CO_2. The suggested anthropogenic warming of the last century is about a half a degree Celsius, or a 2-percent variation on the natural greenhouse. Only about 25 percent of this, and of any projected future warming, is attributed directly to CO_2. The rest is due to feedback from CO_2 on other greenhouse gases such as methane – 25 percent, and water vapor – 50 percent.[17] Yet, if CO_2 is not a driver, the feedback will be mostly from the water to the carbon cycle, rather than the other way around. In that case, both water and CO_2 are to be treated as internal variables of the model, with only the excess "anthropogenic" CO_2 – presently up to about 80 parts per million – considered as an external variable. The real impact of such an external forcing will then be modified by the dominant cycle, water. The usual outcome of increasing complexity is a damping of the signal, in this case of temperature oscillations.

A somewhat exaggerated analogy may perhaps help to understand the difference. Shares of Microsoft are traded on the New York stock exchange, held in Mr. Gates' portfolio, and a few in my own portfolio. Their value is always the same in all three stations, and I may therefore conclude that I am the driver of the stock exchange. Realizing that this is a preposterous claim, the impact on the stock exchange is assumed to be via "feedback" on Mr. Gates. If I sell 30 percent of my shares, Mr. Gates' must sell 60 percent of his. Yet, in reality, not even Mr. Gates is a driver, since he could not stop the large losses in their value in recent months. We are both amplifiers, he a major one, myself a minor one. Now, if someone generously doubles my shares – like doubling the amount of anthropogenic CO_2 – it does not necessarily follow that my portfolio will double in value. It will depend on what Mr. Gates will do and what the market will do. The feedbacks are to me and not from me.

Substituting climate for the stock market, water for Mr. Gates, and CO_2 for myself will give a general idea of the relative importance of CO_2 as a driver of climate change.

From discussions with the modeling community, it is my understanding that it is not yet possible to account for such complex variables and the damping effect of complexity. So, sensitive estimates of potential climate change will depend on developing comprehensive coupled models for atmosphere-ocean-biosphere, and for their physical as well as chemical dynamics.

ARMAGEDDON WHEN?

Considering that we are far from resolving these outstanding issues, should we abandon the generation of predictive scenarios, or even any effort to mitigate the emission of greenhouse gases? This would be an irresponsible attitude. Even if CO_2 has had a minimal effect on climate in the past, the fact remains that other emissions related to the combustion of fossil fuels - such as sulfur or particulates - still result in pollution, much of it due to our wasteful treatment of energy. In addition, anthropogenic greenhouse gases are a likely contributing factor to planetary warming, even if the system damps the signal. For the sake of argument, let us suppose that this damping is 1.5°Celsius. This would negate all lower range models, but if the maximal IPCC scenario of 5.5°Celsius proves the more reliable, such a damping would still yield a temperature rise well within the model predictions. Simple common sense suggests that environmental abatement measures can only help to restore nature's balance.

What is nevertheless disheartening is the deafening silence about the role of water in our public climate debates. The reason perhaps is that the chances of our manipulating the global water cycle are rather minute, except perhaps locally when we enter a hydrogen fuel-cell energy economy with water vapor as the by-product. For now, manipulating the water cycle does not have political appeal. Yet the water cycle, even if it isn't the composer, may be the conductor in the orchestra of nature.

If greenhouse gases, including water vapor, are only temperature amplifiers, they will mostly modify natural trends, enhancing the warming as temperatures rise, and retarding cooling when temperatures fall. Personally, I believe that greenhouse gases are indeed amplifying a natural climate warming, as temperatures rebound from the medieval Little Ice Age, when the Baltic Sea and the canals of Holland were frozen in winter. How much of this warming is natural and how much anthropogenic remains to be resolved.[20]

If neither the CO_2 cycle nor the water cycle is the "master" driver, what is? There may not be a single master driver, although the sun likely plays an important role. Our ability to predict future climates is hampered by the fact that we are dealing with very complex, perhaps "chaotic" systems. Such systems usually do not have a single cause, cannot be predicted in the desired detail, and may jump into a new mode if pushed beyond some threshold level. Since we cannot predict these thresholds, it is only prudent to institute precautionary abatement measures.

The other side of the coin is that such systems also possess many self-regulating feedbacks. In view of this, the shock tactics based on pronouncements of ever-new simplistic Armageddon scenarios may prove counterproductive, resulting in the loss of credibility for

354

environmental and climate agendas in the public consciousness. The issues are complex, and public education that could explain this complexity in search of a consensus is sorely needed. It would be a pity if we would imperil the chance of protecting this planet, the only one we have, by pronouncements that could potentially squander the goodwill of the public.

REFERENCES

1.   1 degree Celsius equals 1.8 degrees Fahrenheit.
2.   V. Ramathan, R.D. Cess, E.F. Harrison, P. Minnis, B.R. Barkstrom, E. Ahmad, and D. Hartmann (1989) "Cloud-radiative Forcing and Climate: Results from the Earth Radiation Budget Experiment," *Science* 243, pp. 57-63.
3.   Assuming a radiative forcing of minus 13.2 versus plus 2.45 watts per square meter ($W m^{-2}$).
4.   J.W. Schopf (1983) *Earth's Earliest Biosphere: Its Origin and Evolution.* Princeton, NJ: Princeton University Press. pp. 543.
5.   S.A. Bowring, I.S. Williams, and W. Compston (1989) "3.96 Ga gneisses from the Slave Province, Northwest Territories, Canada," *Geology* 17, pp. 971-975.
6.   W. Compston and R.T. Pidgeon (1986) "Jack Hills, Evidence of More Very Old Detrital Zircons in Western Australia," *Nature* 321, pp. 766-769.
7.   S.A. Wilde, J.W. Valley, W.H. Peck and C.M. Graham (2001) "Evidence from detrital Zircons for the Existence of Continental Crust and Oceans on the Earth 4.4 Gyr ago," *Nature* 409, pp. 175-178.
8.   M. Schidlowski (1988) "A 3,800–Million–Year Isotopic Record of Life from Carbon in Sedimentary Rocks," *Nature* 333, pp. 313-318.
9.   P.F. Hoffman, A.J. Kaufman, G.P. Halverson, and D.P. Schrag (1998) "A Neoproterozoic Snowball Earth," *Science* 281, pp. 1342-1346.
10.   N.F. Kasting and T.P. Ackerman (1986) "Climate Consequences of Very High CO_2 Levels in Earth's Early Atmosphere," *Science* 234, pp. 1383-1385.
11.   H.-W. Ou (2001) "Possible Bounds on the Earth's Surface Temperature: From the Perspective of a Conceptual Global-Mean Model," *Journal of Climate* 14, pp. 2976-2988.
12.   J. Veizer et al. (1999) "$^{87}Sr/^{86}Sr$, $\_^{13}C$ and $\_^{18}O$ Evolution of Phanerozoic seawater," *Chemical Geology* 161, pp. 59-88.
13.   J. Veizer, Y. Gooddéris, and L.M. François (2000) "Evidence for Decoupling of Atmospheric CO^2 and Global Climate During the Phanerozoic Eon," *Nature* 404, pp. 698-701.
14.   R.A. Berner (1994) "GEOCARB II: A Revised Model of Atmospheric CO_2 over Phanerozoic Time," *American Journal of Science* 294, pp. 56-91.
15.   J.R. Petit et al. (1999) "Climate and Atmospheric History of the past 420,000 Years from the Vostok Ice Core, Antarctica," *Nature* 399, pp. 429-436.
16.   M. Mudelsee (2001) "The Phase Relations among Atmospheric CO_2 Content, Temperature and Global Ice Volume over the past 420 ka," *Quaternary Science Reviews* 20, pp. 583-589.

17. W.F. Ruddiman (2001) *Earth's Climate: Past and Future.* New York, NY: Freeman and Co., 465 pp.

18. K.H. Telmer and J. Veizer (1999) "Carbon Fluxes, pCO_2 and Substrate Weathering in a Large Northern River Basin, Canada: Carbon Isotope Perspective," *Chemical Geology* 159, pp. 61-86.

19. K.H. Telmer and J. Veizer (2000) "Isotopic Constraints on the Transpiration, Evaporation, Energy and GPP Budgets of a Large Boreal Watershed: Ottawa River Basin, Canada," *Global Biogeochemical Cycles* 14, pp. 149-166.

20. U. Berner and H.J. Streif, (2001) *Klimafakten – Der Rückblick, ein Schlüssel für die Zukunft.* Stuttgart: Schweizerbartsche Verlag, 238 pp.

13. SCIENCE AND TECHNOLOGY: DESERTIFICATION—WATER POLLUTION —ALGAL BLOOM

SANDY DESERTIFICATION IN NORTH CHINA

TAO WANG
Cold and Arid Regions Environmental and Engineering Research Institute,
Chinese Academy of Sciences, Lanzhou 730000, China

ABSTRACT

Along with the development of economy and society, desertification exerts increasingly profound influences on natural environment and social-economic advancement and has attracted widespread attention from the world. China, as one of the countries that suffered from severe desertification problems, has made many efforts to research and combat desertification and has progressed in understanding and combating desertification through many years of hard work. Based on existing experiences and research achievements, this paper briefly discusses the causes, developmental processes, damage assessment and control mechanism of desertification in Northern China so as to provide some basic experiences for the further study of desertification in the future.

Keywords: sandy desertification, cause and process, damage assessment, desertification control

INTRODUCTION

According to the UN Convention to Combat Desertification (UNCCD), desertification means land degradation in arid, semi-arid and dry sub-humid areas resulting from various factors, including climatic variations and human activities, which not only results in the destruction of the resource-environment system and poverty but also affects the social stability and economic development. Therefore, it has attracted widespread attention from the international communities. China is one of the countries that has suffered from severe desertification, including wind erosion, water erosion and salinization for many years. Especially the rapid development of desertification and its tremendous influences on the environment, society and economy have received considerable attention. Based on the actual situations in the North China, the sandy desertification is defined as "land degradation characterized by wind erosion mainly resulting from the excessive human activities in arid, semi-arid and partially sub-humid regions." This conception contains the following implications:

1. Temporally, sandy desertification occurred in the human historic period, especially in the past century;
2. Spatially, sandy desertification occurred in the arid, semi-arid and partially sub-humid zones;
3. Genetically, the unreasonable human economic activities (over-cultivation, overgrazing, over cutting and overuse of water resources etc.) are the main cause resulting in desertification. Man is the maker of desertification and also the victim of desertification.
4. Land surface is changed by wind erosion and deposition which are the landscape marks of the desertification processes and indicators of desertification developmental degrees.
5. The developmental trend of desertification is related to desertification intensity, spatial extent, and human and livestock pressure on land.

Desertified land in North China is mainly distributed in the arid, semi-arid, and part of the sub-humid regions, including Inner Mongolia, Ningxia, Gansu, Xinjiang, Qinghai, Tibet, Shaanxi, Shanxi, Hebei, Jilin, Liaoning and Heilonjiang provinces, which are about $37.0\_10^4 km^2$ and form a discontinuously distributed arcuate belt stretched over North China. Of this land 29% is distributed in the mixed farming-grazing regions and rainfed farming regions in the semi-arid and sub-humid regions with wind erosion and sand sheet as the striking features. A further 44% is distributed in the middle and western parts of semi-arid zone and desert steppe regions with reactivated fixed dunes and shifting sand spread as the main features. Another 27% is distributed on the margin of oases in arid zones and lower reaches of inland rivers with reactivation of fixed dunes as the main feature. At present, desertified land area in China is still expanding at high rate: during the period from the 1960s to the 1970s its development rate was $1560 km^2/pa$; in the 1980s was $2100 km^2/pa$ and in the 1990s was $2460 km^2/pa$.[1] Rapid expansion of desertified land not only seriously destroyed the present eco-environmental construction and socio-economic development, but also greatly hinders the ecological construction of the 21st century and the implement of the large development strategy of West China.

Shortly after the 1977 United Nations Conference on Desertification, China officially launched multidisciplinary and comprehensive research and control on sandy desertification. Over the past 20 years, researchers have made some encouraging progress in this field of study, and much work was conducted in the regions with fragile eco-environmental conditions and frequent human activity from the angle of man-land relation.[2-9] Through remote sensing monitoring of desertification, field investigation and mapping in large regions,[4-9] we have achieved a preliminary understanding of desertification and also solved some problems, such as the causes, distribution states, types and damage of land desertification in arid, semi-arid and partially sub-humid regions in Northern China.[15-18] The study included the blown sand dynamic processes, biological processes and anthropogenic processes, the roles of anthropogenic factors and natural factors in the desertification development processes have been established and a multi-level comprehensive indicator system of desertification with blown sand activity as the main indicator has been put forward. In this paper we will give a brief discussion on several important problems concerning desertification research, including desertification causes, processes, damage assessment and control measures etc.

CAUSE OF SANDY DESERTIFICATION

Sandy desertification is land degradation with the processes of land productivity diminution, land resource loss, and desert-like landscape occurrence in arid, semi-arid and partially sub-humid zones resulting from interaction between irrational human economic activities and natural resource environment.

The cause of desertification has always been a basic subject in the research of desertification. Only if the cause of desertification is correctly understood can we put forward effective control measures and thoroughly solve the desertification problem. We divide the causes of desertification into two categories, namely natural causes and anthropogenic causes.

Natural cause

Natural occurrence of desertification is a common phenomenon in arid and semi-arid zones of China as is the natural wind erosion and sand dune encroachment on the river valley terraces and natural vegetation destruction in the wind gap area. The desertification mechanism due to natural causes can be summed up in two points: (1) global climate change, especially climatic warming and aridification in the mid-latitude regions, is a major ecological background favorable for the occurrence of desertification; (2) the presence of some adverse factors such as dry climate, erratic precipitation, sandy soil texture, ollse and erodible ground surface, especially strong and frequent sand-raising wind provides dynamic force for the occurrence of desertification. However, a certain self-regulating capacity in nature and the earth surface system always exists: once the system suffers from slight damage it can be self-regulated by its internal feedback mechanism and thereby maintain the stability of the system. As far as we know, desertification resulting from natural causes is often on a small scale, with low severity and can be easily reversed.

Anthropogenic cause

Desertification mainly occurred in the human historical period but developed rapidly in the past one hundred years. The changes in natural conditions, mainly the climatic fluctuations over a timescale of a century are generally small and therefore insufficient to cause great changes of natural environment. However, rapid increase of population pressure and economic activities in the same period could lead to the serious deterioration of the eco-environment and rapid development of desertification. A lot of archaeological data and field investigations have proved this. When the arid region of China was occupied by nomadic people, almost no eco-environmental pressure existed, but after the nomad was replaced by agricultural production the eco-environment suffered great damage. It is generally accepted that anthropogenic causes, including the rapidly increasing population, induced over-cultivation, over-grazing, over-cutting, over-extracting of groundwater and extensive ecological mismanagement destroyed land-cover and finally led to the rapid development of desertification under adverse environmental background conditions. According to recent studies, man-made destruction of ground cover reduces soil water-holding capacity, suppresses airflow rise and convergence, enhances surface albedo, intensifies descending airflow and finally leads to climatic aridification. Owing to the influence of biological-geophysical feedback mechanism, the desertification induced by anthropogenic causes can bring much faster and more severe direct damage than that induced by natural causes.

According to field investigations and remote data analysis among various types of desertified lands in the North China, over cultivation-induced desertified land area occupied 25.4% of China's total desertified land area; over-grazing 28.3%; over fuel-wood cutting 31.8%; misuse of water resources and vegetation destruction due to industrial construction occupied 9%, and sand dune encroachment 5.5%. So we can say that human factors are the most important and most active factors affecting desertification processes.

OCCURRENCE AND DEVELOPMENT PROCESSES OF DESERTIFICATION

The occurrence and development processes of desertification are practically the processes of blown sand erosion, transport and deposition due to upset of the ecosystem balance by human activities and vegetation degradation or disappearance. The processes study requires elucidation of the occurrence and development laws of surface blown sand activities. It mainly contains such research contents as the dynamics of blown sand movement and the roles of biological and human activities, etc.

Dynamic processes of blown sand movement
The dynamic processes of blown sand movement mainly contain the development processes of sandy surface morphology under wing force, reactivation of fixed dunes and sand dune migration at the margin of sandy desert. The development processes of land surface morphology under the action of wind force deal with the interaction between wind force and exposed ground surface, under the action of wind force, surface particle creep, salinization and suspension take place and form a wind-sand stream, thus initiating the aeolian geomorphologic processes of erosion, transport and deposition. Wind-sand stream is formed by the interaction of two different densities of physical media, i.e. air and sand (or gravel). Once wind velocity reaches the threshold value, surface particles begin to move and form sand-bearing wind to further abrade and erode the surface.

As a result, soil wind erosion is exacerbated and thus leads to topsoil loss, soil quality deterioration and productivity reduction. When wind-sand stream encounters obstacles, the character of underlying surface changes and sand-bearing wind becomes saturated, its velocity drops and many of the particles in the airstream will settle and result in sand accumulation on land and vegetation. According to the dynamical principle of blown sand movement, accumulated sand is in fact an obstacle to blown sand movement, it causes the separation of attachment layer and eddy flow and hence reduces near-surface wind velocity and quickens sand deposition. With further accumulation of sand, shield dune and barchan dune occur. Reactivation of fixed dunes is attributed to the destruction of primary vegetation on sand dunes and the direct action of sand-bearing wind over sand dune surface. It generally appears to be a process of this type: wind-eroded breaches occur on windward slope of sand dunes→blowout→deflation →deflation pit→windward slope of deflation pit becomes gentle; in the meantime on the leeward side of sand dune wind deposition processes occur and appear as spotted shrub-grass sand mound→sand sheet→semifluid sand sheet→moving sand dunes and moving shrub-grass sand mouns→typical moving sand dune landscape; under the action of wind force sand dunes at the margin of sandy desert migrate, namely exposed sand dunes, or newly exposed fixed dune due to vegetation destruction continuously receive sand supply on the windward slope, or continuous wind erosion on the windward slope, thus resulting in the migration of the whole dune body in the prevailing direction. Surface roughness reduction caused by human destruction of ground cover and intensifying blown sand activity are the basic factors affecting the blown sand dynamical processes of desertification.

Biological processes
Biological processes of desertification are mainly manifested in the degraded succession of vegetation i.e. evolution of landscape pattern. Studies in recent years show that the vegetation succession of sandy grassland is different from that of common grassland. Vegetation succession in desert regions is mostly related to the land desertification degrees. Vegetation succession stage and land desertification degree often constitute each other's pre-condition.[19] Vegetation changes in desert regions contain both gradual and sudden changes. They are controlled by land desertification degrees and also dependent on their own structure and function. On the different types of desertified land vegetation changes of ten appear as a sudden change; On the same type of desertified land, vegetation shows a gradual change under slight desertification conditions, but exhibits a sudden change under severe desertification conditions.[20] However, the degradation form and the velocity of vegetation often show a significant difference due to different causes. For grazing-induced grassland desertification, its degradation law is: significant decrease in biodiversity, vegetation cover, grass height and grass yield; perennial grasses firstly disappear from the grassland, followed by palatable annual grasses and finally the grassland will be dominated by unpalatable grasses or toxic grasses. When vegetation cover reduces, a certain degree of small bare spots occur on the grassland surface, with continuous expansion and connection of small bare spots the grassland finally turns into entirely desertified land.[21-23] Grassland desertification processes caused by wind erosion and water shortage are generally similar to those caused by grazing. However, there are also some differences. These are mainly manifested in such a way that from shady slope to sunny slope, from wetland to dryland, and from fixed sand land to mobile sand land the vegetation worsens rapidly. Furthermore, the degradation velocity is significantly faster than that caused by grazing, and both vegetation cover and plant species decrease

rapidly, but vegetation height and output do not necessarily decrease.[24] Under favorable environment conditions degraded vegetation on sand land may occur in positive succession; plant species, vegetation cover and height increase significantly, and the percentage of herbs in the communities also increase.[25-28]

Since vegetation degradation in desertified regions mainly results from human activities and the ecosystem has a self-restoration capacity, once human disturbances are removed, plants in inter-dune depressions or coppice dune areas will invade the surrounding regions and gradually restore the original landscape.

Anthropogenic processes

As described above, desertification is a land degradation process and human economic activities are the main factor responsible for such a process. In the arid, semi-arid and sub-humid zones of northern China the climate is dry, precipitation is sparse and highly variable, strong wind is frequent, the environment is harsh and ecological conditions are fragile. Added to this, people's education level is low, production methods are backward and land productivity is low, hence it has a lower population carrying capacity. With the improvement of people's living standards and public health service, the population rapidly increases and exerts increasingly greater pressure on land. To feed more and more population, people clear vegetation to extend cropland and to find wood for fuel. Under local harsh natural conditions, lands unprotected by vegetation are impossible to restore their original landscape. Once overgrazing, strong cultivation and industrial construction occur in the grassland region, grasses gradually degrade and bare spots occur on the surface. During drought and periods of strong wind, such land is highly susceptible to erosion by wind, further form shifting sand and cause reactivation of sand dunes. As a result, soil becomes coarse and impoverished, the soil's water-holding capacity and moisture content drop, the original forest and grassland landscape is replaced by a desert landscape, exposed ground surface cannot prevent erosion by wind but increases albedo, therefore the climate becomes drier and desertification is further exacerbated. Hence, anthropogenic process of desertification is a vicious cyclic process.

From the above discussion it can be seen that the process of land desertification is closely related to the features of landscape structure. Viewed from a landscape scale, initial small-scale desertification is related to the erosion and deposition processes of a certain site type but does not affect landscape feature. When desertification reaches mid-scale, sand dune stability will change. At this moment landscape features will also change but it does not affect landscape attribute. As large-scale desertification occurs, landscape attribute will change, i.e. landscape elements (for example, patches) of the same attribute will differentiate into landscape elements of different attributes. Therefore, anthropogenic processes appear as a landscape evolution in the desertification development processes. In addition, we also found that three main processes of desertification development complement each other and are closely interrelated. Anthropogenic processes first affect the ground surface and cause the degradation of surface system following the biological processes and finally the original sparse forest landscape changes into desert landscape due to blown sand activities.

DESERTIFICATION DAMAGE AND ASSESSMENT

Desertification not only causes environmental degradation but also affects social and economic development. Although the present assessments on desertification damages are mostly qualitative, they have important significance in understanding desertification issues and to enhance people's urgently felt need to combat desertification. The assessment of desertification's disastrous influence on the environment and socio-economic structures includes the following aspects: (1) Desertification damaged ecological balance, worsened environment, lowered land productivity, threatened people's livelihood, aggravated poverty and even resulted in the appearance of ecological refugees; (2) Desertification caused the loss of usable land resources and decreased the Chinese nation's living space; (3) Desertification seriously threatened the safety and normal operation of communities, traffic lines, water conservancy projects and national defense bases; (4) In China desertification caused a direct economic loss of 54 billion Yuan each year; (5) Sand and dust storms as a mark, and sudden event of desertification are becoming more frequent and stronger. According to statistical data[1] annual dust storm frequency in the last 50 years in Northern China showed a tendency to increase, for example, dust storms occurred 5 times per year in the 1950s, 8 times in the 1960s, 13 times in the 1970s, 14 times in the 1980s and 23 times in the 1990s. The increase in dust storm frequency coincided with the spreading of desertification in China. A single strong dust storm in 1993 resulted in a direct economic loss of 540 million Yuan. Since the spring of 2000, about 12 strong sand-raising events and dust storms have hit Northwest China and even to a certain extent affected large areas of East and South China, in clouding Beijing, Tianjin, Nanjing and Shanghai etc. As compared with previous years, sand and dust storms in the spring of 2001 occurred severely and frequently, affecting extensive regions and causing tremendous economic loss. Their occurrence is not only related to the passage of a cold air mass but also related to the expansion of desertified land and the aggravation of the degree of desertification.

Further research is required for the assessment of desertification damage. It is generally accepted that some indicators concerning natural conditions and socio-economic regimes should be established to reflect the degree of influence of desertification. However, at present there is still no consistency in the indicator and the application and a global indicator system has not been established. According to the actual situation of desertification in Northern China we have put forward a general desertification indicator and severity classification system to assess desertification state and developmental trend, of which surface morphological change is a main indicator, in the meantime other changes in soil, vegetation and ecosystem are also considered. For the monitoring and assessment of desertification in vast regions of Northern China, the selected indicators should have representation. Surface morphological change in the desertification processes has such a character, it is also an obvious landscape indicator.

---

[1] State Forestry Bureau, Northwest China Investigation Group, and Investigation Report on great development of west China and propagation of green homeland construction, 2000.

Many other factors such as vegetation cover, plant community structure, plant species, biomass, soil grain-size composition, organic matter content and soil moisture content are also directly related to surface morphological changes, hence they can be used as additional indicators. We classified various assessment indicators of desertification as follows: (1) Natural indicators include the area changes of wind-eroded land, sand land or sand dune, dust storm frequency, seasonal and annual changes of precipitation, wind velocity and direction, available soil layer thickness, groundwater level and quality and surface albedo etc.; (2) Biological and agricultural indicators include vegetation cover, biomass, dominant plant species and distribution, landuse states (for example, farming, grazing, fuelwood, industry, mining and water resource etc.), crop yield, livestock composition and number, and various economic input etc.; (3) Social and economic indicators include industrial structure, input benefit, population number and structural changes and developmental trend, public health indexes, mandatory plan and special policy etc.

DESERTIFICATION CONTROL

According to natural and economic features of desertified regions and desertification developmental trend in northern China as well as problems and typical experiences in desertification control, the rehabilitation of desertified land should, overall, consider the ecological, economic and social benefits. It should also follow the ecological principles of conservative development and multi-complementarity to contain landuse in the control processes.[29] In order to improve the ecosystem of all the arid and semi-arid zones, we should work out an overall plan and adopt comprehensive rehabilitation strategies. In the area of economic development the principle of diversified economy dominated by forestry should be practiced, in the meanwhile population growth should be effectively controlled. The arrangement of rehabilitation projects can be divided into three levels: 1) research organizations mainly undertake desertification control experiments in experimental plots; 2) research organizations in cooperation with production departments conduct experiments in demonstration plots; and 3) production departments and local people popularize successful techniques. In the mixed farming-grazing desert region where residential areas, cropland and grassland are randomly distributed, with an ecological household as a unit, such measures as prohibiting grazing, readjusting rainfed farming-dominated landuse structure, increasing forest and grassland area, intensive management of the land with better water and fertility conditions, establishing farmland forest net and patchy forest (shrub) in interdune depressions are adopted to control the spread of desertification. This also contributes to economic development. In the grazing grassland a rational stock rate and rotational grazing system should be established. In addition, efforts should be made to construct artificial grassland and forage base, rationally arrange drinking water wells, define grazing density and build roads. In the arid zone an overall plan should be worked out with a basin as an ecological unit, to formulate rational water allocation plans, construct a farmland forest net inside oases and sandbreak, tree-shrub belts around the oases, in combination with mechanical sand fences and sand-fixing plants inside sand fence grids to form a perfect protective system. In addition mechanical sand fences should protect the transport lines in the dense sand dune regions and sand-fixing plants, laying emphasis on fixation in combination with blocks.

Through a series of experiments on different desertification control models in several experiment plots the following successful examples have been found:

Example 1: Sandy land transformed into plastic film-bottomed rice field in Naiman Banner of Inner Mongolia

Desertified land in Naiman Banner occupies 57.6% of its total area, being a typical desert zone in northern China. Owing to a dry climate and serious blown sand disasters agricultural and livestock production outputs are low and unstable, the food problem especially has seriously hindered local economic development. Through many years of exploration and experiments, scientists and local people have successfully developed a rice cultivation technique in plastic film-bottomed sandy land and thus create a new way to control shifting sand. This technique has proved to have a bright future.

Example 2: Sand stabilization by Dinus sylvestris in Zhangguotai Sandy Land of Zhangwu County in Liaoning Province

Zangguotai is located at southeastern part of the Horqin Sandy Land. In view of the serious blown sand disaster in the region, from 1952 onwards people have launched sand stabilization, afforestation and species introduction works. Since then pinus sylvestris has been successfully used in moving dune stabilization. Up to now, some 2130 hm^2 of p. sylvestris forest have been planted in demonstration plots and popularized over 3000 hm^2 in another 6 pilot experiment plots. Long-term observations have proved their obvious ecological, economic and social benefit. Besides Liaoning and Inner Mongolia, P. sylvestris has also been introduced in North China and Northwest China. In addition, about 1000 kg seeds and 30 million seedlings of P. sylvestris are transported each year from the demonstration and pilot plots to "Three-North" regions to be used for the construction of a protective forest system.

Example 3: Wind check and sand stabilization in the Daxing County of Beijing suburb

Dzxing county is located in a suburb of Beijing. Historically eco-environmental conditions in the county were poor, with sparse trees, strong winds and frequent blown sand disasters. In 1981 the county was designated as a key point of Three-North Protective Forest project. After years of hard work a large area of sandy wasteland has been improved. People's living standards have been significantly enhanced and per capita income has increased from 500 Yuan to over 3000 Yuan. The rehabilitation of sandy wasteland improves agricultural production conditions, promotes the development of agriculture, animal husbandry and fishery and creates a new way to eradicate poverty and revitalize the economy.

Example 4: "Four-in-one" household ecological economy in Yutiangao village, Ongniud Banner, Chifeng city, Inner Mongolia

Ongniud Banner, located at the middle of Inner Mongolia and western margin of Horqin Sandy Land, is a part of Horqin Sandy Land. Dry climate, sparse precipitation and frequent blown sand disasters pose a serious threat to local economic development and people's livelihood. In order to shake off poverty, local people launched vegetable production using solar energy in winter in 1992 and later created a "four-in-one" household eco-economic pattern. It has proved to be an effective way to control blown sand damage and to help people to eliminate poverty.

Example 5: "Advance One-Retreat Two-Return Three" sand control strategy in Houshan region, Ulanqab League, Inner Mongolia

Ulanqab League, located to the north of the Yinshan Mountain, include Huade County Shangdu County, Qahar Youyi Middle Banner, Qahar Youyi Rear Banner and Siziwang Banner. Owing to a dry climate, frequent blown sand disasters, severe desertification, impoverished soil and irrational industrial structure,[30] agricultural output in these regions are low: per capita grain share has decreased from 535 kg/yr to 272 kg/yr; per capita income is about 200 yuan. After the National Conference on Sand Control was held in 1991, desertification control in the Houshan region of the league was included in the list of the county's 20 key projects. Local government practiced the "advance one-retreat two-return three" strategy and quickened the pace of comprehensive control of land desertification, thus creating a new way to improve the eco-environmental condition of desertified region and to eradicate poverty.

Example 6: Constructing farmland through washing sand dunes away by water in Yulin region of Shanxi

Yulin region is located at southern margin of Mu Us Sandy Land and includes 7 counties. Natural conditions in the region are harsh, with serious blown sand disasters. Local economy is backward and the people live in poverty. Through 10 years of hard work, 937.5 km^2 of blown sand land were reclaimed by the method diverting water and washing sand dune away. Of this total area, newly reclaimed farmland occupied 10^4 hm^2, soil conservation land 97_10^4 hm^2 and artificia grassland 4_10^4 hm^2. After 10 years of reclamation, vegetation cover increased from 24.5% to 74.3%, per capita grain share increased from 428 kg to 1861 kg, livestock number increase from 137,000 heads to 175,000 heads, and per capita income increased from 497 yuan to 1045 Yuan. The former barren desert has now been changed into fertile land.

CONCLUSION

As described above, desertification is in fact land degradation in arid, semi-arid and sub-humid regions due to the destruction of man-land system balance by irrational human economic activities to such a degree that the system cannot be rapidly restored by its self-organization and feedback mechanism. As a result, various environmental elements degrade and original sparse-tree sandy grassland landscape turns into desert landscape dominated by blown sand activity.

It can be said that the development processes of desertification are dynamic evolution processes of various internal elements of the man-land system and the flow of mass, energy and information of external environment in an arid zone and finally result in structural and functional changes of the system. In order to halt desertification, mankind must actively regulate its own activity, form self-adaptability, establish an interdependent and mutually coordinated man-land relation, and optimize the structure and function of man-land system to reach a new balance and realize a benign cycle.[31]

Owing to its tremendous impact on economy, environment and politics, desertification has attracted world attention. With economic development and the increase of social demands, the pressure on natural resources and eco-environment is increasing. Coupled with the influence of global changes; desertification is posing a serious threat to mankind's existence. Hence, there is an urgent need to understand the mechanism of desertification's occurrence and development and to halt desertification. Although scientists have preliminarily understood the causes and processes of desertification and found some effective measures to control desertification, there are still many questions to be settled. This is because desertification study deals with natural, social and economic issues and belongs to a multidisciplinary research field. It can be said that desertification study is faced with unprecedented challenge and opportunity and great effort should be made in this respect.

For this reason we suggest the following priorities research:

1. Study of the natural and human background of desertification. Include the natural environmental background; temporal and spatial changes and mechanism of desertified land over the past 2000 years; desertified land use and coverage change, process, cause and topsoil feature in the last 50 years; positive and negative influences of natural factors and human effect and their respective contributions.

2. Study of dynamic desertification process and its control. Include physical process and the mechanical principle of desertification; soil-wind erosion law and its control, mechanical mechanism of blown sand movement; mechanical model and the relation of different scales of sand bodies; mechanical principle and numerical imitation of sand control engineering design; dynamic mechanism of sand and dust storms; predication model of soil wind erosion and tolerance limit; indicator system and regionalization for quantitative assessment of soil-wind erosion; dust emission simulation and test from source area; dust transport route, affecting extent and climate-environment effect; frequently occurring area of dust storms, climatic cause, formation and development mechanism; dust storm monitoring, prediction and early warning methods.

3. Biological process of desertification and vegetation re-establishment mechanism including the water consuming law of main plant species; water cycle; stress-resistant mechanism, adaptive strategies and vegetation stability; water balance dynamics in typical regions; and suitable scale of vegetation construction.

4. Comprehensive control strategies and models of desertification. Include cause, state and developmental trend of desertification in northern China; water and land resource carrying capacity and safe landuse patterns in typical regions;

comprehensive control strategies and regionalization of desertification and dust storms in Northern China; harmonious development strategies and patterns of society, economy and environment in desertified regions; comprehensive control optimization models of desertification and technical experiment and demonstration study.

REFERENCES

1. CCICCD, (1996) *China Country Paper to combat desertification*, Beijing, China, Forestry Publishing House, pp. 18-31.
2. Zhou Xingjia, (1993) "Desertification and its control along the corridor of lower Tarim River," *Journal of Desert Research*, 3(1):27-29.
3. Wang Yushan, (1985) "Great attention should be paid to desertification issues in Bashang region in Hebei province," *Journal of Desert Research*, 5(3): 12-14.
4. Ze Ningshu, (1986) "Land use problems in arid and semi-arid zones of China," *Journal of Desert Research,* 6(1):1-5.
5. Zhu Zhenda, (1986) "Land sandification problems in humid and sub-humid regions," *Journal of Desert Research*, 6(4):1-2.
6. Wang Tao, (1986) "Desertification processes and prediction in Alagan region of lower Tarim River," *Journal of Desert Research,* 6(2):16-26.
7. Liu Shu, (1988) "Internal dynamical cause of desertification development in semi-arid regions," *Journal of Desert Research*, 8(1):1-8.
8. Chen Hesheng, (1988) "Influence of water resource development on environment in Shule River basin," *Natural Resources*, 2:12-23.
9. Wang Tao, (1989) "Comparative study of desertification in typical desertified regions of northern China," *Journal of Desert Research*, 9(1):113-137.
10. Zhu Zhenda, (1984) "Principles and methods to compile desertification maps," *Journal of Desert Research*, 4(1): 3-15.
11. Wang Yimu, (1986) *Application of remote sensing technique in the dynamical study of desertification, in MEM of Institute of Desert Research*, Chinese Academy of Sciences, No.3, Beijing, Science Press, pp. 82-88.
12. Wang Zhoulong, Wang Yimu, (1988) "Application of computer mapping in the study of desertification" *Journal of Desert Research*, 8(3):62-68.
13. Wang Yimu, (1988) *Thematic map compilation with TM images as information source, in Wang Yimu, Study of renewable resources*, Beijing, Science Press, pp. 45-47.
14. Zhu Zhenda, Wang Tao, (1990) "Analysis on evolution trend of land desertification in several typical regions of China in recent ton years," *Acta Geographical Sinica*, 45(2):36-49.
15. Zhu Zhenda, Liu Shu, Xiao Longshan, (1981) "Environmental features and restoration of desertification in grassland regions," *Journal of Desert Research*, 1(1):2-12.
16. Zhu Zhenda, Liu Shu, (1982) *Desertification historic processes and resource*

exploitation ways along Great wall in Ningxia and Hexi Corridor region, in MEM of Institute of Desert Research, Chinese Academy of Sciences, No.2, Beijing, Science DRESS, pp. 12-14.

17. Di Xingmin, Zhang Jixian, Liu Yangxuan, (1982) "Land desertification features and control in Ningxia," *Journal of Desert Research*, 2(2):1-8.

18. Zhu Zhenda, Liu Shu, (1982) "Study on agricultural development strategies in agropastoral desertified region of northern China," *Journal of Desert Research*, 2(2):1-5.

19. Wu Wei, (1997) "Remote sensing monitoring methods of desertification dynamics and practice," *Remote sensing Techniques and Application*, 12(4):73-89.

20. Wang Tao, (1998) "Remote sensing monitoring and assessment of desertification — taking desertified land in northern China as example," *Quaternary Research*, (2):108-118.

21. Li Shenggong, Zhao Aifen, Chang Xueli, (1997) "Several problems on vegetation succession in Horqin Sandy Land," *Journal of Desert Research*, 17(Supp.1):25-33.

22. Zhao Halin, (1997) "Study on desertification processes of grazing land of Horqin Sandy Land," *Journal of Desert Research*, 17(Supp.1):15-24.

23. Chang Xueli, Li Shenggong, (1998) "Dynamical change feature of plant diversity in fixed dune field of Horqin Sandy Land," *Journal of Desert Research*, 18(Supp1.2):33-37.

24. Zhao Halin, Zhang Tonghui, Chang Xueli et al., (1999) "Study on differentiation law of plant diversity and ecological niche of Horqin sandy grazing land," *Journal of Desert Research*, 19(Supp1.1):13-20.

25. Liu Xinmin, Zhao Halin, Zhao Aifen, (1996) *Blown sand environment and vegetation of Horqin Sandy Land*, Beijing, Science press, pp. 17-18.

26. Shi Qinghui, (1993) *Succession dynamics of artificial vegetation at northern side of Baolan railway in shapotou area at southeast fringe of Tengger Desert, in Annual Report of Shapotou Desert Experiment and Research station (1991-1992)*, Lanzhou, Gansu Science and Technology press, pp. 45-52.

27. Qin Guoyu, Shi Qinghui, (1993) *Sandy land moisture dynamics and vegetation succession in artificially fixed dunefield in Shapotou region, in Annual Report of shapotou Desert Experiment and Research station (1991-1992)*, Lanzhou, Gansu Science and Technology press, pp. 62-70.

28. Zhao Halin, Li Shenggong, Zhang Tonghui, (1998) "Grazing exclusion effect and assessment of degraded grassland in Horqin Sandy Land," *Journal of Desert Research*, 18(Supp1.2):27-50.

29. Zhu Zhenda, Chen Guangting, (1994) *Land sandy desertification in China*, Beijing, Science press, p. 36.

30. Zhu Junfeng, Zhu Zhenda et al., (1999) *Desertification control in China, Beijing*, China Forestry Publishing House, pp. 45-47.

31. Xue Xian, Wang Tao, (2000) "Desertification and sustainable development problems viewed from the angle of system theory," *Journal of Desert Research*, 20(4):103-201.

THE EXPANDING GLOBAL PROBLEM OF HARMFUL ALGAL BLOOMS

DONALD M. ANDERSON
Biology Department, Woods Hole Oceanographic Institution
Woods Hole, MA 02543 USA

INTRODUCTION

Over the last several decades, countries throughout the world have experienced an escalating and worrisome trend in the incidence of problems associated with blooms of harmful and toxic algae, commonly called "red tides," but now termed "harmful algal blooms" (HABs) by scientists (Anderson[1]). Impacts of these phenomena include mass mortalities of wild and farmed fish and shellfish, human illness and death from contaminated shellfish or fish, death of marine mammals, seabirds, and other animals, and alteration of marine habitats or trophic structure through shading, overgrowth, or adverse effects on life history stages of fish and other marine organisms. Several decades ago, relatively few countries were affected by HABs, but now most coastal countries are threatened, in many cases over large geographic areas and by more than one harmful or toxic species (Anderson;[2] Hallegraeff[3]). It is still a matter of debate as to the causes behind this expansion, with possible explanations ranging from natural mechanisms of species dispersal to a host of human-related phenomena such as pollution-related nutrient enrichment, or transport of algal species via ship ballast water (Anderson;[2] Smayda;[4] Hallegraeff[3]). Whatever the reasons, coastal regions throughout the world are now subject to an unprecedented variety and frequency of HAB events. Many countries are faced with a bewildering array of toxic or harmful species and impacts, as well as disturbing trends of increasing bloom incidence, more impacted resources, larger areas affected, and higher economic losses.

BACKGROUND

HAB events are characterized by the proliferation and occasional dominance of particular species of toxic or harmful algae. In some cases, the cells can increase in abundance until their pigments discolor the water—hence the common use of the term "red tide" to describe these phenomena. There are, however, "blooms" of species which are not in high cell concentrations and which do not discolor the water, but which still cause harm, typically because of the potent toxins produced by those algae. For this reason, the term "harmful algal bloom" is generally used. The term is very broad however, and covers blooms of many types. HABs have one unique feature in common: they cause harm, either due to their production of toxins or to the manner in which the cells' physical structure or accumulated biomass affect co-occurring organisms and alter food-web dynamics.

HAB phenomena take a variety of forms, with multiple impacts. One major category of impact occurs when toxic phytoplankton are filtered from the water as food by shellfish which then accumulate the algal toxins to levels which can be lethal to humans or other consumers. The poisoning syndromes have been given the names paralytic, diarrhetic, neurotoxic, amnesic, and azaspiracid shellfish poisoning (PSP, DSP, NSP, ASP, and AZP). The symptomology and exposure route for each of these are presented in Table 1. Except for ASP, all are caused by biotoxins synthesized by a class of marine algae called dinoflagellates. The ASP toxin, domoic acid, is produced by diatoms that until recently were thought to be free of toxins. A sixth human illness, ciguatera fish poisoning (CFP) is caused by ciguatoxins produced by dinoflagellates that attach to surfaces in many coral reef communities (reviewed in Anderson and Lobel[6]). Ciguatoxins are transferred through the food chain from herbivorous reef fishes to larger carnivorous, commercially valuable finfish. The final human illness linked to toxic algae is called Possible Estuary-Associated Syndrome (PEAS). This vague term reflects the poor state of knowledge of the human health effects of the dinoflagellate *Pfiesteria piscicida* and related organisms that have been linked to symptoms such as deficiencies in learning and memory, skin lesions, and acute respiratory and eye irritation – all after exposure to estuarine waters where *Pfiesteria*-like organisms have been present (Burkholder and Glasgow;[7] Burkholder[8]).

Another type of HAB impact occurs when marine fauna are killed by algal species that release toxins and other compounds into the water. Fish and shrimp mortalities from these types of HABs at aquaculture sites have increased considerably in recent years. HABs also cause mortalities of wild fish, seabirds, whales, dolphins, and other marine animals, typically as a result of the transfer of toxins through the food web. A poorly defined but potentially significant concern relates to sublethal, chronic impacts from toxic HABs that can affect the structure and function of entire ecosystems. Adult fish can be killed by the millions in a single outbreak, with obvious long- and short-term ecosystem impacts (Fig. 1). Likewise, larval or juvenile stages of fish or other commercially important fisheries species can experience mortalities from algal toxins. Impacts of this latter type are far more difficult to detect than the acute poisonings of humans or higher predators, since exposures and mortalities are subtle and often unnoticed. Impacts might not be apparent until years after a toxic outbreak, such as when a year class of commercial fish reaches harvesting age but is in low abundance. Chronic toxin exposure may therefore have long-term consequences that are critical with respect to the sustainability or recovery of natural populations at higher trophic levels. Many believe that ecosystem-level effects from toxic algae are more pervasive than we realize, affecting multiple trophic levels, depending on the ecosystem and the toxin involved.

Non-toxic blooms of algae can cause harm in a variety of ways. One prominent mechanism relates to the high biomass that some blooms achieve. When this biomass begins to decay as the bloom terminates, oxygen is consumed, leading to widespread mortalities of all plants and animals in the affected area. These "high biomass" blooms are sometimes linked to excessive pollution inputs, but can also occur in relatively pristine waters.

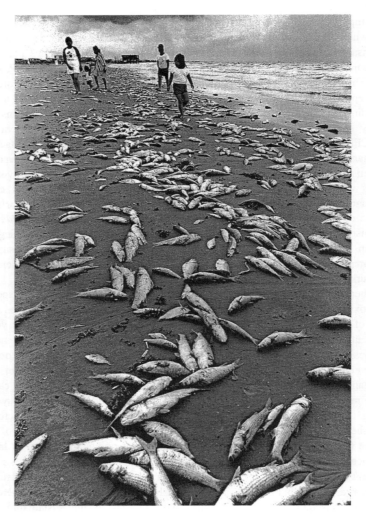

Fig. 1. Dead fish from a Texas red tide. (Credit: Brazosports.)

Large, prolonged blooms of non-toxic algal species can reduce light penetration to the bottom, decreasing densities of submerged aquatic vegetation (SAV). Loss of SAV can have dramatic impacts on coastal ecosystems as these grass beds serve as nurseries for the food and the young of commercially important fish and shellfish. Macroalgae (seaweeds) also cause problems. Over the past several decades, blooms of macroalgae have been increasing along many of the world's developed coastlines. Macroalgal blooms occur in nutrient-enriched estuaries and nearshore areas that are shallow enough for light to penetrate to the sea floor. These blooms have a broad range of ecological effects, and often last longer than "typical" phytoplankton HABs. Once established, macroalgal blooms can remain in an environment for years unless the nutrient supply decreases. They can be particularly harmful to coral reefs (Fig. 2). Under high nutrient conditions, opportunistic macroalgal species outcompete, overgrow, and replace the coral.

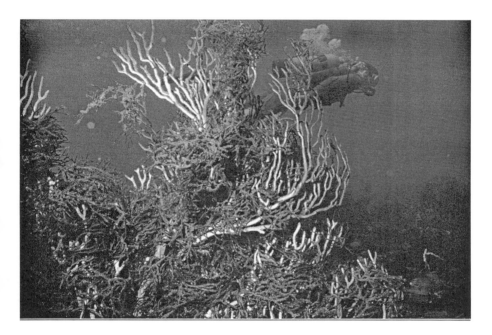

Fig. 2. Sponges and corals overgrown by the seaweed Codium isthmocladum in Southeast Florida. (Credit: B. LaPointe.)

Economic and Societal Impacts

HABs have a wide array of economic impacts, including the costs of conducting routine monitoring programs for shellfish and other affected resources, short-term and permanent closure of harvestable shellfish and fish stocks, reductions in seafood sales (including the avoidance of "safe" seafoods as a result of over-reaction to health advisories), mortalities of wild and farmed fish, shellfish, submerged aquatic vegetation and coral reefs, impacts on tourism and tourism-related businesses, and medical treatment of exposed populations. Estimates of actual impacts are few, in part because these economic losses are difficult to approximate. A conservative estimate of the average annual economic impact resulting from HABs in the U.S. was approximately $49 million over the period 1987 to 1992 (Anderson et al.;[9] Hoagland et al.[10]). Individual blooms, however, can easily exceed this annual average, as occurred for example in 1976 when a massive bloom of the dinoflagellate *Ceratium tripos* led to extensive oxygen depletion in the New York Bight, affecting surf clams, ocean quahogs, sea scallops, and some finfish and lobster. Total lost sales in all sectors combined were estimated to be $1.33 billion in 2000 dollars (Figley et al.[11]).

Losses have been significant in other countries as well. In Japan, for example, fish mortalities due to red tides in the Seto Inland Sea cost fishermen tens of millions of dollars per year, especially during the early 1970s. Even now, after pollution control efforts have decreased bloom incidence (see below), blooms of raphidophytes and dinoflagellates still kill cultured finfish and shellfish, resulting in significant losses (GEOHAB[12]). In China, a widespread red tide in 1989 along the coast of Hebei Province affected 1.5×10^4 hectares of shrimp ponds, resulting in a loss of 10^4 tons of shrimp valued at up to 300 million yuan or $U.S. 40 million (Xu et al.;[13] Wang and Li[14]). This is but one of many similar HAB outbreaks that continue to plague the aquaculture industry along the Chinese coast.

RECENT TRENDS

The nature of the HAB problem has changed considerably over the last three decades throughout the world. Simply judging by participation in international HAB conferences, more than 50 countries are threatened by harmful or toxic algal species, whereas 30 years ago, only a handful of countries were involved. A more definitive view of the expanding global problem is given in Figure 3, which shows the cumulative increase in the recorded distribution of the causative organisms and the confirmed appearance of PSP toxins in shellfish. Clearly, a dramatic expansion in the areas affected by PSP outbreaks has occurred in recent years, and a similar pattern applies to many of the other HAB types. Few would argue that the number of toxic blooms, the economic losses from them, the types of resources affected, and the number of toxins and toxic species have all increased dramatically in recent years throughout the world (Anderson;[2] Smayda;[15] Hallegraeff[3]). Disagreement only arises with respect to the reasons for this expansion.

The first thought of many is that pollution or other human activities are involved. On close inspection, however, many of the "new" or expanded HAB problems have occurred in waters where pollution is not an obvious factor. The organisms responsible for HABs have been on earth for thousands or even millions of years, during which time they had ample opportunities to disperse, assisted by changing climate, movement of tectonic plates, and other global changes. Some new bloom events may thus simply reflect indigenous populations that are discovered because of better detection methods and more observers rather than new species introductions or dispersal events (Anderson[2]). The appearance of ASP along the United States west coast is a good example of this, as the diatom species that are now known to be responsible for that toxin had been observed in those waters many years before the 1991 outbreak (Work et al.[16]). The discovery of ASP toxins in California in 1991 was a direct result of communication with Canadian scientists who had discovered the same toxin four years earlier and developed new chemical detection methods exclusively for domoic acid (see below).

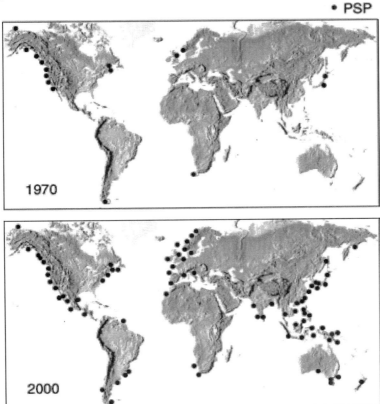

Fig. 3. Expansion of the PSP problem over the past 30 years. Sites with proven records of PSP-causing organisms are noted in 1970, and again in 2000. (Modified from Hallegraeff[3].)

Several other "spreading events" are most easily attributed to natural dispersal via currents, rather than as a result of pollution enhancement or other human activities. The first NSP event ever to occur in North Carolina (Tester et al.[17]) was shown to be a Florida bloom transported over 1500 km by the Gulf Stream to North Carolina waters—a totally natural phenomenon with no linkage to humans. Likewise, a massive

1972 red tide caused by favorable weather problems (including a hurricane) was responsible for transporting dormant cysts of the PSP-producing species *Alexandrium tamarense* to southern New England waters, where it has persisted to this day (Anderson and Wall;[18] Anderson[2]).

It is also clear that man may have contributed to the global HAB expansion by transporting toxic species in ship ballast water (Hallegraeff and Bolch;[19] McMinn et al.;[20] Lilly et al.[21]). In the past, proof of such accidental introductions has relied on inspection of historical plankton records or analysis of sediment cores for the resting stages of certain harmful or toxic species (e.g., McMinn et al.[20]), but the advent of molecular techniques and extensive sequence databases for HAB species now allows researchers to undertake genetic comparisons that provide forensic documentation of introduction events. One example of such a study was for Thau Lagoon in the Mediterranean, where PSP toxicity was first detected in 1998. A variety of chemical and genetic techniques were used to demonstrate that the closest relatives of the Thau Lagoon populations of the toxic dinoflagellate *Alexandrium catenella* were from temperate Asian waters. Thau Lagoon cells show no sequence homology to strains of this organism from western European waters, including the Mediterranean. The most likely scenario is that *A. catenella* was introduced into Thau Lagoon in the ballast water of a ship docked at Sete, France, a shipping port in direct communication with the lagoon. Spreading events of this type have occurred elsewhere and will continue to occur until ballast waters are more carefully regulated and treated.

Another factor underlying the global increase in HABs is the dramatic increase in aquaculture activities that has occurred in many countries. This leads to increased monitoring of product quality and safety, revealing indigenous toxic algae that were probably always there (Anderson[2]). The construction of aquaculture facilities places fish or shellfish resources in areas where toxic algal species occur but were previously unknown, leading to mortality events or toxicity outbreaks that would not have been noticed had the aquaculture facility not been placed there. Another potential linkage is that the pollution from aquaculture facilities may stimulate HABs. A single fish farm can contribute fish feces, urine, and uneaten food equivalent to the pollution loading from a small city.

Of considerable concern, particularly for coastal resource managers, is the potential relationship between the apparent increase in HABs and the accelerated eutrophication of coastal waters due to human activities (Anderson et al.[22]). As mentioned above, some HAB outbreaks occur in pristine waters with no influence from pollution or other anthropogenic effects, but linkages between HABs and eutrophication have been frequently noted within the past several decades (e.g., Lam and Ho;[23] Smayda;[4,15] Riegman;[24] Richardson and Jorgensen;[25] Richardson[26]). Coastal waters are receiving massive and increasing quantities of industrial, agricultural and sewage effluents through a variety of pathways (Vitousek et al.[27]). In many urbanized coastal regions, these anthropogenic inputs have altered the size and composition of the nutrient pool which may, in turn, create a more favorable nutrient environment for certain HAB species. Just as the application of fertilizer to lawns can enhance grass growth, marine algae can grow in response to various types of nutrient inputs. Shallow and restricted coastal waters that are poorly flushed appear to be most susceptible to nutrient-related algal problems. Nutrient enrichment of such systems often leads to excessive production of organic matter, a process known as eutrophication, and increased frequencies and magnitudes of phytoplankton blooms, including HABs. There is no doubt that this is true in certain areas of the world where pollution has increased dramatically. It is perhaps real, but less evident in areas where coastal pollution is more gradual and unobtrusive. A frequently cited dataset from an area where pollution has been a significant factor in HAB incidence is from the Inland Sea of Japan, where visible red tides increased steadily from 44 per year in 1965 to over 300 a decade later, matching the pattern of increased nutrient loading from pollution (Okaichi[28]). Effluent controls were instituted in the mid-1970's, resulting in a 70% reduction in the number of red tides, and that reduction has persisted to this day. A related data set for the Black Sea documents a dramatic increase in red tides up to the mid 1990s, when the blooms began to decline (Bodeanu and Ruta[29]). That decrease, which also has continued to this day, has been linked to reductions in the use of fertilizer in upstream watersheds by former Soviet Union countries that are no longer able to afford large, state-subsidized fertilizer applications to agricultural land (Anderson et al.[22]).

In retrospect, it is now clear that the worldwide expansion of HAB phenomena is in part a reflection of our ability to better define the boundaries of the problem: the nature and extent of toxic or harmful species and their impacts. Those boundaries are, however, also expanding due to natural species dispersal via storms or currents, as well as to enhanced HAB population growth as a result of pollution or other anthropogenic influences. The fact that part of the expansion is simply a result of increased awareness should not temper our concern. The global problem of HABs is serious and large—much larger than we thought.

MANAGEMENT ISSUES

Management options for dealing with the impacts of HABs include reducing their incidence and extent (prevention), minimizing impacts (mitigation), and stopping or containing blooms (control). Where possible, it is preferable to prevent HABs rather than to treat their symptoms, but this is a significant challenge.

Prevention
Since increased pollution and nutrient loading may cause an increased incidence of outbreaks of some HAB species (Smayda;[4] Anderson et al.[22]), these events may be prevented by reducing pollution inputs to coastal waters, particularly industrial, agricultural, and domestic effluents high in plant nutrients. As discussed above, there is evidence from several areas (the Seto Inland Sea and the Black Sea, for example) that major changes in sewage treatment or agricultural fertilization can improve water quality and reduce the number of red tides and algal blooms, but the time-frame for achieving HAB reduction by pollution control policies is long (years to decades) and there is no

guarantee that those actions will actually reduce harmful bloom incidence in other areas. These policy considerations are especially relevant to coastal areas where human activities are having a significant impact on the cycling of nutrients through the input of large quantities of agricultural runoff and domestic sewage. The trends in this regard are indeed alarming. The flux of P to the coastal oceans has increased 3-fold compared to pre-industrial, pre-agricultural levels, and N has increased even more dramatically, especially over the last 4 decades (Caraco;[30] Smil[31]). During that time, the flux of N increased 4-fold into the Mississippi River and more than 10-fold into the rivers entering the North Sea (National Research Council;[32] Smil[31]). Human activity is estimated to have increased N inputs to the coastal waters of the northeastern United States generally, and to Chesapeake Bay specifically, by 6-8-fold (Boynton et al.;[33] Howarth[34]).

These numbers are alarming, but non-point sources of nutrients from agricultural activities, fossil-fuel combustion, and animal feeding operations can be of greater concern than point sources (e.g., sewage treatment plants) because the former are larger and more difficult to control. Fertilizer application on land remains a major contributor to non-point nutrient pollution, and this source is increasing dramatically in many regions (Vitousek[27]). Both industrial and developing nations are using significantly higher loadings of fertilizer in agriculture, with global N and P fertilizer usage increasing 8-fold and 3-fold, respectively, since the early 1960s (Smil[31]). When these nutrient supplies reach rivers, estuaries and coastal waters, they are available for phytoplankton uptake and growth. The nitrate component of fertilizers, in particular, can travel long distances. The "dead zone" of hypoxia in the Gulf of Mexico is a particularly striking example of the long-distance transport of fertilizer nitrogen (Rabalais[35]). Seventeen different states in the Mississippi watershed contribute nutrients that are implicated in enhanced algal growth and the persistent oxygen depletion problem in the Gulf.

Other management strategies that may prevent HAB events include: regulating the siting of aquaculture facilities to avoid areas where HAB species are present, modifying water circulation for those HABs where restricted water exchange is a factor in bloom development, and restricting species introductions (e.g., through regulations on ballast water discharges or shellfish and finfish transfers for aquaculture).

Mitigation

The most effective mitigation tools are monitoring programs that detect toxins in shellfish and/or monitor the environment for evidence of HAB events (e.g., Shumway et al.;[36] Anderson et al.[5]). Numerous monitoring programs have been established worldwide in coastal waters to provide advance warning of outbreaks or to delineate areas that require harvest restrictions. This monitoring is conducted for both HAB species and for their toxins. The latter has become quite expensive in recent times due to the proliferation of toxins and potentially affected resources. The costs of such monitoring programs are significant and growing in parallel with the proliferation of HAB toxins. Molluscs, bivalves and gastropods are typically the primary vectors of algal biotoxins to human consumers, although crustaceans (e.g. crabs and lobsters) can also transfer algal biotoxins through the food chain (reviewed by Shumway[37]). Clearly, the optimum, safest and most commonly used practice involves sampling and testing of wild or cultured product directly from the natural environment, as this allows unequivocal tracking of toxins to their site of origin and targeted regulatory action. A useful review of selected shellfish monitoring programs is given by Anderson et al.[5]

A common mitigation strategy used by fish farms is the towing of fish net pens away from the sites of intense HABs. Though expensive and occasionally costly with respect to lost or damaged fish, this remains one of the primary tools used by fish farmers to combat HABs (Rensel and Whyte[38]). A strategy to mitigate the impact of HAB toxins in shellfish is to process those shellfish in such a way as to reduce toxicity to an acceptable level. A clear example is the removal of scallop viscera and the marketing of only the adductor muscle, which generally contains little or no HAB toxins.

Remote sensing has great potential as a tool to assist in monitoring the development and movement of HAB phenomena over larger spatial and shorter time scales than those accessible through ship- or land-based sampling. This technology has, however, only recently lived up to part of this potential. Although multi-spectral scanners (e.g. Coastal Zone Color Scanner; CZCS) can be used to detect the reflectance of chlorophyll-a and other pigments, these efforts have been constrained by the inability of the sensors to discriminate phytoplankton populations at the species level. This is, of course, a fundamental requirement of HAB programs. Instead, progress has been made by first linking specific water masses to HAB organisms and then identifying and tracking that water mass with an appropriate remote sensing technique (e.g., Keafer and Anderson[39]). In particular, remotely-sensed sea surface temperatures (SST) have been used to follow the movement of fronts, water masses, or other physical features where HAB species accumulate. A coastal current that dominates PSP dynamics in the southwestern Gulf of Maine is easily identified by its temperature signature (Franks and Anderson[40]). Likewise, the long-distance advection of *Karenia brevis* from Florida into the nearshore waters of North Carolina via the Gulf Stream in 1987 was documented with this approach (Tester et al.[17]).

Applying a related type of remote sensing technology, scientists and engineers are now developing automated instruments that can be moored along the coast to detect HAB cells or their toxins while simultaneously measuring the physical and optical characteristics of the water column to provide the complementary information needed to make "algal forecasts" of impending toxicity. These instruments are taking advantage of new molecular and analytical methodologies that allow chemicals (such as HAB toxins) and cells to be detected with great sensitivity and specificity.

A long-term goal of HAB monitoring programs is to develop the ability to forecast bloom development and movement, but predictive models for HABs are only in their infancy (Franks[41]). Prediction of HAB outbreaks requires physical/biological coupled models which account for both the growth and behavior of the toxic algal species, as well as the movement and dynamics of the surrounding water (McGillicuddy et al.[42]). Numerical models of coastal circulation are advancing rapidly, but difficulties arise in incorporating biological and chemical processes into the physics. The growth and accumulation of individual harmful algal species in a mixed planktonic assemblage are exceedingly complex processes involving an array of chemical, physical, and biological interactions. Our level of knowledge about each of the many HAB species varies significantly, and even the best-studied remain poorly characterized with respect to bloom or population dynamics. Resolution of various rate processes integral to the population dynamics (e.g., input and losses due to growth, grazing, encystment, excystment, and physical advection) has not been accomplished, but is fundamental to model formulation. Many of these processes are difficult to quantify in the field because HAB species are often only a small fraction of the planktonic biomass in natural samples. The end result is that despite the proven utility of numerical models in many oceanographic disciplines, there are no predictive models of population development, transport, and toxin accumulation for any of the major harmful algal species. Several are under development, but there is a clear need to increase efforts to formulate realistic physical models for regions subject to HAB events, and to incorporate biological behavior and population dynamics into those simulations.

Control

Human efforts to control insects, diseases, and fungi are common agricultural practices on land, but similar attempts to control unwanted plants or animals in the ocean are rare. The significant public health, economic, and ecosystem impacts of HABs would seem to make these phenomena legitimate targets for control efforts, but research on this topic has been minimal because of concerns about costs, effectiveness, and environmental impacts (Anderson[1]). Potential approaches to controlling HABs are similar to those used to control pests on land – e.g., biological, physical, or chemical treatments that directly target the bloom cells.

Control methodologies can be categorized as either "direct" or "indirect" depending on whether the effort targets the bloom organisms specifically, or strives to reduce impacts, such as through bloom prediction or through alteration of pollution inputs that might stimulate blooms (Boesch et al.;[43] Anderson et al.[5]). General approaches to direct control include: 1) chemicals that kill or disrupt HAB cells during blooms; 2) clays or other materials that flocculate (precipitate) and scavenge cells and other particles from the water column, transporting them to the ocean floor; and 3) biological agents such as viruses, bacteria, or parasites which are lethal pathogens to HAB species.

Despite the significant impacts of HABs on coastal regions, direct intervention efforts to control bloom populations have not been attempted to any significant extent in natural waters, other than large-scale clay treatments used to flocculate and sediment red tide cells in Korea (Na et al.[44]). Research programs on promising control methodologies are needed, concurrent with continued field and laboratory studies to better understand the ecological mechanisms underlying the HABs (Anderson[1]). This would represent a departure from the status quo, as past research activities have been largely focused on monitoring and understanding HAB phenomena, not controlling them.

HABS AS NATURAL DISASTERS

HAB phenomena have all the characteristics of natural disasters, yet they have not typically been viewed as such by government agencies. Disaster assistance is often not provided to areas hit by destructive red tides or HABs, yet the economic and social impacts can be equivalent to, or more severe than storms or other natural phenomena. The following sections provide brief examples of the scales and types of impacts that can be caused by HABs that affect human health, ecosystem health, aquaculture operations, and even the public confidence in seafood quality. These examples are offered to highlight the diverse and significant impacts that can strike a country or region without warning, as is the case with other natural disasters. There are many more outbreaks that could be highlighted under each category of impact, but these few are selected because they best illustrate the nature of the events and their outcomes.

Aquacultural disaster – the Hong Kong red tide of 1998

In March/April 1998, a red tide occurred that caused the most serious fish kill in Hong Kong history, affecting most of the region's aquaculture zones. The alga involved is now known as *Karenia digitata* (Yang et al.[45]), but was previously unknown to science. Most of Hong Kong's mariculture farms (estimates are 1,000 out of 1,500) were affected by the bloom, which appeared first in northeast waters and then proceeded south and then west and northwest through time.

Warnings were given by government officials, but in several locations fish farmers were unaware of the seriousness of the outbreak until fish began to die. The major concern of government departments was to provide warnings of the movement of the red tide, to collect and dispose of the dead fish, and to protect public health. Statements were issued to the public concerning safety aspects of consuming fish and shellfish and about swimming in red tide-affected waters.

The main mitigation measures against the red tide were taken by some of the fish culturists themselves. There are reports of cages being moved and aeration being used, and some culturists managed to harvest their fish before mortalities occurred. The most novel approach involved a group of fishermen who used their boats, outboard motors and water jets to "repel" the incoming algae.

The 1998 Hong Kong red tide was massive in its scale and the extent of its impacts. Estimates of the losses from this event vary dramatically depending on the source of information. The Federation of Hong Kong Aquaculture Association estimated a total, direct loss of U.S. $32 million (Yang and Hodgkiss[46]), though government officials argue that the true loss was lower. The cost of collecting and disposing of dead fish was estimated by the Hong Kong Marine Department to be U.S. $130,000. This does not include staff salaries. Another aspect of the economic impact is that the Hong Kong Government provided low-interest loans for mariculturists. Approximately U.S. $20 million was loaned to farmers at a low interest rate.

Although no direct losses to the capture fisheries can be assumed, monetary losses were incurred due to a phenomenon known as the "halo" effect. This refers to the tendency of consumers to switch to substitute foods or activities because of their concern about the possible toxicity of seafood due to a specific HAB event. Even though only one type of product might be potentially affected, consumers avoid a much broader range of goods and services, over-reacting to the risk and exaggerating the dangers. In Hong Kong, the uncertainty and conflict regarding toxicity of the killed fish contributed to a major decline in the value of all fish sales. The Joint Committee on Hong Kong Fishermen's Organizations estimated that captured fish sold for approximately half their former value during the red tide. Assuming that the average daily earnings for each of 4,000 trawlers decreased by half over a one-month period, the Organization estimates the total loss to be U.S. $77 million. This estimate seems high, however, given that the total annual capture fishery production in 1997 was HK $1.57 billion. Nevertheless, the impact on capture fisheries was significant, and may have exceeded the loss to the mariculturists.

While it would be expected that fish sales and prices would decline during a large-scale HAB event, lack of a consistent or coordinated government response may have exacerbated the problem. As fish and fish products were moved freely about Hong Kong without detailed source and shipping records, wholesale buyers, sellers and consumers were unsure of the source of fish in the markets. There was considerable confusion about whether the dead and dying aquaculture fish should be sold for consumption, since policies on that topic were not well-established in Hong Kong, or worldwide, and government agencies sometimes contradicted each other in their statements. Evidence from other regions of the world suggested that toxin transfer to fish tissues during harmful *Gymnodinium* and *Karenia* blooms does not occur, and thus that freshly killed fish might be safe to eat. Indeed, numerous chemical and bioassay tests of the Hong Kong fish flesh showed no signs of toxin. The government eventually recommended that consumers only buy fish that showed no gill damage or signs of hemorrhage.

The 1998 red tide in Hong Kong was a media event, with reports and speculations filling the newspapers, television, and radio. In many cases, the information that was released was contradictory, incorrect, or misinterpreted, leading to widespread over-reaction to the nature of the problem. One example was cited above as the "halo effect" that halved the price of captured fish even though they were safe to eat. Other impacts include frustrated, angry fishermen and confused retailers and consumers. As a result, a team of HAB experts was hired to evaluate the existing red tide monitoring and management system in Hong Kong, and recommend sweeping modifications in organizational structure and policy (Anderson et al.[47]).

Ecosystem disaster – the Chrysochromulina bloom in Scandinavia – 1988

In May/June 1988, the Kattegat and Skagerrak waters that mark the transition area between the North Sea and the Baltic were the site of an unprecedented bloom of the flagellate *Chrysochromulina polylepis*. This bloom is unusual and noteworthy because of its extent (covering in excess of 75,000 km^2) and the tremendous ecosystem damage it caused (Rosenberg et al.[48]). The toxin produced by *Chrysochromulina* had drastic effects on the marine ecosystem, indiscriminantly killing large numbers of macroalgae, invertebrates, and fish. SCUBA divers reported mass mortalities of invertebrates down to 20 meters, including gastropods, polychaetes, tunicates, anthozoans, and sponges. Many species of fish were killed as well, and those that were not killed were lethargic and easily caught by divers (Rosenberg et al.[48]). Even seaweeds were affected. The red seaweed *Delesseria* was killed or affected in such a way that its color turned from red to orange and finally green, indicating the breakdown of pigments. The brown seaweed *Laminaria* was similarly affected. Caged fish were killed at several sites along the west coast of Sweden (100 tons) and along the southern coast of Norway (500 tons). The economic loss to these fish farming industries was about U.S. \$10 million.

As was the case in Hong Kong, this *Chrysochromulina* bloom attracted considerable public and political attention throughout Europe. Many linked the outbreak to the pollution of the Kattegat and Skagerrak, and subsequent work has confirmed that *Chrysochromulina* toxicity is enhanced by phosphorus limitation (Granéli et al.[49]), as would occur in waters with excess nitrogen inputs. Although other types of HABs were recurrent in that region (including blooms that kill fish and cause shellfish toxicity), this single event precipitated a significant governmental response in the form of research and monitoring funds for HABs that lasted for many years. This *Chrysochromulina* bloom can be credited with opening the eyes of administrators and program managers in Europe to the sudden and devastating impacts of HABs, and the need for research on the factors that stimulate their growth, especially those linked to human activities.

Human health disaster – the 1987 ASP outbreak in Canada
In November 1987, a human poisoning episode took place that highlights the many issues that arise when a new, unknown toxin appears in seafood. This event occurred in northeastern Canada, a region with a long history of PSP outbreaks, and thus with a health system that was familiar with some aspects of marine biotoxin exposure. The outbreak began when hospital emergency rooms began admitting individuals complaining of vomiting, diarrhea and confusion. As the number of patients grew, medical personnel began to search for a source, and soon the illnesses were correlated with consumption of mussels originating in the Prince Edward Island region, the site of a major aquaculture operation (Smith et al.[50]). When the mussels were tested using the standard PSP mouse bioassay, however, the mice did not show typical PSP symptoms, but nevertheless demonstrated that a neurotoxin was present. The entire Canadian Atlantic shellfishery was closed pending investigation, causing millions of dollars in losses, not only in Canada, but in the U.S. as well, especially in Maine and areas immediately to the south of the affected region. There are even reports that seafood sales dropped on the west coast of the U.S. – thousands of miles away. This latter impact is yet another example of the "halo effect" whereby safe fisheries products lose value because of the avoidance of all seafood by wary and poorly informed consumers.

A team of 40 Canadian government scientists was assembled, including chemists and biologists and personnel experienced with PSP issues. In a matter of days, a new toxin (domoic acid) was identified as the causative agent. Ultimately, 150 people had become seriously ill, with 30 hospitalizations and 3 deaths. This caused considerable alarm and fear among the general public, and was a frequent issue in the national news for several weeks (Fig. 4). One important symptom that persisted with those who were poisoned but survived was permanent short-term memory loss. As a result, the new poisoning syndrome was named Amnesic Shellfish Poisoning, or ASP (Todd[51]). The causative organism was subsequently found to be the diatom *Pseudo-nitzschia multiseries,* an organism well-known to science, but previously thought to be non-toxic. As a result of continued monitoring by the Canadian Food Inspection Agency (CFIA) there have been no human poisonings with ASP in Canada since that event.

In response to the 1987 ASP event, Canada's Department of Fisheries and Oceans (DFO) set up new research and monitoring programs and established a Phycotoxin Working Group that continues to coordinate national biotoxin research and monitoring activities. Many other countries have since documented the occurrence of domoic acid in their seafood (typically shellfish and crabs), and there are numerous ASP closures on an annual basis throughout the world. It is clear that this toxin was present in seafood long before the 1987 outbreak. The Canadian episode simply alerted government officials and scientists to the existence of the toxin, which is now regulated in seafood globally.

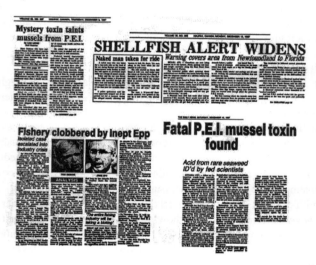

Fig. 4. Newspaper headlines regarding 1987 ASP incident in Canada. (Credit: S. Bates.

Economic disaster – the 1997 Pfiesteria outbreak in Maryland

In 1997, a relatively minor HAB event resulted in a significant economic crisis in the Chesapeake Bay region of the U.S., demonstrating the large impact that even small outbreaks can sometimes have. During that summer, several fish kills occurred in small tributaries along Maryland's eastern shore. Approximately 30,000 fish died - a relatively low number to those experienced with fish mortality events, but sufficient to be alarming to the local population and politicians. Many fish had open lesions on them (Fig. 5), a disturbing image to many, and at the time, thought to be indicative of the involvement of the predator dinoflagellate *Pfiesteria piscicida.* (Burkholder and Glasgow[7,52]). *Pfiesteria* outbreaks had previously been documented in the Albermarle-Pamlico estuary of North Carolina (Burkholder et al.[53]), but had never been reported in the Chesapeake. There the blooms were confined to small areas such as the Pocomoke River, and only a few commercially and recreationally important fish species were affected. The situation attracted considerable attention when a few commercial fishermen complained of health effects – in particular confusion and memory problems. These claims, although initially discounted by some officials, were ultimately confirmed to be medically reliable (Grattan et al.[54]). The state of Maryland closed several Chesapeake tributaries for all recreation and for commercial fishing as a precautionary measure.

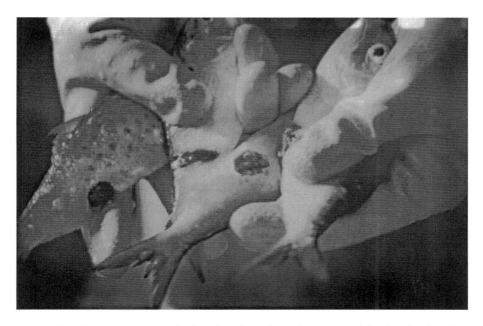

Fig. 5. Lesions on menhaden thought to have been caused by the dinoflagellate Pfiesteria. (Credit: J. Burkholder.)

Tests by the U.S. Food and Drug Administration and other officials consistently failed to demonstrate any toxicity in fish or shellfish from the affected areas. Nevertheless, the high level of attention given the *Pfiesteria* outbreak by the press and the recreation restrictions and fisheries closures by the government contributed to an over-reaction by the general public. Consumers stopped buying seafood of all types and avoided exposure to the water. Some grocery chains went so far as to post signs that they were selling "no Chesapeake Bay seafood products" – greatly exacerbating the concern by consumers, and worsening the economic losses for that regional industry. Based on the differences between the 1996 and 1997 seafood sales, economic losses are estimated at U.S. $43 million to the Chesapeake seafood industry. Further losses were experienced by the recreational fishing industry, bringing the total loss from the event to U.S. $50 million (Lipton[55]).

The consumer panic caused by the *P. piscicida* outbreak in Maryland is yet another striking example of the "halo effect" discussed above. The fish kills were small in size, and only a handful of people were affected medically, yet the economic losses were massive. In general, the halo effect typically affects producers of seafood or providers of recreation and tourist services. Because consumers can switch to other foods or to other recreational activities, the halo effect is not generally serious for consumers, but it can be disastrous for producers.

Another outcome of the *Pfiesteria* outbreak was a substantial inflow of research and monitoring funds. Millions of dollars were committed to these activities, and much of those funds continue to be provided to this day, even though there have not been any major fish kills or human health problems in the Chesapeake region since 1997.

DEFINITION OF 'NATURAL DISASTER'

The foregoing sections highlight the many different types of impacts that can occur with HABs. These were just a few selected examples from a long list of outbreaks and negative consequences. The scale of these impacts can be significant, and many of those who have been impacted have argued that HABs should be considered natural disasters, and thus that they should be given government assistance, as is done after storms or earthquakes, for example. In the U.S., when natural disasters such as hurricanes and floods occur, financial assistance is made available through the Federal Emergency Management Agency (FEMA) provided that the region has been declared a 'disaster area' by the federal government. This allows low-interest loans and other financial assistance to those in need. Following a particularly severe red tide in North Carolina in 1987 (Tester[17]), legislation was enacted that has placed red tides and HABs into the natural disaster category. The definition of 'disaster' has now been modified to be: "a sudden event which causes severe damage including, but not limited to, floods, hurricanes, tornadoes, earthquakes, fires,…, **ocean conditions resulting in the closure of customary fishing waters**, riots,…" (Conference Report on H.R. 4174, SBA Reauthorization and Amendment Act of 1988). This change in the law means that should a red tide or HAB affect fisheries, the federal disaster loan program will be available to aid those who are harmed. Other countries might want to consider enacting similar legislation to provide a much-needed level of protection to fishermen, the tourist industry, and others who are subject to the unpredictable and often devastating effects of an HAB.

CONCLUSION

HABs are increasingly common along the coasts of countries throughout the world. The impacts from these aquatic disasters are substantial, affecting public health, fisheries resources (both wild and farmed), local economies, tourism, ecosystem health, and coastal aesthetics. One alarming aspect of HAB phenomena is that they have been increasing in frequency, areal coverage, and diversity over the past several decades. There are now more algal toxins, more toxic algal species, more fisheries resources affected, larger areas affected, and higher economic losses. Reasons for this expansion are many, and include natural species dispersal via storms or currents, human assisted dispersal (e.g., via ballast water discharge), better detection as a result of increased monitoring and better analytical techniques for toxins, and enhancement of the bloom populations due to nutrients supplied by sewage, agricultural runoff, and other pollution sources. HAB phenomena have all the characteristics of natural disasters, yet they have not typically been viewed as such by government agencies. Disaster assistance has often not been provided to areas hit by destructive red tides or HABs, yet the economic and social impacts can be equivalent to, or more severe than storms or other natural phenomena. Expanded research on management, mitigation, and control of HABs is easily justified in this context, as is legislation to protect fishermen, tourist industries, and others who are subject to their unpredictable and often devastating effects.

Acknowledgments
Work on this paper was supported by NOAA Cooperative Agreement NA17RJ1223 and NOAA National Ocean Service Purchase Order 674-W10197. Contribution No. 10806 from the Woods Hole Oceanographic Institution.

REFERENCES

1.   Anderson, D. 1994. "Red tides." *Scientific American*: 271: 52-58.
2.   Anderson, D.M. 1989. "Toxic algal blooms and red tides: a global perspective." pp. 11-16, in: *Red tides: biology, environmental science, and toxicology*, Okaichi, T., D.M. Anderson, and T. Nemoto (eds.), Elsevier Science Publishing Co., Inc., New York.
3.   Hallegraeff, G.M. 1993. "A review of harmful algal blooms and their apparent global increase." *Phycologia* 32: 79-99.
4.   Smayda, T.J. 1989. "Primary production and the global epidemic of phytoplankton blooms in the sea: A linkage?" pp. 449-484, in: *Novel Phytoplankton Blooms*, Cosper, E.M., V.M. Bricelj, and E.J. Carpenter (eds.), Coastal and Estuarine Studies No. 35, Springer-Verlag, New York.
5.   Anderson, D.M., P. Andersen, V.M. Bricelj, J.J. Cullen and J.E. Rensel. 2001. *Monitoring and Management Strategies for Harmful Algal Blooms in Coastal*

390

Waters. Singapore and Paris, Asia Pacific Economic Program and Intergovernmental Oceanographic Commission, 268 pp.

6. Anderson, D.M. and P.S. Lobel. 1987. "The continuing enigma of ciguatera." *Biol. Bull.* 172: 89-107.

7. Burkholder, J.M. and H.B. Glasgow, Jr. 1997. "*Pfiesteria piscicida* and other *Pfiesteria*-like dinoflagellates: behavior, impacts, and environmental controls." *Limnol. Oceanogr.* 42(5, Pt. 2): 1052-1075.

8. Burkholder, J.M. 1998. "Implications of harmful microalgae and heterotrophic dinoflagellates in management of sustainable marine fisheries. Ecological Applications." *Ecol. Appl.* 8(1, suppl.): S37-S62.

9. Anderson, D.M., P. Hoagland, Y. Kaoru and A.W. White. 2000. *Estimated annual economic impacts from harmful algal blooms (HABs) in the United States*, Woods Hole Oceanographic Institution, 97 pp.

10. Hoagland, P., D.M. Anderson, Y. Kaoru and A.W. White. (in press). "Average annual economic impacts of harmful algal blooms in the United States: some preliminary estimates." *Estuaries.*

11. Figley, W., B. Pyle and B. Halgren. 1979. "Socioeconomic impacts." Chapter 14, in: *Oxygen Depletion and Associated Benthic Mortalities in New York Bight, 1976.* Swanson, R.L. and C.J. Sindermann (eds.), Professional Paper 11, December, NOAA, U.S. Department of Commerce.

12. GEOHAB. 2001. *Global Ecology and Oceanography of Harmful Algal Blooms, Science Plan.* Baltimore and Paris, SCOR and IOC.

13. Xu, Z., X. Gu, Y. Wang, H. Yuan and Y. Chen. 1993. "Analyses of ecological eigenvalue of plankton during red tide occurrence in the Xiangshan Sound, Zhejiang in 1988." Collected oceanic works/Haiyang Wenji. Tianjin 16(1): 83-89.

14. Wang, L. and X. Li. 1998. "Management of shellfish safety in China." *J. Shellfish Res.* 17(5): 1609-1611.

15. Smayda, T. 1990. "Novel and nuisance phytoplankton blooms in the sea: Evidence for a global epidemic." pp. 29-40, in: *Toxic Marine Phytoplankton,* Granéli, E., B. Sundstrom, L. Edler, and D.M. Anderson (eds.), New York, Elsevier.

16. Work, T.M., A.M. Beale, L. Fritz, M.A. Quilliam, M. Silver, K. Buck and J.L.C. Wright. 1993. "Domoic acid intoxication of brown pelicans and cormorants in Santa Cruz, California." pp. 643-650, in: *Toxic Phytoplankton Blooms in the Sea,* Smayda, T. J. and Y. Shimizu (eds.), Elsevier, Amsterdam.

17. Tester, P.A., R.P. Stumpf, F.M. Vukovich, P.K. Folwer and J.T. Turner. 1991. "An expatriate red tide bloom: Transport, distribution, and persistence." *Limnol. Oceanogr.* 36(5): 1053-1061.

18. Anderson, D.M. and D. Wall. 1978. "Potential importance of benthic cysts of *Gonyaulax tamarensis* and *G. excavata* in initiating toxin dinoflagellate blooms." *J. Phycol.* 14(2): 224-234.

19. Hallegraeff, G.M. and C.J. Bolch. 1992. "Transport of diatom and dinoflagellate resting spores in ships' ballast water: Implications for plankton biogeography and aquaculture." *J. Plankt. Res.* 14(8): 1067-1084.

20. McMinn, A., G.M. Hallegraeff, P. Thomson, A.V. Jenkinson and H. Heijnis. 1997. "Cyst and radionucleotide evidence for the recent introduction of the toxic dinoflagellate *Gymnodinium catenatum* into Tasmanian waters." *Mar. Ecol. Prog. Ser.* 161: 165-172.

21. Lilly, E.L., D.M. Kulis, P. Gentien and D.M. Anderson. 2002. "Paralytic shellfish poisoning toxins in France linked to a human-introduced strain of *Alexandrium catenella* from the Western Pacific: Evidence from DNA and toxin analysis." *J. Plankt. Res.* 24(5): 443-452.

22. Anderson, D.M., P.M. Glibert and J.M. Burkholder. (in press). "Harmful algal blooms and eutrophication: nutrient sources, composition, and consequences." *Estuaries.*

23. Lam, C.W.Y. and K.C. Ho. 1989. "Red tides in Tolo Harbour, Hong Kong." pp. 49-52, in: *Red Tides: Biology, Environmental Science and Toxicology,* Okaichi, T., D. M. Anderson, and T. Nemoto (eds.), Elsevier.

24. Riegman, R. 1995. "Nutrient-related selection mechanisms in marine phytoplankton communities and the impact of eutrophication on the planktonic food web." *Water Science and Technology* 32(4): 63-75.

25. Richardson, K. and B.B. Jorgensen. 1996. "Eutrophication: Definition, history and effects." pp. 1-19, in: *Eutrophication in Coastal Marine Ecosystems. Coastal and Estuarine Studies,* Jorgensen, B. and K. Richardson, (eds.), American Geophysical Union, Washington, DC.

26. Richardson, K. 1997. "Harmful or exceptional phytoplankton blooms in the marine ecosystem." *Adv. Mar. Biol.* 31: 301-385.

27. Vitousek, P.M., J.D. Aber, R.W. Howarth, G.E. Likens, P.A. Matson, D.W. Schindler, W.H. Schlesinger and D.G. Tilman. 1997. "Human alteration of the global nitrogen cycle: Sources and consequences." *Ecol. Appl.* 7(3): 737-750.

28. Okaichi, T. 1997. "Red tides in the Seto Inland Sea." pp. 251-304, in: *Sustainable Development in the Seto Inland Sea, Japan - From the Viewpoint of Fisheries,* Okaichi, T. and Y. Yanagi (eds.), Terra Scientific Publishing Company, Tokyo, Japan.

29. Bodeanu, N. and G. Ruta. 1998. "Development of the planktonic algae in the Romanian Black Sea sector in 1981-1996." pp. 188-191 in: *Harmful Algae,* Reguera, B., J. Blanco, M.L. Fernández, and T. Wyatt (eds.), Paris, France, Xunta de Galicia and Intergovernmental Oceanographic Commission of UNESCO.

30. Caraco, N.F. 1995. "Influence of human populations on P transfers to aquatic systems: A regional scale study using large rivers." pp. 235-247 in: *Phosphorus in the Global Environment,* H. Tiessen (ed.), New York, John Wiley & Sons Ltd.

31. Smil, V. 2001. *Enriching the Earth: Fritz Haber, Carl Bosch, and the Transformation of World Food.* MIT Press, Cambridge, MA.

32. National Research Council. 2000. *Clean Coastal Waters: Understanding and Reducing the Effects of Nutrient Pollution.* Washington, DC, National Academy Press.

33. Boynton, W.R., J.H. Garber, R. Summers and W.M. Kemp. 1995. "Inputs, transformations, and transport to nitrogen and phosphorus in Chesapeake Bay and selected tributaries." *Estuaries* 18: 285-314.

34. Howarth, R.W. 1998. "An assessment of human influences on inputs of nitrogen to the estuaries and continental shelves of the North Atlantic Ocean." *Nutrient Cycling in Agroecosystems* 52: 213-223.

35. Rabalais, N.N. 2000. "Hypoxia in the Gulf of Mexico." *J. Environ. Qual.* 30(2): 320-329.

36. Shumway, S.E., S. "Sherman-Caswell and J.W. Hurst. 1988. Paralytic shellfish poisoning in Maine: monitoring a monster." *J. Shellfish Res.* 7: 643-652.

37. sShumway, S.E. 1990. "A review of the effects of algal blooms on shellfish and aquaculture." *J. World Aquacult.* Soc. 21: 65-104.

38. Rensel, J.E. and J.N.C. Whyte. (in press). "Finfish mariculture and harmful algal blooms." in: *Manual on Harmful Marine Microalgae - Revised Edition,* Hallegraeff, G.M., D.M. Anderson and A.D. Cembella,(eds.), IOC, UNESCO.

39. Keafer, B.A. and D.M. Anderson. 1993. "Use of remotely-sensed sea surface temperatures in studies of *Alexandrium tamarense* bloom dynamics." pp. 763-768 in: *Toxic Phytoplankton Blooms in the Sea,* Smayda, T. and Y. Shimizu (eds.), Elsevier, Amsterdam.

40. Franks, P.J.S. and D.M. Anderson. 1992. "Alongshore transport of a toxic phytoplankton bloom in a buoyancy current: *Alexandrium tamarensis* in the Gulf of Maine." *Marine Biology* 112: 153-164.

41. Franks, P.J.S. 1997. "Models of harmful algal blooms." *Limnol. Oceanogr.* 42(5, Pt. 2): 1273-1282.

42. McGillicuddy, Jr., D.J., C.A. Stock, D.M. "Anderson and R.P. Signell. (in press). Hindcasting blooms of the toxic dinoflagellate Alexandrium spp. in the western Gulf of Maine." *Ecological Forecasting Report.*

43. Boesch, D.F., Anderson, D.M., Horner, R.A., Shumway, S.A., Tester, P.A. and Whitledge, T.E. 1997. *Harmful Algal Blooms in Coastal Waters: Options for Prevention, Control and Mitigation.* Silver Springs, MD, NOAA Coastal Ocean Program Decision Analysis Series No. 10, NOAA Coastal Ocean Office, 46 pp.

44. Na, G., Choi, W., and Chun, Y. 1996. A study on red tide control with Loess suspension. J. Aquacult. 9(3): 239-245.

45. Yang, Z.B., H. Takayama, K. Matsuoka and I.J. Hodgkiss. 2000. "*Karenia digitata* sp. nov. (Gymnodiniales, Dinophyceae), a new harmful algal bloom species from the coastal waters of west Japan and Hong Kong." *Phycologia* 39(6): 463-470.

46. Yang, Z.B. and I.J. Hodgkiss. 1999. "Massive fish killing by *Gyrodinium* sp." *Harmful Algae News.* 18: 4-5.

47. Anderson, D.M., P. Andersen, V.M. Bricelj, J.J. Cullen, I.J. Hodgkiss, K.C. Ho, J.E. Rensel, J.T.Y. Wong and R. Wu. 1999. *Red Tide and HAB Monitoring and Management in Hong Kong.* Final Report prepared for the Hong Kong, Agriculture and Fisheries Department, 254 pp.

48. Rosenberg, R., O. Lindahl and H. Blanck. 1988. "Silent spring in the sea." *Ambio.* 17(4): 289-290.

49. Granéli, E., N. Johansson and R. Panosso. 1998. "Cellular toxin contents in relation to nutrient conditions for different groups of phycotoxins". pp. 321-324 in: *Harmful Algae*, Reguera. B., J. Blanco, M.L. Fernández and Wyatt T. (eds.), Xunta de Galicia and Intergovern. Oceanographic Comm. of UNESCO.

50. Smith, J.C., R. Cormier, J. Worms, C.J. Bird, M.A. Quilliam, R. Pocklington, R. "Angus and et al. 1990. Toxic blooms of the domoic acid containing diatom *Nitzschia* pungens in the Cardigan River, Prince Edward Island, in 1988." pp. 227-232, in: *Toxic marine phytoplankton*, Granéli, E., B. Sundström, L. Edler, and D.M. Anderson (eds.), Elsevier Sci. Publ. Co., Inc., New York.

51. Todd, E.C.D. 1990. "Amnesic shellfish poisoning -- a new seafood toxin syndrome." pp. 504-508, in: *Toxic Marine Phytoplankton*, Granéli, E., B. Sundstrom, L. Edler, and D.M. Anderson (eds.), New York, Elsevier.

52. Burkholder, J.M. and H.B. Glasgow, Jr. 1997. "Trophic controls on stage transformations of a toxic ambush-predator dinoflagellate." *J. Eukaryot. Microbiol.* 44(3): 200-205.

53. Burkholder, J.M., E.J. Noga, C.H. Hobbs, and H.B. Glasgow, Jr. 1992. "New "phantom" dinoflagellate is the causative agent of major estuarine fish kills." *Nature*: 407-410.

54. Grattan, L.M., D. Oldach, T.M. Perl, M H. Lowitt, D.L. Matuszak, C. Dickson, C. Parrott, R.C. Shoemaker, C.L. Kauffman, M.P. Wasserman, et al. 1998. "Learning and memory difficulties after environmental exposure to waterways containing toxin-producing *Pfiesteria* or *Pfiesteria*-like dinoflagellates." *Lancet* 352: 532-539.

55. Lipton, D. 1999. *Pfiesteria*'s Impact on Seafood Industry Sales, Sea Grant Extension, University of Maryland.

VIDEO CONFERENCE

EDWARD TELLER
Hoover Institute, Palo Alto, CA; and Lawrence Livermore National Laboratory, Livermore, CA, USA

INTRODUCTION

Professor Zichichi asked me to discuss what scientists can do against terrorists. I accept this assignment with enthusiasm and some doubt.

The United States is the prime objective of terrorists. One reason is envy; another is their basic dislike of science and technology. The United States is behaving in a reasonable manner by taking determined action against any strong center of terrorism, and by being careful in its actions against misguided individuals.

We scientists can be particularly helpful by cutting off any popular support of terrorists, based on their strong opposition to science and progress. We should realize that in this regard the terrorists find some sympathies in the Green Movement. I want to make clear in a few specific examples that science and technology, which are indeed supported by the United States, actually serve everybody.

WEATHER PREDICTION

Involuntary weather modification has become a much-discussed topic, for instance, at the recent Kyoto conference. I shall emphatically avoid discussing weather modification, since it will have different advantages and disadvantages for different countries and would therefore automatically produce disagreements. Good weather prediction, on the other hand, serves the advantage of everybody.

Fifty years ago, reliable weather prediction could be made only for one or two days. Today, reasonably reliable weather predictions can be made for five days. The main reason for this progress is a more than thousand-fold increase in computing capabilities. That progress is not much greater is due to two facts. The first is that small and limited changes of present weather conditions can rather rapidly produce big changes in a short time. The second is that present conditions of the atmosphere are well known in small parts of the world, like United States and Western Europe, while they are poorly known in large parts, such as Africa, South America and huge southern portions of the oceans.

Some of my associates and I have proposed a remedy: deployment and maintenance of a billion inch-sized balloons evenly distributed in the atmosphere, together with a few hundred satellites to emit appropriate infrared radiation to observe the reflection of the balloons. That would lead to accurate measurements of the velocity of the balloons and thereby the wind velocities in every few cubic miles throughout the globe.

Further refinements may give information on moisture and temperature as well. I would like to modify this process by using extremely light inch-sized corner reflectors which deflect light by 180 degrees and will drop very slowly because they weigh much less than air in a few cubic inches. We estimate that the worldwide cost may not greatly exceed one billion dollars a year.

We hope that by these means one could extend weather prediction throughout the world, from the presently valid five days, to as much as two weeks. The benefits would include support for agriculture by determining proper dates for sowing and harvesting in each part of the world, by monitoring air traffic conditions, and also by predicting floods and hurricanes, thus saving lives and property. We estimate that worldwide applications could save a hundred billion dollars annually.

SAFETY OF NUCLEAR REACTORS

Modern civilization strongly depends on ample supply of electricity. This is apt to be limited in times not long compared to a hundred years, particularly if one considers that underdeveloped regions like India, Africa and South America will have to participate more strongly. Other energy sources like solar energy, wind energy, geothermal energy and hydroelectricity which enjoy initial support will suffice only locally. Sufficient worldwide supply can however be had from nuclear reactors for thousands of years to come. Unfortunately, reactor construction has stopped due to fear of the radioactivity released by accidents and also due to worries concerning safe disposal of fission products which remain as a residue of energy production.

At present, the availability of fuel would serve for a longer time than conventional coal and oil. This time could be further extended to thousands of years by using as a basic materials thorium, rather than uranium.

The common thorium, Th232 on top is not readily fissionable, but it can be activated by neutrons from a standard uranium reactor. Neutrons will be absorbed by thorium 232 to yield thorium 233 and this will transform by two beta decays into U233. This is highly fissionable and activates more thorium, so the thorium reactor will function by itself and even have excess neutrons to activate a following thorium reactor. Thus a chain of reactors can be built up as long as we like: uranium reactor thorium reactor do that three times, etc. Thus thorium reactors may supply us well into the future thereby giving us a chance to have the next good idea.

There remains the next question: what to do with reactor products? The old idea is to put them in the least significant place, such as the Yucca Mountain in Nevada. To this all states agree with the peculiar exception of Nevada and myself. My worry is that the decay of products will take thousands of years, and for all I know in 10,000 AD, Nevada will be the center of the universe.

I have a more immediate objection: reactor products are never as dangerous as when they are being transported. One big trouble is that in this particular respect the United States does not stand alone. Even the French have a Nevada in their transportation problem. I propose a very different approach.

So far there have been three major nuclear accidents: in Great Britain in 1957, the Three Mile Island accident in the United States in 1979, and the Chernobyl accident in the Soviet Union in 1986. These three accidents had the same cause: operator error. Indeed, in this respect there seems to be no limit to operator ingenuity. The only exception is Chernobyl, where the Kremlin sent in a completely inexperienced crew, so there is no difficulty in explaining that error. Chernobyl is the only one where there were lives lost (a few hundred). In England and the United States the damage was great in money, but due to the safety of the reactors, no lives were lost. In the Chernobyl incident, the world press, however, was not reticent about the latter point. In addition to the few hundred lives lost locally as an immediate consequence, tens of thousands of unidentified and unproven casualties due to the spread of radioactivity far outside the immediate zone were postulated by the press.[1] But one tragic circumstance must be mentioned. Substantial (but not necessarily harmful) radiation was reported throughout Europe. Consequently people have become exceedingly worried about the effects on unborn children, so that in the following few months 50,000 excess abortions were performed.

I believe that nuclear reactors will not become acceptable unless we manage to exclude the repetition of such a situation. We might construct reactors a few hundred meters underground, rely on expert engineers in their construction and give the reactors a strong negative temperature coefficient so that upon heating they will shut down.

In standard operation the energy will be transferred to a coolant gas (possibly helium) which will transport the energy directly to the electricity generators near or on the surface of the earth. The operators will then be decoupled from the reactors except for operating the coolant gas or performing appropriate and simple shutdown measures. Mistakes of reducing the coolant will, automatically, lead to reactor shutdown rather than an explosion. Of course, one cannot completely exclude a catastrophe such as the impact of a huge meteorite causing an enormous crater or a very unusual eruption of a volcano at precisely the wrong spot. But such catastrophe might in any case lead to casualties. Locating reactors in loose dry earth, not very far from where electricity is needed would appear to lead to sufficient safety. Loose earth may be specified to exclude the propagation of shock of volcanic origin. The use of dry surroundings will exclude the transport to the surface of dissolved radioactivity, and even transport of water from nearby sources will be inhibited by the structure remaining hot before and after shutdown.

Under these conditions the obvious plan should be that after shutdown of the reactors, one should permit the quiet and permanently hot substance to remain in place for tens of thousands of years. Most of the heat may even be used for minor electricity production into the almost indefinite future.

ASTEROID IMPACT

Sixty-five million years ago, the earth was hit by a huge asteroid. Subsequent events, like dense dust throughout the atmosphere, led to remarkable consequences in the biosphere by excluding sunlight, reducing vegetation, and starvation across the entire planet. Specifically, the dinosaurs became extinct. Much more recently, in Tunguska in sub-arctic Siberia a big meteorite hit in 1908 and laid a forest flat for many miles around. Fortunately, we can avoid the fate of the dinosaurs. The big, approaching object will be seen weeks or months in advance and can be shattered or deflected by an explosion (or even a nuclear explosion) appropriately deep under its surface.

CLONING

Progress of biological science has established the feasibility of cloning, its three phases and their quite different stages.

The possibility of animal cloning is an established fact. It is apt to have an enormous impact, as did the domestication of animals. The existing and astonishingly effective method of evolution by mutation did, by mating variation and selection, produce the most amazing variety of animals. Even so, it seems a waste merely to repeatedly mate a particularly productive cow and thereby dilute its advantageous properties by producing mixed progeny. It would certainly help to reproduce it by manifold cloning, and then add to it by with the established process of mating. Of course, present methods still need to be improved to do all this in an economic manner. The second stage is the use of stem cells for medical purposes. A lot will have to happen before out of a human stem cell one can grow functioning, fresh liver tissue in a man's diseased organ. But it appears to be only a matter of time before such procedures can help our contemporaries, particularly in their old age.

In my opinion, cloning of humans must wait until animal cloning and medical cloning are well advanced. It is not justified to multiply human suffering by less than perfect cloning procedures. But in the longer run, human cloning will become practical with many consequences. One must admit that not all of the consequences are desirable. As sexual reproduction is regulated by the institution of marriage, so we shall have to find the rules and practices by which human cloning will be justified from case to case. I have mentioned this last point far ahead of its time to indicate the limitless possibilities of research and its translation into practice.

CONCLUSION

I claim to have given an almost adequate impression of the thorough manner in which research can make big positive contributions. I hope that objections to progress will not prevail, least of all any protest involving violence.

Ten years later an international conference in Vienna discredited these non-local casualties with the possible exception of a few children affected by cancer of the thyroid due to radiation. We now know that this can be prevented by removing the thyroid and providing the individual with available clean thyroid products.

THE IMPACTS OF HARMFUL ALGAL EVENTS

MICHEAL Ó CINNÉIDE
Marine Institute, Marine Environment and Health Services Division, Galway, Ireland

This paper looks at the biological, economic, regulatory and scientific impacts of harmful algal events. As Don Anderson's paper focuses on the global biological aspects, this will look in more detail at stakeholder responses to the HAE and the role of communications.

BIOLOGICAL IMPACTS

Harmful algal events (HAE's) have occurred for centuries and have commonly been described as "Red Tides." There are 5,000 different marine algal species, of which 75 can produce potent toxins. Scientists and the public are concerned that the size and frequency of these events have increased. (Graneli, 1). The biological impacts of HAE's include:

- Contamination and closures of shellfish
- Mass mortalities of wild and farmed fish
- Human illness and in some cases, death from eating shellfish containing biotoxins

When people eat shellfish that have accumulated HAB toxins, there are at least seven different syndromes that can occur such as diarrhetic, amnesic, paralytic or neurotoxic shellfish poisoning (DSP, ASP, PSP or NSP). There is no known antidote and the poisoning can be fatal in certain cases.

ECONOMIC IMPACTS

HAE's have had major economic impacts on coastal communities, including:

- Prolonged closures of commercial shellfish fisheries
- Costs of mortalities in farmed finfish.

The Woods Hole Oceanographic Institution sought to estimate the economic impacts from HABs in the U.S. Their conclusion, based on conservative assumptions, was that the economic costs averaged U.S. $49 million per year in the early 1990s. (Anderson, 2). This was based primarily on public health impacts, commercial fishing losses and recreational/tourism impacts.

To give some concrete examples – in Ireland, rope mussel fisheries were closed for up to 9 months in the years 1995, 2000 and 2001, due to the presence of biotoxins such as *Dinophysis* in the water. The Irish Shellfish Association has estimated the losses in the period 2000/2001 at EU 4 million. The Irish government felt that a multi million remedial aid package was required to help the producers survive the impact of biotoxin losses.

The impacts of HAE through mortalities in farmed finfish have been felt in Japan, Norway, Canada, Chile and in Ireland.

In Japan, blooms of the phytoplankton *Chattonella antiqua* in the Seto inland Sea led to mass mortalities of the cultured yellowtail fish during the 1960s and 1970s.

In 1972, local fishermen lost about 14 million yellowtail at a cost of Y 71 billion, equivalent to U.S. $500 million. (Dale, 3).

In Norway, a bloom in the Skagerrak in May 1988 caused 300 tons of salmon to die near the island of Hidra. A massive rescue operation commenced, which involved moving some 18 million farmed fish from their permanent sites to more inland fjords. This was considered as *"the greatest achievement since the development of the Norwegian fish farming industry."* (Murphy, 4)

In eastern Canada, mortalities of thousands of farmed Atlantic salmon were linked to a bloom of the toxic dinoflagellate *Alexandrium tamarense* in June 2000. Detailed research by Allan Cembella and colleagues showed that dense concentrations of cells were trapped in the mucus of the fish gills. The salmon were killed by direct exposure to the toxic cells and/or to the soluble toxins which were released during the bloom (Cembella, 5).

REGULATORY IMPACTS

The increasing impact of HAE's, especially given the potential consequences for human health, has led to a vigorous response from regulators around the world. *"Experience has shown that awareness of harmful effects of phytoplankton by government officials evolves as a direct response to severe outbreaks of toxic red tides"* (Dale, 6).

There are many examples of this response cycle.

- In Spain, the regional authorities set up a new monitoring laboratory, the Centro de Control de Medio Marino in Pontevedra, after large scale incidents of shellfish poisoning had impacted sales of mussels from the rias of Galicia. The annual budget for the programme is U.S. $1.6 million. (Marino et al., 7)
- In Canada, the deaths and illnesses that were linked with ASP in mussels from Prince Edward Island in the late 1980s triggered a major investment in HAE monitoring and research.

- In New Zealand, the shellfish industry was closed for several months in 1993 following its first marine biotoxin event. Some 180 persons reported illness fitting the description for neurotoxin shellfish poisoning. The Ministry of Agriculture led a fundamental review of the New Zealand biotoxin system and introduced a series of reforms. (Mackenzie, 8). The New Zealand management system is now considered one of the best in the world.

Monitoring programmes have been set up which test for the presence of toxic phytoplankton in the coastal waters and test the shellfish for the presence of biotoxins. HAE monitoring and management programmes are now ongoing in over 50 countries worldwide. (Anderson et al., 9)

The average cost of HAE monitoring and management in 11 coastal U.S. states was estimated at over U.S. $2 million per year (Anderson et al., 10). In six European countries that have invested heavily in the farming of fish and shellfish – France, Spain, Portugal, Scotland, Ireland and Norway – the approximate costs of HAE monitoring is over U.S. $4.5 million dollars per year (Anderson et al., 11).

Most of the monitoring programmes for shellfish are financed by government agencies but a notable exception is New Zealand, where the shellfish industry has paid fully for the biotoxin testing since 1996, at a cost of over NZ 1.45 million pa (U.S. $0.6 million).

SCIENTIFIC RESPONSE

The scientific community has shown a great interest in the HAE issue in recent decades. It offers a fascinating challenge in seeking to understand the factors that control the population dynamics of harmful algae. There are opportunities for multi-disciplinary research involving ecology, physiology, oceanography, toxin chemistry and toxicology.

In the U.S., a call for a concerted national research plan led to the establishment of the ECOHAB programme, which has invested over U.S.$ 40 million in HAE research work since the mid 1990's. The first Symposium on Harmful Marine Algae in the U.S. was held in Woods Hole in December and attracted over 250 scientists. It is expected that the next global HAB conference, due to be held in Florida in October 2002, will be attended by over 1000 scientists.

In the European Union, the EU Commission launched an initiative called EUROHAB in 1998 to generate and coordinate the research needed to manage the effects of harmful micro-algae in the marine and brackish waters of the EU (Graneli, 12).

In the initial three years, funding of 10 million Euros was committed to EUROHAB projects, workshops and studies. This is in addition to the nationally funded research activities on HAEs in the member states of the EU. The latest review of European research concluded that "*major gaps still exist in our understanding the factors that control the population dynamics of harmful algae. Why and how harmful algal blooms develop is not understood at present.*" (Graneli, 13).

In addition to ECOHAB in the U.S. and to EUROHAB in the European Union, there is the GEOHAB programme of international cooperative research. GEOHAB stands for Global Ecology and Oceanography of Harmful Algal Blooms. It had its origin at a workshop held in Denmark in 1998 and is officially endorsed by a commission of UNESCO. GEOHAB defines the central research problem as:

"*To understand and quantify the features and mechanisms underlying the population dynamics of HAB species in a variety of settings. This understanding can be used as a basis for monitoring, modelling and predicting the occurrence, movement, toxicity and environmental effects of HABs*" (GEOHAB, 14)

These are expensive research programmes. While this research into HAE's is a laudable response to a worldwide natural phenomenon, it has not always greeted with enthusiasm by some of the key stakeholders in the marine sector.

STAKEHOLDER RESPONSES

The response of industry and of local communities to the increasing prevalence of HAEs and the growth of regulation in this area has been complex and worthy of reflection.

In Ireland, as in many other countries, it has followed a cycle of initial demands for official action to protect public health, followed by bemusement at the scale of the response, growing distance from the scientific effort and finally frustration and anger at the perceived excesses in regulatory zeal. To quote one mussel producer:

"*Make no mistake, this industry will not survive with the scientific lobby tightening its grip. Levels are squeezed down and the quest for new toxins proves fruitful.*" (O Sullivan, 15)

An official Irish report on regional consultations with shellfish producers and processors said "*The industry has suffered from prolonged closures and has sustained economic losses in 1999/2000. A clear message was received from the shellfish industry at the consultations – they have no confidence in the biotoxin control system in operation.*" (FSAI, 16.)

We have seen evidence of this cycle in various parts of Europe during 2002, as the EU seeks to harmonize the biotoxin testing regime. Most recently in France, the CNC (Comité Nationale de Conchyculture), which represents the interests of shellfish farmers, has called for a national boycott of testing levies in protest at the imposition of new EU decisions on biotoxin testing (Le Marin, 17).

These responses can be interpreted as a classic example of science and/or regulation getting out ahead of the public. Aquaculture producers understand the need for biotoxin monitoring but perceive the growing research/regulatory apparatus as becoming an end in itself.

There is a growing controversy in the United States over funding for HAE research into the species *Pfiesteria piscicida*. This organism was associated with fish kills and fish lesion events in the east coast states of Maryland and North Carolina in the 1990s. A group known as the Waterkeeper Alliance, led by its President, Robert F. Kennedy Jr., has recently called for a public enquiry into the *Pfiesteria* research.

"Over the past 5 years, more than U.S. $16 million in federal funds were allocated to scientists at various institutes to conduct research on the chemistry and impacts of the toxin from this species. Funding was primarily provided by the ECOHAB program. In the past several weeks, researchers who received more than $12 million of this funding reported that they have been unable to find or grow toxic organism. They concluded that Pfiesteria does not make toxin.

We cannot allow limited research dollars to be wasted. When they do wrong, scientists and government agencies must be held accountable, just like corporate executives of ENRON and Worldcom." (Phycotoxins, 18).

TWIN TRACK APPROACH – RESEARCH AND COMMUNICATIONS

A clear lesson from the cycle of stakeholder responses is the need for a "twin track approach" that combines investment in HAE research and monitoring with an active programme of communications. This approach has been seen to work successfully in countries such as New Zealand, Ireland and Chile for example, but it is not always as evident in the UK or the USA.

In New Zealand, the Ministry brings together researchers, regulators and industry leaders every six months in the Marine Biotoxin Science workshops. These sessions have been held twice yearly since 1994. It provides an opportunity for scientists to present their work in progress and to receive early feedback from potential industry user groups.

A delegation of officials from Ireland visited New Zealand in early 2000 to study how they had managed the biotoxin challenge. Following on this visit, the Irish Marine Institute has organized a similar forum for the past two years. Over a hundred industry participants, researchers and regulators have come together to learn about new developments in HAB research and monitoring. In addition, representatives of these groups meet at least 6 times per year in the context of the Molluscan Shellfish Safety Committee. From personal experience, these MSSC meetings provide a forum for strenuously robust exchanges of views. Over the past two years, the investment in dialogue has been paying off in growing awareness and confidence in the system.

In southern Chile, the local agencies set up a Red Tide Programme in the Magellan Region since 1997. The programme has invested in communications and training with groups such as fishermen, public health nurses and journalists. This included workshops, brainstorming sessions, videos and the use of cartoon messages. *"The main objective is to diminish risks to public health and to minimise disturbances to the fisheries sector"* from the threat posed by the PSP toxin, found in the coastal waters. (Guzman, 19).

TRENDS AND CONCLUSIONS

There are three inescapable trends that pose a challenge to all of us that are involved in this area of research or regulatory work:

- The size and frequency of Harmful Algal Events are increasing
- The level and the sophistication of scientific research is growing
- The demand of citizens and industry groups for access to information is increasing.

In HAE's as in other spheres, government functions more effectively with the consent of the governed. Regulators need to ensure that information from the monitoring programmes is made available to user groups – industry, consumers -very quickly. Researchers need to avail of and if necessary, to create opportunities for dialogue and feedback on the HAE issues. Experience has shown that investment in these forms of communication can help to minimize the negative impacts of algal events.

REFERENCES

1. Graneli, E. and Lipiatou, E. (Editors) 2002. EUROHAB Science Initiative – Research and Infrastructural Needs. Directorate General for Research, EU Commission, Brussels.
2. Anderson, D., Kaoru, Y. and White, A. 2000. *Estimated Annual Economic Impact from Harmful Algal Blooms in the United States*, Woods Hole Oceanographic Institution, USA.
3. Dale, B., Baden, D.G., Bary, M., Edler, L., Fraga, S., Jenkinson I.R., Hallegraeff, G.M., Okaichi, T., Tangen, K., Taylor, F.J.R., White, A.W., Yentsch, C.M. and Yentsch, C.S., 1987. "The Problems of Toxic Dinoflagellate Blooms in Aquaculture," *Proceedings. Sherkin Island Marine Station*, Ireland.
4. Murphy, M., Salmon Rescue Operation on the Western Norwegian Coast – Algal Bloom, 1988. Sherkin Island Marine Station, Ireland.
5. Cembella, A, Quilliam, M.A., Lewis, N., Buder, A., Thomas, K., Jellett, J.F., Ferguson, H., Carver, C. and Cusack, R., 2001. "The Toxic Dinoflagellate *Alexandrium tamarense* associated with Mortality of Farmed Salmon in Nova Scotia." *Proceedings of 7th Canadian Workshop on Harmful Marine Algae.*
6. Dale B., *op cit.*
7. Marino, J., Maneiro, J. and Blanco, J. 1998. "The Harmful Algae Monitoring Programme of Galicia: Good Value for Money" in Harmful Algae, Xunta de Galicia and IOC, UNESCO.
8. Mackenzie, "The Evolution of Marine Biotoxin Monitoring Programmes in New Zealand", 2001 in *Proceedings of the Second Irish Marine Science Workshop*, Marine Institute, Ireland.
9. Anderson, D.M., Andersen, P., Bricelj, V.M., Cullen, J.J. and Rensel J.E. 2001. *Monitoring and Management Strategies for Harmful Algal Blooms in the United States*. Asia Pacific Economic Program and International Oceanographic Commission, Paris.
10. Anderson, et al., 2000, *op cit.*
11. Anderson, et al., 2001, *op cit.*

404

12.   Graneli, 2002, *op.cit.*
13.   Graneli, 2002, *op.cit.*
14.   GEOHAB Science Plan, 2001. International Oceanographic Commission, Paris
15.   O Sullivan, F. (pers comm), 2001.
16.   Food Safety Authority of Ireland, 2001. Report on regional consultations with shellfish producers and processors . FSAI, Dublin.
17.   Le Marin, "Durcissement des Normes Sanitairies: le CNC appelle au boycott de l'administration", 7 Juin 2002.
18.   Phycotoxins News Release, August 2002. Phycotoxins @www.agr.ca.
19.   Guzman, L. 2002. "Experiences Gained with Training Activities to Selected Groups to Strengthen Prevention in Areas Affected by PSP outbreaks" in Proceedings of 4th International Conference on Molluscan Shellfish Safety (in press) Xunta de Galicia, Pontevedra, Spain.

14. SCIENCE AND TECHNOLOGY: BRAIN AND BEHAVIOUR DISEASES

THE HUMAN GENOME PROJECT: ITS IMPACT ON COMPLEX DISORDERS

P. MICHAEL CONNEALLY, PH.D.
Department of Medical and Molecular Genetics, Indiana University School of Medicine, Indianapolis, Indiana USA

The human genome has almost been completely sequenced and is expected to be finalized in April 2003, the fiftieth anniversary of the discovery, by Watson and Crick, of the structure of DNA. The completion of the sequence has profound implications in medicine, in the diagnosis, care and treatment of patients with simple Mendelian disorders where the etiology is essentially all genetic and also in complex disorders where both genetic and environmental factors play major roles.

There are over 11,000 unique Mendelian disorders in man. The majority, however, are quite rare. Among the more common ones essentially all have been mapped and with few exceptions the genes and mutation identified.

Unfortunately this is not the case for the vast majority of complex disorders. These disorders unlike Mendelian ones are not due to mutations in a single gene but rather are the result of a combination of many genes and environmental factors. While Mendelian disorders tend to be rare, complex disorders are quite common. Thus the total load of deleterious mutations in the human population is mainly centered in the common complex diseases.

Examples of common complex disorders are Type 2 diabetes, asthma, cardiovascular disease, hypertension, osteoporosis, and most psychiatric disorders. This review will concentrate on the psychiatric disorders and in particular bipolar affective disorder, schizophrenia and alcoholism.

BIPOLAR AFFECTIVE DISORDER

This disorder is highly heritable. Its frequency in the population is approximately one percent, but the risk to first degree relatives is approximately five times greater. Numerous linkage studies have been performed, using various strategies to attempt to locate gene loci involved in the risk for bipolar disorder. Unfortunately the original findings have often been difficult to replicate, a finding common to the majority of complex disorders. However, a number of loci on several chromosomes have been replicated which include 15 chromosomal regions. These include chromosomes 4, 5, 8, 10, 11, 12, 13, 16, 18, 21, 22, and the X chromosome. With the possible exception of the serotonin transporter gene on 17q and the catechol-O-methyltransferase gene on 22q, no other candidate gene studies have been replicated. Since so many loci have been implicated in the etiology of the disorder, it will clearly require a large effort to locate the causative genes. For a summary, see Nurnberger and Foroud.[1]

SCHIZOPHRENIA

Schizophrenia affects approximately one percent of the population and like bipolar illness has a strong genetic component. The incidence in sibs of affected individuals ranges from 6 – 12 percent and the incidence in children of affected is 12 percent. There is clear evidence that multiple susceptibility genes exist for schizophrenia. More loci have been implicated for schizophrenia than for any other complex disorder but many could not be replicated. Presently loci on chromosomes 1, 5, 6, 8, 10, 13, 20 and 22 are being extensively investigated. Recently Kendler and his associates[2] found variation in the DTNBP1 gene on chromosome 6p22.3 to be associated with schizophrenia. This was accomplished using single nucleotide polymorphism (SNP) markers in a study of 270 high-density pedigrees from the west of Ireland. This is the first successful study in behavorial genetics to utilize SNPs. Since there are virtually an unlimited number of SNPs in the human genome, they are proving to be invaluable for fine mapping especially in complex diseases. This gene may play a role in signal transduction. If these results can be replicated in other families, it will be a major breakthrough in the study of this difficult disorder. It also suggests that SNP technology may play a very important role in the study of complex genetic disorders.

ALCOHOLISM

Alcoholism is a leading cause of morbidity and premature death with an incidence as high as ten percent. Family studies show a five-fold increase in the first-degree relatives of alcoholics. This is true for relatives who are adopted and thus in a different environment. Thus it is clear that there is a significant genetic component to alcoholism, which has also been demonstrated using twin studies including twin pairs who were reared apart. A mutation in the aldehyde dehydrogenase gene prevalent in Asians but rare in other populations causes the "flushing response" which acts as a protective factor since imbibing alcohol causes nausea and flushing in mutation carriers.[3]

The first approach to identifying genes for alcoholism was the candidate gene-association studies. The most notable candidate gene, the dopamine D2 receptor on chromosome 11, was found to be associated with alcoholism.[4] This finding is highly controversial since many subsequent studies were negative. This was also true of the serotonin transporter (HTT) gene on chromosome 17. A major problem in association studies is population stratification, where the cases and controls come from different ethnicities that also happen to differ in frequencies at the candidate gene locus.

A more optimum approach is a linkage study using, where possible, extended pedigrees. Most recent studies used a genome-wide approach using approximately 300 polymorphic markers spread across the genome. A major problem is defining alcoholism. Typically DSM-III-R criteria are used. The largest linkage study to date is the Collaborative Study of the Genetics of Alcoholism (COGA) which ascertained, evaluated, and genotyped 105 pedigrees as part of an initial genome screen. This was followed up by a replication data set of 157 pedigrees. Both sets showed evidence for loci for alcoholism on chromosomes 1, 2, 3, and 7.[5] Fine mapping of these regions using SNPs is in progress to locate the causative genes. Hopefully, a number of causative genes will be discovered within the next two years.

REFERENCES

1. Nurnberger, J.I., Foroud, T. (2000) "Genetics of Bipolar Affective Disorder." *Current Psychiatry Reports* 2:147-157.
2. Straub, R.E., Jiang, U., MacLean, C.J., Ma, Y., Webb, B.T., Myakishev, M.V., Harris-Kerr, C., Wormley, B., Sadek, H., Kadambi, B., Cesare, A.J., Gibberman, A., Wang, X., O'Neill, F.A., Walsh, D., Kendler, K.S. (2002) "Genetic variation in the 6p22.3 gene DTNBP1, the human ortholog of the mouse dysbindin gene, is associated with schizophrenia." *American Journal of Human Genetics* 71:337-348.
3. Thomasson, H.R., Edenberg, H.J., Crabb, D.W., Mai, X.L., Jerome, R.E., Li, T-K., Wang, S.P., Lin, Y.T., Lu, R.B., Yin, S.J. (1991) "Alcohol and aldehyde dehydrogenase genotypes and alcoholism in Chinese men." *American Journal of Human Genetics* 48:677-681.
4. Blum, K., Noble, E.P., Sheridan, P.J., Montgomery, A., Ritchie, T., Jagadeeswaran, P., Nogami, H., Briggs, A.H., Cohn, J.B. (1990) "Allelic association of human dopamine D2 receptor gene in alcoholism." *JAMA.* 263:2055-2060.
5. Foroud, T., Edenberg, H.J., Goate, A., Rice, J., Flury, L., Koller, D.L., Bierut, L.J., Conneally, P.M., Nurnberger, J.I., Bucholz, K.K., Li, T-K., Hesselbrock, V., Crowe, R., Schuckit, M., Porjesz, B., Begleiter, H., Reich, T. (2000) "Alcoholism Susceptibility Loci: Confirmation Studies in a Replicate Sample and Further Mapping." *Alcoholism: Clinical and Experimental Research* 24:933-945.

15. THE CULTURAL EMERGENCY — GENERAL DEBATE AND CONCLUSIONS

LANGUAGE, LOGIC AND SCIENCE

ANTONINO ZICHICHI
CERN, University of Bologna, Geneva, Switzerland

THE CULTURE OF OUR TIME AND THE ONE NEEDED

The end of the bipolar world has brought up the need for the Culture of our time to be in phase with the greatest achievements of our intellect. These achievements are not only those originated from Language, as it appears to be the case with the status of our present Culture. Rigorous Logic and Science must be brought into the cultural patrimony of our third millennium. In fact a new Culture is needed in the third millennium, since the number one enemy of humanity is Ignorance.

From the first years of our Erice Seminars on Planetary Emergencies, the Cultural Emergency has been considered. However top priority was given to other emergencies more strictly related to the risk of Nuclear and of Environmental Holocausts. It is the unexpected arrival of **Terrorism** which gives the Cultural Emergency a high priority, since Terrorism and the reaction to Terrorism are strongly correlated to the lack of a Culture, as said above, in phase with the greatest achievements of our Existential Sphere.

We will see that these achievements are not one (Language) but three: Language, Rigorous Logic and Science. While everybody can speak and write and therefore can perfectly understand the existence of Language, not so many people know Rigorous Logic and its achievements; probably even fewer people know Science and its great discoveries. Even worse, Science and Technology are often considered undistinguishable. In the Culture of our time the word "Science" is used in an improper way, as if very many intellectual activities were "Science." If everything is Science, nothing is Science.

We will try to explain why the basic features of our intellectual achievements must be classified in terms of Language, Rigorous Logic and Science, without any confusion. In fact people equate Culture with Language. We will point out the difference which exists between the **"basic"** and the **"applied."** In fact **"basic"** Language, Rigorous Logic and Science can never be against mankind, while **"applied"** Language, Rigorous Logic and Science can be for man and against.

The third millennium needs a Culture where Language, Rigorous Logic and Science are all in. The Erice Seminars have been engaged in the 53 Planetary Emergencies. We have contributed to overcome the risk of the Nuclear Holocaust and have implemented dozens of pilot-projects to overcome the risk of the Environmental Holocaust. The totally unpredicted phase, following the end of the bipolar world, has brought to the first line of our attention the Cultural Emergency, since **Terrorism** brings with it the message that the number one enemy of humanity– as said before – is "Ignorance."

To fight this enemy, we need Culture. Not the old one, which is responsible for the present status, but the new one whose bases will be not only Language but Rigorous Logic and Science, in order to help the North (rich) and the South (poor) to get together and work to combat Ignorance. This paper is a contribution to avoid the risk of a Cultural Holocaust.

THE GREATEST ACHIEVEMENTS OF OUR INTELLECT

Our Existential Sphere has two components. One is in the Immanent, the other is in the Transcendent.

The Existential Sphere in the Transcendent manifests itself in what is called Religion. We will discuss the Immanent only.

A careful study of the Immanent Reality leads to the conclusion that it is based on three pillars: **Language**, **Rigorous Logic** and **Science**, which are the greatest achievements of our intellect.

- **Language**, from which collective and permanent memory are born, thanks to Writing.
- **Rigorous Logic**, which has given rise to the great constructions of Geometry, Arithmetic, Analysis, Algebra, Topology. From now on, Logic will mean "Rigorous Logic."
- **Science** (with its three levels), which allows the certainty that the world is not ruled by chaos but rather by a rigorous Logic with laws that are valid from the heart of a proton (a millionth of a billionth of a centimetre) to the fringes of the Universe (a million billion billion kilometres).

The three levels of scientific credibility:

First Level	Second Level	Third Level
Where there are experiments whose results can be reproduced in the laboratory. Example: *Discovery of the Fundamental Laws*	Where it is not possible to intervene in order to reproduce a result. Example: *Stellar evolution*	A one-off event. Example: *Cosmic evolution*

All the levels must be formulated in a rigorous way, and there should be no contradiction between them.

An example of the link between the three levels of scientific credibility: Cosmic Evolution must be formulated in a rigorously mathematical way, and must be based on the discoveries of the Fundamental Laws made at the first level.

No phenomena known in the Galilean sense (i.e., rigorously reproducible) exist that cannot be explained as a consequence of the Logic of Nature: this represents the greatest conquest of Reason in the Immanent.

This study, undertaken by Galilei just four centuries ago, leads us to the greatest synthesis of all times. Were it not for Galilean Science, we would not be able to say that Fundamental Laws of Nature, Universal and Immutable, exist; nor that these Laws lead to the unification of all the phenomena, as shown in Figure 1, by the convergence of the three straight lines. Each one represents the variation of the so-called "gauge coupling" versus Energy (the horizontal axis in Fig. 1). The fact that these three lines converge towards a unique point is a remarkable result coming from studying all possible phenomena in the visible Universe, which appears to us with just four dimensions.

The Grand Unification brings with it the need for a Superworld, a mathematical structure – at present of purely theoretical nature – with forty-three dimensions: eleven of the "boson" type and thirty-two of a "fermion" type.

The data reported in Figure 1 represent the most extraordinary conceptual synthesis of all time.

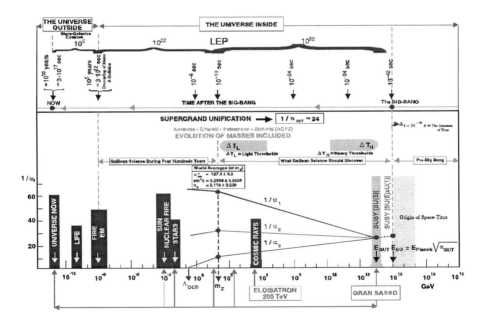

Fig. 1.

The temporal succession of the three pillars – in the history of our Civilisation – is shown in Figure 2.

Language: no-one knows when man started to use this very efficient way of communicating with his fellows. Let us suppose 10^5 years ago. The first written records of human culture date back to about 10^4 years. This is the beginning of collective memory. Here is the Dawn of Civilisation.

Logic started with Epimenide about 2.5×10^3 years ago.

Science with Galileo Galilei 400 years ago.

Science could not arise before **Logic**.

Logic could not arise before (written) **Language**.

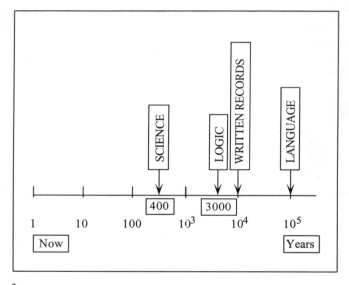

Fig. 2.

Written Language (permanent collective memory) could not arise before the invention of the Spoken Language. Spoken Language very probably came after thousands of years of gesticulation.

When we say **"Language,"** we mean in fact all human activities where the fact that mankind has discovered the **Logic** of Nature **(Science)** plays practically no role.

Thus, for us, **Language** means Poetry, Literature, Music, Arts, Theatre, Economy, Politics and other manifestations of the human intellect such as Philosophy which — I repeat — could exist even if neither **Logic** nor **Science** had ever been discovered.

The Existential Sphere is characterized by Creativity, Leadership, Innovative Leadership, Motivation.

By these terms we mean the following:

1. Creativity is the ability to generate something never before known nor seen nor observed.
2. Leadership is the ability to inspire and motivate people.
3. Innovative Leadership is the ability to inspire and motivate people for creative performance.
4. Motivation is the motor to reach a goal.

In our Immanent Sphere of activities, the three basic pillars, **Language**, **Logic** and **Science** all need Creativity, Leadership and Motivation, the most difficult one being Creativity.

This is why I will concentrate my efforts to discuss Creativity. Let me say that Creativity, no matter where **(Language, Logic, Science)**, needs Memory and Imagination as background. In fact Memory is needed in order not to repeat mistakes and not to restart from **zero** again and again. Imagination is needed because you have to imagine things never thought of before.

Finally, having exploited Memory and Imagination, Creativity corresponds to turning the outcomes of Imagination into Reality.

We will now discuss the three pillars; in §4 the Creativity in them and in §6 the distinction between "basic" and "applied."

LANGUAGE, LOGIC AND SCIENCE

In Figure 3 there is a synthetic representation of the sequence needed to arrive at the three pillars. The Universe could have existed without Life. Life without Conscience. Conscience without Creativity. Creativity without Reason. We are the only form of living matter with the extraordinary privilege of possessing Reason.

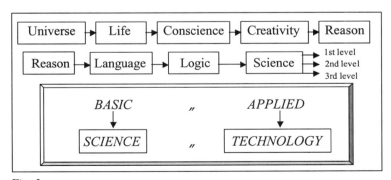

Fig. 3.

418

It is thanks to this privilege that Language, Logic and Science have been discovered. We will see later (§6) that "basic" Science must be distinguished from "applied" Science (Technology) as well as "basic" Logic and Language must be distinguished from their applications.

In Figure 4 the sequence Language, Logic, Science is shown as it did happen.

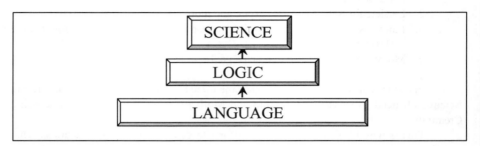

Fig. 4.

Figure 5 synthesizes the content of Language, Figure 6 the content of Logic with its sequence of Arithmetic, Algebra, Analysis and Topology. In Arithmetic, thanks to Cantor, it has been discovered that there are two levels of Infinite, aleph-zero α_0 and aleph-one α_1 . The third level of Infinite, α_3 , is present in the theory of functions. We use the Greek symbols α instead of aleph.

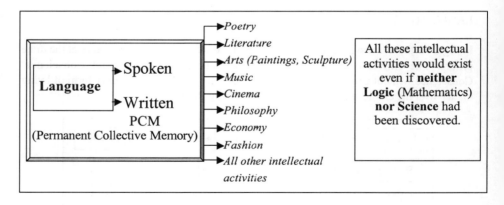

Fig. 5.

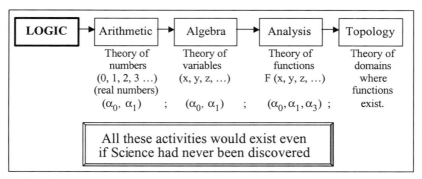

Fig. 6.

In Figure 7 the three levels of Science are exemplified in terms of the Galilean inventions, discoveries and basic measurements for the first two; the third one refers to the XXth century invention, discovery and measurement of what happened to the cosmic evolution 300.000 years after the Big-Bang (see also Fig. 1 – upper part).

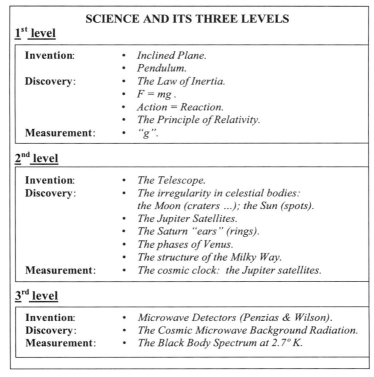

Fig. 7.

Following Galilei, Enrico Fermi emphasized in the XXth century that even the most advanced frontier of Physics needs – as ever – inventions, discoveries and measurements (of the fundamental quantities). Fermi – the greatest Galilean of the XXth century – pointed out that no one should be considered a "physicist" if he has never invented anything, nor discovered anything nor measured a basic quantity.
This is illustrated in Figure 8.

ENRICO FERMI

Physics
- Inventions
- Discoveries
- Measurements of basic quantities

No fellow can be called a Physicist
if he has never
invented, discovered, measured.

Fig. 8.

And now Creativity.

CREATIVITY IN THE THREE PILLARS

Creativity has distinctive features in the three pillars of our Immanent Sphere.
In **Basic Language, Creativity** has the following parameters: aesthetics, beauty, to end up with something which has to be "magnificent". That is why it is necessary to corroborate the concept of **Creativity** with other parameters such as, "satisfy specific formal-aesthetic standards," "be fascinating." We will see in §6 that the **Applied** part of **Language** needs public appeal, success and "be of value to society". In all cases, **Creativity** corresponds to turning the new form of art or music or literature (or all others) into reality.
In **Basic Logic, Creativity** has just one parameter: non-contradiction. A logical structure that leads to self-contradiction cannot exist. The existence of a logical structure corresponds to demonstrating that the new logical structure invented does not lead to self-contradiction. The most impressive and fascinating example is the Infinite.

In **Basic Science**, **Creativity** has one and only one parameter. No matter how elegantly they may be expressed, there are no beautiful or ugly ideas in Science, just true or false ones. By ideas we mean theories. Here Creativity needs not only to rely on a logical structure which avoids self-contradiction, but **it must overcome** the **reproducible experimental proof**. In other words, a theory logically rigorous and non self-contradictory does not necessarily fulfil the requirements of being scientifically proven.

There are many logical theoretical structures which are not found in Nature, e.g. a space with infinite dimensions does not lead to any self-contradiction. It therefore exists from a mathematical point of view, but the space where we live has a finite number of dimensions (probably forty-three, if the Superworld exists). Space with an infinite number of dimensions does not exist for Science. A theory that can be corroborated by the baptismal fire of experimental proof enters into the logic structure of Galilean Science: one that cannot, is discarded.

Creativity in Basic Science thus corresponds to establishing a truth by **experimental reproducibility**, exactly as advocated by Galileo Galilei.

As mentioned before, the background needed for **Creativity** is **Memory** and **Imagination**.

Memory has a common role in the three pillars and it is essential in order not to repeat what has already been "created".

Imagination in **Basic Language** corresponds to inventing new forms of poetry, of music, of art and of other intellectual activities.

Imagination in **Basic Logic** means to invent new mathematical structures with their axioms and their rules.

Imagination in **Basic Science** corresponds to thinking of a new principle, of a new phenomenon, of a new law and to imagining a new experiment. Let me point out that the greatest steps in Science have been originated from the **"totally unexpected"** results of reproducible experiments (Radioactivity $\Rightarrow$Fermi Forces; Strange Particles $\Rightarrow$Flavour Charges, Stability of Matter; Lamb-shift $\Rightarrow$Virtual Phenomena etc. ...).

It is very important to make a clear-cut distinction between **Science** and **Technology**.

For this to be done, it is necessary to have a look at the Technology from the dawn of civilisation to Galilei, and at the Technology from Galilei to our days.

TECHNOLOGY

Let us call the former "pre-Galilean Technology" and the latter "post-Galilean Technology." The pre-Galilean Technology was based on trial and error, and not on the understanding of Fundamental Laws which could give rise to applications such as the wheel or the fire.

This is why, during the ten thousand years that preceded Galileo Galilei, there were two, and only two, inventions: the fire and the wheel. No-one knows who was the man who first succeeded in deliberately producing a spark to start a fire. And no-one knows who was the man who invented the wheel. What we do know, for sure, is that the

wheel and the **fire** have been understood after the discovery of **Science**: the wheel by Galilei and the fire by Einstein. The post-Galilean Technology has its roots in well-understood Fundamental Laws of Nature.* **

Post-Galilean Technology requires our intellect to work in such a way as to produce an **"invention:"** it covers all the activities that arise from the applications of the great scientific discoveries.

Basic Science requires our intellect to work in such a way as to produce a "discovery." **Science** cannot **invent** a new Law of Nature. **Science** can only **discover** a new Law of Nature. On the other hand, technological progress is based on a new idea which puts together, in an original way, different "structures" or "pieces" and uses them in a way which no-one had ever tried before. This is the meaning of a technological **"invention."**

Since each product of our intellect has to be defined in a way which distinguishes it from others, we should not confuse "invention" and "discovery."

Technology "invents" while **Science** "discovers."

The myth of equivalence between **Science** and **Technology** has to be fully discredited.

There is another myth too which needs to be discredited: the myth of the strong correlation between Science and war-weapons. This myth claims that, if the world is stuffed with H-bombs, this is due to Science.

The Stone Age produced peace-tools and war-weapons. The Iron Age produced the scalpel and the sword. The choice of using either scalpel or sword was a cultural one. The choice of producing either peace-tools or war-weapons could not have been scientific, since Galilean Science did not yet exist.

Post-Galilean Technology, through "inventions," is the means by which the Fundamental Laws of Nature discovered by Science can be given meaning and application in our daily lives.

These applications should not be attributed to Science.

From now on, post-Galilean Technology will be simply referred to as Technology.

Technology is the element of rupture that opens our eyes, confronting us with the choice of using it for the benefit or the detriment of man and society.

EXAMPLES OF BASIC AND APPLIED IN THE THREE PILLARS

Science is neither good nor evil. Unfortunately, people currently use the word "science" to mean the "use of science" (i.e. technology) which is no longer "science," just as the "use of language" is no longer "language" and the "use of logic" is no longer "logic."

---

* The invention of the "Steam Machine" precedes the discovery of Thermodynamics. However it is thanks to Thermodynamics that this technology has been fully understood and has given rise to vast technological inventions in this field.

** The optical instruments existed before the understanding of the "dual nature" of light.

Let me elaborate further on this point. An example of **Creativity** in **Basic Science** is the discovery of the "Standard Model," i.e. the superb synthesis that can. explain all phenomena of our world in terms of three Fundamental Structures (called the three families of elementary particles) and three Fundamental Forces of Nature.

An example of **Creativity** in **Basic Logic** is the invention of the rigorous and formidable logical structure called the Infinite.

Examples of **Creativity** in **Basic Language** are the *Pietà* by Michelangelo, the *Primavera* by Botticelli, the Ninth Symphony by Beethoven, the Fifth Symphony by Mahler, the *Divina Commedia* by Dante.

All these achievements are for mankind.

Examples of **Applied Science**, **Logic** and **Language** do exist. These "applications" can be **for** and **against** mankind.

For example, **Creativity** against mankind in the **Use of Science**, also called **Applied Science (Technology)**, corresponds to war technology.

Creativity against mankind in **Applied Logic** corresponds to the invention of computer technology applications for the control of billions of people, thus destroying individual freedom.

Creativity against mankind in **Applied Language** corresponds to the invention of ideologies like Stalinism and Nazism.

Examples, which are for mankind, do indeed exist in the domain of **Applied Science**, **Language** and **Logic**.

Peace technology, instruments to help mankind in Medicine, Agriculture and Meteorology, correspond to **Creativity** for mankind in **Applied Science**.

Creativity for mankind in **Applied Logic** corresponds to the invention of new robots to avoid dangerous and unpleasant work for man, of specialised computer-based applications for medicine, for weather forecasting, etc.

In **Applied Language**, the creative power for mankind corresponds to the performance of pieces of poetry, of music and of art, plus all other activities designed to **help increase the quality of every-day life** in all sectors that would exist even if **Logic** and/or **Science** would have never been discovered.

The components for mankind in **Applied Logic** and **Applied Science** contribute enormously to improve the quality of life. The three pillars have a common task and reach the same goal in their applied part **for man**, i.e. to improve the quality of every-day life, as shown in Table 1.

It is evident that with all three pillars, **Language**, **Logic** and **Science**, **their use** can be for mankind and against mankind. The **Use of Science (Technology)** — as we have already emphasized — is the most spectacular way to distinguish the **"basic"** from the **"applied"** part of the same pillar. The terrible weapon able to destroy a metropolis as big as New York — the H-bomb — is not the result of **Creativity** in **Basic Science** but in **Applied Science**. Nazism and Stalinism are not the result of **Creativity** in **Language** but in **Applied Language**.

424

Table 1.

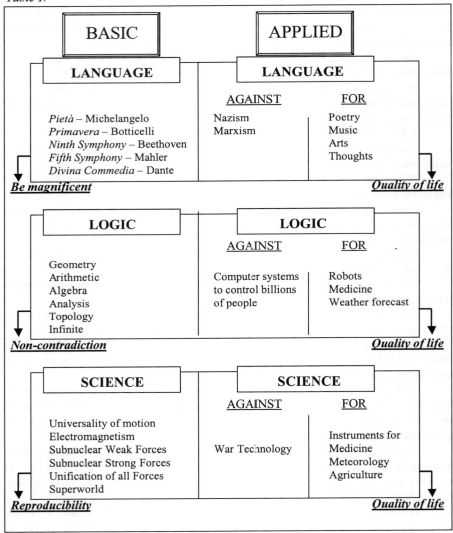

Science, in the Immanent (therefore without appealing to any existential topics connected with the Sphere of the Transcendent), is the source of a new hope, well-rooted in the Fundamental Laws of Nature so that the components mentioned above can all aim at good and never at evil.

In order that the above may happen, it is necessary that the **Applied Science** (i.e. the technological applications of the great scientific discoveries) be entrusted not to political bodies but to the scientific community itself. This is in flagrant conflict with Democracy. A scientist is in fact not elected to be a scientist.

It has never been that way because political activity belongs to **Applied Language**. And this can be for man (Democracy) and against (Dictatorship). Nevertheless everybody considers we scientists as responsible for the **Applied Science**. Worse than this, people think that **Science** was born of Technology. Some would even say that we scientists would not be here, if it were not for the technological development.

The claim, by the fellows responsible for the Culture of our time, that Technology precedes **Basic Science** is due to the fact that the "fire" and the "wheel" were invented before Galilei discovered **Science**. To corroborate this claim they put forward the invention of the telescope, as we will see in §7.

As mentioned above, the "fire" and the "wheel" were understood after **Basic Science** had been discovered by Galilei. To "invent" a new instrument does not necessarily mean to understand "why" it works. The spectacular successes in the construction of Pyramids and of other masterpieces of Architecture, all over the world, did not give rise to the discovery of the first pieces of the Logic of Nature, such as the Principle of Inertia and the other two laws of Mechanics.

A discovery in **Basic Science** corresponds to "understanding" all possible instruments that can be invented. For example, the discovery of a Fundamental Force of Nature, the electromagnetic force, has allowed us to understand that all our senses, sight, hearing, smell, taste and touch, are manifestations of the same and unique fundamental force. This force originates from a unique entity, called "the electric charge." If we could switch off this "charge", our five senses would cease to exist.

Thus all present and future "inventions" connected with sight, hearing, smell, taste and touch are understood, even before they are really implemented.

Before **Basic Science** was discovered thanks to Galileo Galilei, it was the other way round. Since the Fundamental Laws of Nature did not exist, the technological inventions were always rotating around the same two original ones, the "fire" and the "wheel". Since neither the "fire" nor the "wheel" were "understood," the technological development could not produce anything really new.

THE GALILEAN TECHNOLOGY

It is said that the great discoveries by Galileo Galilei were the results of an important technological invention, the "telescope." In fact, it is thanks to the telescope that Galilei discovered that the Sun and the Moon were not "perfect" bodies, despite being **celestial**. The Sun had "sunspots" and the Moon very many irregularities: mountains and craters. Jupiter had satellites, like our Moon. And Saturn had "ears," better known as rings nowadays.

If it were not for a peculiar feature of our Solar System, namely the existence of an immense number of Asteroids, the surface of the Moon might have been less battered, and at first sight might have appeared nearly perfect to Galilei's telescope. Jupiter could have been without satellites and Saturn without rings. The irregularities of the Sun's surface could have been much weaker and nearly undetectable by the primitive telescope invented by Galilei. In other words, all the astronomical discoveries of Galilei are "irrelevant" details when compared with the great achievements of Galilei. Let me recall some of these.

The Law of Inertia; the discovery that acceleration — not velocity — is proportional to a force; the *Principle of Relativity*: "No matter what you do, under no circumstances will you ever detect an effect (experimentally reproducible) that depends on the velocity of a system, if this system travels at constant rectilinear velocity." Notice that this formulation of the principle of relativity includes "all possible effects," not only those due to the motion of material objects. In fact, the principle of relativity as formulated by Galilei includes all phenomena and therefore the Electromagnetic ones which gave rise to the invariance for Lorentz transformations, better known as Einstein's "restricted" relativity.

All these discoveries by Galilei needed neither the technological development of the telescope, nor any technological instrument whatsoever.

All Galilei started to do was to take a piece of stone, tie it up with a string and study its oscillations. He took another piece of stone, as much as possible looking like a sphere, and studied how it rolls down a piece of wood. Then he varied the angle of the plane of the wood.

He discovered that motion obeys the law of constant acceleration and this is how Galilei measured "g": the acceleration due to the gravitational attraction of the earth on all material bodies.

He discovered that a "feather" would fall down like a "hammer" if it were not for the resistance due to the "air." On the Moon, where there is no "air", both the **feather** and the **hammer** would fall down in exactly the same way. During Galilei's time there were no planes, nor missiles, and to think of the man on the Moon was not so easy. "Galilei was right" David Scott exclaimed, when 400 years later he let a feather and a hammer fall down on the Moon.

The great contribution of Galilei to human knowledge is not due to the telescope, i.e. to a technological invention, but to the firm conviction that Fundamental Laws of Nature had to exist. He discovered that this is indeed the case, using the most simple elements of our world: a **stone**, a **piece of wood** and a **string**. And his heart-beat as a **clock**. Can this be **called Technology**?

Galilei was convinced that each piece of matter must carry the imprints of the fellow who created the Universe, with its Laws, rigorous and valid everywhere in Space and Time. Galilei could have discovered neither the laws of the pendulum nor the laws of the "inclined plane" but the chaos. Galilei opened the human intellect to a new horizon. We are, among the many thousands of forms of living matter, the only one to whom a great privilege has been granted. The privilege of being able to understand the **Logic** of **Nature**. Among all possible logical structures, one has been chosen. The task of **Basic Science** is to discover this **Logic**.

In this task we have reached the most incredible synthesis of all times.

I have already mentioned the synthesis: it gives us the feeling that we have understood almost everything about the world. And this, thanks to the so-called Standard Model from where the new theoretical frontier called the Superworld emerges.

If there is the Light, there must be the Superlight. If there is the Electron, there must be the Superelectron. If there are the Stars (ashes of the world), there must also be the ashes of the Superworld, i.e. the Superstars (if they exist, we would not see them because they cannot emit Light). Despite two decades of intensive research, we have not been able to detect any evidence for the existence of the Superworld. I believe that it should exist. But this is a "philosophical" dream corroborated by a mathematical structure. What is missing is the experimental proof. In other words the Logic is there, the Galilean proof is not.

CONCLUSIVE SUMMARY

To sum up, it is **Creativity** in **Applied Language**, **Logic** and **Science** that can be for, but **also** against, mankind. On the other hand, **Creativity** in **Basic Language**, **Basic Logic** and **Basic Science** can never be against mankind. Let us recapitulate.

Creativity in **Basic Language** needs **neither** to obey the principle of "non-self-contradiction" **nor** to overcome the baptism of fire of the experimental proof.

Creativity in **Basic Logic** needs to fulfil the principle of "non-self-contradiction" but no experimental proof is needed.

Creativity in **Basic Science** needs to overcome the principle of the reproducible experimental proof. And this means to check our imagination with the fellow who created the **three Basic Structures** (three families of elementary particles) and the **three Fundamental Laws** of the Universe. As Isidor I. Rabi used to say, "he is smarter than all of us".

Thus **Creativity** in **Basic Science** is the most difficult one, when compared to **Basic Logic** and **Basic Language**, since **Basic Science** means the Logic of Nature and this **Logic** has been chosen by a fellow who is "smarter than all of us".

A synthesis of how the three pillars could be expressed in terms of a possible set of formulae is shown in the following figures. In Figure 9 we refer to Language which is a function F_{La} of the various components R, Cr, Co, Li and U. In turn, each component has a series of functional structures, such as f_{La}^j (R) where the index j runs over a finite number of inputs according to the various contributions so far known. The meaning of the various symbols like Σ, Π, $\oplus$, $\otimes$ and the indices (j, k, l, m, n,) is not the standard one. Their purpose is to recall that many different possible combinations either simple (Σ) or complicated (Π) exist where the various parts of the achievements in Language can all contribute to some original structure of the Language itself.

As it appears from Figure 9, Language is very complex in its structure. The "basic" part of Language must have as final purpose to be "magnificent" and therefore this is the "condition" to be compared with that of Basic Logic and of Basic Science.

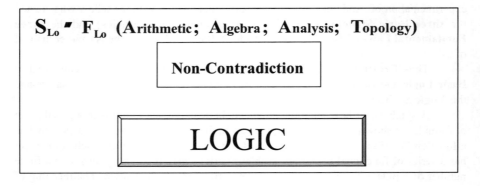

$$La \equiv F_{La}(R, Cr, Co, Li, U) \equiv \sum_{j,k,l,m,n} \left[f^j_{La}(R) \oplus f^k_{La}(Cr) \oplus f^l_{La}(Co) \oplus f^m_{La}(Li) \oplus f^n_{La}(U) \right] \oplus$$

$$\oplus \prod_{j,\,k,\,l,\,m,\,n} \left[f^j_{La}(R) \otimes f^k_{La}(Cr) \otimes f^l_{La}(Co) \otimes f^m_{La}(Li) \otimes f^n_{La}(U) \right] \Rightarrow$$

$$\Rightarrow \boxed{\text{Be Magnificent}}$$

Reason	$\equiv$	R	$\Rightarrow$	j =	1, 2
Creativity	$\equiv$	Cr	$\Rightarrow$	k =	1, 2
Self Conscience	$\equiv$	Co	$\Rightarrow$	l =	1, 2
Life	$\equiv$	Li	$\Rightarrow$	m =	1, 2
Universe	$\equiv$	U	$\Rightarrow$	n =	1, 2

LANGUAGE

Fig. 9.

Logic is much simpler, as shown in Figure 10. It depends on Arithmetic, Algebra, Analysis and Topology. As repeatedly emphasized, Logic must satisfy one and only one condition: non-contradiction.

$$\mathbf{S_{Lo}} \cdot \mathbf{F_{Lo}} \ (\textbf{Arithmetic; Algebra; Analysis; Topology})$$

Non-Contradiction

LOGIC

Fig. 10.

In Figure 11 there is the structure of Science which depends on, and therefore needs, – as previously emphasized – inventions, discoveries and measurements. The only condition being reproducibility.

Applied Language, Logic and Science in their components for man have a common condition, i.e. to improve the quality of life, as already shown in Table 1.

The quantitative measurement of this is our average lifetime which has reached – in the most developed parts of our Earth – the value of 80 years.

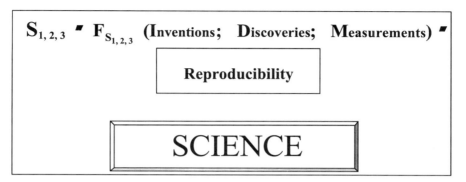

Fig. 11.

Finally we have in Figure 12 the complete structure of all sequences.

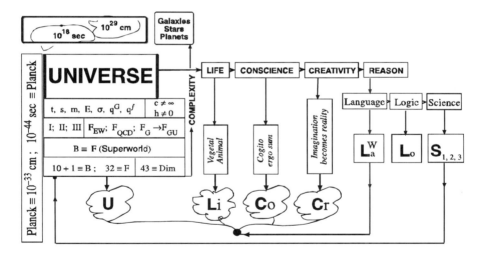

Fig. 12.

Language can discuss in all possible ways, including the totally irrealistic ones, the Universe, the Life, the Conscience, the Creativity, without any boundary condition, but one: to be "magnificent". The most genuine expression of Language is Poetry. In fact with Language, we can say anything and its opposite, the total being zero. Following Borgés, Poetry should be totally deprived of any meaning but be "magnificent." It is the "magnificent" nature of Basic Language which makes Poetry to be the best and most significant part of the first intellectual achievement of our Existencial Sphere in the Immanent.

Logic stands in its box totally isolated from the rest since it deals with axioms and rules and its existence needs only the condition of "non-self-contradiction." Logic is the purest and most rigorous form of thought which is totally invented by our intellect without any reference to the chain illustrated in the upper part of Figure 12.

Science studies the Universe using the three levels and obeying the condition that all measurements must be reproducible. The achievements of **Basic Science** give man a great intellectual dignity and must generate an awareness in mankind in order that Motivation, Creativity, Innovation, Leadership, Innovative Leadership, be all turned in the **Applied Science** to good and never to evil.

ACKNOWLEDGMENTS

I would like to express my warmest thanks to my co-Presidents Professors Tsung-Dao Lee and Kai Siegbahn for having discussed with me the content of this paper and to our colleagues, shown below, for their contribution – during this Seminar – to the items of interest in the various components of this paper.

LANGUAGE:	Alain Peyraube
CREATIVITY:	Norbert Kroo
POETRY:	Senator Josef Jarab
POETS AND DREAMERS:	A. Adamishin
RELIGION:	Eda Sagarra
THE CHARM OF SCIENCE AND ITS VALUES:	Edward Teller
TOTAL LACK OF VALUES FOR GENOCIDES:	Richard Garwin
ROMAN EMPIRE:	William Shea
HIGH-TECH TERRORISM:	Karl Rebane

SOCIETY AND STRUCTURES WORKING GROUP A: CULTURE, IDEOLOGY, HUMAN RIGHTS, FREEDOM AND DEMOCRACY

WILLIAM R. SHEA
Institut d'histoire des sciences, Universite Louis Pasteur de Strasbourg, Strasbourg, France

In the 1980s, the Erice Seminars successfully confronted the international threat of nuclear warfare. In the 1990s they addressed issues related to environmental problems. Now, at the beginning of the twenty-first century, the Seminars are providing a forum for the discussion of new planetary emergencies. Several of these have political, economic, cultural and ethical implications. The First Working Group described these new situations and addressed some of the related concerns in the hope that once they are understood the Scientific Community will be in a better position to respond creatively and decisively.

The tragic and reprehensible events of 11 September 2001 have stirred the consciousness of mankind, and we have the duty to study both the causes and the remedies of terrorism. But we must not forget the more serious planetary problems of poverty, illiteracy, drug abuse, and the widespread disregard for human rights.

The 2002 Erice Seminar recognized that the challenges posed by globalization constitute the most alarming cultural planetary emergency that we have to face. Globalization seems inevitable. What is a matter of disquiet is the way it is being implemented. At one level, globalization holds the potential for a common planetary awareness and a general improvement of the quality of life throughout the world. Unfortunately, the benefits of globalization are not being felt everywhere. Disparities in wealth, in access to health services, and in overall well-being are deeply troubling. They not only pose a threat to security, they are a matter of deep concern for all those who know that there can be no lasting peace without justice. As members of the Scientific Community we are accustomed to work at the international level, and we are therefore in a position to channel globalization into positive channels. Indeed the Scientific Community is the most successful example of globalization. This is why we call on the best scientific minds to address the social and cultural implications of globalization in order to create a world where intellectual and material resources are shared in a more equitable way, and where human dignity and mutual respect are not reserved for a privileged few. The conceptual tools, the rigour of analysis, and the impressive technological resources of our Scientific Community must continue to be developed, but they must also be made available to all the inhabitants of our planet. Peace, security and international understanding can only be secured at this price. The Scientific Community can respond to this challenge, and we are confident that it will.

SOCIETY AND STRUCTURES WORKING GROUP B: ECONOMY, NATIONAL AND REGIONAL GEOPOLITICAL ISSUES

K.C. SIVARAMAKRISHNAN
Centre for Policy Research, New Delhi, India

OVERVIEW

- Terrorism, criminality, violence or insurgency share many characteristics. It is not possible to define a clear typology or make suggestions specific for each type.
- 9/11 is a dramatic manifestation of terrorism but only one such.
- Militancy and terrorism cover a wide spectrum: eg. Separatism–LTTE, IRA; Drugs and arms–Columbia, Economic and social discontent–Nepal, Religion or ethnicity–Middle East, Kashmir, Philippines.
- We share the current anguish and anger about all these events but recognize we need to know much more to be able to respond wisely.

PROBLEMS OF POVERTY AND DEVELOPMENT AS A ROOT CAUSE

- Not exclusive to underdeveloped countries per se (e.g. yesterday's sub-saharan Africa is today's Argentina).
- **Poverty** leads to **frustration** and **fragmentation** – Conducive ground for terrorism and new recruits.
- Poverty causes more deaths than terrorism.
- May not be a direct cause of terrorism but poverty, inequity and the discontent it breeds cannot be ignored.
- Continuing independent cause for dealing with poverty and inequities–violence makes issue more relevant, not less.

ECONOMIC ISSUES AND LINKAGES

- Terrorism and organized violence financed on large, continuous scale.
- Sources of funding are many and interconnected with other criminal activities (drugs, arms; e.g., Columbia).
- Remittances and other forms of support from the Diaspora are an important source.

- Ever-present and increasing shadow economies sustain terrorism.
- Repressive financial regimes and trade restrictions aggravate national economic problems.
- Repressive measures also alienate people: International economic order insensitive and slow to respond to problems (e.g., Argentina).

Recommendations
- Need better understanding of how shadow economies function and their linkages to real economy; changes in one (e.g., globalization) lead to adjustments in the other.
- Need good governance, more effective policing for dealing with new actors in the economy.
- More responsive international economic order to reduce disparities and despair.

POLITICAL STRUCTURES, LEADERSHIP, AND AUTONOMY

- Good Governance has to be a basic, continuing response to terrorism and violence.
- Ingredients of good governance:
  - Representativeness
  - Inclusiveness (e.g., minorities), not exclusiveness
  - Participative processes, e-government
  - Electoral systems and formal systems of democracy
  - Respect for human rights – indivisible.
- Effectiveness depends on transparency and accountability (e.g., free press).
- Realistic taxation and financial systems; paying tax is one concrete proof of participation (no taxation without representation; per contra no representation without taxation).
- Examples of concern: Degeneration of secular states formed after WWII into sectarian states in which cultural, religious, and linguistic identities created; specialized, exclusive systems of education and conditioning of people from a very young age.

Suggested approach
Rather than shut down sectarian schools, establish standards to augment curricula with tolerant, broad-based elements of science, mathematics, history, and so forth; past experience with "colonial" type broadening may not help.

SENSITIVE GEOPOLITICAL REGIONS: THE PALESTINE QUESTION

- Intractable because of the existence of two interlinked wars:
  - War of the Palestinians to **obtain** sovereignty like Israel

— War of militants to **take away** sovereignty from Israel.

Recommendation

- As Bertrand Russell says, *Placing intractable problems in a different framework may reduce animosity, fanaticism and the suspicions involved* Thus, creating a scientific framework in the context of Eirce to address these issues may offer new analyses and concepts into a political void of ideas, such as the concpt of neutrality.
- **A truly neutral** Israel or Palestine may be an answer: to look forward beyond short term political goals, a long term vision is needed: scientists can help shape such a vision.
- For such a vision framework scientists from both Israel and the Palestine diaspora should be sought.
- Window of opportunity if UN, US, Russia, and EU act in concert.

SENSITIVE GEOPOLITICAL REGIONS: RESOURCE MANAGEMENT AS A SOLUTION

- **Water** is both produced and distributed regionally.
- To varying degrees, water (both supply and quality) may be related to regional stability and economic concerns in many areas, including:
  - Middle East (water problems are acute)
  - Central Asia
  - South Asia (Indus, Ganges, etc.).
- **Oil** is produced regionally and distributed globally.
- To varying degrees, **oil** production and consumption may be related to interconnected social and economic stresses on a global level.
- Regional stability problems in production areas will have global implications:
  - Middle East
  - Central Asia
  - South Asia.
- Sudan, North Africa has another sensitive region; need to engage scientists and intellectuals to explore links between instability and terrorism.

Recommendations

- Conflicts over oil and water resource issues may be ameliorated by improved science-based resource assessments and better management strategies and the development of improved consumption efficiencies.
- OECD countries (particularly the US) should endeavor to reduce oil dependency to moderate political, societal, and economic stresses.
- Erice discussions on transboundary water conflicts (2001) to be developed further as initiatives for conflict resolution.

ROLE OF SCIENCE AND TECHNOLOGY

Note: We do not refer to "countermeasure" S&T issues here.

- Science and technology is important for education:
    - Better standard of living tied to better economy and educated workforce
    - Economy is increasingly based on science and technology
    - Education can address regional asymmetries in science and technology capabilities (talent, institutions, etc.).
- Cooperation and collaboration in science and technology can be important in solving critical regional problems :
    - Oil and transboundary water resource problems
    - Environmental contamination problems
    - Identification and mitigation of natural hazards.
- Science and technology collaboration offers a pathway for engagement that may have collateral diplomatic and political benefits:
    - Contribute to fill the present void in diplomatic and political ideas.

Recommendation
- Erice can play a role in fostering regional scientific collaborations among participants from important regions of the world:
    - Middle East
    - Central Asia
    - South Asia.

CONFRONTATION AND COUNTERMEASURES WORKING GROUP

R.A. MASON
University of Birmingham, Birmingham, UK

INTRODUCTION

The Working Group was directed to identify the main issues and consequences associated with confrontation and countermeasures and to make specific recommendations for their resolution and mitigation through actions of the international scientific community in general and the World Federation of Scientists in particular. The Group concluded that while many sources of previous confrontation continued, the appearance of a new generation of global terrorism had created a most serious planetary emergency. Terrorism as a phenomenon is not new, but its most recent manifestation combined a number of features in a novel way: scale, suicide, lack of warning, indiscriminate targeting, ambiguous objectives, media manipulation, and transnational organization and funding that exploits developments in information and communication technologies (ICTs) and vulnerabilities of networked societies. This report will therefore examine the impact of global terrorism. It is recognized that cultural resource, ethnic, and other factors are associated with terrorism, but these ongoing problems will not be examined in this report.

DISCUSSION AND RECOMMENDATIONS

Unchecked, this form of global terror will have very serious consequences. No single nation state can effectively respond to this situation. The situation is further complicated when nation states provide breeding grounds and sanctuary for terrorism, thereby creating regional instability. It is in the security interests of the international community to co-operate and remove factors that contribute to and cause terrorism. Humanitarian aid only is insufficient. What is required is assistance directed at long-term sustainable development.

The scientific study of vulnerability is critical. This includes the vulnerabilities of communities, governments, industry, and information infrastructure. Vulnerability has become a transnational concern and the interdependencies of vulnerabilities must be considered. This transnational threat can come in a variety of forms, including the threat of nuclear, chemical, and biological weapons of mass destruction (WMD). An existing problem of proliferation and defence against missiles has also been aggravated with the advent of the new generation of terrorism. International co-operation should be sought to reduce the vulnerability to terrorist activity by WMDs. All countries, including developing nations, must address this threat and control access to WMD weapons and materials.

A further transnational problem lies in the association between organized crime and terrorism. Measures to curtail organized criminal activities, including restricting drug and human trafficking, money laundering, counterfeiting, and smuggling, require immediate attention from the international community. Countries must address "comprehensive security" within their own borders and communities. Contingency planning within the armed forces should give a higher priority to contributions to support civil power in combating terrorism.

Additional efforts are needed to facilitate international co-operation of information and intelligence to help counter these activities. Therefore, priority should be given to systems that can enable the tracking and identification of communications and the security of information and communications infrastructure.

However, actions in response to these transnational activities raise profound legal and policy considerations on both the national and international levels. For example, ample evidence exists that terrorists and organized crime are using sophisticated technologies, including steganography. In governments' actions to counter these activities, consideration must be given to personal privacy, human rights, and individual liberties. Indeed, the balance between antiterrorist measures and the preservation of individual liberties and the quality of democratic life is delicate. Therefore, scientific research should follow two tracks: (1) the contribution to the development of technologies which seek to both clarify the origin and destination of communications and protect individual rights, and (2) the evaluation of the impact of such, measures on human rights, individual liberties, and the quality of democratic life. We question whether the body of international law is adequate to provide generally acceptable transnational responses to terrorism. Therefore, we invite our scientists and jurisprudence colleagues to examine the relevant bodies of law and technologies to identify legal processes and technologies for a swift response to terrorism. A further question arises in the application of current international law to this new, global terrorism.

In considering all aspects of global terrorism, there is a need for additional scientific study of complexity and risk, taking into account developments in information and communication technologies. It is important to develop new methodologies of risk assessment that integrate technical expertise and political, legal, and social analysis. Further engagement of the scientific community is needed to ensure effective prevention, detection, deterrence, and response to terrorism, keeping in mind that actions taken should not enhance the risk of further terrorism. Despite changes in circumstances there is a need to maintain the fundamental principles of discrimination and proportionality. Research on the intended and unintended consequences of countermeasures is needed. A list of suggested initiatives is included in Annex A.

ANNEX A

FOURTEEN OF THE MOST IMPORTANT TECHNICAL INITIATIVES
(of the U.S. National Academies report on Science and Technology to Counter Terrorism, June 2002)

Immediate Applications of Existing Technologies:

1. Develop and utilize robust systems for protection, control, and accounting of nuclear weapons and special nuclear materials at their sources.
2. Ensure production and distribution of known treatments and preventatives for pathogens.
3. Design, test, and install coherent layered security systems for all transportation modes, particularly shipping containers and vehicles that contain large quantities of toxic or flammable materials.
4. Protect energy distribution services by improved security of supervisory control and data acquisition (SCADA) systems and provide physical protection of key elements of the electricity distribution system.
5. Reduce vulnerability and improve effectiveness of air filtration in building ventilation systems.
6. Deploy known technologies and standards for allowing emergency responders to reliably communicate with each other.
7. When the technical aspects of an emergency are dominant in the public's concerns, ensure that trusted spokespersons will be able to inform the public promptly and with technical authority.

Urgent Research Opportunities:

1. Develop effective treatments and preventatives for known pathogens for which current responses are unavailable or inadequate, and for potential emerging pathogens.
2. Develop, test, and implement an intelligent, adaptive electric-power grid.
3. Advance the practical utility of data fusion and data mining for intelligence analysis and enhance information security against cyber attacks.
4. Provide emergency responders with new and better technologies (e.g. protective gear, sensors, communications.)
5. Advance engineering design technologies and fire-rating standards for blast and fire resistant buildings.
6. Develop sensor and surveillance systems (for a wide range of targets) that create useful information output to emergency officials and decision makers.
7. Develop new methods and standards for filtering air against both chemicals and pathogens as well as better methods and standards for decontamination.

16. PERMANENT MONITORING PANEL REPORTS

MOTHER AND CHILD PERMANENT MONITORING PANEL: MANIFESTO

NATHALIE CHARPAK
Kangaroo Mother's Foundation, Bogota, Columbia

MATERNAL AND INFANT MORTALITY IS A PLANETARY EMERGENCY

Situation
Every year, complications arising from pregnancy and childbirth cause the deaths of half a million women, and over 4 million newborns. Most of these deaths result from poorly managed pregnancies, deliveries and neonatal care. However, the role of environment, i.e. water and pollution and unexpected events such as natural disasters, wars, terrorism, on this situation is virtually unexplored.

Mission
- Decrease mortality and morbidity of mother and infant (less than one year) and secure quality of life.
- Investigate the impact of the other planetary emergencies on Maternal and Infant mortality and morbidity through an efficient and effective network with the International Scientific Community in general and the World Federation of Scientists in particular.

Specific Objectives
- Review and analyze the major factors responsible for this emergency and identify preventive measures.
- Recommend specific steps that could be done with the involvement of relevant partners in the scientific community taking into account religious and sociocultural differences.

Targets
Some major causes of mother and infant mortality had been identified and could be tackled in small workshops involving professionals from different disciplines and origins:

- LBW infants
- HIV
- Toxemia

- Birth asphyxia
- Other infectious diseases
- Maternal and Infant Nutrition
- Reproductive Health Education at school
- Primary perinatal health care
- Birth control

Activities

- HIV and Mother to Child Transmission: two joint PMP workshops were held in Erice in 2000 and 2001 (Mother and Child, and Infectious diseases PMPs). Recommendations were made and published in the international pediatric journal (Acta Paediatrica) and are now adopted in many parts of the world.
- LBW infants and Kangaroo Mother Care Method: Since the first scientific evaluation of the method in 1989 funded by the World Laboratory, KMC training, education and implementation are spreading all over the world (more than 30 countries). WHO adopted the method, collaborates with the Kangaroo Network and is publishing guidelines for November 2002.
- LBW infants, KMC and monitoring the impact of the program. A small workshop will be held during this session to build a practical database in 3 languages that will be sent to all teams implementing KMC.

REPORT BY PERMANENT MONITORING PANEL ON MISSILE PROLIFERATION AND DEFENSE

ANDREI PIONTKOVSKY
Strategic Studies Centre, Moscow, Russia

The Panel notes that the principles expressed in its Statement at Erice in Spring 1998 have been vindicated in subsequent years. A key statement in that declaration was "The relationship between the USA and Russia should not be based on adversarial principles, as the current paradigm based on mutual assured destruction is not adequate to address emerging security concerns of Russia and the West." The Bush-Putin joint declaration on a new strategic relationship clearly reflects the sentiment of the Erice declaration.

The emphasis of the Erice Statement on international cooperation in the construction of global and regional defence systems has become even more urgent since the tragedy of 11 September. The threat from international terrorist organisations has now been added to that from "rogue states."

Terrorist organisations do not need to develop the capability to construct ballistic or other missiles to deliver weapons of mass destruction. They may be provided with the means for launching missile attacks by rouge states trying to avoid the political cost that come with an attack and minimize the risk of having to suffer immediate retaliation. Moreover, short of rogue support terrorists only need to seize, or be given access to, existing systems anywhere. It is therefore essential to ensure that all states which have deployed ballistic missiles safeguard them on the ground against asymmetric terrorist activity. Such measures should include the security of all personnel associated with weapon authorisation and release.

During the Cold War and in several states in the last decade, speed of response to authorisation for weapon delivery has been balanced with protection against accidental or unauthorised release by variations of a two key system located with the missile, and external authorisation. Now however, the security of the missile and crew against terrorist threat should be given priority. One possible procedure would be to remove one key to another location, so that both authorisation and release would require action from two different locations. Knowledge of such a procedure would inhibit terrorist attempts to seize any single missile or site.

International response should be establishing internationally acceptable and verifiable security and release procedures.

The Monitoring Panel welcomes the news that the USA is seeking international cooperation to establish a global Battle Management Command and Control System so that ultimately defense systems for all regions would fit in. Consultations are already taking place between the Missile Defence Agency (MDA) and Japanese and European governments. We look forward to the extension of such consultation to governments in South and East Asia, and to constructive proposals for international cooperation aimed at evolving a global protection system through a process that takes advantage of existing capabilities and opportunities.

For example, the principle of cooperation between U.S. and Russian ground forces against international terrorism has already been established. There seem to be opportunities for extending such cooperation into the construction of ballistic missile early warning and detection systems, together with bases for the deployment of such systems as the USAF Airborne Laser. Such deployment would provide a valuable complement to the proposed U.S. naval BMD systems, constantly enlarging BMD cover of the Middle East. South and East Asia providing cooperative access otherwise inaccessible to the U.S. and the West.

In conclusion, the U.S. commitment to a global BMD system could be not only a major contribution to the protection of the U.S., its friends and their deployed forces but also provide the framework for a truly cooperative global system generating a wider impetus to international stability and security thus finally overcoming, on a global scale, the paradigm of mutual assured destruction in favour of mutual assured protection.

LIMITS OF DEVELOPMENT PERMANENT MONITORING PANEL REPORT

HILTMART SCHUBERT
Fraunhofer Institute for Chemical Technology, Pfinztal, Germany

LAST MEETING CONCLUSIONS

EMERGENCY RELATED TO DEVELOPMENT LIMITS

To speak with one language, the following definition of "Limits of Development" was agreed:

> *Limits of development are the observance of limitations of ecological, economical and social developments in order to avoid emergencies to human beings in a global or regional sense.*

The PMP has adopted to keep the title "Limits of Development" for the PMP but adding the expression **"Sustainability"** to it. The main aspects shall be in the same category, as shown in the following graphic:

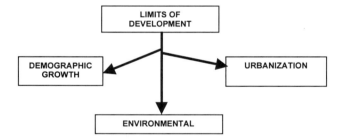

Monitoring the Scientific Results of Research
The PMP has proposed to monitor scientific results on the objects:

- Use of renewable resources
- Development of substitutes and technologies for *non-renewable resources*

- Development of technologies to reduce emission, recycle or make disposal of pollutants harmless
- Demographic growth
- Urbanization

Organization of a Data Bank
The PMP intends to feed in a permanent manner a data bank on relevant findings in the field mentioned above and will produce an annual report evaluating the progress made.

2002 Session Theme
Especially for the year 2002, *Urban Waste* should be the topic. The objective is monitoring the state of the art and science in this subject, what means gathering information and interpretation taking into account various countries, development stages and available technologies.

2003 Session Theme
For the year 2003 the State of the Art and Science of the topic *Urban Mobility* is proposed taking the following items in consideration:

- Moving people, material, waste, information and energy
- Organization of urban mobility

Other Conclusions
As can be seen in the 2001 Meeting Report, many other aspects were considered during the PMP sessions that can be considered as guidelines for future developments.

SCOPE OF THIS YEAR MEETING

The theme of this year meeting is solid urban waste. The task of collecting, transporting and disposal of urban waste grows more and more complex, particularly regarding the trend of modern societies to generate ever larger quantities of solid waste. Nowadays, in large urban areas it is more and more difficult to find disposal space. The main tasks of our PMP are the definition of the emergency character of this problem and to monitor the scientific and technological results conducted in the field of urban and territorial planning and management to solve it. Therefore, at our meeting we intend to gather information on the situation of this problem and its solutions in several countries and cities. To suggest a general approach to member's contributions, we present hereafter a set of items on the subject. A few questions should be answered (with suggestions of Prof. Siva):

- What is the amount of waste generation in a city or a country? What is the extent of increase?

- What broadly is the composition of the waste? How much of it is biodegradable, inorganic, combustible, non-degradable etc.? Do we have an adequate approximation?
- What has been the effort in minimizing or reducing waste?
- What is the approach to recycling? How extensive is the effort? What are the present methods of recycling?
- What is the position regarding hazardous waste?
- How much of the problem is internal and how much of it is imported? In other words is the city or country a dump for hazardous waste from other cities and countries?
- To what extent is the solid waste problem and the understanding of it in the city and country being reported?
- What is the degree of public awareness about solid waste as a major urban problem? What are the innovations, initiatives at the city or the community level?

Prof. Siva proposes that we "should go beyond the technology aspects, raise questions of sustainability and to what extent the solid waste problem impinges on that sustainability."

An approach proposed by Prof. Borthagaray is presented hereafter.

A very interesting aspect of our meetings was the two sided aspect of our aims: one concerning the state-of-the-art solutions available to cope with an essential megacity problem, and another how this scientific and technological potentiality was sailing or sinking in the ferocious storms of misgovernance, mafias, corruption, collapse of states, threats of nuclear conflict, murder and kidnapping of decision makers, etc.

We should keep this duality in our database or databases. One should monitor the state-of-the-art and another the actual application of them in real megacities cases. I am inclined to think that the first aspect offers a smoother path than the second one. Nevertheless, in my opinion, if we are to monitor anything, we should have a critical mass of actual cases of megacities dealing with the problems, of successes and failures, and some explanation of those.

The Waste Chain

Origin of Solid Waste

In the first place, solid waste is either manufactured or cultivated, as packaging, non-usable parts of food, or disposable products, discarded semi-durable or durable goods.

What can be done in order to minimize manufactured or cultivated loads of waste to enter the industrial, commercial or domestic cycle? How much do they represent of the waste load? A glimpse into the frontiers of minimization is needed.

As to the products, from the disposable to the more durable, what is desirable from the economic, as well as ethical point of view? Of course, not only from the point of view of the business results of the manufactures and seller, but for society as a whole. What cultural changes are needed? This product complex should be broken down in order to estimate the potential social benefits of operating upon each of the possible items.

Domestic Handling of Waste

This aspect is a grass roots' one and has deep cultural implications. What can be expected through changes in the way waste is handled between production and recollection? Quantification of the impact of changes.

Industrial Handling of Waste

Not easy to typify. Quantification is also imperative.

Recollection and Transport of Waste

All the former have very strong consequences in this very important link of the waste chain. Frequency, type of vehicles, discrimination of materials, and distances have direct impacts in transport and land uses.

Treatment and Final Disposal

At this point, we may have the crowd of vendors, but what we should need to examine are not the patents in the private domain, but the most desirable general process specifications and characteristics to be expected. Environment and land use considerations are paramount, but the magnitudes of the problem can be very substantially changed if we can operate efficiently upon the former variables.

Actual Examples of City Solid Waste Managements

What has been said may be one aspect of our reflections. The other should be real cases in existing cities, in which the whole of the problematic of the waste chain, all the explicit intentions, and also the deviations could be observed, so that the successes and failures of each particular case could be properly assessed.

WORLD FEDERATION OF SCIENTISTS PERMANENT MONITORING PANEL ON INFORMATION SECURITY

HENNING WEGENER
Madrid, Spain

The Panel met on August 19th and continued its work in the days thereafter, including in the framework of a larger Working Group on Information Security on August 24th.

Its work was based on a number of drafts for the various chapters of its planned comprehensive interdisciplinary report, prepared on the basis of an agreed work schedule adopted last year. These drafts will now be revised by their respective authors, in the light of the Panel's discussions, and additional chapters will be included.

The group concentrated its work on a package of recommendations addressed to the international community, which already at this stage could be extracted from the draft texts. In the group's view, these recommendations, although not reflecting its whole work program, or fully covering the subject matter, should already at this juncture be published. They should be given wide distribution through the channels of the World Federation of Scientists, in light of the urgency of action on the international level to combat the dangers of cyber crime, preferably before the end of 2002. Recipients should include the President of the UN General Assembly (UNGA); the Chairmen of the First, Second, and Sixth Committees of the UNGA; the Secretary-General of the UN; and the heads of other relevant UN agencies.

The Panel decided to proceed to a second phase of its work, which will consist in the completion of its comprehensive interdisciplinary report and the elaboration of additional recommendations. Revised and additional drafts of the report will be considered at a meeting to be held at Erice in the early spring of 2003. The report containing the full set of recommendations, should then be published in book form and addressed to a wide international audience, including the member organizations of the United Nations system, prior to the next annual session of the International Erice Seminars.

MEETING OF THE PERMANENT MONITORING PANEL ON DEFENCE AGAINST FLOODS AND UNEXPECTED METEOROLOGICAL EVENTS

ROBERT A. CLARK
University of Arizona, Tucson, Arizona. USA

A meeting of the Permanent Monitoring Panel was held in Erice in the San Francesco Center (Eugene P. Wigner Institute) on 19 August 2002.

Participants in the meeting included:

Robert A. Clark, University of Arizona, USA
Margaret S. Petersen, University of Arizona, USA
William A. Sprigg, University of Arizona, USA
Slobodan Nickovic, University of Malta, Malta
Nafia Al-Shalabi, Meteorological Department of Syria, Damascus, Syria
Wang Hui-jin, Chinese Academy of Sciences, Beijing, China
Alfred Grove, Cambridge University, U.K.

TOPICS DISCUSSED

The meeting opened with a discussion by Professor Clark on the primary goal of the working group this year, i.e., the development of a "Proposal on Modeling and Prediction of Dust and Sand Storms in the Arab Countries" for presentation at the Annual Meeting of the World Federation of Scientists (WFS) in Geneva in November 2002.

1999 WL Proposal for Dust and Sand Storm Modeling
The World Laboratory (WL) made a proposal in 1999 to the WFS to provide assistance to the League of Arab States to improve forecasts of dust and sand storms. Objectives of the 1999 proposal were to:

1. Improvement of existing numerical models for dust and sand storms in the Arab region.
2. Develop operating programs.
3. Develop verification programs.
4. Prepare training programs in:

a. Basic forecasting.
b. Advanced forecasting.
c. Use of geographic information systems and remote sensing technology.

Current Status
The status of dust and sand storm forecasting was discussed by Dr. Nafia Al-Shalabi, Director, Meteorology Department, Syria. Little has changed since 1999 with regard to capability for forecasting dust in the Arab Region. In March 1996 the League of Arab States (LAS) proposed ASAPRO (ARab SAnd PROject) to the World Meteorological Organization, but it was never initiated or funded. The 1999 World Laboratory (WL) proposal was designed to help solve this problem. Unfortunately, funding was not available by WL to initiate the program.

The ASAPRO program is chaired by the Syrian Meteorology Department Director, Dr. Al-Shalabi. It is now hoped that, through initiation of a pilot program in Syria by the WL, additional funding can be obtained from various sources to eventually expand the program in line with the original ASAPRO proposal.

Some initial steps have taken place recently through training programs in Egypt with active support of the WL. However, additional training and equipment are still needed to strengthen the national capability of Syria (and other Arab League countries) in limited-area numerical weather forecasting as a scientific basis for dust and sand storm prediction.

We were also presented with a brief statement from the Lebanese Meteorological Service prepared by Dr. Abdo Bejjani, Meteorological Department, Lebanon. Since 1995 their local meteorological network has been rehabilitated, including some personnel training, installation of forecasting work stations, some telecommunications systems, and a wind profiler. Sixteen synoptic meteorological stations have been installed and cover Lebanon adequately. The meteorological stations are interrogated hourly via telephone. Thirteen climatological stations report manually on a monthly basis. However, an adequate data backup and archiving system and training for personnel in forecasting and meteorological equipment maintenance are still lacking.

Dr. Nickovic reviewed current activities of his meteorological forecasting group at the University of Malta. They have been preparing daily forecasts of blowing dust using the ETA model (developed for the U.S. National Center for Environmental Prediction (NCEP), National Weather Service (NWS), Washington, D.C.) and daily meteorological analytical input from NCEP obtained on the internet. The Malta group has developed some models to predict areas of blowing dust based on surface conditions. The results to date have been very promising. Dr. Nickovic also showed recent forecasts of precipitation for eastern Sicily using grid lengths as small as four kilometers. The results were very impressive. The University of Malta is prepared to assist the Syrians in the implementation of a numerical prediction dust model plus providing training in use of the model.

Dr. Sprigg apprised the group of the new WL Center for Soil and Water Conservation and Environmental Protection in Yangling, China. The Center is a focal point for collaboration on wind erosion of soil and for development of dust-storm forecasts and remedial actions. The Center works on this issue with the Chinese Academy of Sciences in Beijing, Yangling, and Lanzhou; the Chinese Meteorological Administration in Beijing; and the U.S. National Weather Service and U.S. Department of Agriculture.

Dr. Wang Huijin discussed current activities in China related to dust storms. China has experienced a marked increase in dust storms in the North China Plain in the recent decade, and is currently developing several models in cooperation with the U.S. NWS. The Chinese are willing to cooperate on any program related to dust.

Subsequent to the meeting, we were furnished a proposal from Dr. M. M. Arafa, Egyptian Meteorological Authority and the WL Research Center, Cairo, Egypt, for a continuation into 2003 of their Collaborative R&D and Educational programme on Numerical Prediction of Extreme Atmospheric Events. The proposal summarized recent activities of that Center in the past year and proposed further activities in 2003. Unfortunately, we were unable to discuss this proposal at our meeting. We consider the courses in Cairo to be very important to development of meteorological forecasting in the Arab League countries. However, those attending the Cairo programme need to be well educated, or have a good background, in scientific meteorological forecasting to obtain maximum benefit.

Current WL Proposal

The concensus of the panel was that a pilot program should be initiated to assist Syria in improving their meteorological program to forecast dust and sand storms. The current WL proposal, developed subsequent to the Erice meeting and based on discussions at that meeting, includes a very basic program that will assist the Syrians in initiating a viable program to help solve their forecasting problems. The proposed program includes:

A. Year One.
1. Training and technology transfer.
   a. Review of Syrian problems by a staff member from the University of Malta related to existing computer facilities, current training requirements, and access to data. One week.
   b. Two fellowships at the University of Arizona for one year of specialized training in atmospheric science.
   c. Two short-term scholarships for specialized training in remote sensing and geographical information systems (GIS) at the University of Arizona.
2. Purchase of hardware, software, and peripherals.
B. Year Two.
1. Training and Technology Transfer.
   a. Training in Malta for two Syrian forecasters for four weeks using specialized dust and sand storm forecasting programs.

    b. Training of two Syrian specialists in data archiving at the U.S. National Climate Data Center.

    c. Initiate training in another Arab country.

2. Transfer of hardware, software, and peripherals from Malta to Damascus.

WATER; CLIMATE, OZONE AND GREENHOUSE EFFECTS; AND DESERTIFICATION

ROBERT A. CLARK
University of Arizona, Tucson, AZ, USA

A meeting of the Permanent Monitoring Panels on Defence against floods and unexpected meteorological events; Water; Climate, ozone and greenhouse effects; and Desertification was held in Erice in the San Francesco Center (Eugene P. Wigner Institute) on 24 August 2002.

Participants in the meeting included:

Robert A. Clark, University of Arizona, USA
Margaret S. Petersen, University of Arizona, USA
William A. Sprigg, University of Arizona, USA
Slobodan Nickovic, University of Malta, Malta
Anton Micallef, University of Malta, Malta
Larry L. Tieszen, EROS Data Center, USA
Mbareck Diop, Advisor to the President, Dakar, Senegal
Alfred T. Grove, Cambridge University, U.K.
Tao Wang, Chinese Academy of Sciences, Lanzhou, China
Andrew Warren, University College, London, U.K.
Aaron Yair, Hebrew University, Jerusalem, Israel
Claude Manoli, World Laboratory, Lausanne, Switzerland

TOPICS DISCUSSED

The meeting opened with a discussion by Robert Clark on the primary goal of the working groups, i.e., a discussion and development of information concerning scientific and technological expertise of the various Permanent Monitoring Panels (PMPs) represented at the meeting. Primary emphasis was on expertise applicable to the Mediterranean region.

When one examines the expertise of the various PMPs, it is evident that most of them center about the central theme of water.

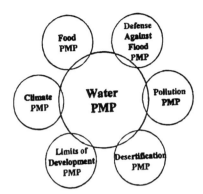

It was apparent from the ensuing discussions that several specific topics encompass some or all of the PMPs, as illustrated by the above diagram. Numerous areas of expertise related to water were listed by the various panel members present. These include:

Water (surface and groundwater)
Coastal zone problems
Sustainable management of water resources
Capacity building (modeling education and training)
Drought
Desertification (including combating and socio-economic impacts)
Deforestation
Wildfires
Extreme events
Meteorology (operational forecasting)
Climate change
Water pollution
Vulnerability and Risk Assessment
Contingency plans
Environmental observations, protection, and impact assessment
Database development
Remote sensing applications

It is apparent from the above not all-inclusive listing that the various PMPs are capable of studies and implementation of a large range of studies pertaining to water and its various related fields.

A "white paper" was prepared for President A. Zichichi defining in more detail the capabilities of the above PMPs.

POLLUTION PERMANENT MONITORING PANEL

RICHARD C. RAGAINI
Department of Environmental Protection, University of California, Lawrence Livermore National Laboratory, Livermore, CA, USA

The continuing environmental pollution of earth and the degradation of its natural resources constitutes one of the most significant planetary emergencies today. This emergency is so overwhelming and encompassing, it requires the greatest possible international East-West and North-South co-operation to implement effective ongoing remedies.

It is useful to itemize the environmental issues addressed by this PMP, since several PMPs are dealing with various overlapping environmental issues. The Pollution PMP is addressing the following environmental emergencies:

- degradation of surface water and ground water quality
- degradation of marine and freshwater ecosystems
- degradation of urban air quality in mega-cities
- impact of air pollution on ecosystems.

Other environmental emergencies, including global pollution, water quantity issues, ozone depletion and the greenhouse effect, are being addressed by other PMPs. The Pollution PMP coordinates its activities with other relevant PMPs as appropriate. Furthermore, the PMP will provide an informal channel for experts to exchange views and make recommendations regarding environmental pollution.

PRIORITIES IN DEALING WITH THE ENVIRONMENTAL EMERGENCIES

The PMP on Pollution monitors the following priority issues:

- clean-up of existing surface and sub-surface soil and ground-water supplies from industrial and municipal waste-water pollution, agricultural run-off, deforestation, and military operations
- reduction of existing air pollution and resultant health and ecosystem impacts from long-range transport of pollutants and trans-boundary pollution
- prevention and/or minimization of future air and water pollution

- training scientists & engineers from developing countries to identify, monitor and clean-up pollution

ATTENDEES

The following scientists listed below attended the August 2002 Pollution PMP meeting:

Chairman Dr. Richard C. Ragaini, Lawrence Livermore National Laboratory, USA
Dr. Lorne G. Everett, University of California at Santa Barbara, USA
Prof. Vittorio Ragaini, University of Milan, Italy
Dr. Andy Tompson, Lawrence Livermore National Laboratory, USA
Prof. Joseph Chahoud, University of Bologna, Italy

HISTORICAL AREAS OF EMPHASIS OF THE POLLUTION PMP

The following areas listed below have been addressed by the Pollution PMP since its beginning in 1997 in order to more effectively monitor global and regional impacts of pollution in developing countries:

1998: Workshop on Impacts of Pharmaceuticals and Disinfectant Byproducts in Sewage Treatment Wastewater Used for Irrigation
1999: Memorandum of Agreement (MOA) between WFS and the US Department of Energy
1999: Seminar Talks on Contamination of Groundwater by Hydrocarbons
1999: Workshop on Black Sea Pollution
2000: Seminar Talks on Contamination of Groundwater by MTBE
2000: Workshop on Black Sea Pollution by Petroleum Hydrocarbons
2001: Workshop on Caspian Sea Pollution
2001: Seminar Talks on Trans-boundary Water Conflicts
2001: Workshop on Water and Air Impacts of Automotive Emissions in Mega-cities
2002: Seminar Talk on Radioactivity Contamination of Soils and Groundwater
2002: Seminar Talk on Environmental Security in the Middle East and Central Asia

FUTURE ACTIVITIES PLANNED BY THE POLLUTION PMP

August, 2003
Organize a two-day workshop on "Long-Term Stewardship of Radioactive and Chemical Contamination of Soils and Groundwater" following the International Seminars. It will include talks on the US program to stabilize and monitor the Department of Energy sites in the US, which are contaminated with radioactivity. It will also include talks on other

international sites, including nuclear sites of the U.S., Soviet Union and France, such as the Nevada Test Site, Semipalatinsk, Mayak, French Polynesia, etc.

Four themes will be addressed:

1. Contamination, Containment and Control;
2. Monitoring and Sensors;
3. Decision Making and Institutional Performance;
4. Safety Systems and Institutional Controls.

We anticipate 25 speakers, and the Workshop Director will be Steven Kowall of the Idaho National Environmental and Engineering Lab. A final report containing conclusions and recommendations for future governmental actions will be produced.

August, 2003

Organize a two-day workshop on "Water Management in the Middle East" following the International Seminars. Trans-boundary water issues are a very contentious issue in the Middle East, as well as in many other regions around the globe. We believe that a concrete step forward for regional stability can be made by convening a meeting in Erice

The scientific topics would include what is known about the subsurface water aquifers in the Middle East, the availability of surface waters, irrigation issues, issues concerning recharging the Dead Sea, issues concerning the Jordan River, technologies for producing drinking water, and technologies for cleaning up contaminated aquifers.

We anticipate 25 speakers, and the Workshop Director will be Andy Tompson of Lawrence Livermore National Lab. The goal of the meeting will be to make recommendations for achieving consensus water management in the Middle East based on sound science.

REPORT OF THE ENERGY PERMANENT MONITORING PANEL

KAI SIEGBAHN

Institute of Physics, University of Uppsala, Uppsala, Sweden

The session was opened by the Chairman, Professor Kai Siegbahn, at 9:30 am. Professor Siegbahn started off the meeting with the topic of the PMP purpose and Mission. Coordinator Stram stated that the official mission of PMP was to share information and keep members up to date with regard to scientific and public policy events related to the concerns of the PMP, and then for the PMP to undertake action when it concluded there was a chance to improve the situation and no similar group was already engaged. Professor Siegbahn pointed out that energy related issues were highly controversial and that he thought the PMP should take a long term rather than short term focus. He also suggested that it was important to have a broad focus and resist the tendency to overly emphasize nuclear energy and fusion. Prof Richard Wilson agreed, but stated that the PMP should also identify some key issues for special emphasis, discussion and study. He cited trying to understand the public's aversion to nuclear power as one example of a key issue.

The PMP then turned to some organizational matters. Stram recommended that subcommittees be appointed to cover key subject areas of interest to the PMP so that at future meetings someone would have clear responsibility to update and inform the PMP on those topics. He indicated that a subcommittee had been formed for fusion energy. Professor Francois Waelbroeck proposed that the PMP organize a workshop, inviting experts in various areas to give the PMP members a broad perspective on energy topics. Stram suggested that such broad surveys have already been done, and that the PMP could utilize one or more of these as a basis for organizing a workshop rather than gathering information from scratch.

Dr. P.K. Iyengar pointed out that much of the energy technology discussion had related to energy issues as they affected the US, Japan and Western Europe rather than issues facing developing countries. For example, development of low pollution central power stations, a western issue, would do nothing to alleviate the key problem of inefficient and inadequate power distribution that plagues many developing countries.

The PMP agreed to establish the following subcommittees: Fusion, fission, renewable energy and efficiency, developing country issues, transportation issues, and carbon sequestration.

Fusion Report from Jef Ongena: The last 2 years research on magnetic fusion has been characterized by the preparations needed in view of the ITER project. Fusion research has been reorganized in Europe and Fusion Technology R&D, the EU participation in ITER, and the collective use of the Joint European Torus (JET) are now brought together under EFDA, the European Fusion Development Agreement. This Agreement started in January 2000, and is at currently signed up to the end of 2004, with further extensions expected and depending on the details of the future Framework Programmes of the European Commission. The collective use of JET under EFDA is a totally new way of operating this facility. Instead of having a fixed technical and scientific team operating JET, they have now have implemented a team consisting of members of all fusion associations, which propose, execute and analyze fusion experiments on JET, and which remain at JET only for the time needed for the preparation and execution of their experiment. Analysis and planning of the experiment is done remotely by intensive use of modern telecommunication techniques, such as telephone and video conferencing. In this way, all EU fusion associations are now collaborating even more intensively as before 2000 in a coordinated way for a common goal on JET, in view of further preparations for ITER. This has been a real endeavor, but has resulted in a wealth of new results, mainly due to a much enhanced exchange of ideas between the fusion researchers of all laboratories in Europe and the rest of the world. For the standard operational scenario of ITER, the so-called "ELMy H-Mode" model plasmas have been made at JET where most of the normalized parameters as needed for ITER operations are realized simultaneously; for the so-called "Advanced Operations Phase" of ITER, they have been able to nearly double the fusion output for a given heating power in plasmas with a so-called "Internal Barrier."

Important progress has also been obtained in the political preparations for ITER. Since May 2002 the ITER program now has 4 official host countries, which presented a site for ITER: France, Spain, Japan and Canada. In addition, US fusion researchers expressed interest to rejoin the ITER project last July. A group of so-called "negotiators" (with members from EU, Russian Federation, Japan and Canada) has been established and the EU members have received the mandate from the EU Council of Ministers to start negotiations for the siting of ITER. A decision is realistically expected (and hopefully will be made) in about one year. ITER is ready to be built, scientifically (confirmed again by the latest results of JET) and technically (all main components – some of them requiring new technologies have been built and tested with intensive international collaboration). The main aim of ITER is to show the scientific and technological feasibility of fusion. A fast track plan for fusion has been proposed in the UK by Prof. David King, science advisor to Prime Minister Blair, including an increase in funding and building in parallel to ITER a Facility for Fusion Material Research (IFMIF).

Akira Miyahara provided an update on fusion events from Japan:

1. Important Items:
   1-1 On May 1, 2002, Japanese Government decided to invite ITER to candidate Japanese site.
   1-2 LHD Stellarator in National Institute for Fusion Science (NIFS)

achieved excellent plasma parameters of Ti=6keV, Te=3keV(10keV as maximum value), ne=8*1019/m3 and energy confinement time=0.9sec.

1-3 JT-60U Tokamak in Japan Atomic Energy Research Institute (JAERI) are operated in remarkably good confinement time. It is a good back-up for ITER.

1-4 Universities are keeping their activities as TRIAM-Tokamak in Kyushu and Gekko-Laser in Osaka, to increase populations of Fusion Scientists for future fusion activities.

1-5 International Conference on Plasma Surface Interactions in Fusion Devises was held with 300 participants (200 foreign, 100 domestic).

1-6 International Conference on Fusion Reactor Materials will be held in Kyoto in next spring and preparations are being made now.

2. Personal Comments:

2-1 ITER design has made great progress since a day of INTOR through the efforts of Drs. Shimomura, Rebut and Dietz, namely, blanket structure was installed inside vacuum vessel. Cost reduction efforts were done at the later phase of EDA. I appreciated the efforts but it seems to be not sufficient. Because cost issue is a social science matter, we need to ask for a third party's criticism. The mission of the ITER must be rechecked, because quite often fusion scientist say that ITER is International Thermonuclear Experimental Reactor. The naming of Experimental Reactor is correct?

Or it is simply the device after TFTR, JET and JT-60 but with a blanket to produce neutrons?

2-2 Compatibility of ITER with other projects must be discussed in an international framework, because the impact of the ITER budget is enormous. Not only the Japanese project, but also the German Wendelstein, Culham and PPPL activities will suffer a serious impact. These projects are not yet considered, including blanket or other methods of energy conversion studies, but are still seriously directed to achieve reasonable long pulse, enhanced plasma parameters operations to reduce the size of the devices to realize an easy design of the Reactor.

2-3 Unexpected large numbers of participants of PSI Conference indicated that core plasma studies including plasma facing component are not yet completed for ITER and other fusion devices. The situations must be critically discussed.

2-4 Concerning fusion material studies, it is necessary to establish well defined problems. Because the studies are not only near term related but also medium and long term oriented. Since it takes a long time to develop materials, research direction must be critically discussed in order to meet the requirements of the 21st and later centuries.

3. Conclusions:

    3-1   ITER is an excellent project for international scientists to contribute to, and to solve the future energy demands together with environmental impact. However, necessity of serious discussions of compatibility with other fusion projects is urgent. ITER has some priority because blanket studies are included. We should define the mission of each project clearly in the framework of the magnetic fusion communities.

    3-2   Social acceptance issues must be analyzed and discussed internationally from a social sciences aspect, because they will impact stongly on future fusion reactor studies.

Current and future technologies for producing and using hydrogen were reviewed by Carmen Difiglio with a particular emphasis on carbon emissions, cost and technological uncertainty. Three different approaches to produce carbon-free hydrogen were discussed – nuclear, renewables and fossil fuels with carbon capture and storage. Data were presented that suggested that these three carbon-free sources might be more profitably used to displace higher-carbon sources in the production of electricity. But firm conclusions would require more specific data that reflect regional circumstances, technology development and climate change policies. Nonetheless, an analytic link was established between the hydrogen-using transport sector and the power generation sector since the same carbon-free technologies needed to produce hydrogen are also required to reduce power-sector emissions.

The environmental community appears to be converging on renewable energy and hydrogen as the long-term answer to climate change. However, it is unlikely that enough carbon-free electricity and hydrogen can be produced without also developing other technologies to produce carbon-free power. Analysis to provide a better understanding of the entire energy economy was proposed that would focus on the interdependencies among the various technologies needed to solve the climate-change problem. With this information, a more integrated policy strategy can be developed.

Richard Wilson commented on developments per acceptance of nuclear fission energy in the US over the past decade. In 1991 the nuclear fission proponents had become very pessimistic. Some existing nuclear plants had become so costly to operate that their power often did not generate enough revenue to cover operating costs. Capacity factors had typically declined to 60%. White House policy makers and NRC regulators exacerbated this situation by blocking the Ward Valley low level waste site (Hillary Clinton), and reacting to even relatively minor operational problems with shutdown orders under Chairperson Shirley Jackson. (Maine Yankee, Connecticut Yankee, Trojan and San Onofree 1).

However a key change improved the situation: the appointment of NRC Chairman Richard Meserve, perhaps driven by Al Gore's realization that shutting down nuclear plants would make attainment of Global Climate Change Goals much more difficult.

Under Meserve, the NRC adopted a risk guided regulation that by prioritizing oversight according to risk, actually yielded safer operation of plants, while substantially reducing operational disruption. Thus industry was encouraged to improve operations and the consequence has been dramatically improved capacity factors (90%-92%) and reduced operating cost. License renewal has become more tractable, unopposed by greens, and less costly.

Consequently new investors in existing, operating nuclear facilities have reaped large profits and the price of such plants has significantly increased.

Other positive developments have led to a much more optimistic view:

- WIPP operational.
- Yucca Mountain has green light.
- 4-year construction using new license procedures.
- One-stop licensing has been authorized, but has not been tried. This may lead to building new facilities based on new technology:
  - Light-water evolutionary reactors.
  - GE boiling water reactor (4-5 cents/kWh).
  - Pebble-bed reactor, 200 MW. South Africa for the first project. An outstanding issue is whether a containment vessel is necessary. If not, they could be economic but not with a containment vessel.
  - Fast-neutron reactor (do not call it a breeder-reactor) to demonstrate safety.
  - Generation IV program.

Of course these positive developments are highly dependent on NRC regulation. The switch from Shirley Jackson to Richard Merserve could be reversed.

Zenonas Rudzikas provided written recommendations that the PMP: 1) Take effective measures to improve public perception of nuclear energy; 2) Emphasize that wider use of nuclear energy will mitigate global warming effects; and 3) Try to achieve a high priority for fusion and solar and renewable energy sources. Juras Pozela provided similar written recommendations.

Action Proposal: Bruce Stram made an action proposal for the PMP. He addressed the problem of reduced expenditures for energy R and D, that was noted by the Energy PMP in 2000, and suggested this was inconsistent with the concern over Global Warming and other concerns, such as pollution, geopolitical conflict, and depletion, thought to be associated with continued fossil fuel use. Bruce Stram specifically proposed that the energy PMP organize an effort to develop a suggested worldwide budget for energy R and D. The purpose of this budget is to give the governments of the world a basis to judge their efforts against what a learned group of scientists, who have done some significant homework, think is appropriate.

Key emergencies: The members of the PMP agreed to focus efforts for the upcoming year around two themes that rise to the level of planetary emergencies: 1) the lack of access to energy resources by much of the developing world particularly electricity; and 2) the potential need of the world economy to switch from fossil fuel over the next century. Members agreed to communicate regularly over the course of the next year to refine these issues, develop greater understanding on the part of the PMP members, and suggest specific actions.

Administrative decisions: The PMP agreed that Richard Wilson will be Chairman.

The PMP agreed to initiate the following Subcommittees with suggested membership: Fusion with J. Ongena, F. Waelbrooke, A. Miyahara, and W. Barletta; Fission with R. Wilson and D. Bodansky; Renewables and efficiency with B. Stram and R. Rosenfeld; Developing country issues with J. Chahoud and P.K. Iyengar; Transportation with C. Difiglio; and Carbon sequestration which is open. All members of the PMP are invited and encouraged to participate in these subcommittees and should inform either the Chairman, R. Wilson, or Coordinator, B. Stram, if they wish to do so.

The PMP agreed that Stram should initiate his project by contacting other groups such as the Moore Foundation and Pugh Foundation in order to develop financial support for the "homework" exercise, and well as intellectual support. B. Stram is to report back to the PMP as to progress before the PMP will commit itself. Several participants have volunteered to help in the effort: C. Difiglio, B. van der Zwann, and W. Fulkerson. Other members are of course invited to volunteer.

MINUTES OF DESERTIFICATION PERMANENT MONITORING PANEL, ERICE

Present:

Larry L.Tieszen, Chair, EROS Data Center, Sioux Falls, SD
Andrew Warren, Rapporteur, University College London/Lund University
Mbareck Diop, Environmental Advisor to President, Senegal
Wang Tao, Institute of Desert Research, Lanzhou
Aaron Yair, Hebrew University, Jerusalem
Dick Grove, University of Cambridge.

Apologies: Paul Bartel, Petra Tchakert, Lennart Olsson

INTRODUCTION

The Chair introduced the meeting and participants.

HOMEPAGE

The homepage was briefly discussed. It has become the responsibility of Lennart Olsson at Lund. It exists in outline, but it was agreed that more links should be made from the existing homepage to others in which work by PMP participants was reported. These links will be accompanied by short paragraph introductions, which provide a direct linkage with the WFS and the PMP. Andrew Warren undertook to convey this decision to Lennart Olsson.

COOPERATION WITH FAO

Like the other projects reported below, this project has evolved out of cooperation at the Erice meetings of the desertification PMP. Andrew Warren reported briefly on this project. It is financed by FAO and involves Lund University and the University of Essex. The project aims to compile information on existing projects in Asian and African drylands in which carbon sequestration is a major aim. It will produce web-based information, including the analysis of a questionnaire, and a review of the literature, both technical and organisational. Training workshops are also planned. One of these may be combined with Larry Tieszen's workshop in Dakkar in February-March 2003 (see below). Larry and Andrew have produced a draft outline for this workshop, to be presented to Lennart Olsson for discussion.

SENEGAL PROJECT

Larry Tieszen reported on the progress in the Senegal carbon-sequestration project. Its main achievements to date have been the production of a manual of field methods, a series of training workshops on biogeochemical modelling, land cover monitoring for land degradation and improvement by remote sensing, ground observations and socio-economic surveys of three sites chosen to represent a climatic spectrum in Senegal. Surveys have been made of land degradation/improvement, potentials for carbon sequestration, and the possible management impacts of carbon sequestration projects. A major synthesis will occur in early 2003, in the workshop mentioned above.

SENEGAL PRESENTATION AT THE WORLD SUMMIT FOR SUSTAINABLE DEVELOPMENT, JOHANNESBURG 2002

Mbareck Diop reported on the development of the NEPAD proposal, in which environmental concerns and specifically desertification play prominent roles. This will provide a framework for the Senegal presentation at the World Summit on Sustainable Development conference in Johannesburg in August 2002. One initiative will be the cooperative development of environmental information systems by several African countries. There will also be an emphasis on carbon sequestration.

WFS IN SUDAN

Andrew Warren reported on progress in Sudan. A climate station had been established, beside which the Agricultural Research Corporation of Sudan has begun a series of long-term experiments on the effects of land use on carbon sequestration. Research on socio-economic controls on land use is nearing completion. It is based on very detailed field work in two villages, in conjunction with biogeochemical modelling and sampling. A proposal is being developed for a project which will develop a prototype sequestration programme that might interest corporate investors. It is being developed in cooperation with an international NGO (the Near-East Foundation), the Agricultural Research Corporation of Sudan and UNDP, Khartoum.

INPUT TO THE ERICE MEETING OF WFS, 2003

The PMP will propose a session on desertification for the plenary meetings at the Erice in 2003. It will propose three presentations: one on remote sensing applications related to land cover change, land cover performance, and carbon sequestration; one on carbon sequestration as a possible method of attracting funding to combat land degradation/desertification in the Sahel; and one on the socio-economic implications of such projects.

THE "SICILY PROJECT"

An outline of the PMP's input was discussed. This was presented to the meeting on the 24th of August 2002, at which WFS contributions to studying a variety of environmental problems in Sicily was discussed. This resulted in an integrated approach to project implementation and capacity development from a variety of PMPs. These integrated topics and the premises under which they were developed along with "1 page" descriptions will be forwarded to Mr. Manoli and are to be incorporated by Mr. Robert Clark. A joint list of WFS/WL capabilities, as concerns Sicily, was prepared by a joint committee including other PMPs. The recommended integrated approaches and list were to be presented to professor Zichicci for discussion with the Governor of Sicily.

PRESENTATION TO THE MEETING OF THE PARTIES OF THE CONVENTION TO COMBAT DESERTIFICATION

Aaron Yair and Dick Grove had been invited to Erice in 2002, specifically so that they could participate in the discussion of a "Sicily Project" ("9" above), but, even more urgently, because they, along with Larry Tieszen, had been asked to make a presentation to the CCD meeting, to be held in Sicily in November 2002. The status of the invitation was discussed, and clarification sought from the WFS secretariat.

PRESENTATION OF THE DESERTIFICATION PROJECT IN CHINA

Wang Tao presented a comprehensive review of the work carried out at his institute in Lanzhou. The work demonstrates both the ability to document the magnitude and spread of desertification and, especially, sand movement, and the ability to intervene successfully. Although sand encroachment has been successfully curtailed in some areas, other problems remain, including major and severe dust storms over large parts of China. The potential contribution to an integrated project in Sicily was discussed.

17. BRAIN AND BEHAVIOUR DISEASES WORKSHOP

UNRAVELLING THE MYSTERIES OF SCHIZOPHRENIA: ADVANCES FROM GENETIC STUDIES

ANNE S. BASSETT, M.D., FRCPC
Professor, Department of Psychiatry, University of Toronto, and Director, Clinical Genetics Research Program, Centre for Addiction and Mental Health, Toronto, Ontario

EVA W.C. CHOW, M.D., FRCPC
Assistant Professor, Department of Psychiatry, University of Toronto, and Centre for Addiction and Mental Health, Toronto, Ontario

ROSANNA WEKSBERG, M.D., PH.D., FRCPC
Professor, Department of Paediatrics, University of Toronto, Clinical Genetics and Metabolic Genetics & Research Institute, Hospital for Sick Children, Toronto, Ontario

LINDA BRZUSTOWICZ, M.D.
Associate Professor, Department of Genetics, Rutgers University, Piscataway, and Department of Psychiatry, University of Medicine and Dentistry of New Jersey, Newark/Piscataway, New Jersey, USA

ABSTRACT

Schizophrenia is a serious psychiatric illness involving changes in thinking, behaviour and emotions, that affects 1 in 100 people worldwide. The precise causes and disease mechanisms are currently unknown. It is likely that many people carry genes predisposing to schizophrenia but only some are expressed as the severe illness. Genetic subtypes of schizophrenia are helping to reveal genetic and other factors involved in disease expression.

Several susceptibility genes for schizophrenia have now been localized from studies of large families with familial forms of the illness, using methods successful for isolating genes for other complex conditions. Although no susceptibility gene for schizophrenia has yet been identified, the chromosomal "neighbourhoods" containing these genes have been found. These studies are also beginning to reveal factors, such as childhood head injury, that may modify expression of schizophrenia. Another research strategy has focussed on identifying physical genetic abnormalities associated with schizophrenia. An under-recognized genetic syndrome, 22q Deletion Syndrome (22qDS) associated with a microdeletion on chromosome 22, appears to comprise an identifiable subtype of schizophrenia involving 1-2% of all patients with the illness. This research has had immediate clinical relevance, since 22qDS can be diagnosed using clinical screening criteria and a blood test. The syndrome also provides a useful model for the neurodevelopmental mechanism believed to be involved in schizophrenia.

Genetic studies promise to provide a better understanding of the biological mechanisms that result in schizophrenia. This could lead to improved treatments for schizophrenia and significant reduction of the stigma that is associated with mental illness.

INTRODUCTION

Schizophrenia is a serious neuropsychiatric disorder affecting ~1% of the world's population, and with substantial impact on a much larger proportion of the population, including family members and society at large. The illness has significant associated mortality and morbidity and high costs to society, but, like other mental illnesses, schizophrenia is highly stigmatized in most societies.

There is substantial evidence that the principal etiology of schizophrenia involves genetic factors that predispose an individual to develop the disorder; indeed, multiple genetic and non-genetic factors are likely to be involved.[1,2] No individual susceptibility gene for schizophrenia has yet been identified. Recently, however, there has been much progress and several new developments in the genetics of schizophrenia. These include the identification of the first clinically relevant genetic subtype of schizophrenia that is detectable by clinical and laboratory evaluations, advances in our understanding of possible mechanisms, and multiple localizations of potential susceptibility genes.

A GENETIC SUBTYPE OF SCHIZOPHRENIA: 22Q DELETION SYNDROME

One of the most exciting developments in recent years is the identification of 22q Deletion Syndrome (22qDS) as a clinically detectable genetic subtype of schizophrenia that may serve as a model to study the etiopathogenesis of schizophrenia, including the neurodevelopmental process involved. 22qDS, also known as velocardiofacial or DiGeorge syndrome, is a genetic syndrome associated with a high (~25%) rate of schizophrenia [3-5] and microdeletions in the long or "q" arm of chromosome 22. This means that individuals with a chromosome 22q11.2 deletion have a higher genetic risk for schizophrenia than any other group of individuals except for individuals with two parents with schizophrenia or monozygotic (identical) co-twins of individuals with schizophrenia.[5]

22q Deletion Syndrome - an under-recognized condition
The estimated rate of 22q11.2 microdeletions in the general population is about 1/4000 live births, making it the most common of all microdeletion syndromes, and the second most common genetic syndrome after Down syndrome. The rate of chromosome 22q11.2 microdeletions in a population of individuals with schizophrenia, however, is about 80 times more frequent than that in the general population, occurring in up to 1 in 50 patients.[5,6]

22qDS is therefore several times more prevalent than childhood onset schizophrenia, and is much more common in the general population than Huntington disease.

In specific sub-populations of schizophrenia, 22qDS is even more prevalent. For example, as many as 40% of adults with schizophrenia who meet clinical screening criteria for 22qDS have a detectable 22q11.2 deletion.[7,8] The prevalence of 22qDS also appears to be high in patients with dual diagnoses of schizophrenia and mental retardation (~9%),[9] and in childhood onset schizophrenia.[10] However, several features conspire to make 22qDS ascertainment incomplete, and this genetic subtype of schizophrenia may therefore be misperceived as rare. A set of clinical criteria designed to increase the rate of detection of 22qDS in adults may be helpful in this regard.[7]

Table 1. Major clinical features of adults with 22q11.2 Deletion Syndrome.

Clinical Features	Cohen et al., 1999[11] Maximum n = 126		Murphy et al., 1999[3] Maximum n = 48	
	Subjects with the clinical feature			
	n	(%)	n	(%)
Physical				
Facial anomalies (variable)	120	(99)	-	-
Palatal anomalies (any)	92	(88)	13	-
Overt or submucous cleft palate	43	(41)	13	(27)
Congenital heart defects (major, e.g., tetralogy of Fallot, ventricular septal defect)	36	(30)	19	(40)
Neuropsychiatric				
Learning difficulties (any)	104	(94)	-	-
Mental retardation (IQ < 70)	-	-	16	(33)
Borderline intellectual functioning (IQ 71 - 85)	-	-	19	(40)
Psychiatric disorders (any)	45	(36)	20	(42)
Schizophrenia and other psychoses	-	-	15	(31)

Clinical features

The physical and neurobehavioural features of 22qDS are highly variable and are often so mild that the condition goes unrecognized, particularly in adults (see Table 1).[11] The facial features are subtle and variable,[7,12,13] reducing the index of suspicion for a genetic syndrome. Palatal problems are common, but usually take the form of velopharyngeal insufficiency, a neuromuscular problem, or submucous cleft palate, both of which result in a variable degree of hypernasal speech; overt cleft palate is uncommon.[11] The majority of individuals with 22qDS have learning difficulties, but these are most commonly subtle and may not be detected by local school systems. About 35-40% have intellectual functioning in the mild range of mental retardation, and there are case reports of more severe mental retardation.[14]

Platelet counts are usually in the low normal to below normal range, which may be a useful adjunctive feature in screening patients for 22qDS.[15]

Family history

The fact that the 22q11.2 deletion is usually (>90% of newly identified cases)[16] a spontaneous (de novo) mutational event may also make the syndrome difficult to recognize because there is no family history of 22qDS or its component features. The term "genetic" is sometimes interpreted as equivalent to "inherited". However, 22qDS is a transmissible genetic condition that is not usually inherited, because most patients have a deletion that arises from a *de novo* mutation. Even in the minority of cases with an inherited deletion, the transmitting parent often has such subtle manifestations that a genetic condition has never been suspected[17].

Molecular testing

Clinical testing for 22qDS only became widely available in about 1995. Specialized testing is required; routine karyotyping does not detect the 22q11.2 microdeletion. The most commonly associated deletions are identifiable with standard molecular cytogenetic studies, now available in clinical laboratories, using a fluorescence *in-situ* hybridization (FISH) technique and 22q11.2 probes (D22S75 or TUPLE1)[18] (Fig. 1). These common deletions include a 3 million base pair (Mb) deletion (>85%) and a 1.5 Mb deletion (8-14%) nested within the 3 Mb deletion region.[16,19] 22qDS therefore represents the first genetic subtype of schizophrenia detectable using a blood test. The main limitation to the available clinical FISH testing is that it cannot detect rare, atypical deletions, though these appear to account for very few 22q11.2 deletions.[19]

Typical schizophrenia

Recent studies of individuals with a 22qDS subtype of schizophrenia (22qDS-SZ) suggest strong similarities in clinical, demographic, neurocognitive, and structural brain features to other forms of schizophrenia. Age at onset, major signs and symptoms of schizophrenia, level of functioning, profile of cognitive deficits, and structural brain findings are similar.[12,20-22] Possible differences from other forms of schizophrenia include: a lower rate of comorbid substance use, lower rate of family history of schizophrenia, higher rate of physical congenital anomalies, lower mean IQ, and equal sex distribution.

Research advantages

The relative genetic homogeneity of 22qDS makes this an especially powerful model in which to study other etiopathogenetic factors because individuals with 22qDS all share the primary genetic predisposition for schizophrenia: a 22q11.2 deletion. This makes 22qDS different from other genetic high risk groups available for study. For example, most samples of first degree relatives or monozygotic co-twins of individuals with schizophrenia are genetically heterogeneous since they derive from multiple different families with various, unknown genetic predispositions. A further advantage of 22qDS is the capability of molecular testing for the 22q11.2 deletion, both to identify this sub-group with elevated genetic risk for schizophrenia and to characterize the specific predisposing DNA alteration (primary genetic lesion). Chromosome 22 was the first chromosome to be sequenced, and its interesting genomic structure[23,24] has intrigued researchers attempting to understand the non-Mendelian genetic mechanisms that may underlie the 22qDS phenotype.

Immediate clinical relevance
22qDS is a syndromic form of schizophrenia of immediate clinical relevance.[5,7] There is insufficient information yet with respect to optimal psychiatric treatments. Individuals with 22qDS appear to respond to the symptomatic medications currently available but, as for other patients with schizophrenia and cognitive dysfunction, may be more susceptible to neurologic side effects. Diagnosis of a 22qDS subtype of schizophrenia may however significantly alter medical management. For example, regular assessment for known associated conditions such as hypocalcemia and hypoparathyroidism is important since hypocalcemia can arise at any time and can lower the seizure threshold. This may have significant implications to medication management if a seizure ascribed solely to psychotropic medications is actually precipitated by undetected hypocalcemia. A diagnosis of 22qDS also has important genetic counselling implications.[25]

FAMILIAL FORMS OF SCHIZOPHRENIA

Evidence for genetic heterogeneity - multiple plausible localizations
Recent findings from genetic linkage studies of families with several affected family members (familial schizophrenia) add substantially to the longstanding body of work implicating genetic factors in the cause of schizophrenia.[2,26] Linkage studies serve to narrow down a region where a gene for schizophrenia may be localized. This is like finding the city or neighbourhood a susceptibility gene is in, though not actually identifying which gene it is, nor precisely what genetic change has occurred to predispose to the illness. Prior to 2001 there was convincing evidence for schizophrenia susceptibility loci on the long arm of both chromosome 1[27] and chromosome 13.[28,29] These studies involved multigenerational Canadian[27,28] and nuclear (small) and multigenerational American families,[29] and found significant[28,29] or highly significant[27] genome-wide linkage.[30]

Significant linkage results
Now there is further evidence helping to confirm a chromosome 1q21-q22 schizophrenia susceptibility locus from British and Icelandic families[31] and several new localizations of possible schizophrenia susceptibility genes (see Table 2). There is significant evidence for linkage of schizophrenia to three different genomic regions from three different genetic isolate populations: the short ("p") arm of chromosome 2 (2p13-14) in large Palauan families,[32] chromosome 2q37 in Finnish nuclear and larger families,[33] and chromosome 6q25 in a very large northern Swedish pedigree[34]. A locus on chromosome 15q14 also reached a genomewide level of significance in a reanalysis of small European-American and African-American families.[35]

Suggestive linkage results

Several other chromosomal regions show evidence from multiple suggestive linkage findings to support their possible involvement in schizophrenia susceptibility. A recent review found that three of these regions (6p24-p23, 8p21-p22, and 10p14-p11) had four or more genome scan studies with suggestive linkage findings, and are therefore consistent with regions where true schizophrenia susceptibility loci are most likely to be located.[36] The 5q22-qter region should probably now be added, given recent studies with similar suggestive linkage results.[31-33,37] We now await further laborious steps to narrow down these regions of interest, and hopefully identify susceptibility genes.

Challenges to replication

Unambiguous (e.g., lod score >10) linkage findings that are frequent in Mendelian disorders are unlikely to occur in complex disorders such as schizophrenia, where a significant finding needs to be differentiated from a false positive error.[38] While specific ascertainment strategies and careful methods likely play a role, significant linkage results in complex disorders may be due in part to the draw of a "lucky hand" - a set of families with disease attributable to a specific locus.[39] This provides a partial explanation for difficulties in replicating susceptibility loci for complex disorders after initial significant results.[30,39] The reason is low power secondary to the genetic heterogeneity inherent in complex disorders.[39,40] Indeed, when there are multiple genes for a disorder, the _more_ representative a data set is of the illness in the general population, the _less_ likely that data set will be to confirm an initial finding of linkage.[39] Furthermore, small nuclear families or affected sib pairs may generate different results from more densely affected, larger families due to different susceptibility genes segregating.[39-41]

Phenotype issues

The significant linkage findings in schizophrenia to date have used conservative diagnostic categorization, a narrow definition of illness usually comprising schizophrenia and schizoaffective disorders or a broader definition including other related disorders (see Table 2). Use of diagnostic categorization provides some comfort that the susceptibility loci localized to date are relevant to expression of a schizophrenic illness. However, it is likely that other phenotypic features are involved in the full range of expression of a susceptibility genotype. Interestingly, there is a suggestion that there may be overlap of susceptibility loci for some familial forms of schizophrenia and bipolar disorder.[42] For example, there are significant[43] and suggestive[44] linkage results for bipolar disorder involving the same region of chromosome 13 (13q32) as that for schizophrenia.[27,29] These findings are consistent with the likelihood of variable expression in schizophrenia, as in most other genetic disorders.

Identifying features characterizing individual susceptibility loci could significantly increase power for localizing genes. Alternative phenotypes, often termed "endophenotypes" in psychiatry, that consistently subtype the illness in a genetically meaningful way with respect to schizophrenia may be helpful in this regard. These may be more identifiable now that there are significant linkage results using a schizophrenia phenotype.

SPONTANEOUS MUTATIONS AND SCHIZOPHRENIA

As noted above, there are high rates of new mutations with respect to 22q11.2 deletions in 22qDS. Identification of 22qDS patients with transmitted deletions is 10 times less common than identification of patients with deletions due to spontaneous mutations in germ cells (i.e., both parents with normal chromosomes).[16] There is now new evidence,[45] added to that from several previous studies, which supports the possibility of spontaneous mutations in other forms of schizophrenia, an idea first advanced by Böök in 1953.[46] This possibility is supported by the observation that rates of schizophrenia are slightly higher with advancing paternal age (i.e., older age of fathers at the birth of individuals who eventually develop schizophrenia).[45,47] The likelihood of mutations in sperm increases with age,[48] thus association of illness with advancing paternal age provides indirect evidence for possible spontaneous mutations. This finding may have more resonance with the general public today since older parents are more common than in previous decades. However, the clinical relevance of a small association between advanced paternal age and risk of schizophrenia is uncertain.

The relevance to research is more tangible. This advancement of an old idea is timely given the possibility that identifying unstable mutations or other genomic instabilities that could underlie an increased frequency of spontaneous mutations has become plausible.[1] For example, large unstable nucleotide repeats have been found to be responsible for several neuropsychiatric disorders. Large repeats do not appear to be involved in schizophrenia,[49] although smaller repeats or other genomic instabilities remain a possible etiology and source of new mutations. A mechanism that included a high rate of spontaneous mutations predisposing to schizophrenia would be consistent with the low rate of family history of schizophrenia usually found in individuals with the illness and apparent "sporadic" schizophrenia.[26] A high rate of spontaneous mutations could help explain the maintenance of the illness prevalence despite low reproductive fitness.[50] And the possibility of spontaneous mutations re-emphasizes the idea, also noted above, that "genetic" does not equate with "inherited."

NEW RECOMMENDATIONS FOR GENETIC COUNSELLING IN SCHIZOPHRENIA

Genetic counselling in schizophrenia is an area that has received little recent attention.[25] Genetic counselling, the process through which knowledge about the genetics of illnesses is shared, provides information on the inheritance of illnesses and their recurrence risks, addresses the concerns of patients, their families and their health care providers, and supports patients and their families dealing with these illnesses. Empiric risks for schizophrenia are available, but must be used in the context of the individual's family history, in order to tailor the risk assessment to the individual. For example, detailed family history and medical history are necessary to determine whether there is an "isolated" case of schizophrenia within a family, a more complex family structure with schizophrenia and/or other psychiatric disorder(s) in several members, or evidence for 22qDS. Access to genetic counselling should be available to all individuals with schizophrenia, and is particularly important for family planning, although this service is not routinely offered in most clinical settings today.

An important addition to genetic counselling issues in recent years is the ability to identify individuals with a 22qDS subtype of schizophrenia. If 22qDS or another genetic syndrome is suspected, a referral to a geneticist would be appropriate. Transmission of a 22q11.2 deletion follows a Mendelian autosomal dominant pattern. Thus, an individual with 22qDS has a 50% chance of having a child with 22qDS with each pregnancy. As with most Mendelian conditions however, the severity of the condition or any of its physical or neurobehavioural manifestations cannot be predicted. Genetic counselling regarding the syndrome, its variable expression, available testing, and future pregnancies is an essential component of the comprehensive medical management of patients with 22qDS. In 22qDS, as in other forms of schizophrenia, there may be varying levels of learning disabilities. Genetic counselling for these patients may therefore require unique approaches to help convey the information.[25]

Parents of an individual with 22qDS are also routinely tested for the deletion since in about 10% of newly diagnosed cases the deletion has been inherited from one of the parents, who often has a mild presentation of the syndrome. In the majority of newly diagnosed cases of 22qDS, however, the deletion has occurred as a *de novo* mutation. Counselling regarding the chance nature of this occurrence, likely during gametogenesis, may relieve parents of guilt or inappropriate blame they may have felt over the years, particularly about behavioural and developmental features.[25]

Future issues
New findings in the genetics of schizophrenia and related disorders may have important clinical implications to patients and their families in the near future. Identifying susceptibility genes will likely have an impact on our understanding of pathophysiology, and may in the future alter what information will be available to patients and families for genetic counselling. Guided by experience being gained in other neuropsychiatric disorders,[51] consideration of ethical issues related to genetic testing for schizophrenia will be essential to determine the most appropriate implementation of services for genetic testing.[25,52]

A NEURODEVELOPMENTAL PATHWAY FROM GENETIC SUSCEPTIBILITY TO SCHIZOPHRENIA

It has long been recognized that genetic factors are involved in a pathway from an initial causal event (susceptibility) to clinical expression of schizophrenia.[1,2] A model of etiopathogenesis has recently been proposed that brings molecular genetic and other etiologic factors together with the popular neurodevelopmental hypothesis of schizophrenia.[1] This model emphasizes the dynamic nature of genetic effects and their role in pathogenetic processes that likely include changes in neurodevelopment.

Individual genes are an important component in eventual illness expression, but increased understanding from the human genome project has clarified that other genomic or epigenetic mechanisms may also be important and may explain the non-Mendelian segregation patterns observed in schizophrenia[1]. In addition, there is some evidence for gene-gene interactions, stochastic (chance) factors, and non-genetic factors playing a role in expression, likely as modifying factors.[1,26] For example, there is preliminary evidence for genetic factors being involved in modifying age at onset of schizophrenia,[53] as has been recently found in Alzheimer disease and Parkinson's disease.[54] Also, our group has found that mild childhood head injury (age 10 years or younger) is associated with younger age at onset in familial schizophrenia.[55XXXX]

Even single gene Mendelian disorders show evidence of complex genetic mechanisms and interacting factors likely to influence expression.[56] Indeed, it is the norm in the genetics of human disorders to have reduced penetrance (a genetic susceptibility that in some individuals is not expressed) and variable expression (a genetic condition that is expressed with variable severity). Schizophrenia will be no exception to this,[1] as illustrated by studies of offspring of discordant monozygotic twins.[57,58] Even the genetic heterogeneity of schizophrenia will likely prove advantageous in developing an understanding of the pathogenesis of the disorder, and in providing multiple targets for new treatment possibilities.

CONCLUSION

Gene discoveries, aided by the Human Genome Project, are predicted to revolutionize medicine[59] and these genetic advances will encompass psychiatry as well as other disciplines. The advances in the past several years in the genetics of schizophrenia promise that further advances will soon be forthcoming, leading to identification of molecular subtypes of schizophrenia[60] and eventually an initial understanding of the pathogenesis of the disease.[1]

Correspondence to be addressed to: Dr. Anne Bassett, Clinical Genetics Research Program, Centre for Addiction and Mental Health, 1001 Queen Street West, Toronto, Ontario, M6J 1H4 Canada, phone: (416) 535-8501 ext. 2731, fax: (416) 535-7199. E-mail: anne.bassett@utoronto.ca

ACKNOWLEDGMENTS

Funded in part by Medical Research Council of Canada grants MT-1225 and MOP-38099, Ontario Mental Health Foundation, and by an Independent Investigator Award from the National Alliance for Research on Schizophrenia and Depression (ASB), and by the National Institute of Mental Health grant R01 MH62440 and an Independent Investigator Award from the National Alliance for Research on Schizophrenia and Depression (LMB).

REFERENCES

1.   Bassett, A.S., Chow, E.W.C., O'Neill, S. and Brzustowicz, L. (2001) "Genetic insights into the neurodevelopmental hypothesis of schizophrenia. "*Schizophr Bull* **27**, 417-430.

2.   Gottesman, I.I. (2001) "Psychopathology through a life span - genetic prism." *Am Psychologist* **56**, 864-878.

3.   Murphy, K.C., Jones, L.A. and Owen, M.J. (1999) "High rates of schizophrenia in adults with velo-cardio-facial syndrome." *Arch Gen Psychiatry* **56**, 940-945.

4.   Pulver, A.E. et al. (1994) "Psychotic illness in patients diagnosed with velo-cardio-facial syndrome and their relatives." *J Nerv Ment Dis* **182**, 476-478.

5.   Bassett, A.S., Chow, E.W.C. and Weksberg, R. (2001) "Chromosomal abnormalities and schizophrenia." *Am J Med Genet (Semin Med Genet)* **97**, 45-51.

6.   Karayiorgou, M. et al. (1995) "Schizophrenia susceptibility associated with interstitial deletions of chromosome 22q11." *Proc Natl Acad Sci USA* **92**, 7612-7616.

7.   Bassett, A.S. and Chow, E.W.C. (1999) "22q11 Deletion Syndrome: a genetic subtype of schizophrenia." *Biol Psychiatry* **46**, 882-891.

8.   Bassett, A.S., Chow, E.W.C., Waterworth, D. and Brzustowicz, L. (2001) "Genetic insights into schizophrenia." *Can J Psychiatry* **46**, 131-137.

9.   Murphy, K.C., Jones, R.G., Griffiths, E., Thompson, P.W. and Owen, M.J. (1998) "Chromosome 22q11 deletions. An under-recognised cause of idiopathic learning disability." *Br J Psychiatry* **172**, 180-183.

10.   Nicolson, R. et al. (1999) "Clinical and neurobiological correlates of cytogenetic abnormalities in childhood-onset schizophrenia." *Am J Psychiatry* **156**, 1575-9.

11.   Cohen, E., Chow, E.W.C., Weksberg, R. and Bassett, A.S. (1999) "Phenotype of adults with the 22q11 Deletion Syndrome: A review." *Am J Med Genet* **86**, 359-365.

12.   Bassett, A.S. et al. (1998) "22q11 deletion syndrome in adults with schizophrenia." *Am J Med Genet (Neuropsychiatr Genet)* **81**, 328-337.

13.   Scutt, L., Chow, E.W.C., Weksberg, R., Honer, W.G. and Bassett, A.S. (2001) "Patterns of dysmorphic features in schizophrenia." *Am J Med Genet (Neuropsychiatr Genet)* **105**, 713-723.

14.   Swillen, A. et al. (1997) "Intelligence and psychosocial adjustment in velocardiofacial syndrome: a study of 37 children and adolescents with VCFS." *J Med Genet* **34**, 453-458.

15.   Lazier, K. et al. (2001) "Low platelet count in 22q11 Deletion Syndrome and schizophrenia." *Schizophr Res* **50**, 177-180.

16.   Kerstjens-Frederikse, W.S. et al. (1999) "Microdeletion 22q11.2: clinical data and deletion size." *J Med Genet* **36**, 721-723.

17.   McDonald-McGinn, D.M. et al. (2001) "Phenotype of the 22q11.2 deletion in individuals identified through an affected relative: Cast a wide FISHing net!" *Genet Med* **3**, 23-29.

18.   Lindsay, E.A. et al. (1995) "Velo-cardio-facial syndrome: Frequency and extent of 22q11 deletions." *Am J Med Genet* **57**, 514-522.

19.   Edelmann, L. et al. (1999) "A common molecular basis for rearrangement disorders on chromosome 22q11." *Hum Mol Genet* **8**, 1157-1167.

20.   Chow, E.W.C., Zipursky, R.B., Mikulis, D.J. and Bassett, A.S. (2002) "Structural brain abnormalities in patients with schizophrenia and 22q11 Deletion Syndrome." *Biol Psychiatry* **51**, 208-215.

21.   Chow, E.W.C. et al. (1999) "Qualitative MRI findings in adults with 22q11 Deletion Syndrome and schizophrenia." *Biol Psychiatry* **46**, 1436-1442.

22.   Chow, E.C. et al. (1999) "Neuropsychological functioning in adults with 22q11 Deletion Syndrome and schizophrenia (abstract)." *Schizophr Res* **36**, 88-89.

23.   Collins, J.E., Mungall, A.J., Badcock, K.L., Fay, J.M. and Dunham, I. (1997) "The organization of the g-glutamyl transferase genes and other low copy repeats in human chromosome 22q11." *Genome Res* **7**, 522-531.

24.   Dunham, I. et al. (1999) "The DNA sequence of human chromosome 22." *Nature* **402**, 489-495.

25.   Hodgkinson, K., Murphy, J., O'Neill, S., Brzustowicz, L. and Bassett, A.S. (2001) "Genetic counselling for schizophrenia in the era of molecular genetics." *Can J Psychiatry* **46**, 123-130.

26.   McGuffin, P., Asherson, P., Owen, M. and Farmer, A. (1994) "The strength of the genetic effect: Is there room for an environmental influence in the aetiology of schizophrenia?" *Br J Psychiatry* **164**, 593-599.

27.   Brzustowicz, L.M., Hodgkinson, K.A., Chow, E.W.C., Honer, W.G. and Bassett, A.S. (2000) "Location of a major susceptibility locus for familial schizophrenia on chromosome 1q21-q22." *Science* **288**, 678-682.

28.   Brzustowicz, L. et al. (1999) "Linkage of familial schizophrenia to chromosome 13q32." *Am J Hum Genet* **65**, 1096-1103.

29.   Blouin, J.-L. et al. (1998) "Schizophrenia susceptibility loci on chromosomes 13q32 and 8p21." *Nat Genet* **20**, 70-73.

30.   Lander, E. and Kruglyak, L. (1995) "Genetic dissection of complex traits: Guidelines for reporting and interpreting linkage results." *Nat Genet* **11**, 241-247.

31.   Gurling, H.M.D. et al. (2001) "Genomewide genetic linkage analysis confirms the presence of susceptibility loci for schizophrenia, on chromosomes 1q32.2, 5q33.2, and 8p21-22 and provides support for linkage to schizophrenia, on chromosomes 11q23.3-24 and 20q12.1-11.23." *Am J Hum Genet* **68**, 661-673.

32.   Tavtigian, S.V. et al. (2001) "A candidate prostate cancer susceptibility gene at chromosome 17p." *Nat Genet* **27**, 172-180.

33.   Ekelund, J. et al. (2001) "Chromosome 1 loci in Finnish schizophrenia families." *Hum Mol Genet* **10**, 1611-1617.

34.   Lindholm, E. et al. (2001) "A schizophrenia-susceptibility locus at 6q25, in one of the world's largest reported pedigrees." *Am J Hum Genet* **69**, 96-105.

35.   Freedman, R. et al. (2001) "Evidence for the multigenic inheritance of schizophrenia." *Am J Med Genet (Neuropsychiatr Genet)* **105**, 794-800.

36.   Bassett, A.S., Chow, E.W.C. and Brzustowicz, L.M. (2001) "The genetics of schizophrenia." *Neurosci News* **4**, 20-26.

37.   Straub, R.E., MacLean, C.J., O'Neill, F.A., Walsh, D. and Kendler, K.S. (1997) "Support for a possible schizophrenia vulnerability locus in region 5q22-31 in Irish families." *Mol Psychiatry* **2**, 148-155.

38.   Xu, J., Weisch, D.G., Eugene, W.T. and Meyers, D.A. (1999) "Evaluation of replication studies, combined data analysis, and analytical methods in complex

diseases." *Genet Epidemiol* **17**, S773-S778.

39. Ostrander, E.A. and Stanford, J.L. (2000) "Genetics of prostate cancer: Too many loci, too few genes." *Am J Hum Genet* **67**, 1367-1375.

40. Goddard, K.A.B., Witte, J.S., Suarez, B.K., Catalona, W.J. and Olson, J.M. (2001) "Model-free linkage analysis with covariates confirms linkage of prostate cancer to chromosomes 1 and 4." *Am J Hum Genet* **68**, 1197-1206.

41. IBD International Genetics Consortium. (2001) "International collaboration provides convincing linkage replication in complex disease through analysis of a large pooled data set: Crohn disease and chromosome 16." *Am J Hum Genet* **68**, 1165-1171.

42. Berrettini, W.H. (2000) "Are schizophrenic and bipolar disorders *related?* A review of family and molecular studies." *Biol Psychiatry* **48**, 531-538.

43. Detera-Wadleigh, S. et al. (1999) "A high-density genome scan detects evidence for a bipolar-disorder susceptibility locus on 13q32 and other potential loci on 1q32 and 18p11.2." *Proc Natl Acad Sci USA* **96**, 5604-5609.

44. Kelsoe, J.R. et al. (2001) "A genome survey indicates a possible susceptibility locus for bipolar disorder on chromosome 22." *Proc Natl Acad Sci USA* **98**, 585-590 (2001).

45. Malaspina, D. et al. "Advancing paternal age and the risk of schizophrenia." *Arch Gen Psychiatry* **58**, 361-367.

46. Böök, J.A. (1953) "Schizophrenia as a gene mutation." *Acta Genetica* **4**, 133-139.

47. Hare, E.H. & Moran, P.A.P. (1979) "Raised parental age in psychiatric patients: evidence for the constitutional hypothesis." *Br J Psychiatry* **134**, 169-177.

48. Evans, H.J. (1988) "Mutation as a cause of genetic disease." *Philos Trans R Soc Lond B Biol Sci* **319**, 325-340.

49. Vincent, J.B. et al. (2000) "An unstable trinucleotide-repeat region on chromosome 13 implicated in spinocerebellar ataxia: a common expansion locus." *Am J Hum Genet* **66**, 819-829.

50. Bassett, A.S., Bury, A., Hodgkinson, K.A. and Honer, W.G. (1996) "Reproductive fitness in familial schizophrenia." *Schizophr Res* **21**, 151-160.

51. Steinbart, E.J., Smith, C.O., Poorkaj, P. and Bird, T.D. (2001) "Impact of DNA testing for early-onset familial Alzheimer disease and frontotemporal dementia." *Arch Neurol* **58**, 1828-1831.

52. Burke, W., Pinsky, L.E. and Press, N.A. (2001) "Categorizing genetic tests to identify their ethical, legal, and social implications." *Am J Med Genet (Semin Med Genet)* **106**, 233-240.

53. Cardno, A. et al. (2001) "A genomewide linkage study of age at onset in schizophrenia." *Am J Med Genet (Neuropsychiatr Genet)* **105**, 439-445.

54. Li, Y. et al. (2002) "Age at onset in two common neurodegenerative diseases is genetically controlled." *Am J Hum Genet* **70**, 985-993.

55. AbdelMalik, P., Husted, J.A., Chow, W.C. and Bassett, A.S. "Childhood head injury and expression of familial schizophrenia in multiply affected families." *Arch Gen Psychiatry* (in press).

56. Dipple, K.M. and McCabe, E.R.B. (2000) "Phenotypes of patients with 'simple'

mendelian disorders are complex traits: thresholds, modifiers, and systems dynamics." *Am J Hum Genet* **66**, 1729-1735.

57. Gottesman, I.I. and Bertelsen, A. (1989) "Confirming unexpressed genotypes for schizophrenia: Risks in the offspring of Fischer's Danish identical and fraternal discordant twins." *Arch Gen Psychiatry* **46**, 867-872.

58. Kringlen, E. and Cramer, G. (1989) "Offspring of monozygotic twins discordant for schizophrenia." *Arch Gen Psychiatry* **46**, 873-877.

59. Hyman, S.E. (2000) "The genetics of mental illness: Implications for practice." *Bull WHO* **78**, 455-463.

60. Cowan, W.M. and Kandel, E.R. (2001) "Prospects for neurology and psychiatry." *JAMA* **285**, 594-600.

61. Camp, N.J. et al. (2001) "Genomewide multipoint linkage analysis of seven extended Palauan pedigrees with schizophrenia, by a Markov-Chain Monte Carlo method." *Am J Hum Genet* **69**, 1278-1289.

62. Paunio, T. et al. (2001) "Genome-wide scan in a nationwide study sample of schizophrenia families in Finland reveals susceptibility loci on chromosomes 2q and 5q." *Hum Mol Genet* **10**, 3037-3048.

63. Faraone, S.V. et al. (1998) "A genome scan of European-American schizophrenia pedigrees: results of the NIMH genetics initiative and millennium consortium." *Am J Med Genet (Neuropsychiatr Genet)* **81**, 290-295.

64. Kaufmann, C.A. et al. (1998) "NIMH genetics initiative millennium schizophrenia consortium: Linkage analysis of African-American pedigrees." *Am J Med Genet (Neuropsychiatr Genet)* **81**, 282-289.

GENETICS OF SUBSTANCE DEPENDENCE

C. ROBERT CLONINGER, M.D.
Department of Psychiatry, Washington University School of Medicine,
Campus Box 8134, 660 So. Euclid, St. Louis, MO 63110
Phone 314-362-7005, email clon@tci.wustl.edu

Twin and adoption studies have recently distinguished the effects of genes that influence the initiation of drug use from those that influence the transition from use to abuse and dependence. The genes that influence the initiation of drug use are related to antisocial personality traits, particularly high Novelty Seeking. The same genes have a strong influence on the initiation of a wide variety of substances, including stimulants, opiates, psychedelics, sedatives, marijuana, alcohol, and nicotine. In contrast, the transition from drug use to abuse or dependence is weakly influenced by heritable traits, such as low Self-directedness and low P300 amplitude. However, the transition to abuse is largely influenced by factors unique to the experiences of each individual. Linkage and association studies have identified several chromosomal regions and specific genes that influence initiation of substance use and the transitions to abuse and dependence. For example, several genes influencing dopaminergic and serotonergic neurotransmission have been implicated in the initiation of drug abuse. These include genetic polymorphisms influencing the activity of the dopamine and serotonin transporters, the dopamine DRD4 receptor and the serotonin 5HT1B receptor.

GENETIC EPIDEMIOLOGY OF SUBSTANCE ABUSE

Family, twin, and adoption studies have consistently confirmed the importance of genetic influences on the risk of substance abuse. However, clinicians observed that the same individual often abused several classes of substances, and different individuals in the same family sometimes abused different substances despite similar opportunities for drug use. A variety of explanations were offered for such polysubstance abuse and individual differences in drug preferences. For example, some hypothesized that readily available substances, such as marijuana and cigarettes, served as a gateway that may or may not lead to subsequent use of less often used drugs, such as stimulants, opiates, and psychedelics. Others suggested that vulnerability to each drug had specific genetic antecedents, but that environmental influences common to siblings (such as availability in particular neighborhoods) favor the use of the same drugs by members of a family.

However, recent data from twins and adoptees indicate that neither the gateway hypothesis nor the common environment hypothesis can explain the heritability of polysubstance abuse (Tsuang et al., 1998). Recent findings clearly show that the strongest genetic influences on risk of drug abuse are the genes that influence drug initiation. The genes that influence initiation of use have a strong effect on the ultimate risk of abuse, and they are largely non-specific for the class of drug. For example, heritable personality traits, such as high Novelty Seeking, increase the risk of experimentation with a wide variety of drugs (Cloninger et al., 1988; Howard et al., 1997; Comings et al., 2000). The ease of availability largely explains what particular drugs are used if there is any experimentation. Once there is an opportunity to use a drug, the genetic factors for initiation of use are largely the same for all classes of drugs except opiates (see Table 1).

Table 1. Common and unique genetic variance by type of drug in the Vietnam Era Twin Study (adapted from Tsuang et al., 1998).

	Heritabilities	
Drug Type	**Common**	**Unique**
Marijuana	2	11
Stimulants	24	9
Sedatives	22	5
Opiates	16	38
Hallucinogens	26	0

The genes uniquely involved in use of specific drugs are unknown. Even the alcohol dehydrogenase (ADH3) and mu-opioid receptor genes appear to influence susceptibility to polysubstance abuse (Uhl et al., 2001). This non-specificity of gene effects is not explained by indiscriminant drug use due to intoxication because cigarette smoking, which is not intoxicating, shares most of its genetic variance with alcoholism (True et al., 1999) and hence probably with other forms of substance abuse.

Different genes influence the transition from use to abuse or dependence than those that influence initiation (Sigvardsson et al., 1996; Tsuang et al., 1998; Kendler et al., 1999 & 2000). Furthermore, once there is initiation of drug use, the factors that influence the transition from initiation to repeated use, abuse, or dependence are largely non-genetic factors unique to each individual. This is shown in a sample of veteran twins (Tsuang et al., 1998) in Table 2. In other words, the heritability of the transition from use to abuse is weak. The greater heritability of initiation compared to that of the transition to abuse was also observed in a large sample of female twins in Virginia (Kendler et al., 1999).

PERSONALITY ANTECEDENTS OF SUBSTANCE ABUSE

Antisocial personality traits in a person's biological parents predict an increased risk of early-onset alcoholism and substance abuse (Cadoret et al., 1995). This is true even if children are adopted away at an early age (Cloninger, 1987; Cadoret et al., 1995; Sigvardsson et al., 1996). Adopted men whose biological fathers were early-onset antisocial alcoholics had a nine-fold increased risk of type 2 alcoholism (18% versus 2%) compared to those without such genetic predisposition regardless of the quality of the adoptee's home placement (Sigvardsson et al., 1996). In contrast, severe type 1 alcohol dependence was only weakly heritable in the absence of environmental influences that encouraged heavy drinking. These adoption findings are consistent with the recent twin findings of strong heritability for initiation of substance abuse (as seen in type 2 alcoholism) in contrast to the weak heritability of the transition from drug use to abuse or dependence (as seen in severe type 1 alcoholism).

Table 2. Genetic (H) and unique environmental (E) influences on the transition from any drug use to using five or more times by class of drug (Vietnam Era twin study, Tsuang et al., 1998).

Drug Type	H	E
Amphetamines	0	75
Cocaine	28	72
Heroin	1	99
Marijuana	53	47
Psychedelics	1	99
Sedatives	33	62

Likewise, antisocial personality traits in a person's own childhood and adolescence predict the early onset of substance abuse. The only prospective study is a study of the onset of alcoholism before age 28 years (Cloninger et al., 1988). Personality was rated at age 11 years prior to any substance use. High Novelty Seeking (impulsive-aggressive traits) and low Harm Avoidance (risk-taking) were most strongly predictive of early-onset alcohol abuse. These two childhood variables distinguished boys who had nearly 20-fold differences in their risk of alcohol abuse: the risk of alcohol abuse varied from 4 to 75% depending on childhood personality. Likewise, reviews of the personality correlates of substance abusers confirm that Novelty Seeking, as measured by reliable personality inventories, predicts early onset alcoholism, criminality, and other substance abuse (Howard et al., 1997).

In addition to the association with Novelty Seeking, severe alcohol dependence, as measured by the ICD-10 criteria for alcohol dependence in the Collaborative Study of the Genetics of Alcoholism (COGA), is also strongly correlated with the personality trait of low Self-directedness and low P300 amplitude in evoked potential studies. Self-directedness and P300 amplitude are themselves moderately correlated. The personality traits with the largest effect sizes in distinguishing subjects with severe alcohol dependence from those with no alcohol dependence are low Self-directedness (-0.85), high Novelty Seeking (+0.79), and low Cooperativeness (-0.79). Individuals who are low in Self-directedness are described as irresponsible, goal-less, helpless, and undisciplined.

They have difficulty controlling their emotional impulses to accomplish long-term goals such as sobriety. Individuals who are low in Cooperativeness are described as prejudiced, selfish, hostile, revengeful, and unprincipled. In other words, individuals who are high in Novelty Seeking, low in Self-directedness, and low in Cooperativeness have impulsive (cluster B) personality disorders, which are at high risk for comorbid substance abuse. These individuals are most frequently diagnosed as having antisocial or borderline personality disorders. These individuals are characterized by their inability to delay gratification, leading to both early initiation of drug experimentation and frequent transition to substance abuse or dependence.

GENOME SCANS FOR DETECTING LINKAGE & ASSOCIATION

Four large-scale genome scans have been carried out to identify chromosomal regions containing susceptibility genes for substance dependence (see review by Uhl et al., 2001) and personality traits related to substance dependence (Cloninger et al., 1998). Despite the difficulty of replicating linkage findings for complex phenotypes like substance dependence, some findings about linkage to alcohol dependence have been replicated in independent samples (Foroud et al., 2000): high risk for mild dependence on chromosome 1 (LOD 2.6) and for severe dependence on chromosome 7 (LOD 2.9). In addition there is replicated evidence (LOD 2.5) that a region on chromosome 4 near the alcohol dehydrogenase ADH3 locus has a protective effect against the development of alcoholism in Americans of European or African descent. This is consistent with other evidence that the high activity isoforms of ADH2 and ADH3, as well as low activity isoforms of acetaldehyde dehydrogenase ALDH2, protect against alcoholism in East Asians (Chen et al., 1999). These variant enzymes lead to accumulation of high levels of acetaldehyde, which causes unpleasant flushing and decreases the risk of alcohol dependence.

A gene for the serotonin 5HT1B receptor has been linked to type 2 alcoholism in two independent samples (see review by Uhl et al., 2001). In further work, this gene was associated with Harm Avoidance, which mediated its effect on alcohol dependence.

Although alcohol and nicotine dependence share most of their genetic variance according to twin studies, little overlap in specific chromosomal regions has been identified in preliminary genome scans of cigarette smokers (Straub et al., 1999). However, a polymorphism of the dopamine transporter is associated with individual differences in initiating and continuing to smoke cigarettes, an effect which is mediated by the joint association of cigarette smoking and the dopamine transporter with Novelty Seeking (Sabol et al., 1999).

A genome scan of 1494 single nucleotide polymorphisms (SNPs) in 667 substance abusers and 327 controls identified 42 associations with substance abuse that replicated in blacks and whites (Uhl et al., 2001). Nine loci were also replicated in the four prior genome scans of substance abusers. These nine replicated loci included the chromosome 4 region nearby the ADH3 locus and the locus for brain-derived neurotropic factor (BDNF), which is known to regulate dopamine and serotonin neurotransmitters that are strongly associated with substance dependence.

Genetic factors that influence the risk of specific end-organ complications have been examined, particularly for alcoholic liver disease. The risk of liver disease in alcoholics depends on individual differences in genes regulating specific cellular processes involving cytokines and cytochromes (Savolainen et al., 1996; Reed et al., 1997; Grove et al., 2000).

These replicated findings are very encouraging. However, it is not possible to identify specific genes that are necessary or sufficient to cause substance dependence. In complex behaviors like substance abuse that have a multifactorial etiology, the effects of individual genes are small and dependent on non-linear interactions with other genes and environmental events. For example, the dopamine receptor DRD4 exon III 7-repeat allele has been associated with high Novelty Seeking and increased risk of opiate dependence (Kotler et al., 1997). However, high Novelty Seeking has also been reported to be associated with the 10 repeat allele of the dopamine transporter DAT1, but only when the DRD4 7-repeate allele is absent (Van Gestel et al., 2002). Consequently, it may be necessary to identify and evaluate sets of several genes simultaneously in order to predict risk of a complex behavior like substance use or abuse in a particular individual (Comings et al., 2000).

IMPLICATIONS FOR TREATMENT OF SUBSTANCE ABUSE

At the present time there is insufficient knowledge to individualize treatment according to a person's genetic profile. However, as more specific molecular targets are identified, therapies can be developed to influence susceptibility and thereby prevent abuse or relapse into abuse.

What is most important to observe, however, is that the transition from substance use to abuse is largely influenced by non-genetic events that are unique to each individual. This suggests that individual self-efficacy, not genetic predisposition, is the most important factor in determining success in cessation of substance abuse. Accordingly, therapy must encourage a person to accept responsibility for substance abuse rather than blaming their genetic predisposition or external influences.

REFERENCES

1. Chen, C.C., Lu, R.B., Chen, Y.C., et al. (1999) "Interaction between the functional polymorphisms of the alcohol-metabolism genes in protection against alcoholism." *Am J Hum Genetics* 65:795-807.
2. Cloninger, C.R. (1987) "Neurogenetic adaptive mechanisms in alcoholism." *Science* 236:410-416.
3. Cloninger, C.R., Sigvardsson, S., Bohman, M. (1988) "Childhood personality predicts alcohol abuse in young adults." *Alcohol Clin Exp Res* 12:494-504.

4.   Cloninger, C.R., Van Eerdewegh, P., Goate, A., et al. (1998) "Anxiety proneness linked to epistatic loci in genome scan of human personality traits." *Am J Med Genetics* 81:313-317.

5.   Comings, D.E., Gade-Andavolu, R., Gonzalez, N., et al. (2000) "A multivariate analysis of 59 candidate genes in personality traits: the temperament and character inventory." *Clin Genet* 58:375-385.

6.   Foroud, T., Edenberg, H.J., Goate, A., et al. (2000) "Alcoholism susceptibility loci: confirmation studies in a replicate sample and further mapping." *Alcohol Clin Exp Res* 24:933-945.

7.   Van Gestel, S., Forsgren, T., Claes, S., et al. (2002) "Epistatic effect of genes from the dopamine and serotonin systems on the temperament traits of Novelty Seeking and Harm Avoidance." *Molecular Psychiatry* 7:448-450.

8.   Grove, J., Daly, A.K., Bassendine, M.F., et al. (2000) "Interleukin 10 promoter region polyorphisms and susceptibility to advanced alcoholic liver disease." *Gut* 46:540-545.

9.   Howard, M.O., Kivlahan, D., Walker, R.D. (1997) "Cloninger's tridimensional theory of personality and psychopathology: applications to substance use disorders." *J Stud Alcohol* 58:48-66.

10.   Kendler, K.S., Karkowski, L.M., Neale, M.C., et al. (2000) "Illicit psychoactive substance use, heavy use, abuse, and dependence in a US population-based sample of male twins." *Arch Gen Psychiatry* 57:261-269.

11.   Kendler, K.S., Karkowski, L.M., Corey, L.A., et al. (1999) "Genetic and environmental risk factors in the aetiology of illicit drug initiation and subsequent misuse in women." *British J Psychiatry* 175:351-356.

12.   Reed, T., Page, W.F., Viken, R.J., et al. (1996) "Genetic predisposition to organ-specific endpoints of alcoholism." *Alcohol Clin Exp Res* 20:1528-1533.

13.   Sabol, S.Z., Nelson, M.L., Fisher, C., et al. (1999) "A genetic association for cigarette smoking behavior." *Health Psychology* 18:7-13.

14.   Savolainen, V.T., Pajarinen, J., Perola, M., et al. (1997) "Polymorphism in the cytochrome P450 2E1 gene and the risk of alcoholic liver disease." *J Hepatology* 26:55-61.

15.   Sigvardsson, S., Bohman, Cloninger, C.R. (1996) "Replication of the Stockholm Adoption Study of alcoholism: confirmatory cross-fostering analysis." *Arch Gen Psychiatry* 53:681-687.

16.   Straub, R.E., Sullivan, P.F., Ma, Y., et al. (1999) "Susceptiblity genes for nicotine dependence: a genome scan and followup in an independent sample suggest that regions on chromosomes 2,4,10, 16, 17, and 18 merit further study." *Molecular Psychiatry* 4:129-144.

17.   True, W.R., Xian, H., Scherrer, J.F., et al. (1999) "Common genetic vulnerability for nicotine and alcohol dependence in men." *Arch Gen Psychiatry* 56:655-661.

18.   Tsuang, M.T., Lyons, M.J., Harley, R.M., et al. (1999) "Genetic and environmental influences on transitions in drug use." *Behavior Genetics* 29:473-479.

19. Tsuang, M.T., Lyons, M.J., Meyer, J.M., et al. (1998) "Co-occurrence of abuse of different drugs in men: the role of drug-specific and shared vulnerabilities." *Arch Gen Psychiatry* 55:967-972.

20. Uhl, G.R., Liu, Q., Walther, D., et al. "Polysubstance abuse—vulnerability genes: Genome scans for association, using 1,004 subjects and 1,494 Single-nucleotide polymorphisms." *Am J Hum Genet* 69:1290-1300, 20.

HUNTINGTON DISEASE AND OTHER CAG REPEAT DISORDERS

P.MICHAEL CONNEALLY, PH.D.
Department of Medical and Molecular Genetics, Indiana University School of Medicine, Indianapolis, Indiana USA

In 1991 Fischbeck and colleagues described the first CAG repeat disorder.[1] This created great excitement in the scientific community since it was a novel mutational mechanism leading to excess CAG repeats in the coding region of the gene, which was in turn expressed as extra polyglutamines in the functional protein. The disease they described was the motor neuron disease spinal and bulbar muscular atrophy also known as Kennedy's disease.

Two years later the Huntington Disease gene was cloned by the Huntington Disease Collaborative Research Group[2] as was the spinocerebellar ataxia type 1 genes by Orr and his colleagues;[3] both mutations were also found to be CAG repeat expansions in the coding regions of the respective genes. All three disorders are neurodegenerative. The latter two have variable onset, the greater the number of CAG repeats in the expansion, the earlier the onset of symptoms. With large repeats (>60) onset can occur at early as two years of age, fewer repeats can delay onset into the seventies with the mean age of onset in the late thirties.

Previous to these discoveries mutations were in general thought to be limited to a base-pair substitution or small insertions or deletions in a gene. Expanded CAG repeats have now been discovered in approximately 15 disorders, all of which have neurological deficits.

The proteins involved in these disorders have an independent function that, with the exception of Kennedy's disease and two others, are unknown. The gene involved in Kennedy's disease codes for the androgen receptor. A typical mutation in this X-linked gene causes testicular feminization, that is XY individuals who are phenotypically females. However, as with the genes involved in the other disorders there is a CAG triplet repeat in the coding region of the androgen receptor gene, which when expanded causes a very different type of disorder namely Kennedy's disease.

This review will briefly describe Huntington Disease (HD). With the exception of the clinical and pathological findings most of the characteristics of HD are similar to the other CAG repeat disorders.

Huntington Disease was first described in 1872 by George Huntington, an American physician. The cardinal features are choreiform movements and psychiatric symptoms leading to progressive dementia and premature death. The age of onset is variable with a mean of 38 years and an average duration, from onset to death, of 18 years. There is selective death of striatal and cortical neurons. Neuronal intranuclear inclusions containing the huntingtin protein are found both in HD patients and in mouse models of HD.[4]

The disease is inherited as an autosomal dominant and is due to a toxic gain of function in the mutant protein. The huntingtin gene has been transferred into a number of organisms. Transgenic mice exhibit neurological symptoms approximating those found in humans and are an ideal model system for studying the etiology of the disorder and also possibly useful for therapeutic intervention.[5]

An interesting aspect of these polyglutamate disorders is the paternal transmission found in the vast majority of juvenile (>20 years) onset of HD.[6] The reason eluded researchers until the discovery of the CAG repeat tract. During male meiosis there is expansion of CAGs in the huntingtin gene. The greater the length of the CAG repeat, the more likely there will be an expansion. The amount is positively correlated with the length of the original repeat. This does not occur during oogenesis and the precise reason for this disparity is unknown.

Once a number of these CAG repeat diseases were discovered, it became clear that a common pathogenic mechanism related to the extra polyglutamines in the tract of the mutant genes existed. The proteins containing these expanded polyglutamine tracts appear to have no homology to one another. In all cases, however, the length of the tract determines the age of onset and severity. In all of these disorders, the tract contains approximately 38 or more glutamine residues. Individuals with 36 or fewer repeats are clinically unaffected. The length of the repeat explains approximately 50 percent of the variability in age of onset suggesting that other factors are also involved. Examining the residual variance (after correcting for CAG repeat length) there is a familial component still present. Two other loci have been found to modulate onset with the possibility of others being involved.

A cardinal pathological feature of these disorders is the appearance of inclusions containing polyglutamate and ubiquitin in neurons and neuronal processes (neutrophils) in the affected area of the brain. The areas differ for each disorder.

The huntingtin protein is reported to co-localize to other cellular proteins to form the nuclear inclusions. It is not clear what causes these inclusions. However, the most prominent hypothesis for HD and other polyglutamine extended tract diseases is that their aggregation with other proteins, such as CREB binding protein, is the primary cause of the pathology and thus the disease state.[7,8]

A major goal to be achieved is therapeutic intervention. This would be most appropriate before onset of the disease since it is unlikely that any drug could repair damage already occurring in individuals after onset. Studies are underway to more precisely define onset. These studies will result in more precise evaluation of double blind intervention studies designed to prolong onset.

In a recent study to suppress polyglutamine aggregation and pathogenesis in drosophila, the expression of suppressor polypeptides delayed and limited the appearance of aggregates and protected photoreceptor neurons.[9] Should such findings eventually be useful in humans, this would be a major step forward in the search for a cure for this fatal neurodegenerative disorder.

ACKNOWLEDGMENTS

This work was supported by Public Health Service contract number N01-NS82398.

REFERENCES

1. LaSpada, A.R., Wilson, E.M., Lubahn, D.B., Harding, A.E., Fishbeck, K.H. (1991) "Androgen receptor gene mutations in X-linked spinal and bulbar muscular atrophy." *Nature* 352:77-79.
2. Huntington's Disease Collaborative Research Group (1993) "A novel gene containing a trinucleotide repeat that is unstable on Huntington's disease chromosomes." *Cell* 72:971-983.
3. Orr, H.T., Chung, M-Y., Banji, S., Kwiatkowski, Jr., T.J., Servadio, A., Beaudet, A.L., McCall, A.E., Dunick, L.A., Ranum, L.P.W., Zoghbi, H.Y. (1993) "Expansion of an unstable trinucleotide CAG repeat in spinocerebellar ataxia type 1." *Nat Genet* 4:221-226.
4. Reddy, P.H., William, M., Tale, D.A. (1999) "Recent advances in understanding the pathogenesis of Huntington's disease." *Trends Neurosci* 22:248-255.
5. Menalled, L.B., Chesselet, M-F. (2002) "Mouse models of Huntington's disease." *Trends Pharmacol Sci* 23:32-39.
6. Merritt, A.D., Conneally, P.M., Rahman, N.F., Drew, A.L. (1969) *Juvenile Huntington's chorea. In: Progress in Neuro-Genetics*, Barbeau A, Burnette JR (eds), pp 645-650, Excerpta Medica, Amsterdam.
7. Steffan, J.S., Karzantsev, A., Spasic-Boskovic, O., Greenwald, M., Ya-Zhen, Z., Gohler, H., Wanker, E.E., Bates, G.P., Housman, D.E., Thompson, L.M. (2000) "The Huntington's disease protein interacts with p53 and CREB-binding protein and represses transcription." *Proc Natl Acad Sci USA* 97:6763-6768.
8. Nucifora, F.C., Sasaki, M., Peters, M.F., Huang, H., Cooper, J.K., Yamada, M., Takahashi, H., Tsuji, S., Troncoso, J., Dawson, V.L., Dawson, T.M., Ross, C.A. (2001) "Interference by huntingtin and atrophin-1 with CBP mediated transcription leading to cellular toxicity." *Science* 291:2423-2428.
9. Kazantsev, A., Walker, H.A., Slepko, N., Bear, J.E., Preisinger, E., Steffan, J.S., Zhu, Y-Z., Gertler, F.B., Housman, D.E., Marsh, J.L., Thompson, L.M. (2002) "A bivalent Huntingtin binding peptide suppresses polyglutamine aggregation and pathogenesis in Drosophila." *Nat Genet* 30:367-376.

DEMENTIA FROM BRAIN VASCULAR DISEASE: THE SILENT EPIDEMIC

CHARLES DECARLI, M.D.
Professor of Neurology, Associate Director, Alzheimer's Disease Center, Department of Neurology, University of California at Davis, Davis, CA, USA

INTRODUCTION

Improved health has led to a growing population of older individuals at risk for later life cognitive impairment. This is particularly true of the oldest old (age greater than 85 years), whose segment of the population is growing the fastest (Fig. 1).

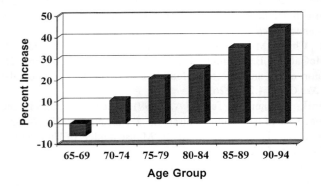

Fig. 1. Increase in Oldest Old for the United States, 1990-2000.

Such demographic changes have striking consequences for the population distribution in industrialized countries where this effect is greatest (Fig. 2). Previous population statistics show an age distribution where the vast majority of the population is less than 65 years of age and the proportion of older individuals declines with each 5-year increase in age similar to figures for less-developed nations (Fig. 2, right). Current predictions of aging demographics deviate substantially from this model and predict a nearly box-like age structure with as many individuals above the age of 65 years as those younger than 65 (Fig. 2, left). Since age is the single greatest risk factor for dementia

(Fig. 3), increasing numbers of older individuals within the population will have pronounced consequences for public health within our society.

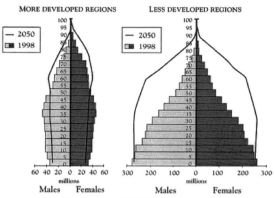

Source: United Nations Population Division, *World Population Prospects: The 1998 Revision*.

Fig. 2. Aging in Industrialized versus Developing Nations.

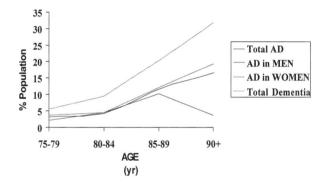

Fig. 3. Age-Specific Prevalence of Dementia.

While much attention has focused on the rising prevalence of older individuals and their risk for Alzheimer's disease,[1,2] the potential impact of cerebrovascular risk factors (CVRFs)—which can be treated—on later life cognitive function is just being recognized[3-7] (Fig. 4). Moreover, CVRFs may interact with Alzheimer's disease to increase the prevalence of late life dementia[8,10] (Fig. 5). Brain imaging techniques, in particular MRI, are able to detect cerebral injury in the absence of stroke, broadening our concept of cerebrovascular-related brain injury and the impact of potentially treatable CVRFs on brain aging and cognitive impairment. Further understanding of these relations, particularly with regard to the potential impact that CVRFs may have on progressive cognitive decline, could lead to new strategies designed to alleviate asymptomatic cerebrovascular brain injury and improve later life cognitive function.

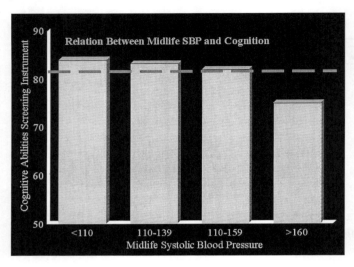

Fig. 4. Relation between Midlide SBP and Cognition.

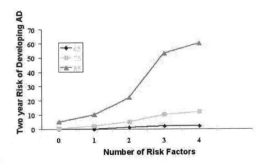

Fig. 5. Cerebrovascular Risk Factors and AD Incidence.

The Spectrum of Vascular Brain Changes

Stroke or symptoms of transient brain ischemia have long been viewed as the hallmark expression of cerebrovascular disease. Multiple studies conclusively show that the two most significant risk factors for stroke, advancing age and hypertension, are also the most common risk factors for cardiovascular and peripheral vascular disease, suggesting that these disorders share a common mechanism of vascular injury.[11-16] Unfortunately, less attention had been paid to the possible spectrum of brain injury resulting from hypertension or other CVRFs. Fortunately, the advent of neuroimaging has given rise to an era of rapid growth in studies examining the relation between CVRFs and brain structure. For example, early work showed that a considerable number of cerebral infarcts are clinically silent,[17-22] and more recent studies show that these apparently clinically silent brain infarctions are associated with significant behavioral changes.[23,24] In addition, the hallmark observations of Hachinski and colleagues that related abnormalities of cerebral white matter to CVRFs and diminished cognitive performance have been confirmed and extended.[30-36] Finally, the association between[25-29] CVRFs and accelerated cerebral atrophy has been explored.[37-40] The fact that white matter hyperintensities (WMH) significantly predicts future stroke[41] and mortality[42] lends further support to the notion of that WMH and other brain changes in the absence of clinically apparent stroke are part of a spectrum of vascular related brain injury.[36] Even in this brief review, it is apparent that CVRFs lead to a spectrum of brain injury including accelerated brain atrophy, abnormalities of cerebral white matter and even brain infarction without symptoms of stroke. Each of these brain changes likely affect behavior in a variety of ways, further expanding the clinical relevance of CVRFs.

THE IMPACT OF CEREBROVASCULAR RISK FACTORS ON THE BRAIN

CVRFs and Global Brain Atrophy

Early studies using x-ray computed tomography (CT) were the first to note brain atrophy in individuals with hypertension.[25,43,44] These observations were later confirmed by MRI[37] and extended to include evaluation of regional brain changes.[38,39] Salerno et. al. also were the first to note a significant correlation between the duration of hypertension.[37] Follow-up metabolic studies found significant regional metabolic changes with hypertension[37] in a pattern consistent with end-arterial distributions.[45] While it has been assumed that the vascular changes associated with chronic hypertension are the processes by which brain atrophy occurs, only limited work has been done to explore this relation.[46-48]

A recent longitudinal study of the NHLBI Twins, however, sheds further light on a possible relation between brain atrophy and the extent of vascular disease.[35] In this study, 31% had symptomatic cardiovascular disease (CHD), 11% had symptomatic cerebrovascular disease (CVD) and 8% had symptomatic peripheral vascular disease (PAD). Lifetime systolic blood pressure (SBP) was significantly correlated with brain volume (Fig. 6). In addition, lifetime SBP also was significantly associated with the extent of concurrent vascular disease measured at the time of brain imaging, with the prevalence of symptomatic CHD, CVD and PAD doubling for those individuals with a lifetime pattern of high BP.[35] While this association does not prove a causal relation between vascular injury and brain atrophy, it does support the notion of common processes that need further investigation.

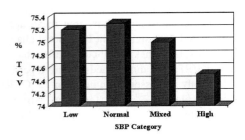

Fig. 6. Blood Pressure Pattern and Brain Volume.

A second study examining 1147 offspring of the original Framingham Heart Study, explored the relation between stroke risk factors and brain atrophy more directly.[49] In this study, Framingham Stroke Risk Scale scores were related to brain volume. The Framingham Stroke Risk Scale is a formula that can be used to predict 10-year risk for symptomatic stroke.[50,51] Subjects of this study were approximately 60 years of age at the time of MRI, but ranged in age from 40-84 years. Individuals with symptomatic stroke or dementia were excluded from the analysis. Importantly, Stroke Risk Scale Scores were determined approximately 5-8 years prior to brain MRI. There was a strong and highly significant relation between increasing Stroke Risk Scale scores and decreasing total brain volume after correcting for age and gender effects.[49] Secondary analyses found that the elevated systolic blood pressure, diabetes and smoking components of the Stroke Risk Scale where the most significant predictors. These results suggest that CVRFs known to predict clinically apparent stroke also predict significant reductions in brain volume and these effects appear to begin relatively early in life.

CVRFs and Hippocampal Volume

While extensive WMH and brain infarction are nearly always seen in the presence of VaD[52] or subcortical ischemic vascular disease,[53-55] it is generally assumed that hippocampal atrophy is specific to the AD process.[56-58] Recent work by Fein et al.,[59] however, found reduced hippocampal volumes in VaD. They reported WMH volumes twofold greater in a demented group with lacunes (representing subcortical ischemic vascular dementia) versus a cognitively normal group with lacunes, whereas WMH volumes were not significantly different in an AD versus cognitively normal group. Hippocampal volumes for both dementia groups were significantly smaller than controls, with the mean hippocampal volume being slightly, but not significantly larger in the VaD group.

The etiology of hippocampal and neocortical atrophy associated with vascular cognitive impairment remains unknown. Several potential and possibly overlapping possibilities may be considered. First, the presence of atrophy in VaD may reflect concomitant AD. Pathological study of three cases with VaD and hippocampal atrophy revealed the presence of neurofibrillary tangles (albeit mild) in each case.[59] Second, vascular brain injury may lead to secondary (deafferentation) neuronal degeneration or third, hippocampal atrophy may result directly from the ischemic process. It is clear that asymptomatic neuronal or axonal loss can occur from ischemic processes[60,61] and patients with severe WMH (i.e., Binswanger type vascular dementia) may be at particular risk for subclinical ischemia. Deficient autoregulatory reserve[62] and increased oxygen extraction fraction[63,64] occur in the presence of extensive WMH. Extensive WMH, therefore, may serve as a marker for impaired subcortical perfusion resulting in brain atrophy, including hippocampal atrophy.

From this evidence, I conclude that the pathogenesis of hippocampal atrophy in subcortical vascular impairment is variable and may reflect a combination of degenerative and ischemic pathologies. Unfortunately, our understanding of the pathological processes leading to global and regional brain atrophy remains unclear and more studies addressing the pathophysiology atrophy in VaD, including its relation to dementia, are needed.

CVRFS and WMH

In 1986, Hachinski, coined the term 'Leukoaraiosis' to describe abnormal cerebral white matter as seen on CT.[26,27] At nearly the same time, Awad reported 'Incidental Subcortical Lesions' seen on MRI.[65] In both instances, abnormalities of cerebral white matter were more prevalent and severe with advancing age and cerebrovascular disease. Since that time, an extensive literature examining various CVRFs associated with abnormal white matter (WMH) has developed.

The Cardiovascular Health Study (CHS) is currently the largest study to examine risk factors for WMH based on qualitative ratings.[66] Results from this study found that the strongest predictors of WMH were age, stroke, diastolic blood pressure, diuretic use and internal carotid artery thickness as measured from duplex ultrasonography.[67-69] Interestingly, however, if individuals with evidence of cerebral infarction are removed from the analyses, gender and orthostatic hypotension were significantly associated with WMH scores. A number of important conclusions can be drawn from these studies. First, approximately one-third of the CHS subjects were identified as having clinically silent cerebral infarctions. Second, there appeared to be a greater increase in WMH scores with age for women than for men. Third, WMH are significantly associated with other evidence of cerebral atherosclerosis, including extracranial carotid disease. Finally, the authors noted a strong relation between orthostatic hypotension and WMH score.

This unique observation, later confirmed in an independent sample,[36] suggests the potential for multiple causes of WMH. In particular, changes in vascular reactivity from long-standing hypertension may impair cerebral autoregulation resulting in transient hypoperfusion of the vulnerable end-artery supplied territories of cerebral white matter.[48]

The Rotterdam Scan Study comprising 1077 European subjects is another large population study with results similar to those found with the CHS.[70] Brain MRIs were qualitatively measured in a manner similar to the CHS. In an initial report of 111 subjects 65-84 years of age, 27% had evidence of WMH that increased in prevalence significantly with age.[70] Elevated blood pressure, hypertension and elevated cholesterol levels were significantly associated with the presence and severity of WMH only for those individuals 65-74 years of age. A history of stroke or myocardial infarction, and elevated factor VIIc activity, and fibrinogen levels were significantly and independently associated with the presence of WMH across the entire age range. Atrial fibrillation and carotid artery atherosclerosis were additionally found to be associated with increased WMH[71,72] and WMH were associated with reduced vasomotor reactivity.[48] Finally, these authors found a strong association between WMH determined in later-life and evidence of abdominal aortic atherosclerosis identified as the presence of aortic calcification seen on abdominal x-ray almost 20 years earlier.[73] The authors also showed that WMH were significantly more severe in women.[74] In addition to age and hypertension, other CVRFs such as atrial fibrillation and increased coagulation factors as well as female gender are also associated with WMH. These findings support previous observations that WMH may represent another general measure of vascular disease,[69,71,75.76] more common in older women.[68]

Both the CHS and Rotterdam studies focused primarily on individuals of European heritage. The Athersclerosis Risk in Communities (ARIC) study focused on a slightly younger, but bi-racial population of 1,920 individuals.[33,34] Using the same rating scale devised for the CHS, the ARIC study examined demographic, ethnic and CVRFs associated with WMH. In all ethnic and gender groups, prior history of hypertension was associated with significantly more severe WMH. A second important finding related to ethnic differences in WMH. African Americans consistently had greater WMH severity scores than European Americans. Importantly, however, this difference was moderated significantly when WMH severity scores were adjusted for significant mean differences in blood pressure between the two ethnic groups, implying an ethnic difference in hypertension and its treatment as the principal cause for ethnic differences in WMH. These findings have important public health consequences.

While these epidemiological studies have contributed significantly to our understanding of CVRFs associated with WMH, all have been principally cross-sectional studies, unable to assess the potential impact of lifetime trends in CVRFs, especially blood pressure, on WMH. As noted earlier, the National Heart Lung and Blood Institute (NHLBI) Twin Study is a longitudinal study designed to examine the potential genetic influences on cardiovascular disease allowing examination of the association between middle-life CVRFs and later-life brain injury. The 414 subjects of this study were an average of 72.5 ± 2.9 years of age at the time of MRI. There were strong correlations between middle life systolic blood pressure and later life WMH volume. In addition, orthostatic differences in systolic blood pressure were also significantly correlated with WMH volume.[36] Importantly, individuals with extensive WMH volumes (> 0.5% of intracranial volume) had significantly higher systolic blood pressure measures and significantly higher incident CVD and CAD as compared to individuals with normal WMH volumes, despite no significant differences in use of antihypertensive medications.[36] Results of this study suggested that WMH are associated with incident (and clinically relevant) vascular disease and may be the consequence of blood pressure changes beginning in middle age. The authors suggest that early and aggressive treatment of elevations in blood pressure in middle age might significantly reduce later life vascular disease.[36] A follow-up study, examined the vascular disease consequences of four lifetime patterns of systolic blood pressure.[35] In this analysis, individuals were identified as having low (<120 mmHg), normal (120-139 mmHg) and High (≥140 mmHg) systolic blood pressure measures at each of the first three examinations spanning approximately 15 years. Analysis of the relation between lifetime pattern of systolic blood pressure and WMH revealed a significant linear trend (Fig. 7). This suggested that blood pressure values were significantly associated with increased WMH volume, even when they were in the normal range confirming previous observations[77] and consistent with previous observations of the ARIC study.[33,34] This study also showed that the lifetime pattern of blood pressure for most individuals is relatively stable and that both the magnitude and the duration of blood pressure are likely important factors for the development of WMH.

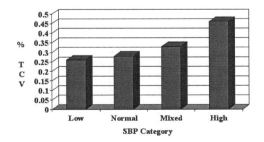

Fig. 7. Blood Pressure Pattern and WMHI Volume.

In conclusion, a large number of cross-sectional and longitudinal studies show strong relations between age, a variety of CVRFs, and the severity of WMH. These age-related changes may be worse for women and African Americans, although African

American increases in WMH probably reflect higher mean blood pressure during life. Importantly, it appears that the magnitude and duration of blood pressure elevation is most significant to WMH formation. This is particularly true if blood pressures remain elevated after treatment.[33,34,77] Moreover, it appears that the extent of brain WMH likely reflects the extent of vascular disease throughout the body, and that this process may begin in middle age. Finally, the degree of blood pressure considered abnormal might need to be reevaluated in light of the fact that even mild increases in blood pressure within the normal range are associated with increased WMH and incident vascular disease. Strategies aimed at aggressive treatment of blood pressure beginning in middle age may, therefore, be warranted.[36]

CVRFs and Clinically Silent Brain Infarction

Recent large-scale imaging and pathologic studies suggest that clinically asymptomatic cerebral infarction is present in approximately 15-25% of individuals over 65 years of age[17-22,24] (Fig. 8). Elevated systolic blood pressure is universally found in individuals with asymptomatic cerebral infarction,[17,19,20,22,24] but other studies also show that these individuals share many of the same cerebrovascular risk factors as those with clinically apparent stroke.[17,20-22,24] Cerebral infarctions seen on MRI are also significantly associated with WMH measures.[36,68] While not surprising, this association does reinforce the notion that WMH can be one manifestation of cerebrovascular disease.

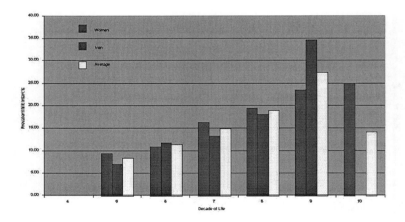

Fig. 8. Age and MRI Infarcts.

The major differences between individuals with stroke and those with silent cerebral infarction appear to relate to the size, location and number of infarcts found.[17-22,24] Patients with clinically apparent strokes generally have larger, cortically located infarcts,[17,18,20-22,24] or multiple cerebral infarcts,[22,24] although even small infarcts involving the thalamus are likely to be symptomatic.[24]

It is important to note, however, that while patients with clinically silent cerebral infarction fail to recognize their symptoms, these infarctions are often associated with neurological abnormalities. Results of the Cardiovascular Health Study[23,24] and the NHLBI Twin Study[78] reliably show that clinically silent cerebral infarcts are associated with moderate functional impairment. These studies most commonly found slowed or unbalanced gait as well as pyramidal type motor dysfunction. The impact of silent cerebral infarctions on cognition are discussed below.

Summary

In this section, I note that CVRFs are associated with a wide spectrum of brain changes in the absence of clinical stroke. The extent of WMH and possibly brain atrophy are often associated with other evidence of systemic atherosclerosis, such as coronary artery disease, peripheral vascular disease and increased carotid intimal wall thickness.[40,68-70] While the pathological processes that may cause generalized or regional brain atrophy are yet still poorly understood, there is considerable evidence to support the notion that WMH are the likely result of ischemic processes in most older individuals. These observations confirm that structural brain imaging, particularly with MRI, can be used as measure of clinically silent cerebrovascular injury.

With this understanding in mind, I next review the relation between these MRI findings and cognition in normal individuals, individuals with MCI and patients with dementia.

CVRFs, STRUCTURAL BRAIN CHANGES AND COGNITIVE IMPAIRMENT

Impact of CVRFs on Cognition in Community Dwelling Normal Individuals

A number of epidemiological studies show strong associations between elevations in middle life blood pressure and the prevalence of later life cognitive impairment and dementia.[5-7,79] The mechanisms by which CVRFs lead to cognitive impairment remain unclear, but a number of cross-sectional epidemiological studies as well as longitudinal prospective studies suggest that CVRF-related brain changes are associated with these cognitive changes.

Large epidemiological studies, while sometimes limited in the extent of cognitive testing available, consistently show moderate associations between brain atrophy or WMH volumes and diminished cognitive impairment.[68,80-84] A number of smaller, cross-sectional studies consistently suggest deficits in tests of attention and mental processing,[70,77,85,86] although impairments in memory and general intelligence are also seen.[70,77] A number of these studies also show a threshold effect where extensive amounts of WMH are necessary before cognitive impairments are seen.[77,85,86]

Two studies from the CHS have examined the relation between cognitive impairment and clinically silent cerebral infarction.[23,24] While Price et al. focused primarily on the neurological manifestations of silent cerebral infarcts, they did note a significant increase in the number of individuals with a history of memory loss amongst those with silent cerebral infarction.[23] Longstreth et al. examined cognitive function in more detail and noted a significant association between silent cerebral infarctions and diminished performances on the modified Mini-Mental State Examination and the Digit-Symbol Substitution Test.[24] These findings are remarkably similar to their previously reported effect of WMH on cognition.[68]

Unfortunately, these studies did not examine the impact of lifetime cerebrovascular risk on brain structure and cognition. Recent results from the NHLBI Twin Study, however, confirm the suspected link between CVRFs, brain injury and decline in cognitive performance over time.[35] Lifetime patterns of SBP were significantly associated with differences in brain atrophy, WMH volume and 10- year changes in MMSE and DSS scores.[35] Importantly, however, even after correcting for age, education, baseline cognitive performance and incident cerebrovascular disease, there were strongly significant associations between WMH volume, DSS, Benton Visual Retention Test (BVRT) and a Verbal Fluency Test (VFT). These results suggest that the cognitive changes associated with elevations in midlife blood pressure may be mediated by the brain injury induced by prolonged elevations of blood pressure (and possibly other CVRFs). A follow-up study of the same subjects explored the pattern of cognitive changes in association with midlife blood pressure patterns more carefully.[40] Cognitive tests selected for this study fell into the two broad functional categories of memory and psychomotor speed. Subjects with combined brain atrophy and WMH were significantly older and had a higher prevalence of CVRFs[40] and performed more poorly on all tests of psychomotor speed even after correcting for age, educational achievement and incident cerebrovascular disease, whereas group differences on memory tests were small. These results confirm the notion that the cognitive changes associated with CVRFs generally impact frontal executive functioning.[40]

Longitudinal studies offer the advantage of examining lifetime CVRFs influences on brain behavior relations. Unfortunately, these studies have generally focused on older individuals,[35,40] while epidemiological studies show that the impact of CVRFs—especially diabetes and hypertension—may occur at a considerably younger age.[3] Seshadri et al.[49] recently examined the relation between stroke risk factors, brain volume and cognition in a younger group of individuals with an average age of 62 years. Age-corrected differences in brain volume were significantly and positively associated with performance on tests of attention and executive function (e.g. Trails A and B), new learning (e.g. Paired Associates) and visuospatial function (e.g. delayed visual reproduction and Hooper visual organization test), but not with performance on tests of verbal memory or naming. While these results are consistent with those of Swan et al.,[40] they suggest that the impact of CVRFs on brain structure and function may begin shortly after midlife.

In summary, subtle cognitive deficits in community dwelling essentially normal individuals are associated with CVRFs and appear to be mediated by CVRF-related brain injury. CVRFs appear to effect brain structure and function relatively early in life, as cognitive impairment and brain injury are present to some degree even in individuals 60 years of age or younger. Frontal lobe mediated cognitive domains of attention, concentration and psychomotor speed appear to be most affected in subjects free of dementia or stroke. Given that CVRFs can cause brain injury and cognitive impairment, it is possible that these changes may contribute to later life dementia. In the following two sections, I explore the impact of cerebrovascular disease on clinically significant cognitive impairment.

CVRFS and Mild Cognitive Impairment

Mild Cognitive Impairment (MCI) has become increasingly recognized as common to later life.[87] Usually defined as isolated memory impairment in an otherwise healthy individual, MCI is associated with a yearly risk for Alzheimer's disease (AD) that varies from 1% to 25%.[88] Given that CVRFs, such as hypertension, are often associated with late-life brain abnormalities and cognitive impairment, DeCarli et al examined the potential contribution of CVRFs to MCI in the NHLBI Twin Study.[89] Using a standard definition of MCI, 37 of 369 or 10% of subjects were identified as having MCI. Univariate comparisons revealed that MCI subjects were significantly older, consumed significantly less alcohol and had significantly greater WMH volumes than subjects with normal memory. The prevalence of apolipoprotein E4 genotype (ApoE4) was marginally increased in the MCI group (31.4% versus 19.2%). WMH volume, ApoE4 and midlife blood pressure were associated with significantly increased risk for MCI in subjects free of symptomatic cerebrovascular disease. From these results, the authors concluded that CVRFs increase the risk for the MCI. This study is somewhat limited by its focus on older male veteran twins who may not adequately reflect the general population and did not assess the possible contribution of AD pathology (e.g. by measuring hippocamapus volume). In a second study, similar relationships between WMH and cognition were found in a community based, population study that also included measurement of hippocampal volume.

In this study, a sample of 122 subjects was selected from the Sacramento Area Latino Study on Aging (SALSA), and subjects were categorized into four groups of increasing levels of cognitive impairment: normal, memory impaired (MI), cognitively impaired but not demented (CIND), and demented.[90] Hippocampal volume was quantified using a region of interest approach and WMH were rated on a semi-quantitative scale. The authors found that hippocampal volume was significantly reduced in CIND and demented individuals, and WMH were significantly increased in demented subjects. The risk for developing dementia was significantly and comparably increased in subjects with either hippocampal atrophy or high WMH. However, the risk for dementia increased dramatically in subjects with both hippocampal atrophy and high degree of WMH (Figs. 9 and 10). From this data, the authors conclude that reductions in hippocampal volume may be present before dementia, but not until cognitive impairment is relatively severe. Furthermore because of the synergistic effect between high WMH and hippocampal atrophy, interactions between vascular and degenerative processes may be important determinants of CIND and dementia.

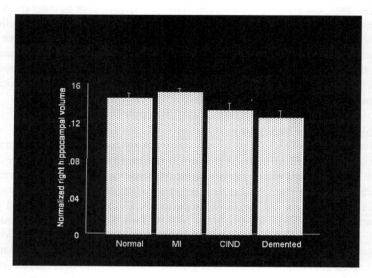

Fig. 9. Cognitive State and Hippocampal Volume.

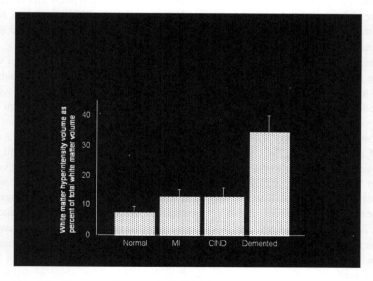

Fig. 10. Cognitive State and WMH Volume.

While these data support a significant synergistic effect for CVD on AD leading to MCI or CIND, follow-up evaluations of these individuals with brain vascular injury and MCI will be necessary to determine whether they progress to dementia and if so, the type of dementia they develop. A preliminary report suggests that WMH may increase the likelihood of conversion to AD.[91]

CVRFS and Dementia

The relative impact of cerebrovacular disease on dementia occurrence has a long and debatable history.[92,93] While there is a well developed literature with regard to dementia after stroke,[94-101] it remains quite common to identify individuals who have a slowly progressive dementing illness, multiple CVRFs and extensive WMH or lacunar infarction detected by brain imaging. Currently, the impact of this asymptomatic cerebrovascular brain injury remains unclear, but accumulating evidence suggests that CVRFs and the accompanying brain injury associated with them may significantly increase the likelihood to develop dementia.[8,91] In this section, I review possible anatomical substrates that may be necessary for the development of dementia in the setting of cerebrovascular disease.

It is clear that CVRFs influence cognition through brain injury. It is unclear, however, why some individuals with cerebrovascular injury in the absence of clinical stroke develop dementia, whereas others do not. Certain anatomical brain differences amongst demented patients with CVRFs suggest a possible explanation. For example, early studies of incident dementia after stroke found that brain atrophy at the time of stroke was a significant predictor of dementia.[95] Fein et al., also noted striking brain atrophy—greater than in the AD group—amongst individuals with dementia and lacunar infarcts.[59] Importantly, Fein et al.,[59] also noted significant hippocampal atrophy in the same group. As noted above with the SALSA study, a possible interaction between AD and CVD may significantly increase the likelihood to develop dementia.[90] In this study, the authors noted that the presence of extensive WMH and hippocampal atrophy were each independently associated with an increased risk for dementia, but this effect was additive in the presence of both brain changes.[90] While these data come from a population study of Hispanics and may not directly generalize to other ethnic populations,[3] it does suggest that anatomical brain changes associated with AD and cerebrovascular disease may interact to create dementia.[8,102]

The independent impact of WMH on dementia incidence in the absence of CVRFs, however, remains controversial. For example, WMH are common in AD,[103-109] but may be the consequence of amyloid deposition in cerebral vessels.[110] While some studies find significant relationships between WMH and certain cognitive functions or dementia severity,[111-117] other studies[77,103-105,107-109,118-131] do not. Differences in study populations and the heterogeneity of white matter changes may explain the inconsistency amongst these studies. For example, selection of AD patients without vascular risk factors may result in excluding individuals with extensive WMH,[119] therefore minimizing their effects (i.e. the vascular impact of amyloid deposition in the absence of CVRFs may be small). In patients with CVRFs and dementia, small subcortical infarcts also frequently accompany WMH[132,133] obscuring the independent effects that WMH confer to the dementia.[124] Although I note that Fein et al.[59] found no effect of the number of lacunes or the location of the lacunes on dementia prevalence in their study. The type of neuroimaging technique used to detect WMH may also be an important factor in defining the relation between WMH and dementia given that MRI is more sensitive to WMH than CT.[134-137] It may also be that extensive WMH are necessary to convey injury[77,86] and many negative studies fail to take this possibility into account. Finally, as noted earlier, the impact of brain atrophy on dementia prevalence is probably very large, but rarely considered[116,138] although some studies[103,113,122] have analyzed cerebrospinal fluid volumes. Importantly, Fein et al.,[59] noted significant correlations between the extent of WMH and gray matter volume across dementia groups. It is therefore possible that diffuse brain atrophy in association with extensive WMH may be an index of neuronal and synaptic loss and increase the risk for dementia, although the ultimate impact of WMH on dementing processes remains to be completely understood.

In summary, it appears that the presence of generalized brain and hippocampal atrophy are important anatomic substrates for dementia irrespective of cause.[59] White matter injury resulting in WMH may lead to brain atrophy, but this relation has been incompletely studied. Interestingly, the independent role of asymptomatic lacunar infarcts is less clear,[59] with the possible exception of those involving the thalamus.[24,139] Moreover, while it is clear that individuals may have a slowly progressive dementing illness caused by CVD,[59] most individuals with this type of clinical history probably have some component of AD pathology as part of their dementia. The relative importance of finding brain structural evidence of cerebrovascular disease in a demented individual clearly needs further study.

Summary

In this section, I note that CVRFs impact on cognition through brain injury. Community dwelling individuals with CVRFs have modest cognitive impairment related primarily to the presence of WMH and accelerated brain atrophy. Frontal mediated cognitive processes appear disproportionately affected in these individuals. WMH also appear associated with mild cognitive impairment, but more extensive generalized atrophy and the presence of hippocampal atrophy may be necessary before dementia is manifest. Within demented individuals with CVD, frontal mediated processes may be affected,[140,141,142] but differences in specific cognitive domains are often obscured by the generalized cognitive impairments of the dementia. The role of concurrent AD is likely important to the genesis of dementia in many individuals with asymptomatic CVD and dementia, explaining, in part, the possible mechanism by which CVRFs increase the prevalence of AD.[10,31,81,84,102,143-147]

PATHOPHYSIOLOGY

The exact mechanism by which CVRFs might increase the rate of cognitive decline in AD is unclear and may have multiple explanations. For example, brain injury from CVD might enhance the clinical expression of AD in an additive or synergistic manner.[8]

Alternatively, CVD and AD may share genetic (e.g. apolipoprotein _ 4 genotype) or other risk factors that make an individual susceptible to both disorders. Finally, CVD may actually work in some way to increase AD pathology.

The possibility of an additive or synergistic effect of CVD on AD has the most compelling scientific support. Post-mortem studies suggest that the presence of even small amounts of infarcted brain tissue can substantially amplify the effects of AD neuropathology on cognition,[8,148-150] particularly when the AD changes are mild,[149] although not all studies support this finding.[151] Behavioral data also indicate that small strokes often cause cognitive impairment.[99,152-155] Moreover, cognitive impairment with stroke may result from dysfunction of different brain systems than those initially affected by AD,[141] suggesting that stroke and AD may have synergistic effects on cognition because they combine to compromise multiple functional systems.

Epidemiological data offer further support for a synergistic relationship between CVD and AD. For example, several epidemiological studies show strong associations between middle life blood pressure elevation and later life dementia[5,7,79,156-159] (Fig. 4) including increased risk for AD specifically[4,160,161] (Fig. 5). Whether these shared risk factors increase the incidence of AD by causing CVD, thus amplifying the effects of AD pathology and increasing the likelihood of expressed disease[8] is unknown at this time. An alternative is that certain risk factors for CVD are additionally pathogenic for AD neuropathology. This may particularly be true for apolipoprotein _ 4 (ApoE4), which not only increases the risk for AD, but also modulates the effects of vascular disease on the brain.[160,162] For example, ApoE4 polymorphisms enhance the extent of neuronal damage from cerebral ischemia,[163,164] the vascular complications of diabetes,[165] and the risk of dementia in relation to smoking.[166-168] ApoE4 and CVD also may have a synergistic effect on cognition. Studies show that the combined presence of CVD and ApoE4 diminishes late life cognitive performance[169,170] and increases the prevalence of AD[145] significantly more than expected from the independent effects of CVD or ApoE4 genotype alone. A similar relation between elevated levels of serum homocysteine, vascular disease and increased risk for AD has been found as well. Finally, a number of provocative studies suggest that CVD may even play a pathogenetic role in the development of AD.[9,171-173]

TREATMENT

While this review has focused primarily on the effects of CVRFs and their possible interaction with AD, it is important to recognize that most CVRFs are currently treatable. Although little information is available regarding the cognitive effects of treating all CVRFs, early evidence suggests considerable success with treating hypertension amongst the elderly.[174-176] In the Syst-Eur trial,[174] cognition was primarily assessed by the mini-mental state examination.[177] Treatment with a calcium channel blocking antihypertensive was associated with a nearly 50% reduction in incident dementia amongst approximately 2,000 elderly with isolated systolic hypertension.[174] Given the high percentage of elderly suffering with untreated hypertension,[178] secondary prevention treatment trials such as

Syst-Eur may have a substantial impact on cognitive impairment amongst the elderly. Of course, further work regarding treatment of other CVRFs such as diabetes is also necessary to fully realize the potential impact.

CONCLUSIONS

In this review I have examined a large and growing body of literature that seeks to understand the impact of CVRFs on brain structure and behavior. I note that a broad spectrum of brain injury may result in response to asymptomatic CVD. Brain atrophy, WMH and silent cerebral infarction appear to be manifestations of brain injury due to CVD in the absence of stroke. Each of these brain changes in response to CVRFs also mirror diseases of other bodily systems, supporting the notion that asymptomatic brain injury may reflect systematic vascular disease. I also note that accelerated brain atrophy is a common response to CVRFs and may occur relatively early in life. While a number of studies suggest brain atrophy may result from ischemic processes, this conclusion is far from proven and further work is necessary, particularly with regard to regional brain changes such as hippocampal atrophy. WMH also consistently occur in the setting of CVRFs and are strongly associated with vascular disease in other organ systems. Finally, I note that WMH, brain atrophy and brain infarction appear to result from similar processes, and yet, these processes not highly correlated in magnitude. This may reflect distinct, but currently unknown processes by which these types of brain injury occur, also deserving further study.

Despite the need for further understanding of the pathophysiology by which CVRFs lead to brain injury, it is clear from this review that these types of brain injury are associated with a spectrum of cognitive impairment. Subtle brain injury, generally manifest as brain atrophy and increased WMH, is often associated with only subtle cognitive impairment that appears to disproportionately affect frontal mediated cognitive function. These subtle brain changes may also place an individual at risk for symptomatic memory impairment such as that seen with MCI as well as increases the risk of an individual with MCI to develop dementia. More severe brain injury appears to accompany dementia. Individuals with dementia often have extensive WMH and significant brain atrophy, particularly hippocampal atrophy. Surprisingly, from my review, it appears that lacunar infarcts (with the possible exception of those in the thalamus) may not predict an individual's risk for cognitive impairment when brain and WMH volumes are known. Unfortunately, a clear understanding of the impact of CVD on dementia remains somewhat allusive as many older individuals with CVD also have concomitant AD. I postulate, however, that these two diseases likely interact in a synergistic manner to increase the likelihood of expressed dementia and possibly accelerate the course of the disease (Fig. 11).

While further research regarding the impact of clinically silent CVD on brain structure and behavior remains to be done, available evidence strongly suggests that CVRFs lead to pernicious brain injury and cognitive impairment. The public health consequences of this observation are potentially enormous, but rectifiable as CVRFs remain the most common, but easily treatable cause of morbidity and mortality for our aging population.

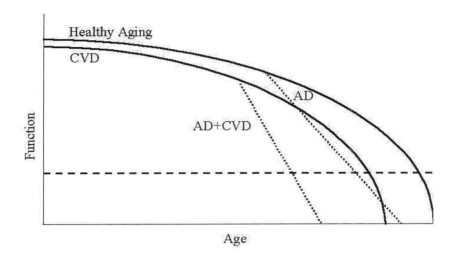

Fig. 11.

   In conclusion, improved health has led to a growing population of older individuals at risk for later life cognitive impairment. While much attention has focused on the rising prevalence of Alzheimer's disease,[1,2] the impact of CVRFs on later life cognitive function is just being recognized.[3,7] Importantly, CVRFs may interact with Alzheimer's disease to increase the prevalence of late life dementia.[8,10] Brain imaging techniques, particularly MRI, are sensitive to cerebral injury in the absence of stroke, broadening our concept of cerebrovascular-related brain injury and the impact of potentially treatable CVRFs on brain aging and cognitive impairment. Further understanding of these relations, particularly with regard to the potential impact that CVRFs may have on progressive cognitive decline, could lead to new strategies designed to alleviate asymptomatic cerebrovascular brain injury and improve later life cognitive function.

REFERENCES

1.   Beiser, A., et al., "Computing estimates of incidence, including lifetime risk: Alzheimer's disease in the Framingham Study. The Practical Incidence Estimators (PIE) macro." *Statistics in Medicine,* 2000. **19**(11-12): p. 1495-522.

2. Fratiglioni, L., et al., "Incidence of dementia and major subtypes in Europe: A collaborative study of population-based cohorts. Neurologic Diseases in the Elderly Research Group." *Neurology,* 2000. **54**(11 Suppl 5): p. S10-5.

3. Knopman, D., et al., "Cardiovascular risk factors and cognitive decline in middle-aged adults." *Neurology,* 2001. **56**(1): p. 42-48.

4. Launer, L.J., et al., "Midlife blood pressure and dementia: the Honolulu-Asia aging study." *Neurobiology of Aging,* 2000. **21**(1): p. 49-55.

5. Elias, M.F., Wolf, P.A, D'Agostino, R.B., Cobb, J., White, L.R., "Untreated blodd pressure level is inversely related to cognitive functioning: the Framingham Study."*Am J Epidemiology,* 1993. **138**: p. 353-364.

6. Elias, M.F., et al., "Neuropsychological test performance, cognitive functioning, blood pressure, and age: the Framingham Heart Study." *Experimental Aging Research,* 1995. **21**(4): p. 369-91.

7. Elias, P.K., et al., "Blood pressure, hypertension, and age as risk factors for poor cognitive performance." *Experimental Aging Research,* 1995. **21**(4): p. 393-417.

8. Snowdon, D.A., et al., "Brain infarction and the clinical expression of Alzheimer disease. The Nun Study." *JAMA,* 1997. **277**(813-817).

9. Petrovitch, H., et al., "Midlife blood pressure and neuritic plaques, neurofibrillary tangles, and brain weight at death: the HAAS. Honolulu-Asia aging Study." *Neurobiology of Aging,* 2000. **21**(1): p. 57-62.

10. Breteler, M.M., et al., "Risk factors for vascular disease and dementia." *Haemostasis,* 1998. **28**(3-4): p. 167-73.

11. Weber, M.A., "Role of hypertension in coronary artery disease." *American Journal of Nephrology,* 1996. **16**(3): p. 210-6.

12. Gillum, R.F., "Coronary heart disease, stroke, and hypertension in a U.S. national cohort: the NHANES I Epidemiologic Follow-up Study. National Health and Nutrition Examination Survey." *Annals of Epidemiology,* 1996. **6**(4): p. 259-62.

13. Zheng, Z.J., et al., "Associations of ankle-brachial index with clinical coronary heart disease, stroke and preclinical carotid and popliteal atherosclerosis: the Atherosclerosis Risk in Communities (ARIC) Study." *Atherosclerosis,* 1997. **131**(1): p. 115-25.

14. Papademetriou, V., et al., "Influence of risk factors on peripheral and cerebrovascular disease in men with coronary artery disease, low high-density lipoprotein cholesterol levels, and desirable low-density lipoprotein cholesterol levels. HIT Investigators. Department of Veterans Affairs HDL Intervention Trial." *American Heart Journal,* 1998. **136**(4 Pt 1): p. 734-40.

15. Cooper, R., et al., "Trends and disparities in coronary heart disease, stroke, and other cardiovascular diseases in the United States: findings of the national conference on cardiovascular disease prevention." *Circulation,* 2000. **102**(25): p. 3137-47.

16. Antikainen, R., P. Jousilahti, and J. Tuomilehto, "Systolic blood pressure, isolated systolic hypertension and risk of coronary heart disease, strokes, cardiovascular

disease and all-cause mortality in the middle-aged population." *Journal of Hypertension*, 1998. **16**(5): p. 577-83.

17. Boon, A., et al., "Silent brain infarcts in 755 consecutive patients with a first-ever supratentorial ischemic stroke. Relationship with index-stroke subtype, vascular risk factors, and mortality." *Stroke*, 1994. **25**(12): p. 2384-90.

18. Brott, T., et al., "Baseline silent cerebral infarction in the Asymptomatic Carotid Atherosclerosis Study." *Stroke*, 1994. **25**(6): p. 1122-9.

19. Ezekowitz, M.D., et al., "Silent cerebral infarction in patients with nonrheumatic atrial fibrillation. The Veterans Affairs Stroke Prevention in Nonrheumatic Atrial Fibrillation Investigators." *Circulation*, 1995. **92**(8): p. 2178-82.

20. Jørgensen, H.S., et al., "Silent infarction in acute stroke patients. Prevalence, localization, risk factors, and clinical significance: the Copenhagen Stroke Study" [see comments]. *Stroke*, 1994. **25**(1): p. 97-104.

21. Kase, C.S., et al., "Prevalence of silent stroke in patients presenting with initial stroke: the Framingham Study." *Stroke*, 1989. **20**(7): p. 850-2.

22. Shinkawa, A., et al., "Silent cerebral infarction in a community-based autopsy series in Japan. The Hisayama Study." *Stroke*, 1995. **26**(3): p. 380-5.

23. Price, T.R., et al., "Silent brain infarction on magnetic resonance imaging and neurological abnormalities in community-dwelling older adults. The Cardiovascular Health Study. CHS Collaborative Research Group." *Stroke*, 1997. **28**(6): p. 1158-64.

24. Longstreth, W.T., Jr., et al., "Lacunar infarcts defined by magnetic resonance imaging of 3660 elderly people: the Cardiovascular Health Study." *Archives of Neurology*, 1998. **55**(9): p. 1217-25.

25. Steingart, A., et al., "The significance of white matter lucencies on CT scan in relation to cognitive impairment." *Canadian Journal of Neurological Sciences*, 1986. **13**(4 Suppl): p. 383-4.

26. Hachinski, V.C., P. Potter, and H. Merskey, "Leuko-araiosis: an ancient term for a new problem." *Canadian Journal of Neurological Sciences*, 1986. **13**(4 Suppl): p. 533-4.

27. Hachinski, V.C., P. Potter, and H. Merskey, "Leuko-araiosis." *Archives of Neurology*, 1987. **44**(1): p. 21-3.

28. Steingart, A., et al., "Cognitive and neurologic findings in subjects with diffuse white matter lucencies on computed tomographic scan (leuko-araiosis)." *Archives of Neurology*, 1987. **44**(1): p. 32-5.

29. Steingart, A., et al., "Cognitive and neurologic findings in demented patients with diffuse white matter lucencies on computed tomographic scan (leuko-araiosis)." *Archives of Neurology*, 1987. **44**(1): p. 36-9.

30. Yue, N.C., et al., "Sulcal, ventricular, and white matter changes at MR imaging in the aging brain: data from the cardiovascular health study [see comments]." *Radiology*, 1997. **202**(1): p. 33-9.

31. Ott, A., et al., "Diabetes mellitus and the risk of dementia: The Rotterdam Study [see comments]". *Neurology*, 1999. **53**(9): p. 1937-42.

32. Manolio, T.A., Kronmal, R.A., Burke, G.l.,et.a., "Magnetic resonance abnormalities and cardiovascular disease in older adults: the Cardiovascular Health Study." *Stroke*, 1994. **25**: p. 318-327.

33. Liao, D., et al., "Presence and severity of cerebral white matter lesions and hypertension, its treatment, and its control. The ARIC Study. Atherosclerosis Risk in Communities Study." *Stroke*, 1996. **27**(12): p. 2262-70.

34. Liao, D., et al., "The prevalence and severity of white matter lesions, their relationship with age, ethnicity, gender, and cardiovascular disease risk factors: the ARIC Study." *Neuroepidemiology*, 1997. **16**(3): p. 149-62.

35. Swan, G.E., et al., "Association of midlife blood pressure to late-life cognitive decline and brain morphology." *Neurology*, 1998. **51**(4): p. 986-93.

36. DeCarli, C., et al., "Predictors of brain morphology for the men of the NHLBI twin study." *Stroke*, 1999. **30**(3): p. 529-36.

37. Salerno, J.A., et al., "Brain atrophy in hypertension. A volumetric magnetic resonance imaging study." *Hypertension*, 1992. **20**(3): p. 340-8.

38. Strassburger, T.L., et al., "Interactive effects of age and hypertension on volumes of brain structures." *Stroke*, 1997. **28**(7): p. 1410-7.

39. Garner, J., et al., "Regional brain differences after sustained elevations of systolic blood pressure: 25 year follow-up of the NHLBI Twins." *Neurology*, 1998. **50**(Supplement 4): p. A196.

40. Swan, G.E., et al., "Biobehavioral characteristics of nondemented older adults with subclinical brain atrophy." *Neurology*, 2000. **54**(11): p. 2108-14.

41. Miyao, S., et al., "Leukoaraiosis in relation to prognosis for patients with lacunar infarction." *Stroke*, 1992. **23**(10): p. 1434-8.

42. Streifler, J.Y., Eliasziw, M., Fox, A.J., et. al., "Prognostic importance of leukoaraiosis in patients with ischemic events and carotid artery disease." *Stroke*, 1999. **30**: p. 254.

43. Hatazawa, J., et al., "Association of hypertension with increased atrophy of brain matter in the elderly." *J Am Geriatr Soc*, 1984. **32**: p. 370-374.

44. Inzitari, D., et al., "Vascular risk factors and leuko-araiosis." *Archives of Neurology*, 1987. **44**(1): p. 42-7.

45. Mentis, M.J., et al., "Reduction of functional neuronal connectivity in long-term treated hypertension." *Stroke*, 1994. **25**(3): p. 601-7.

46. Tajima, A., et al., "Smaller local brain volumes and cerebral atrophy in spontaneously hypertensive rats." *Hypertension*, 1993. **21**(1): p. 105-11.

47. Gesztelyi, G., et al., "Parenchymal microvascular systems and cerebral atrophy in spontaneously hypertensive rats." *Brain Research*, 1993. **611**(2): p. 249-57.

48. Bakker, S.L., et al., "Cerebral vasomotor reactivity and cerebral white matter lesions in the elderly." *Neurology*, 1999. **52**(3): p. 578-83.

49. Seshadri, S., Wolf, P.A., Beiser, A., Elias, M.F., Au, R., Kase, C.S., D'Agostino, R.B., DeCarli,C., "Stroke risk profile predicts brain volume and cognitive function in stroke-free subjects: the Framingham Study." *Stroke*, 2001. **32**(1): p. 321-c.

50. D'Agostino, R.B., et al., "Stroke risk profile: adjustment for antihypertensive medication. The Framingham Study." *Stroke*, 1994. **25**(1): p. 40-3.

51. Wolf, P.A., et al., "Probability of stroke: a risk profile from the Framingham Study." *Stroke*, 1991. **22**(3): p. 312-8.

52. Liu, C.K., et al., "A quantitative MRI study of vascular dementia." *Neurology*, 1992. **42**(1): p. 138-43.

53. Fukuda, H., et al., "Age-related changes in cerebral white matter measured by computed cranial tomography." *Computerized Medical Imaging and Graphics*, 1990. **14**(1): p. 79-84.

54. Corbett, A., H. Bennett, and S. Kos, "Cognitive dysfunction following subcortical infarction." *Archives of Neurology*, 1994. **51**(10): p. 999-1007.

55. Sultzer, D.L., et al., "Cortical abnormalities associated with subcortical lesions in vascular dementia. Clinical and position emission tomographic findings." *Archives of Neurology*, 1995. **52**(8): p. 773-80.

56. Jack, C.R., Jr., et al., "Medial temporal atrophy on MRI in normal aging and very mild Alzheimer's disease [see comments]." *Neurology*, 1997. **49**(3): p. 786-94.

57. Jack, C.R., Jr., et al., "Rates of hippocampal atrophy correlate with change in clinical status in aging and AD." *Neurology*, 2000. **55**(4): p. 484-89.

58. Jack, C.R., et al., "Antemortem MRI findings correlate with hippocampal neuropathology in typical aging and dementia." *Neurology*, 2002. **58**: p. 750-757.

59. Fein, G., et al., "Hippocampal and cortical atrophy predict dementia in subcortical ischemic vascular disease." *Neurology*, 2000. **55**: p. 1626-1635.

60. Garcia, J.H., "The evolution of brain infarcts. A review." *Journal of Neuropathology and Experimental Neurology*, 1992. **51**(4): p. 387-93.

61. Garcia, J.H. and G.G. Brown, "Vascular dementia: neuropathologic alterations and metabolic brain changes." *Journal of the Neurological Sciences*, 1992. **109**(2): p. 121-31.

62. Kuwabara, Y., et al., "Cerebrovascular responsiveness to hypercapnia in Alzheimer's dementia and vascular dementia of the Binswanger type [see comments]." *Stroke*, 1992. **23**(4): p. 594-8.

63. Yao, H., et al., "Leukoaraiosis and dementia in hypertensive patients." *Stroke*, 1992. **23**(11): p. 1673-7.

64. Hatazawa, J., et al., "Subcortical hypoperfusion associated with asymptomatic white matter lesions on magnetic resonance imaging." *Stroke*, 1997. **28**(10): p. 1944-7.

65. Awad, I.A., et al., "Incidental subcortical lesions identified on magnetic resonance imaging in the elderly. I. Correlation with age and cerebrovascular risk factors." *Stroke*, 1986. **17**(6): p. 1084-9.

66. Bryan, R.N., et al., "A method for using MR to evaluate the effects of cardiovascular disease on the brain: the cardiovascular health study." *American Journal of Neuroradiology*, 1994. **15**(9): p. 1625-33.

67. Manolio, T.A., et al., *Magnetic resonance abnormalities and cardiovascular disease in older adults. The Cardiovascular Health Study.* Stroke, 1994. **25**(2): p. 318-27.

68. Longstreth, W.T., Jr., et al., "Clinical correlates of white matter findings on cranial magnetic resonance imaging of 3301 elderly people. The Cardiovascular Health Study [see comments]." *Stroke*, 1996. **27**(8): p. 1274-82.

69. Manolio, T.A., et al., "Relationships of cerebral MRI findings to ultrasonographic carotid atherosclerosis in older adults : the Cardiovascular Health Study. CHS Collaborative Research Group." *Arteriosclerosis, Thrombosis, and Vascular Biology*, 1999. **19**(2): p. 356-65.

70. Breteler, M.M., van Amerongen, N.M., van Swieten, J.C., Claus, J.J., Grobbee,D.E., van Gijn, J., Hofman, A.,van Harskamp, F., "Cognitive correlates of ventricular enlargement and cerebral white matter lesions on MRI: the Rotterdam Study." *Stroke*, 1994. **25**: p. 1109-1115.

71. de Leeuw, F.E., et al., "Carotid atherosclerosis and cerebral white matter lesions in a population based magnetic resonance imaging study." *Journal of Neurology*, 2000. **247**(4): p. 291-6.

72. de Leeuw, F.E., et al., "Atrial fibrillation and the risk of cerebral white matter lesions." *Neurology*, 2000. **54**(9): p. 1795-801.

73. de Leeuw, F.E., et al., "Aortic atherosclerosis at middle age predicts cerebral white matter lesions in the elderly." *Stroke*, 2000. **31**(2): p. 425-9.

74. de Leeuw, F.E., et al., "Prevalence of cerebral white matter lesions in elderly people: a population based magnetic resonance imaging study. The Rotterdam Scan Study." *J Neurol Neurosurg Psychiatry*, 2001. **70**: p. 9-14.

75. O'Leary, D.H., et al., "Thickening of the carotid wall. A marker for atherosclerosis in the elderly? Cardiovascular Health Study Collaborative Research Group.." *Stroke*, 1996. **27**(2): p. 224-31.

76. O'Leary, D.H., et al., "Carotid-artery intima and media thickness as a risk factor for myocardial infarction and stroke in older adults. Cardiovascular Health Study Collaborative Research Group [see comments]." *New England Journal of Medicine*, 1999. **340**(1): p. 14-22.

77. DeCarli, C., et al., "The effect of white matter hyperintensity volume on brain structure, cognitive performance, and cerebral metabolism of glucose in 51 healthy adults." *Neurology*, 1995. **45**(11): p. 2077-84.

78. Carmelli, D., et al., "Silent brain infarction on MRI and neurological deficits in older male twins from the NHLBI Twin Study." *Neurology*, 2000. **54**(Suppl 3): p. A97.

79. Launer, L.J., Masaki, K., Petrovich H., Foley D., Havlik, R.J., "The association between mid-life blood pressure levels and late-life cognitive function. The Honolulu-Asia Aging Study." *JAMA*, 1995. **274**(1846-1851).

80. Longstreth, W.T., Jr., et al., "Clinical correlates of ventricular and sulcal size on cranial magnetic resonance imaging of 3,301 elderly people. The Cardiovascular

Health Study. Collaborative Research Group." *Neuroepidemiology*, 2000. **19**(1): p. 30-42.

81. Breteler, M.M., "Vascular involvement in cognitive decline and dementia. Epidemiologic evidence from the Rotterdam Study and the Rotterdam Scan Study." *Annals of the New York Academy of Sciences*, 2000. **903**(11 Suppl 5): p. 457-65.

82. de Groot, J.C., et al., "Cerebral white matter lesions and cognitive function: the Rotterdam Scan Study [see comments]." *Annals of Neurology*, 2000. **47**(2): p. 145-51.

83. de Groot, J.C., F.E. de Leeuw, and M.M. Breteler, "Cognitive correlates of cerebral white matter changes." *Journal of Neural Transmission. Supplementum*, 1998. **53**(1): p. 41-67.

84. Ott, A., et al., "Association of diabetes mellitus and dementia: the Rotterdam Study." *Diabetologia*, 1996. **39**(11): p. 1392-7.

85. Schmidt, R., et al., "Magnetic resonance imaging cerebral abnormalities and neuropsychologic test performance in elderly hypertensive subjects. A case-control study." *Archives of Neurology*, 1995. **52**(9): p. 905-10.

86. Boone, K.B., Miller, B.L., Lesser, I.M., Mehringer, C.M., Hill,E.,Berman, N., "Cognitive deficits with white-matter lesions in healthy elderly." *Arch Neruol*, 1992. **49**: p. 549-554.

87. Petersen, R.C., et al., "Mild cognitive impairment: clinical characterization and outcome." *Arch Neurol*, 1999. **56**(3): p. 303-8.

88. Dawe, B., Procter,A.,Philpot,M., "Concepts of mild cognitive impairment in the elderly and their relationship to dementia: a review." *Int J Geriatr Psychiatry*, 1992. **7**: p. 473-479.

89. DeCarli, C., Miller, B.L., Swan, G.E., Reed, T., Wolf, P.A., Carmelli, D., "Cerebrovascular and brain morphologic correlates of mild cognitive impairment in the National Heart, Lung, and Blood Institute Twin study" *Arch Neruol,* 2001. **58**(4).

90. Wu, C.C., et al., "Structural Brain Changes and Cognitive Impairment in a Community Sample: The SALSA Study." *Neurology*, 2002.

91. Wolf, H., et al., "Do white matter changes contribute to the subsequent development of dementia in patients with mild cognitive impairment? A longitudinal study." *Int J Geriatr Psychiatry*, 2000. **15**(9): p. 803-12.

92. O'Brien, M.D., "Vascular dementia is underdiagnosed." *Archives of Neurology*, 1988. **45**: p. 797-798.

93. Brust, J.C.M., "Vascular dementia is overdiagnosed." *Archives of Neurology*, 1988. **45**: p. 799-801.

94. Tatemichi, T.K., "How acute brain failure becomes chronic: A view of the mechanisms of dementia related to stroke." *Neurology*, 1990. **40**: p. 1652-1659.

95. Tatemichi, T.K., et al., "Dementia in stroke survivors in the stroke data bank cohort. Prevalence, incidence, risk factors, and computed tomographic findings." *Stroke*, 1990. **21**: p. 858-866.

96.   Tatemichi, T.K., et al., "Dementia after stroke: Baseline frequency, risks, and clinical features in a hospitalized cohort." *Neurology*, 1992. **42**: p. 1185-1193.

97.   Tatemichi, T.K., et al., "Dementia associated with bilateral carotid occlusions: neuropsychological and haemodynamic course after extracranial to intracranial bypass surgery." *Journal of Neurology, Neurosurgery and Psychiatry*, 1995. **58**(5): p. 633-6.

98.   Moroney, J.T., et al., "Risk factors for incident dementia after stroke. Role of hypoxic and ischemic disorders." *Stroke*, 1996. **27**(8): p. 1283-9.

99.   Tatemichi, T.K., D.W. Desmond, and I. Prohovnik, "Strategic infarcts in vascular dementia. A clinical and brain imaging experience." *Arzneimittel-Forschung*, 1995. **45**(3A): p. 371-85.

100.   Moroney, J.T., et al., "Dementia after stroke increases the risk of long-term stroke recurrence." *Neurology*, 1997. **48**(5): p. 1317-25.

101.   Moroney, J.T., et al., "Cerebral hypoxia and ischemia in the pathogenesis of dementia after stroke." *Annals of the New York Academy of Sciences*, 1997. **826**(3): p. 433-6.

102.   Skoog, I., R.N. Kalaria, and M.M. Breteler, "Vascular factors and Alzheimer disease." *Alzheimer Disease and Associated Disorders*, 1999. **13 Suppl 3**(6): p. S106-14.

103.   Mirsen, T.R., et al., "Clinical correlates of white-matter changes on magnetic resonance imaging scans of the brain." *Archives of Neurology*, 1991. **48**(10): p. 1015-21.

104.   McDonald, W.M., et al., "Magnetic resonance findings in patients with early-onset Alzheimer's disease." *Biological Psychiatry*, 1991. **29**: p. 799-810.

105.   Scheltens, P., et al., "White matter lesions on magnetic resonance imaging in clinically diagnosed Alzheimer's disease: evidence for heterogeneity." *Brain*, 1992. **115**: p. 735-748.

106.   Waldemar, G., et al., "White matter magnetic resonance hyperintensities in dementia of the Alzheimer type: morphological and regional cerebral blood flow correlates." *Journal of Neurology, Neurosurgery and Psychiatry*, 1994. **57**: p. 1458-1465.

107.   Scheltens, P., et al., "Histopathologic correlates of white matter changes on MRI in Alzheimer's disease and normal aging." *Neurology*, 1995. **45**: p. 883-888.

108.   Fazekas, F., et al., "The relation of cerebral magnetic resonance signal hyperintensities to Alzheimer's disease." *Journal of the Neurological Sciences*, 1996. **142**(1-2): p. 121-5.

109.   Barber, R., et al., "White matter lesions on magnetic resonance imaging in dementia with Lewy bodies, Alzheimer's disease, vascular dementia, and normal aging." *Journal of Neurology, Neurosurgery and Psychiatry*, 1999. **67**: p. 66-72.

110.   Alonzo, N.C., et al., "Progression of cerebral amyloid angiopathy: accumulation of amyloid-beta40 in affected vessels." *Journal of Neuropathology and Experimental Neurology*, 1998. **57**(4): p. 353-9.

111. Kertesz, A., M. Polk, and T. Carr, "Cognition and white matter changes on magnetic resonance imaging in dementia." *Archives of Neurology*, 1990. **47**: p. 387-391.

112. Bondareff, W., et al., "Quantitative magnetic resonance imaging and the severity of dementia in Alzheimer's disease." *Am J Psychiatry*, 1988. **145**: p. 853-856.

113. Bondareff, W., et al., "Magnetic resonance imaging and the severity of dementia in older adults." *Arch Gen Psychiatry.*, 1990. **47**: p. 47-51.

114. Harrell, L.E., et al., "The relationship of high-intensity signals on magnetic resonance images to cognitive and psychiatric state in Alzheimer's disease." *Arch Neurol*, 1991. **48**: p. 1136-1140.

115. Diaz, J.F., et al., "Improved recognition of leukoaraiosis and cognitive impairment in Alzheimer's disease." *Archives of Neurology*, 1991. **48**(10): p. 1022-5.

116. Stout, J.C., et al., "Association of dementia severity with cortical gray matter and abnormal white matter volumes in dementia of the Alzheimer type." *Arch Neurol*, 1996(53): p. 742-749.

117. Ott, B.R., et al., "A SPECT imaging study of MRI white matter hyperintensity in patients with degenerative dementia." *Dement Geriatr Cogn Disord.*, 1997. **8**: p. 348-354.

118. Fazekas, F., et al., "MR signal abnormalities at 1.5 T in Alzheimer's dementia and normal aging." *Am J Neuroradiol*, 1987. **8**: p. 421-426.

119. Kozachuk, W.E., et al., "White matter hyperintensities in dementia of Alzheimer's type and in healthy subjects without cerebrovascular risk factors: a magnetic resonance imaging study." *Arch Neurol.*, 1990. **47**: p. 1306-1310.

120. Leys, D., et al., "Periventricular and white matter magnetic resonance imaging hyperintensities do not differ between Alzheimer's disease and normal aging." *Arch Neurol.,* 1990. **47**: p. 524-527.

121. Lopez, O.L., et al., "Neuropsychiatric correlates of cerebral white-matter radiolucencies in probable Alzheimer's disease." *Arch Neurol.,* 1992. **49**: p. 828-834.

122. Schmidt, R., "Comparison of magnetic resonance imaging in Alzheimer's disease, vascular dementia and normal aging." *Eur Neurol.,* 1992. **32**: p. 164-169.

123. Bennett, D.A., et al., "Clinical correlates of high signal lesions on magnetic resonance imaging in Alzheimer's disease." *J Neurol.*, 1992. **239**: p. 186-190.

124. Bennett, D.A., et al., "White matter changes: neurobehavioral manifestations of Binswanger's disease and clinical correlates in Alzheimer disease." *Dementia*, 1994. **5**: p. 148-152.

125. Wahlund, L., O,, et al., "White matter hyperintensities in dementia: does it matter?" *Magn Reson Imaging*, 1994: p. 387-394.

126. Brilliant, M., et al., "Rarefied white matter in patients with Alzheimer disease." *Alzheimer Dis Assoc Disord*, 1995. **9**: p. 39-46.

127. Marder, K., et al., *"*Clinical correlates of Alzheimer's disease with and without silent radiographic abnormalities." *Arch Neurol,* 1995. **52**: p. 146-151.

128. Lopez, O.L., et al., "Computed tomography-but not magnetic resonance imaging-identified periventricular white-matter lesions predict symptomatic cerebrovascular disease in probable Alzheimer's disease." *Arch Neurol*, 1995. **52**: p. 659-664.

129. Starkstein, S.E., et al., "Neuropsychological, psychiatric, and cerebral perfusion correlates of leukoaraiosis in Alzheimer's disease." *J Neurol Neurosurg Psychiatry*, 1997. **63**: p. 66-73.

130. Doody, R.S., et al., "Cognitive consequences of subcortical magnetic resonance imaging changes in Alzheimer's disease: comparison to small vessel ischemic vascular dementia." *Neuropsychiatry Neuropsychol Behav Neurol*, 1998. **11**: p. 191-199.

131. Teipel, S.J., et al., "Dissociation between corpus callosum atrophy and white matter pathology in Alzheimer's disease." *Neurology*, 1998. **51**: p. 1381-1385.

132. Roman, G.C., "Senile dementia of the Binswanger type: a vascular form of dementia in the elderly." *JAMA*, 1987. **258**: p. 1782-1788.

133. Caplan, L.R., "Binswanger's disease-revisited. Neurology, 1995. **45**: p. 626-633.

134. Johnson, K.A., et al., Comparison of magnetic resonance and roentgen ray computed tomography in dementia." *Arch Neurol*, 1987. **44**: p. 1075-1080.

135. Erkinjuntti, T., et al., "Do white matter changes on MRI and CT differentiate vascular dementia from Alzheimer's disease?" *J Neurol Neurosurg Psychiatry*, 1987. **50**: p. 37-42.

136. Kobari, M., et al., "Leukoaraiosis: correlation of MR and CT findings with blood flow, atrophy, and cognition." *Am J Neuroradiol*, 1990. **11**: p. 273-281.

137. Lechner, H., et al., "Nuclear magnetic resonance image white matter lesions and risk factors for stroke in normal individuals." *Stroke*, 1988. **19**(263-265).

138. DeCarli, C., et al., "Comparison of positron emission tomography, cognition, and brain volume in Alzheimer's disease with and without severe abnormalities of white matter." *Journal of Neurology, Neurosurgery and Psychiatry*, 1996. **60**(2): p. 158-67.

139. Swartz, R.H., et al., "Quantification of brain hyperintensities and atrophy on MRI: The Sunnybrook Dementia Study." *Neurology*, 2001. **56**(Suppl 3): p. A263-A264.

140. Reed, B.R., et al., "Frontal lobe hypometabolism predicts cognitive decline in patients with lacunar infarcts." *Arch Neurol*, 2001. **58**: p. 493-497.

141. Reed, B.R., et al., "Memory failure has different mechanisms in subcortical stroke and Alzheimer's disease." *Annals of Neurology*, 2000. **48**(3): p. 275-84.

142. Royall, D.R. and G.C. "Roman, Differentiation of vascular dementia from AD on neuropsychological tests [letter]." *Neurology*, 2000. **55**(4): p. 604-6.

143. Stolk, R.P., et al., "Insulin and cognitive function in an elderly population. The Rotterdam Study." *Diabetes Care*, 1997. **20**(5): p. 792-5.

144. Ott, A., et al., "Atrial fibrillation and dementia in a population-based study. The Rotterdam Study." *s*, 1997. **28**(2): p. 316-21.

145. Hofman, A., et al., "Atherosclerosis, apolipoprotein E, and prevalence of dementia and Alzheimer's disease in the Rotterdam Study [see comments]." *Lancet*, 1997. **349**(9046): p. 151-4.

146. van Kooten, F., et al., "The Dutch Vascular Factors in Dementia Study: rationale and design." *Journal of Neurology*, 1998. **245**(1): p. 32-9.

147. Breteler, M.M., "Vascular risk factors for Alzheimer's disease: an epidemiologic perspective." *Neurobiology of Aging*, 2000. **21**(2): p. 153-60.

148. Heyman, A., et al., "Cerebral infarcts in patients with autopsy-proven Alzheimer's disease: CERAD, part XVIII. Consortium to Establish a Registry for Alzheimer's Disease." *Neurology*, 1998. **51**: p. 159-162.

149. Esiri, M.M., G.K. Wilcock, and J.H. Morris, "Neuropathological assessment of the lesions of significance in vascular dementia." *J Neurol Neurosurg Psychiatry*, 1997. **63**(6): p. 749-53.

150. Nagy, Z., et al., "The effects of additional pathology on the cognitive deficit in Alzheimer disease." *J Neuropathol Exp Neurol*, 1997. **56**(2): p. 165-70.

151. Lee, J.H., et al., "Small concomitant vascular lesions do not influence rates of cognitive decline in patients with Alzheimer disease." *Arch Neurol*, 2000. **57**(10): p. 1474-1479.

152. Lafosse, J.M., et al., "Fluency and memory differences between ischemic vascular dementia and Alzheimer's disease." *Neuropsychology*, 1997. **11**(4): p. 514-22.

153. Wolfe, N., et al., "Frontal systems impairment following multiple lacunar infarcts." *Arch Neurol*, 1990. **47**(2): p. 129-32.

154. Cummings, J.L., et al., "Neuropsychiatric aspects of multi-infarct dementia and dementia of the Alzheimer type." *Arch Neurol*, 1987. **44**(4): p. 389-93.

155. Tatemichi, T.K., et al., "Confusion and memory loss from capsular genu infarction: a thalamocortical disconnection syndrome?" *Neurology*, 1992. **42**(10): p. 1966-79.

156. Elias, P.K., et al., "NIDDM and blood pressure as risk factors for poor cognitive performance. The Framingham Study." *Diabetes Care*, 1997. **20**(9): p. 1388-95.

157. Elias, M.F., et al., "A longitudinal study of blood pressure in relation to performance on the Wechsler Adult Intelligence Scale." *Health Psychology*, 1998. **17**(6): p. 486-93.

158. Elias, M.F., "Effects of chronic hypertension on cognitive functioning." *Geriatrics*, 1998. **53 Suppl** 1(6): p. S49-52.

159. Swan, G.E., D. Carmelli, and A. LaRue, "Relationship between blood pressure during middle age and cognitive impairment in old age: the Western Collaborative Group Study." *Aging Neuropsychol Cognition*, 1996. **3**: p. 241-250.

160. Slooter, A.J., et al., "Apolipoprotein E genotype, atherosclerosis, and cognitive decline: the Rotterdam Study." *J Neural Transm Suppl*, 1998. **53**: p. 17-29.

161. Skoog, I., et al., "15-year longitudinal study of blood pressure and dementia." *Lancet*, 1996. **347**(9009): p. 1141-5.

162. Slooter, A.J., et al., "Risk estimates of dementia by apolipoprotein E genotypes from a population-based incidence study: the Rotterdam Study." *Archives of Neurology*, 1998. **55**(7): p. 964-8.

163. DeCarli, C., et al., "Impact of apolipoprotein E epsilon4 and vascular disease on brain morphology in men from the NHLBI twin study." *Stroke*, 1999. **30**(8): p. 1548-53.

164. Laskowitz, D.T., et al., "Apolipoprotein E-deficient mice have increased susceptibility to focal cerebral ischemia." *J Cereb Blood Flow Metab*, 1997. **17**(7): p. 753-8.

165. Ukkola, O., et al., "Apolipoprotein E phenotype is related to macro- and microangiopathy in patients with non-insulin-dependent diabetes mellitus." *Atherosclerosis*, 1993. **101**(1): p. 9-15.

166. Ott, A., et al., "Smoking and risk of dementia and Alzheimer's disease in a population- based cohort study: the Rotterdam Study." *Lancet*, 1998. **351**(9119): p. 1840-3.

167. Dufouil, C., et al., "Influence of apolipoprotein E genotype on the risk of cognitive deterioration in moderate drinkers and smokers." *Epidemiology*, 2000. **11**(3): p. 280-4.

168. Carmelli, D., et al., "The effect of apolipoprotein E epsilon4 in the relationships of smoking and drinking to cognitive function." *Neuroepidemiology*, 1999. **18**(3): p. 125-33.

169. Carmelli, D., et al., "Midlife cardiovascular risk factors, ApoE, and cognitive decline in elderly male twins." *Neurology*, 1998. **50**(6): p. 1580-5.

170. Haan, M.N., et al., "The role of APOE epsilon4 in modulating effects of other risk factors for cognitive decline in elderly persons." *JAMA*, 1999. **282**(1): p. 40-6.

171. Sparks, D.L., et al., "Increased incidence of neurofibrillary tangles (NFT) in non-demented individuals with hypertension." *J Neurol Sci*, 1995. **131**(2): p. 162-9.

172. Sparks, D.L., "Coronary artery disease, hypertension, ApoE, and cholesterol: a link to Alzheimer's disease?" *Ann N Y Acad Sci*, 1997. **826**: p. 128-46.

173. Sparks, D.L., et al., "Link between heart disease, cholesterol, and Alzheimer's disease: a review." *Microsc Res Tech*, 2000. **50**(4): p. 287-90.

174. Forette, F., et al., "Prevention of dementia in randomised double-blind placebo-controlled Systolic Hypertension in Europe (Syst-Eur) trial." *Lancet*, 1998. **352**(9137): p. 1347-51.

175. Hansson, L., "Antihypertensive treatment and the prevention of dementia: further insights from the Syst-Eur trial." *J Hypertens*, 1999. **17**(3): p. 307-8.

176. Birkenhager, W.H., et al., "Blood pressure, cognitive functions, and prevention of dementias in older patients with hypertension." *Arch Intern Med*, 2001. **161**(2): p. 152-6.

177. Folstein, M.F., S.E. Folstein, and P.R. McHugh, " 'Mini-mental state'. A practical method for grading the cognitive state of patients for the clinician." *J Psychiatr Res*, 1975. **12**(3): p. 189-98.

178. Barker, W.H., J.P. Mullooly, and K.L. Linton, "Trends in hypertension prevalence, treatment, and control: in a well-defined older population." *Hypertension*, 1998. **31**(1 Pt 2): p. 552-9.

NONCOGNITIVE SYMPTOMS OF DEMENTIA: RIGOR AND RELEVANCE

MARSHAL F. FOLSTEIN, M.D.
Tufts University Medical School, New England Medical Center Hospital
Boston, MA USA

"In science one tries to tell people, in such a way as to be understood by everyone, something that no one ever knew before. But in poetry, it's the exact opposite."
—Paul Dirac, Quoted in H. Eves, *Mathematical Circles Adieu* (Boston 1977).

INTRODUCTION

Dementia is a syndrome characterized by deterioration of memory and other cognitive impairments in clear consciousness. Alzheimer disease, Parkinson disease, Huntington disease, as well as Diffuse Lewy Body disease are pathological conditions that cause dementia. A great deal is known about the cognitive impairment in these disease states and in comparable normal populations. For example, the Mini-Mental Status Examination, a cognitive screening test used in many countries, has been applied to 18,000 representative community-dwelling adults. From this work it was determined that cognitive impairment was related to disease and education levels, but less related to age (Crum, Anthony et al., 1993).

Demented patients also suffer from hallucinations, depression, and other noncognitive symptoms (NCS) (Deutsch, Bylsma et al., 1991; Deutsch and Rovner, 1991). These NCS are clinically relevant because they cause suffering in both the patient and the patient's family and other caregivers. Therefore, patients with untreated NCS are more likely to be admitted to nursing homes (Steele, Rovner et al., 1990). NCS are also heuristically relevant to thinking about neural mechanisms. For example, patients with NCS have a more rapid decline, and the frequency and type of NCS differ according to the type and location of neuropathology. Research involving NCS, as well as their detection and documentation for clinical care, requires clear concepts, clear definitions, and reliable and valid methods for measurement. More research is needed to determine their relationship to selective neuronal vulnerability in particular brain regions and to determine their relationship to the process of cell death.

DETECTION AND MEASUREMENT OF THE NON-COGNITIVE SYMPTOMS OF DEMENTIA

The non-cognitive symptoms that are commonly seen in dementia are delusions, hallucinations, depression, apathy, and irritability and aggression, and over-activity that can resemble mania. The particular symptoms seen in patients with particular dementing disorders depend on the pattern of neuropathological abnormalities in that condition and the duration of illness at the time of examination.

Despite their importance, NCS have not been studied frequently in persons with cognitive impairment, and most of the existing studies are limited by small sample sizes and by use of unsatisfactory methods for detection and measurement.

The only method currently available for assessing NCS is a conversation with the patient and an informant to determine if the patient experiences and reports any of the symptoms. Because patients often have different words for the same feeling or perception, they must be asked culturally familiar questions in language that their experience, education, and intelligence enable them to understand. Since patients might not recognize their own symptoms or have a distorted view of them, another informant who knows the patient well greatly improves the validity of the information. However, in some kinds of research, such informants are not available.

Two general methods are used to assess NCS, rating scales and interviews. Rating scales that subjects fill out about themselves or rating scales that observers fill out about the subject are widely used (Devanand, Miller et al., 1992; Cummings, Mega et al., 1994). Because rating scales specify the questions to be answered by subject, observer reliability is high and administration is inexpensive since experienced clinicians are not required. Rating scales produce a score, a single number that indicates the severity of the symptom being rated and thus, if valid, should provide a measure of the severity the NCS being rated. However, rating scales have several limitations, particularly when used for patients with cognitive impairment. First, they are not very useful in detecting syndromes that have an intermittent course (and thus may or not be present at the time the questionnaire is completed). Second, the patients or informants completing the scale may not be clear about the intended meaning of the words used in the questionnaire. And third, many demented patients cannot accurately complete such rating scales either because of poor attention or language difficulties.

There are two types of interviews. The first type is a highly structured interview in which the questions are read to the subject by the interviewer who is not an experienced clinician. In many ways such an interview is really a questionnaire. Semi-structured interviews provide the opportunity, indeed the requirement, for the interviewer to discuss the symptoms with the patient or the informant to be sure that they understand the definition of the symptom. The examiner has a glossary that provides definitions for each item, but the interview does not specify the language to be used to inquire about the symptoms. Rather, the examiner accommodates the question to the subject's culture, language, education and intelligence. This is the method used in clinical psychiatry in the clinical situations where psychiatrists originally identified and defined NCS (Jaspers,

1963). The limitations of semi-structured interviews are the clinical experience required of the interviewer and the greater effort needed to assure reliability between interviewers. They are also of course more time consuming to administer and score than questionnaires. Their advantage is that the information obtained has much higher validity, and it can thus be used with more confidence for both clinical and research purposes.

The Dementia Symptom Scale is a semi-structured interview derived from The Present State Examination of Wing Sartorius and Cooper, an interview developed for use in general psychiatric patients. It has been shown to be reliable between raters, and has been extensively validated . (Loreck, Bylsma et al., 1994). This scale has several unique features. First, it is the only scale suitable for measuring NCS in demented patients that includes questions about mania. This is important because of the frequency of manic symptoms in several dementing syndromes, particularly stroke and Huntington disease. Second, ratings based on information from the subject, the informant, and opinion of the examiner are recorded separately.

When we compared the ratings made by patients with those of informants who knew them well, we learned that patients almost always report fewer symptoms than their informants do. Thus, for demented patients, the principle derived from the survey research field that subjects more accurate than proxy informants, does not hold (Loreck, Bylsma et al., 1994). However, as described above, such semi-structured interviews are time consuming and require skilled interviewers. So the investigator must trade off between thoroughly examining a relatively small sample of cases and applying rating scales to much larger populations. The first sacrifices representativeness of the sample and the power to analyze subsamples. The second sacrifices some aspects of validity of assessment. There is evidence that the two methods do not detect and assess the same symptoms (Anthony, Folstein et al., 1985; Folstein, Romanoski et al., 1985).

NONCOGNITIVE SYMPTOMS IN FOUR DEMENTING ILLNESSES

Even though there is not yet the same rigor for psychopathological investigation as for pathological or etiological studies, interesting results are emerging which indicate that NCS are indeed relevant for care and research. I will discuss depression, delusions, and hallucinations as they occur in Alzheimer disease, Diffuse Lewy Body Disease, Parkinson disease and Huntington disease. The definitions follow Jaspers (Jaspers, 1963).

DEPRESSION

The normal variation in mood is considerable. Normal individuals have moods that differ in their set point; some people have overall more sunny dispositions than others. Normal moods can change from hour to hour or not at all. Depressed mood outside the range of normal variation may occur as an isolated symptom, or as part of a relatively stereotyped cluster of symptoms called a syndrome. This syndrome has three characteristic features:

low mood, loss of self confidence, sometimes with hopelessness, and a change in the sense of vitality toward feeling ill, sluggish and lacking energy.

Sufferers describe their negative affect with a variety of terms, such as low, low spirits, blue, nervous, tense or just feeling bad. Depression can be responsive to encouragement or unresponsive to even treasured family members. People with a depressive syndrome are often pessimistic, lack confidence, feel hopelessness, and sometimes worthless and inappropriately guilty. Mood is sometimes is connected to 24-hour circadian rhythms that regulate sleep and hormones; it can be worse in the morning and then improve as the day goes on, or it can be worse at night. Depressed mood is sometimes connected to cognition, particularly in the elderly and in people with pre-existing brain disease. As mood improves, so does thinking ability. Mood also affects memory so that depressed people recall less pleasant memories.

Depression can arise de novo out of the blue or following a perceived stimulus such as loss, death, or physical events like trauma, infection, intoxication, lowered thyroid or elevated cortisol or cytokines. Depression is common in many brain diseases that have a variety of types and locations of neuropathology, including brain tumor, stroke, Parkinson's disease and Alzheimer disease. Even in brain diseases, depression can have a waxing and waning course, appearing suddenly or gradually and subsiding in the same way. Depression is often rated using rating scales, which have the strengths and weaknesses referred to above.

HALLUCINATIONS

Hallucinations are *perceptions* without a stimulus. Modes of hallucinations are visual, auditory, tactile, olfactory and proprioceptive (Berrios, 1982) and to some extent, these different forms have been associated with specific brain regions. Hallucinations vary tremendously in their complexity. For example, visual hallucinations can be simple geometric figures or complex scenes. The content of hallucinations is usually related to the patient's life experience. A fisherman's visual hallucinations might be of fishing line, while an auto salesman might have hallucinations of pink or blue Toyotas. The form is the visual hallucination and the content is the line or car. Etiology and pathology determine the form but life history and memory supply the content. Some kinds of hallucinations are normal, such as those that occur on falling asleep (hypnogogic) or awakening (hypnopompic) or those that occur in association with some concurrent sensation, e.g., hearing voices when the water is running.

Many causes of hallucinations are recognized. Visual hallucinations can be associated with eye disease; mescaline produces simple hallucinations of color and shapes whereas alcohol withdrawal can produce complex hallucinations auditory or visual. Cocaine produces tactile hallucinations. Grief can induce hallucinations as can the depressive syndrome. Mood-related, or mood-congruent, hallucinations are usually auditory. People hear a single voice telling them to commit suicide or that they are evil or worthless. Auditory hallucinations are also characteristic of schizophrenia, but the content is not related to the patient's mood.

Documentation of hallucinations requires interviewing the patient by an experienced clinician usually a psychiatrist. who has examined and followed pateints with NCS. Hallucinations must be differentiated from imagery, vivid thoughts and dreams. Since subjects do not know the difference the examiner must explain the difference. Rating of hallucinations as severe or mild is problematic because a hallucination is either present or not, although severity can be graded according to time (present for hours or days or years). Because it is often difficult to be certain whether or not patients have hallucinations, ratings should also include a notation of the examiner's certainty that the symptom is present.

DELUSIONS

Delusions are false fixed *ideas* that are idiosyncratic and ego preoccupying (Cummings, 1985). Delusions arise in isolation, ("authocthonus" delusions) or are secondary to mood or hallucinations. For example, a person with severe depression may have an auditory hallucination saying that he/she is a bad person and develop a secondary delusion that he/she is bad.

Delusions can only be assessed by interview. This is because patient's often do not readily admit to them and because several questions are required in order to differentiate them from emotion-laden ideas that Wernicke called "overvalued ideas". Overvalued ideas are not idiosyncratic since other members of the culture share them. Examples include fanaticism, religiosity, even sports and stamp collecting. Delusions must also be distinguished from repetitive sometimes false ideas that intrude on the mind of the patient in spite of the patient's resistance to the idea; these are called obsessions.

DEPRESSION, DELUSIONS, AND HALLUCINATIONS IN DEMENTIAS

Depression, delusions, and hallucinations vary in prevalence in dementing diseases that are differentiated from each other by the distribution of the pathology. Although none of these diseases are caused by pathology in one only location, there is a predominant location. Alzheimer disease is primarily cortical. Diffuse Lewy Body disease is primarily cortical but more subcortical. Huntington disease is primarily subcortical with some cortical distribution. Parkinson disease is almost entirely subcortical with minimal cortical involvement.

Studies from the published literature were reviewed for prevalence rates of NCS in these four disorders. The median frequency is seen in the figure. Depression is more prevalent in primarily subcortical diseases (McHugh and Folstein, 1979; Burns, Folstein et al., 1990; Lyketsos, Steele et al., 1997; Mindham, Steele et al., 1985; Rovner, Broadhead et al., 1989). Delusions are more prevalent in primarily cortical disease (Binetti, Padovani et al., 1995; Rovner, Kafonek et al., 1986; Bassiony, Steinberg et al., 2000). Hallucinations occur in association with both cortical and subcortical pathology (Aarsland, Larsen et al., 1999).

Lewy Body disease may be a special case. It causes a much higher prevalence of NCS than any of the other dementing diseases. (Aarsland, Ballard et al., 2001; Ballard, O'Brien et al., 2001). Patients with Lewy Body Disease are also very sensitive to the effects of antidepressants and psychotropic medications. They become delirious and even stuporous when taking doses that are well tolerated by the other patient with dementia.

NEUROPATHOLOGICAL CORRELATES OF HALLUCINATIONS AND MOOD DISORDERS

Lesions in nearly every part of the brain can cause hallucinations. The form of the hallucinations (visual, auditory, tactile) depends on the location of the pathology. Hallucinations follow lesions of peripheral nerves, (paresthesia, tinnitus and phantom limb phenomena), spinal cord (shooting pains of tabes), diencephalon (peduncular hallucinosis of L'Hermitte), striatum (visual hallucinations of Parkinson's disease), and cortex (both auditory and visual hallucinations in parietal stroke).

An important cause of depression in dementing conditions is any lesion affecting the frontal-striatal circuits. Depression is very common with left frontal lesions or left striatal lesions in stroke, and mania with right-sided lesions in either of these same brain regions. Either depression or mania can be the first symptom of Huntington disease, and often precede the movement disorder and cognitive decline by several years (Folstein, 1989). The mood disorders begin at a time when the neuropathology is limited to the caudate and putamen, and within these structures, to the striosomes. The striosomes receive their input mainly from the limbic cortex, and have different connections with the substantia nigra (Hedreen and Folstein, 1993). Depression also occurs in Alzheimer disease, in some cases as the first sign of trouble. The prevalence is variously reported because samples differ in severity of disease and methods of examination. The relationship to neuropathology is also controversial.

It has not been possible to uncover any neuropathological correlates with delusions.

NCS AND COURSE OF ILLNESS

NCS are relevant to the course of illness. Depression often occurs prior to the onset of cognitive decline in Alzheimer disease and Huntington disease. Perhaps the brain circuits mediating depression are the most vulnerable for the pathological process of Huntington and Alzheimer disease. Later in the course of Alzheimer disease NCS predict a more rapid decline in cognition (Stern, Mayeux et al., 1987;Chui, Lyness et al., 1994).

TREATMENT OF NCS

The NCS of dementias respond to same medications as the NCS in manic-depressive disease or schizophrenia. Antidepressants improve depression, mood stabilizers mitigate bipolar disorder and manic-like symptoms, and psychotropics improve delusions and hallucinations (Steele, Lucas et al., 1986; Devanand, Marder et al., 1998; Cummings, Street et al., 2002). In addition, the new cholinesterase inhibitors designed for stabilization of cognition also improve NCS (Rojas-Fernandez, 2001).

SUMMARY

Patients differentiated from one another by the presence of NCS are also differentiated by pathology, treatment, and prognosis. Complete explanation of the mechanism of dementing diseases will necessarily need to account for noncognitive as well as cognitive symptoms.

REFERENCES

1. Aarsland, D., C. Ballard, et al. (2001). "A comparative study of psychiatric symptoms in dementia with Lewy bodies and Parkinson's disease with and without dementia." *Int J Geriatr Psychiatry* **16**(5): 528-36.

2. Aarsland, D., J.P. Larsen, et al. (1999). "Prevalence and clinical correlates of psychotic symptoms in Parkinson disease: a community-based study." *Arch Neurol* **56**(5): 595-601.

3. Anthony, J.C., M. Folstein, et al. (1985). "Comparison of the lay Diagnostic Interview Schedule and a standardized psychiatric diagnosis. Experience in eastern Baltimore." *Arch Gen Psychiatry* **42**(7): 667-75.

4. Ballard, C.G., J.T. O'Brien, et al. (2001). "The natural history of psychosis and depression in dementia with Lewy bodies and Alzheimer's disease: persistence and new cases over 1 year of follow-up." *J Clin Psychiatry* **62**(1): 46-9.

5. Bassiony, M.M., M.S. Steinberg, et al. (2000). "Delusions and hallucinations in Alzheimer's disease: prevalence and clinical correlates." *Int J Geriatr Psychiatry* **15**(2): 99-107.

6. Berrios, G.E. (1982). "Tactile hallucinations: conceptual and historical aspects." *J Neurol Neurosurg Psychiatry* **45**(4): 285-93.

7. Binetti, G., A. Padovani, et al. (1995). "Delusions and dementia: clinical and CT correlates." *Acta Neurol Scand* **91**(4): 271-5.

8. Burns, A., S. Folstein, et al. (1990). "Clinical assessment of irritability, aggression, and apathy in Huntington and Alzheimer disease." *J Nerv Ment Dis* **178**(1): 20-6.

9. Chui, H.C., S.A. Lyness, et al. (1994). "Extrapyramidal signs and psychiatric symptoms predict faster cognitive decline in Alzheimer's disease." *Arch Neurol* **51**(7): 676-81.

10. Crum, R M., J.C. Anthony, et al. (1993). "Population-based norms for the Mini-Mental State Examination by age and educational level." *Jama* **269**(18): 2386-91.

11. Cummings, J.L. (1985). "Organic delusions: phenomenology, anatomical correlations, and review." *Br J Psychiatry* **146**: 184-97.

12. Cummings, J.L., M. Mega, et al. (1994). "The Neuropsychiatric Inventory: comprehensive assessment of psychopathology in dementia." *Neurology* **44**(12): 2308-14.

13. Cummings, J.L., J. Street, et al. (2002). "Efficacy of olanzapine in the treatment of psychosis in dementia with lewy bodies." *Dement Geriatr Cogn Disord* **13**(2): 67-73.

14. Deutsch, L.H., F.W. Bylsma, et al. (1991). "Psychosis and physical aggression in probable Alzheimer's disease." *Am J Psychiatry* **148**(9): 1159-63.

15. Deutsch, L.H. and B.W. Rovner (1991). "Agitation and other noncognitive abnormalities in Alzheimer's disease." *Psychiatr Clin North Am* **14**(2): 341-51.

16. Devanand, D.P., K. Marder, et al. (1998). "A randomized, placebo-controlled dose-comparison trial of haloperidol for psychosis and disruptive behaviors in Alzheimer's disease." *Am J Psychiatry* **155**(11): 1512-20.

17. Devanand, D.P., L. Miller, et al. (1992). "The Columbia University Scale for Psychopathology in Alzheimer's disease." *Arch Neurol* **49**(4): 371-6.

18. Folstein, M.F., A.J. Romanoski, et al. (1985). "Brief report on the clinical reappraisal of the Diagnostic Interview Schedule carried out at the Johns Hopkins site of the Epidemiological Catchment Area Program of the NIMH." *Psychol Med* **15**(4): 809-14.

19. Jaspers, K. (1963). *General Psychopathology*. Manchester, University of Manchester Press.

20. Loreck, D.J., F. Bylsma, et al. (1994). "The Dementia Symptom Scale." *American Journal of Geriatric Psychiatry* **2**: 60-74.

21. Lyketsos, C.G., C. Steele, et al. (1997). "Major and minor depression in Alzheimer's disease: prevalence and impact." *J Neuropsychiatry Clin Neurosci* **9**(4): 556-61.

22. McHugh, P.R. and M.F. Folstein (1979). "Psychopathology of dementia: implications for neuropathology." *Res Publ Assoc Res Nerv Ment Dis* **57**: 17-30.

23. Mindham, R.H., C. Steele, et al. (1985). "A comparison of the frequency of major affective disorder in Huntington's disease and Alzheimer's disease." *J Neurol Neurosurg Psychiatry* **48**(11): 1172-4.

24. Rojas-Fernandez, C.H. (2001). "Successful use of donepezil for the treatment of dementia with Lewy bodies." *Ann Pharmacother* **35**(2): 202-5.

25. Rovner, B.W., J. Broadhead, et al. (1989). "Depression and Alzheimer's disease." *Am J Psychiatry* **146**(3): 350-3.

26. Rovner, B.W., S. Kafonek, et al. (1986). "Prevalence of mental illness in a community nursing home." *Am J Psychiatry* **143**(11): 1446-9.

27. Steele, C., M.J. Lucas, et al. (1986). "Haloperidol versus thioridazine in the treatment of behavioral symptoms in senile dementia of the Alzheimer's type: preliminary findings." *J Clin Psychiatry* **47**(6): 310-2.

28. Steele, C., B. Rovner, et al. (1990). "Psychiatric symptoms and nursing home placement of patients with Alzheimer's disease." *Am J Psychiatry* **147**(8): 1049-51.

29. Stern, Y., R. Mayeux, et al. (1987). "Predictors of disease course in patients with probable Alzheimer's disease." *Neurology* **37**(10): 1649-53.

CAN WE FIND GENES FOR COMMON DISORDERS?

SUSAN E. FOLSTEIN, M.D.
Tufts-New England Medical Center, Boston, MA, USA

The genetic disorders that are prevalent enough and severe enough to constitute planet-wide public health problems are caused by the interaction of several genes, which in turn interact with environmental factors. The genes that, in aggregate, cause these conditions generally do not, individually, cause serious disease. Rather they are likely to be alleles that are normally distributed in the population and act as susceptibility factors. Only when they combine with additional genes or environmental factors do they cause conditions with enough morbidity to come to clinical attention. Likewise, the environmental risk factors with which they are hypothesized to interact are probably also commonly experienced by many people in the population without untoward effects. We hypothesize that morbid conditions occur only when they are experienced by persons who have one or more of the genetic alleles that render them less tolerant, or more susceptible, to develop the illness.

In this paper, I will use autism as an example of a disorder that is likely caused in this manner. I will describe some studies that lead us to this causal hypothesis and describe the strategies we are using to identify some of these genetic and environmental factors.

INTRODUCTION

Autism was first described by Leo Kanner, one of the founders of Child Psychiatry and its first Professor in the United States (at the Johns Hopkins University School of Medicine). In 1943, Kanner described eleven children, mostly boys, whose condition he distinguished from mental retardation on the basis of the children's social isolation.[1] He named the syndrome "infantile autism" because the children's lack of social interaction resembled the criterion that Eugene Bleuler used for schizophrenia that indicates loss of social interest. One year later, Hans Asperger in Germany described similar patients and termed the condition "autistic psychopathy."[2] The sex ratio is usually estimated at 4:1 male to female, and the prevalence, using Kanner's criteria, is 2-5 per 10,000. However, recent changes in diagnostic criteria and how they are applied have resulted in increased prevalence estimates.[3,4]

Both Kanner and Asperger reasoned from the early age of onset that the disorder had a neuropathological origin. However, during the 1950s this formulation was questioned because the children "seemed intelligent" (although uncommunicative), because they did not appear to have the dysmorphic features or histories of serious birth trauma typical of most neurologically impaired children, and also because their parents were frequently socially reticent. There was a widespread bias in American psychiatry at that time toward explaining all psychiatric disorders as resulting from deficiencies in parenting and early life experiences. In this atmosphere, Bruno Bettelheim pronounced, without evidence, that the social reticence observed in the parents created an environment that caused autism.[5] The mothers were labeled "refrigerator mothers" even though social reticence was more common in fathers.[6] Eventually, studies that tested biological hypotheses put forward by Rimland[7] and by Rutter,[8] established empirically that the parents of autistic children were no different in their parenting from the parents of nonautistic controls,[9] and, further, that neurobiological explanations for the condition were compelling.

EVIDENCE FOR A GENETIC ETIOLOGY

More than twenty years after Kanner's original description, investigators finally recognized that genetics had an important part to play in the etiology of autism. In the early case series, approximately 2-3% of the families had more than one autistic child. Rutter[8] noted that this was 50 to 100 times greater than expected by chance, given the population prevalence. When the first twin study[10] revealed significantly higher concordance for autism among monozygotic twins than among dizygotic twins, researchers began to recognize the genetic basis of autism, even though it did not follow simple Mendelian inheritance patterns.

Twin studies
In the three epidemiologically based twin studies of autism,[10-12] all twins (one or both of whom were affected with autism) who lived in a geographically defined population were sought out. This method is important for reducing bias in ascertainment, because twins found through advertisements for volunteers yield more monozygotic (MZ) twin pairs than expected from the population frequency, and parents whose twins are concordant for a disorder or trait are also more likely to volunteer for such studies.

Autism twin studies have also only used same sex twin pairs because the skewed male:female ratio in autism leads to greater rates of discordance in opposite sex twin pairs. However, the combined number of pairs studied in the three autism twin studies is only 66, with 36 MZ pairs and 30 dizygotic (DZ) pairs. The average MZ concordance rate is 70% compared with a DZ rate of 0%. The observed rate of 0% is undoubtedly a chance finding resulting from the small number of DZ pairs that have been studied. The DZ concordance rate should be about the same as the recurrence risk in siblings, which is 6-8%. The recurrence risk, or the risk to siblings born after the proband, is higher than the prevalence in siblings because parents, are less likely to have subsequent child.

The concordance of autism in the MZ pairs cannot be accounted for by shared prenatal or perinatal difficulties, and so the large MZ:DZ difference in concordance suggests that autism is highly heritable. The heritability estimate, calculated from the recurrence risk and the MZ:DZ concordance ratio, is over 90%. However, this does not necessarily imply that the environment has little influence on the autism phenotype. It may simply mean that very little environmental variation existed in populations studied.

When concordance is examined for a phenotype consisting of *either* autism *or* milder cognitive or social deficits, 82% of MZ twins, compared with approximately 10% of DZ pairs, are concordant.[10] Most of the non-autistic MZ co-twins had language-based learning disabilities, and several were also socially reticent. The social reticence was even more striking when the twins were re-examined in adulthood.[11]

Studies of non-autistic relatives

The finding by Folstein and Rutter[10] that many of the non-autistic co-twins had cognitive and social deficits similar to autism was not anticipated, although perhaps it should have been. As early as 1957, Eisenberg and Kanner[6] reported that many of the fathers of autistic children had unusual personality traits, such as rigidity and a lack of interest in social interaction. These men were married, mostly successful professionals who were clearly able to socialize adequately, but in their free time they preferred solitary activities and tended to follow set routines. The article was actually published in response to the outpouring of psychoanalytic speculation that autism was caused by "refrigerator mothers."[5] Eisenberg wanted to point out that if either parent fit that description, it was more likely to be the father.

Following the Folstein and Rutter twin study, several groups resumed the study of families, this time with a genetic hypothesis and with the goal of using the information to establish the genetic mechanism by which autism might be inherited. Taken as a whole, the studies of parents and siblings have clearly demonstrated that several characteristics are found more often in the parents of autistic children than the parents of controls. These include social reticence, communication difficulties (pragmatic aspects of language), preference for routines and difficulty with change. These three traits are conceptually the same as the defining criteria for autism, but are much milder and have come to be known as the broader autism phenotype (BAP).[13,14] They are not usually associated with difficulties in functioning (although they can be) and may be associated with high achievement. Folstein and Rutter hypothesized that these features are manifestations of the genetic liability to autism.[15]

Delayed onset of speech and difficulty with reading are also more common in family members of persons with autism,[16] as are recurrent depression, anxiety disorders,[17] elevated platelet serotonin,[18] and increased head circumference.[19,20] Mental retardation in the absence of autism has not been found in siblings of autistic children more often than expected by[21] (see also review by Santangelo and Folstein[22]).

Based partly on the family studies and the striking similarity between autism and the milder social deficits seen in some children, autism is now considered to encompass a spectrum of similar, probably genetically related phenotypes. The spectrum includes severely mentally retarded individuals with epilepsy and no speech, classical autism, milder Asperger syndrome with normal intelligence and structural language capability, and the even milder broader autism phenotype seen in family members of autistic probands.

GENETIC MECHANISMS FOR AUTISM

There are several different genetic disorders where those affected have higher rates of autism than expected, and the literature contains numerous case reports of autism associated with cytogenetic abnormalities. These cases are one important reason for the increased prevalence of autism as measured in recent epidemiological studies. Cases with translocations, deletions and duplications have occasionally been heuristically important in suggesting chromosomal regions that may harbor susceptibility genes for autism.

Studies to find genetic mechanisms that underlie autism have tried to include only cases that were idiopathic, i.e., of unknown cause. It is important to understand that the cases included as idiopathic have varied over time. For Kanner, this meant cases that were not only of unknown cause, but also without dysmorphic features that might suggest a neurologic syndrome, even if the cause of that syndrome was unknown. A recent analysis of a case series of autistic children illustrates the value of this approach for genetic studies. When only cases without minor congenital anomalies were included, the male:female sex ratio was nearly 10:1 and there was a much higher rate of autism cases in the families.[23] This was also true of Kanner's cases.[24] While modern studies have excluded cases with known etiologies, they have not excluded cases with mild dysmorphic features of unknown origin.

For autism judged by the examiners to be idiopathic, the most parsimonious genetic model is one in which several genes interact with one another to produce the autism phenotype. In an analysis of family history data, Pickles and colleagues rejected a single-locus model and heterogeneity models in favor of a multilocus epistatic model involving anywhere from 2 to 10 loci, with 3 loci being most plausible.[25] Using a different approach, Van Eerdewegh obtained similar results: he found that a model with 3 to 6 epistatic (interacting) loci was the simplest model consistent with the data (Van Eerdewegh, unpublished analysis). According to these models, autism is most likely to occur in a child who inherits 3 or 4 genes from his/her parents, with each gene contributing to the phenotype. The models cannot specify whether these are always the *same* 3 or 4 genes, or whether several combinations of 3 or 4 genes, from a larger array of predisposing genes, could cause autism. The models are consistent with the variation in severity of autism in sibling pairs and with the fact that in families ascertained through an autistic proband, other members are found with Asperger syndrome or other milder manifestations of autistic-like phenotypes. The milder phenotypes in relatives of probands with autism could reflect the inheritance of a subset of the genes that predispose to autism.

While this model is the most parsimonious, it is only a model, and there are other possibilities, perhaps the most likely being that there is no one model that will be relevant to all the cases currently judged idiopathic. Another possible explanation for the spectrum of severity within families is that autism is caused by the confluence of genetic predisposition to language disorder or social reticence, along with a second hit from an environmental or immunogenetic risk factor.

<u>An Immunogenetic Connection?</u>

Considerable indirect evidence suggests a role for autoimmunity in autism. One study found more family members with autoimmune diseases in the families of autistic compared with control probands.[26] A few studies have reported that some children with autism, or their mothers, have haplotypes at the major histocompatibility complex (MHC) locus that may predispose their autistic children to autoimmunity.[27] In two studies, more children with autism than controls had auto-antibodies to certain brain tissues, including myelin basic protein, neurofilament proteins, and vascular endothelium.[28-30] The immunogenetic findings vary across studies, and most reports describe small samples from a single laboratory. Most of these findings could conceivably be explained by functional deficit of MHC molecules. However, none of the genome screens (see below) have signals anywhere near the MHC locus on chromosome 6p. Nevertheless, enough circumstantial evidence exists to support a role for autoimmunity in the etiology of autism that larger, well-controlled studies as well as a consideration of immune-related genes on other chromosomes are warranted. In a thoughtful and scholarly review of the evidence, Korvatska et al.[31] suggest that the hypothesis most consistent with variety of immunological findings in autism is one in which a primary CNS defect leads secondarily to immune abnormalities. However, they suggest other possible scenarios.

HOW CAN WE FIND SPECIFIC SUSCEPTIBILITY GENES?

Numerous linkage signals on numerous chromosomes have been reported, but few are in exactly the same place, as shown in the cartoon below, and none are large. The field of autism genetics has reached what has proved to be a difficult point for investigators of disorders that have "complex" genetic mechanisms. It is not easy to replicate linkage findings in multiplex disorders, even when loci are truly present,[32] and the ability to localize true signals is poor.[33]

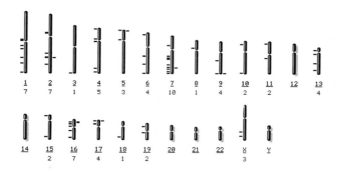

Fig. 1.

"Suggestive" signals from the published genome screens. (Each red line indicates a reported signal; numerals below the chromosome numbers indicate total number of signals reported on that chromosome.)

There are several possible next steps, all of which may need to be pursued iteratively in order to localize the linkage signals enough to decrease the number of candidate genes to a reasonable number, although what is a "reasonable number" will increase with advances in technology.

As a first step, we need larger samples. Several consortia are now working toward this end. It may be possible to tease larger signals and more precise localization of signals from a "mega-analysis" of several hundred families although this approach is limited when the genotypes have been carried out in different laboratories and using different sets of markers. It is possible that even using very large samples, locus heterogeneity will limit the power of such analyses.

Thus, a second step is to carefully reconsider all included families in order to minimize phenocopies of the autism phenotype. As the definition of autism has become broader, many of the cases no longer resemble the highly familial disorder Kanner described in 1943. He did not diagnose any child who had dysmorphic features, and he also required a rich array of autistic features, particularly "a preoccupation with the maintenance of sameness."[1] The children thus diagnosed had a highly familial disorder.[24] Dysmorphic features are particularly common in trios, but they also occur in sib pairs. Omitting such families from linkage and association studies should reduce the phenocopy rate somewhat, but much heterogeneity will remain.

Third, therefore, we need to take advantage of the phenotypic heterogeneity in autism, rather than be hampered by it. Evidence is accumulating that (a) autism is not the best phenotype to use to find its genes, and that (b) it is possible to dissect autism into genetically relevant components. For some years, considerable research has focused on defining genetically relevant phenotypes that can increase the power to find susceptibility loci for autism. As mentioned above, these can be noticed as variation within the autism phenotype, and they are also evident in non-autistic family members.

We made an initial test of the genetic value of dissecting the phenotype by subsetting families based on proband language development and including as "cases" those parents with language abnormalities. The linkage signals improved on 7q,[34] 13q and 2q (2q data are unpublished). This has been replicated on 7q and 2q.[35-37] The same marker that gave the peak score on 13q (D13S800) provided a LOD of more than 3 in families with developmental language disorder.[38]

Other traits are also candidates for subsetting families, including symptom clusters documented in the Autism Diagnostic Interview-Revised (ADI-R), head size, platelet serotonin and a history of autoimmune disease.

GENES TO STUDY IN DETAIL

Plausible candidate genes for autism are frighteningly numerous. However, integration of evidence from a variety of fields should increase the likelihood of choosing relevant genes. Evidence comes from several types of studies. (1) Biochemical analyses of peripheral blood from patients and their families have repeatedly implicated the serotonin system and, more recently, other neurotransmitter systems and neuropeptides (e.g., oxytocin.[39-41] (2) Positron emission tomography (PET)-based studies have provided more direct evidence that serotonin synthesis is altered and $GABA_A$ receptor binding is decreased in various brain structures in autism probands.[42] Parents with the BAP have unusual patterns of spiperone binding (a serotonin agonist).[43] (3) MRI and autopsy studies of neuroanatomy and neuropathology point to developmental abnormalities in the limbic system and cerebellum,[44-48] as well as macrocephaly.[4,49-52] The autistic brain appears to overgrow early in life and then to grow too slowly later in life. Neuronal size, packing, and migration abnormalities have also been identified.[44,47,53] Correlation of these findings with observations of similar neuropathology in mouse models may be helpful in identifying genes and systems that may play a similar role in the human. (4) Radiolabeled ligand binding analysis of autopsy material suggests abnormalities in $GABA_A$ receptors in hippocampus.[39] (5) Studies of animal social behavior have also provided clues. Differences in social behavior between montane and prairie voles is caused by a variation in the promoter of the oxytocin receptor gene (*Oxtr*).[54,55] Social abnormalities in the *Disheveled* mouse (a knock-out of the *Dvl1* gene) point to genes in that system.[53] (6) Cytogenetic abnormalities occur throughout the genome, but most commonly involve maternal duplications on 15q11-q13. Translocations and deletions have identified areas on 7q, 2q and Xq among others that may harbor genes whose disruption leads to autism phenotypes.[56-59]

When these data are considered together with the evidence for linkage either in our complete dataset or in phenotypically defined subsamples, a far more manageable number of candidates emerge.

RELN

For example, autopsy studies of brains of persons with autism have found consistent profound decreases in Purkinje cells in cerebellar hemispheres. Naturally occurring mouse mutants, including *Reeler*,[60] have developmental abnormalities of these neurons. A positive association has been reported between the *RELN* gene on human 7q and autism.[61] Reelin, located within 5 cM of the most consistent and highest linkage signal for autism, is a secreted glycoprotein that acts as a signaling molecule with significant roles in neurodevelopment.[62] The serotonin receptor 2A gene (*HTR2A*) maps within a 13q region linked in our dataset. Given the likely involvement of serotonergic systems, this gene is an excellent functional candidate.

WNT2

It had been observed that the mouse knockout of the dvl1 gene displays abnormal social behavior - no grooming of cage mates and failure to sleep in a communal pile. The interval with the strongest linkage signal on 7q in autism families contains a gene, *WNT2*, which depends for its function on the DVL family of proteins. Wassink et al reported two families with non-conservative mutations as well as significant association in the larger sample to an allelic variation in the gene.

For the language subsetting study and the analyses of *WNT2*, we used only a single variable, onset of phrase speech, to divide the families. We speculated that we could identify more homogeneous subsets for genetic analysis by developing factors of the many items in the Autism Diagnostic Interview. We developed these factors without the imposition of pre-existing diagnostic concepts. We used ADIs (the original version of the interview) and ADI-Rs from 293 subjects (only one proband was used per family) who met criteria for autism. The best solution included 6 factors. Items were retained in each factor that correlated at least $r^2=0.40$ with other items in the factor and that had low correlations with the next "closest" factor. We then validated these factors in an independent sample of 68 autistic children from a different study of language in autism (Table 3). For five of the six factors, the within-sib pair correlation (using both sibs from 165 multiplex families) were highly significant, suggesting that they are genetically relevant. Social Intentionality has not shown sib-sib correlations in two other datasets.[63,64]

Table 1: ADI factors.

FACTOR	VALIDATING TEST	CORRELATION (Spearman ρ)	PARTIAL CORR	SIB-SIB CORR (Pearson r)
1. Spoken Language	Expressive Vocabulary Test	ρ =-0.28, p= .020	for IQ, ρ = -0.30, p=.013	r=.21 p=.008
2. Social Intentionality	Vineland socialization standard score	ρ = -0.37 p = .002	For IQ, ρ =-.40, p=.001	r=.11 p=.142
3. Compulsions	KSADS Impairment and time spent on compulsions	ρ = 0.57 p = .000		r=.25 p=.001
4. Developmental Milestones	Vineland total score Full scale IQ	ρ = -. 27 p = .026 ρ = -.26 p = .029		r=.29 p=.0001
5. Splinter skills	Composite score of performance on backward word and block span	ρ =.38, p=.017		r=.39 p<.0001
6. Sensory Aversions	Phobia score derived from KSADS ADOS unusual sensory reactions	ρ = 0.26 p = .054 ρ = -0.27 p = .001		r=.26 p=.002

We used the ADI factors as part of a multi-step process to choose chromosomal intervals to analyze in greater detail. Our multi-step process was as follows.

1. Using autism as the phenotype, we selected seven chromosomal intervals that demonstrated HLODs of >1 and that had also been implicated in at least one other study or in which there were highly plausible candidate genes.

2. We then repeated the analyses using the 6 factor scores. For this illustration, we used a simple approach. For each of the 6 analyses (one using each factor) at each of the selected intervals, the average score for a given factor was determined for each sib pair. The families were then divided into two subsamples, split at the median factor score. Simple dominant and recessive models were used, and disease susceptibility allele frequencies set at q = 0.01 and q = 0.1, respectively. Phenocopy rates were set at P(+/+) = 0.0005 (where "+" denotes the wild-type allele), and all non-trivial penetrance rates were set at 50%.

3. When the affected phenotype was defined as one of the ADI-based factors, there was a substantial increase in the HLOD and the proportion of linked families for 4 of the 7 intervals chosen.

542

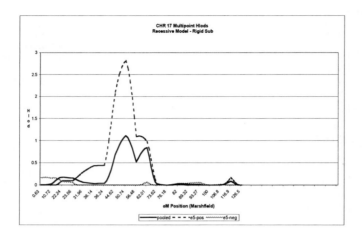

Fig. 2. Effect of subsetting on linkage signal on Chromosome 17.

In the Boston/AGRE dataset (N = 97 families for this interval), linkage on chromosome 17 showed a modest multipoint HLOD of 1.11 (α = 0.20) under a recessive model at D17S1294 (51 cM) with a NPL score of 2.13 (P = 0.014). Linkage has also been reported for this region in the IMGSAC families.[65] The serotonin transporter (*SLC6A4* or *5-HTT*) has long been considered a candidate because of consistent abnormalities in autism in the serotonin system.[18,40] The selective serotonin reuptake inhibitors (SSRIs) reduce compulsions and anxiety seen in children with autism.[66,67] Analysis for the subset of families with high factor scores on the compulsions factor (N = 52) revealed a recessive HLOD of 2.82 (α = 0.44), again at D17S1294 at 51 cM, with a NPL of 2.82 (P = 0.0026). Association studies of the *SLC6A4* gene have been mixed, although this is of limited significance as only two polymorphisms have been examined in the vast majority of studies.[68-71] One of these markers is an insertion/deletion polymorphism in the promoter (5-HTTLPR), speculated to affect gene expression.[72] One study analyzed a number of SNP and microsatellite markers and corresponding haplotypes across the gene; they found significant LD effects at three markers.[73] We have also found highly significant association with alleles in the gene, but only in the subset of families where probands had high compulsion scores.

HEAD CIRCUMFERENCE AND WIDTH AS A FAMILIAL TRAIT IN AUTISM FAMILIES

There are numerous other phenotypic aspects of autism that vary from case to case and are also seen in family members. In his original description of autism, Kanner[8] noted that the children tended to have large heads. This has been rediscovered in recent years and documented in several studies. The head circumference (HC) in probands is normally distributed, but skewed to the right, and more children than expected meet criteria for macrocephaly (1.88 standard deviations from mean; 97th percentile)[19,20,74,75] (Appendix I, reprint 3) confirmed this and showed, using our Boston multiplex families, that the HC of parents and sibs also tends to be large, with 9.8% of parents with HC> 97th percentile (N=41; Chi square = 6.4; p<.02). We had only 15 unaffected sibs (these are few in multiplex autism families); 2/15 had macrocephaly. We now have HC on probands and both parents for 46 families. At least one proband is more likely to be macrocephalic if one parent is macrocephalic than if neither parent is macrocephalic (p=0.056). Like the ADI factor scores, HC can be analyzed in autism families as a quantitative trait, and parents can be included in the phenotype.

EPIGENETIC EFFECTS

The field has focused mainly on direct genetic effects in the etiology of autism; that is, effects on development that result from the genes that are present in the child. However, epigenetic effects are also being explored. For example, the level of maternal dopamine-beta hydroxylase (DBH) has been reported to be lower in the mothers of multiplex autism families than in controls (ref). Dopamine beta-hydroxylase is an enzyme that converts dopamine to norepinephrine. The dopaminergic system has been implicated in a number of psychiatric disorders including schizophrenia, social anxiety disorder, addiction, and attention deficit hyperactivity disorder. Maternal DBH levels may play a role in the development of autism by altering the pre-natal intra-uterine concentrations of neurotransmitters and morphogens; specifically, dopamine and norepinephrine. DBH levels are in part regulated by two promoter alleles: a 19 base-pair insertion/deletion (+/-) polymorphism and a -1021 C/T transition (ref). The 19 b.p +/+ allele and the -1021 C/C allele are associated with increased levels of DBH.

We examined DBH levels in 100 mothers of children with autism. We have found that the children of mothers with the 19 b.p. +/+ allele have statistically significant worse outcomes with respect to obsessive-compulsive behaviors than children of mothers with the 19 b.p. -/- allele. Children of mothers with the -1021 C/C genotype may have worse outcomes with respect to spoken language than did the children of mothers with the -1021 T/T genotype.

Another epigenetic effect may result from gene-environment interactions. In a small case series we collected in Tanzania (Mankoski and Folstein in preparation), half the 16 cases that met criteria for autism had the onset of symptoms immediately following their first attack of falciparum malaria (Table 2). These cases were phenotypically indistinguishable from the non-infectious cases, but there was an equal male:female ratio and only one case had cranial dysmorphology.

Of the eight post-infectious cases, three were developing normally prior to the malaria, which was extremely severe, with extremely high fevers, seizures and loss of consciousness lasting for several days. The other five had mild developmental delays and family histories other features more similar to typical non-infectious cases (Table 3). We thus speculate that very severe cerebral malaria is sufficient to cause autism, without other risk factors. However, in the presence of genetic risk factors, which by themselves were not sufficient to cause full blown autism, milder infection may serve as a "second hit" that causes the autism phenotype to appear.

Table 2.

	Infectious Etiology N = 8	Non-infectious Etiology N = 8
m:f ratio	4:4	7:1
Language present (verbal)	1	2
Positive family history of developmental difficulties	4	3
Cranial dysmorphology	1	4
Head circumference $\geq 75^{th}$ percentile	4 (N = 7)	4
Non-febrile seizures	4	2

Table 3.

	Severe infection N = 3	Mild infection N = 5
Agent	Plasmodium, Salmonella, unknown	Plasmodium
Abnormal developmental background prior to infection	0	3
Positive family history of developmental difficulties	1	3 (3)
Head circumference $\geq 75^{th}$ percentile	0	3 (2)
Non-febrile seizures	2	2 (1)
* Parentheses indicate number of subjects with an abnormal developmental background		

WHAT IS THE LIKELY NATURE OF THE GENES AND ALLELES INVOLVED IN CAUSING AUTISM?

When several to many genes interact to cause a moderately common phenotype, the relevant alleles of these genes will be very common, and thus, not likely to cause disease unless they are paired with other susceptibility alleles or environmental risk factors. This idea is consistent with the traits that make up the broader autism phenotype. They are traits in the normal range, albeit at the extreme of that range, and they usually do not interfere enough with functioning to result in clinical referral. Indeed, several studies of the siblings of children with autism have indicated that they may have unusually high intelligence, and there are many examples of parents who make important contributions to their fields.

It is thus of interest that variations in genetic regions that regulate gene expression, such as promotors, have been significantly associated with autism for several of the candidates for which some positive evidence of involvement has been reported.

In conclusion, it seems likely that while individual children with autism may be caused by the interaction of a few common susceptibility alleles, which on their own have phenotypes. Large numbers of genes may be involved that impose both genetic and possibly epigenetic effects. Once genes that cause autism have been found, it will be possible to study their timing and mechanisms of action in the hope of finding a way of intervening that would prevent or treat autism or decrease the severity of its symptoms.

REFERENCES

1.   Kanner, L. (1943) "Autistic disturbances of affective contact". *Nervous Child*, **2**: p. 217-250.
2.   Asperger, H. (1944) "Die autistischen psychopathen im kindesalter." *Archiv fur Psychiatrie und Nervenkrankheiten*, **117**: p. 76-136.
3.   Gillberg, C. and L. Wing (1999) "Autism: not an extremely rare disorder". *Acta Psychiatr Scand*, **99**(6): p. 399-406.
4.   Fombonne, E. "The epidemiology of autism: a review." *Psychological Medicine*, **29**: p. 769-786.
5.   Bettelheim, B. (1967) *The empty fortress; infantile autism and the birth of the self*. New York: Free Press.
6.   Eisenberg, L. (1957) "The fathers of autistic children." *American Journal of Orthopsychiatry*, **127**: p. 715-724.
7.   Rimland, B. (1964) *Infantile autism: the syndrome and its implications for a neural theory of behavior*. New York: Appleton-Century-Crofts.
8.   Rutter, M. (1968) "Concepts of autism: a review of research. [Review]." *Journal of Child Psychology & Psychiatry & Allied Disciplines*, **9**(1): p. 1-25.
9.   Cantwell, D.P., L. Baker, and M. Rutter (1979) "Families of autistic and dysphasic children. I. Family life and interaction patterns". *Archives of General Psychiatry*, **36**(6): p. 682-7.
10.   Folstein, S. and M. Rutter (1977) "Infantile autism: a genetic study of 21 twin pairs". *Journal of Child Psychology & Psychiatry & Allied Disciplines*, **18**(4): p. 297-321.
11.   Bailey, A., et al. (1995) "Autism as a strongly genetic disorder: evidence from a British twin study". *Psychological Medicine*, **25**(1): p. 63-77.
12.   Steffenburg, S., et al. (1989) "A twin study of autism in Denmark, Finland, Iceland, Norway and Sweden." *Journal of Child Psychology & Psychiatry & Allied Disciplines*, **30**(3): p. 405-16.

13. Fombonne, E., et al. (1997) "A family study of autism: cognitive patterns and levels in parents and siblings". *Journal of Child Psychology and Psychiatry*, **38**(6): p. 667-684.

14. Pickles, A., et al. (2000) "Variable expression of the autism broader phenotype: findings from extended pedigrees." *J Child Psychol Psychiatry*, **41**(4): p. 491-502.

15. Folstein, S.E. and M.L. Rutter (1988) "Autism: familial aggregation and genetic implications." [Review]. *Journal of Autism & Developmental Disorders*, **18**(1): p. 3-30.

16. Folstein, S.E., et al. (1999) "Predictors of cognitive test patterns in autism families." *J Child Psychol Psychiatry*, **40**(7): p. 1117-28.

17. Piven, J., et al. (1991) "Psychiatric disorders in the parents of autistic individuals." *Journal of the American Academy of Child & Adolescent Psychiatry*, **30**(3): p. 471-8.

18. Cook, E.H. and B.L. Leventhal (1996) "The serotonin system in autism". *Curr Opin Pediatr*, **8**(4): p. 348-54.

19. Lainhart, J.E., et al. (1997) "Macrocephaly in children and adults with autism." *J Am Acad Child Adolesc Psychiatry*, **36**(2): p. 282-90.

20. Deutsch, C.K., et al. "Macrocephaly and cephalic disproportion in autistic probands and their first-degree relatives." *American Journal of Medical Genetics*, In Press.

21. Freeman, B.J., et al. (1989) "Psychometric assessment of first-degree relatives of 62 autistic probands in Utah." *American Journal of Psychiatry*, **146**(3): p. 361-4.

22. Santangelo, S.L. and S.E. Folstein (1999) *Autism: A Genetic Perspective*, in *Neurodevelopmental Disorders*, H. Tager-Flusberg, Editor. MIT Press: Cambridge. p. 431-447.

23. Miles, J.H. and R.E. Hillman (2000) "Value of a clinical morphology examination in autism". *Am J Med Genet*, **91**(4): p. 245-53.

24. Piven, J., et al. (1990) "A family history study of neuropsychiatric disorders in the adult siblings of autistic individuals". *Journal of the American Academy of Child & Adolescent Psychiatry*, **29**(2): p. 177-83.

25. Pickles, A., et al. (1995) "Latent-class analysis of recurrence risks for complex phenotypes with selection and measurement error: a twin and family history study of autism." *American Journal of Human Genetics*, **57**(3): p. 717-26.

26. Comi, A.M., et al. "Familial clustering of autoimmune disorders and evaluation of medical risk factors in autism." *J Child Neurol*, **14**(6): p. 388-94.

27. Burger, R. and R. Warren (1998) "Possible immunogenetic basis for autism." *Mental Retardation and Developmental Disabilities Research Reviews*, **4**: p. 137-141.

28. Singh, V.K., et al. (1993) "Antibodies to myelin basic protein in children with autistic." *Brain, Behavior, & Immunity*, **7**(1): p. 97-103.

29. Connolly, A.M., et al. (1999) "Serum autoantibodies to brain in Landau-Kleffner variant, autism, and other neurologic disorders." *J Pediatr*, **134**(5): p. 607-13.

30. Weizman, A., et al. (1982) "Abnormal immune response to brain tissue antigen in the syndrome of autism." *Am J Psychiatry*, **139**(11): p. 1462-5.
31. Korvatska, E., et al. (2002) "Genetic and immunologic considerations in autism". Neurobiol Dis, **9**(2): p. 107-25.
32. Suarez, B., C. Hampe, and P. Van Eerdewegh, (1994) *Problems of replicating linkage claims in psychiatry*, in *Genetic Approaches to Mental Disorders*, E. Gershon and C. Cloninger, Editors. American Psychiatric Press, Inc.: Washington, DC. p. 23-46.
33. Altmuller, J., et al. (2001) "Genomewide scans of complex human diseases: true linkage is hard to find." *Am J Hum Genet*, **69**(5): p. 936-50.
34. Folstein, S.E. and R.E. Mankoski (2000) "Chromosome 7q: where autism meets language disorder?" *Am J Hum Genet*, **67**(2): p. 278-81.
35. Liu, J., et al. (2001) "A genomewide screen for autism susceptibility loci.." *Am J Hum Genet*, **69**(2): p. 327-40.
36. Buxbaum, J.D., et al. (2001) "Evidence for a susceptibility gene for autism on chromosome 2 and for genetic heterogeneity." *Am J Hum Genet*, **68**(6): p. 1514-20.
37. Shao, Y., et al. (2002) "Phenotypic homogeneity provides increased support for linkage on chromosome 2 in autistic disorder." *Am J Hum Genet*, **70**(4): p. 1058-61.
38. Bartlett, C.W., et al. (2001) "Linkage analysis of chromosome 3 in families selected for specific language impairment." *American Journal of Human Genetics*, **69**(4): p. 506.
39. Blatt, G.J., et al. (2001) "Density and distribution of hippocampal neurotransmitter receptors in autism: an autoradiographic study." *J Autism Dev Disord*, **31**(6): p. 537-43.
40. Tordjman, S., et al. (2001) "Role of the serotonin transporter gene in the behavioral expression of autism." *Mol Psychiatry*, **6**(4): p. 434-9.
41. Green, L., et al. (2001) "Oxytocin and autistic disorder: alterations in peptide forms." *Biol Psychiatry*, **50**(8): p. 609-13.
42. Chugani, D.C., et al.(2001) "Postnatal maturation of human GABAA receptors measured with positron emission tomography." *Annals of Neurology*, **49**(5): p. 618-26.
43. Goldberg, J., et al. (2001) *Brain Serotonin 2A (5HT2A) Receptor Density in Parents of Autistic Probands*. in *International Meeting for Autism Research (IMFAR)*. San-Diego, CA.
44. Courchesne, E. (1997) "Brainstem, cerebellar and limbic neuroanatomical abnormalities in autism." *Current Opinion in Neurobiology*, **7**(2): p. 269-78.
45. Kemper, T.L. and M. Bauman (1998) "Neuropathology of infantile autism." *J Neuropathol Exp Neurol*, **57**(7): p. 645-52.
46. Saitoh, O. and E. Courchesne (1998) "Magnetic resonance imaging study of the brain in autism." *Psychiatry & Clinical Neurosciences*, **52**(Suppl): p. S219-22.

47. Aylward, E.H., et al. (1999) "MRI volumes of amygdala and hippocampus in non-mentally retarded autistic adolescents and adults." *Neurology*, **53**(9): p. 2145-50.

48. Sweeten, T.L., et al. (2002) "The amygdala and related structures in the pathophysiology of autism." *Pharmacology, Biochemistry & Behavior*, **71**(3): p. 449-55.

49. Miles, J.H., et al. (2000) "Head circumference is an independent clinical finding associated with autism." *Am J Med Genet*, **95**(4): p. 339-50.

50. Fidler, D.J., J.N. Bailey, and S.L. Smalley (2000) "Macrocephaly in autism and other pervasive developmental disorders." *Developmental Medicine & Child Neurology*, **42**(11): p. 737-40.

51. Fraser, F.C. and L.A. Arbour (2001) "Association of non-syndromic macrocephaly with autism." *American Journal of Medical Genetics*, **104**(4): p. 342.

52. Bolton, P.F., et al. (2001) "Association between idiopathic infantile macrocephaly and autism spectrum disorders." *Lancet*. **358**(9283): p. 726-7.

53. Lijam, N., et al. (1997) "Social interaction and sensorimotor gating abnormalities in mice lacking Dvl1." *Cell*, **90**(5): p. 895-905.

54. Young, L.J., et al. (2001) "Cellular mechanisms of social attachmentHormones & Behavior, **40**(2): p. 133-8.

55. Young, L.J. (2002) "The neurobiology of social recognition, approach, and avoidance." *Biological Psychiatry*, **51**(1): p. 18-26.

56. Gillberg, C. (1998) "Chromosomal disorders and autism." *Journal of Autism & Developmental Disorders*, **28**(5): p. 415-25.

57. Lauritsen, M., et al. (1999) "Infantile autism and associated autosomal chromosome abnormalities: a register-based study and a literature survey." *Journal of Child Psychology & Psychiatry & Allied Disciplines*, **40**(3): p. 335-45.

58. Wassink, T.H. and J. Piven (2000) "The molecular genetics of autism." *Current Psychiatry Reports*, **2**(2): p. 170-5.

59. Wassink, T.H., J. Piven, and S.R. Patil (2001) "Chromosomal abnormalities in a clinic sample of individuals with autistic disorder." *Psychiatric Genetics*. **11**(2): p. 57-63.

60. Sotelo, C. (1990) "Cerebellar synaptogenesis: what we can learn from mutant mice." *Journal of Experimental Biology*. **153**: p. 225-49.

61. Persico, A.M., et al. (2001) "Reelin gene alleles and haplotypes as a factor predisposing to autistic disorder." *Molecular Psychiatry*. **6**: p. 150-159.

62. Magdaleno, S.M. and T. Curran (2001) "Brain development: integrins and the Reelin pathway." *Current Biology*, **11**(24): p. R1032-5.

63. Silverman, J.M., et al. (2002) "Symptom domains in autism and related conditions: evidence for familiality". *Am J Med Genet*, **114**(1): p. 64-73.

64. MacLean, J.E., et al. (1999) "Familial factors influence level of functioning in pervasive developmental disorder." *J Am Acad Child Adolesc Psychiatry*, **38**(6): p. 746-53.

65. IMGSAC, (1998) "A full genome screen for autism with evidence for linkage to a region on chromosome 7q. International Molecular Genetic Study of Autism Consortium." *Human Molecular Genetics*, **7**(3): p. 571-8.

66. Pigott, T.A. and S.M. Seay (1999) "A review of the efficacy of selective serotonin reuptake inhibitors in obsessive-compulsive disorder." *Journal of Clinical Psychiatry*, **60**(2): p. 101-6.

67. McDougle, C.J., L.E. Kresch, and D.J. Posey (2000) "Repetitive thoughts and behavior in pervasive developmental disorders: treatment with serotonin reuptake inhibitors." *Journal of Autism & Developmental Disorders*, **30**(5): p. 427-35.

68. Klauck, S.M., et al. (1997) "Serotonin transporter (5-HTT) gene variants associated with autism?" *Hum Mol Genet*, **6**(13): p. 2233-8.

69. Maestrini, E., et al. (1999) "Serotonin transporter (5-HTT) and gamma-aminobutyric acid receptor subunit beta3 (GABRB3) gene polymorphisms are not associated with autism in the IMGSA families. The International Molecular Genetic Study of Autism Consortium." *American Journal of Medical Genetics*, **88**(5): p. 492-6.

70. Yirmiya, N., et al. (2001) "Evidence for an association with the serotonin transporter promoter region polymorphism and autism." *American Journal of Medical Genetics*, **105**: p. 381-386.

71. Betancur, C., et al. (2002) "Serotonin transporter gene polymorphisms and hyperserotonemia in autistic disorder." *Mol Psychiatry*, **7**(1): p. 67-71.

72. Lesch, K.P., et al. (1996) "Association of anxiety-related traits with a polymorphism in the serotonin transporter gene regulatory region." *Science*. **274**: p. 1527-1531.

73. Kim, S.J., et al. (2002) "Transmission disequilibrium mapping at the serotonin transporter gene (SLC6A4) region in autistic disorder." *Mol Psychiatry*. **7**(3): p. 278-88.

74. Piven, J., et al.(1995) "An MRI study of brain size in autism." *Am J Psychiatry*. **152**(8): p. 1145-9.

75. Piven, J., et al. (1996) "Regional brain enlargement in autism: a magnetic resonance imaging study." *J Am Acad Child and Adolescent Psychiatry*, **35**(4): p. 530-536.

NEUROPATHOLOGY AT THE CROSSROADS OF NEUROPSYCHIATRY AND GENETICS: NEW INSIGHTS INTO NEUROSERPIN ENCEPHALOPATHY

BERNARDINO GHETTI, MASAKI TAKAO, MASAHIDE YAZAKI, MARTIN R. FARLOW, FREDERICK W. UNVERZAGT, PEDRO PICCARDO, JILL R. MURRELL, MERRILL D. BENSON
Indiana Alzheimer Disease Center, Indiana University School of Medicine, Indianapolis, IN, USA

INTRODUCTION

Neuronal or perineuronal protein aggregates are a characteristic feature of several forms of dementia as for example deposits of amyloid-β in Alzheimer disease and prion protein in prion encephalopathies. In sporadic and familial Parkinson disease, α-synuclein accumulates within neurons to form discrete Lewy bodies; similarly, deposits of aggregated tau protein are present in some forms of familial frontotemporal dementia and in progressive supranuclear palsy.

We studied an Indiana family in which three subjects across two generations have been diagnosed with progressive myoclonus epilepsy. Neuropathologic studies in two of these patients revealed neuronal protein aggregates in most gray matter regions of the central nervous system and in neurons of the dorsal root ganglia. The neuropathologic investigation carried out with a multidisciplinary approach using morphologic, biochemical and molecular genetic methods lead to the understanding of the genetic etiology and molecular pathogenesis of this disease.

We found that intraneuronal deposition of the protein neuroserpin causes severe disfunction of the central nervous system and the accumulation of the protein is the result of a mutation in the *PI12 (Neuroserpin)* gene. In addition, some questions were raised on the basis of our findings. Is protein structure or its effects on protein function the immediate cause of neurodegeneration? In this autosomal dominant disease, is the neuroserpin protein coded by the normal allele involved in the disease process and present in the intraneuronal inclusions in conjunction with the mutant neuroserpin? Are there identifiable changes in the composition of the mutant neuroserpin (e.g. glycosylation, which render the protein resistant to normal degradation or to extracellular transport)? To address these questions, we have biochemically characterized neuroserpin from intracellular inclusions isolated from the brain of the proband, postmortem.

Using a multidisciplinary approach, we have provided novel insights into the correlates between clinical phenotype, molecular pathology and genetics relevant to progressive myoclonus epilepsy caused by neuroserpin mutations.[1,2] Taken together the results of our studies underlie the central role of neuropathology in the discovery of the etiology and pathogenetic mechanisms of hereditary neurodegenerative diseases.

RESULTS

Clinical History

Two Caucasian male siblings, one year apart in age, had been healthy and had conducted uneventful lives until they were 24 years of age. Both individuals presented progressive myoclonus epilepsy during the third decade of life and died at the age of 43.

The mother of the two individuals presented seizures at 25 years of age and was diagnosed as having progressive myoclonus epilepsy as well. She died at 37 years of age following third degree burns. One of the mother's paternal uncles is reported to have been institutionalized in a mental hospital and diagnosed as having epilepsy, psychosis and cerebral arteriosclerosis. He died at age 57.

The proband worked as an architectural drafter. According to information obtained from family members, he had frequent episodes of somnambulism since adolescence and was often found profusely sweating following these episodes. At 24-years of age, he had an episode of generalized seizures during the night and periodically thereafter continued to have action myoclonus. His performance at work deteriorated and he had difficulties with memory, occasionally being unable to write his own name.

At age 27 seizures reappeared; they were myoclonic, complex partial, and tonic-clonic seizures. In spite of aggressive treatment with phenytoin, carbamazepin, valproic acid and clonazepam, his seizures were difficult to control and there were several episodes of status epilepticus.

A neurological examination at age 29 revealed slow speech, diplopia, vertical and horizontal directional nystagmus, dysarthria and myoclonus in the extremities. The tendon reflexes of the extremities were increased, except for the Achilles tendon reflex, which could not be elicited. Sensory examination showed hypoalgesia in a glove and stocking distribution. A neuro-opthamologic examination was negative for both a cherry red spot in the fundus oculi and a Kayser-Fleischer ring in the cornea. Routine laboratory tests were normal.

Neuropsychology

The patient was tested five times over a ten-year interval. He was first examined in the context of a disability evaluation at age 28. The proband had stopped working and his daily activities consisted of keeping house, going to church, and caring for his 4-year-old son. He was described as somewhat depressed. Intelligence was measured in the borderline defective range on Wechsler Adult Intelligence Scale - Revised (WAIS-R, Full Scale IQ = 73, Verbal IQ = 78, Performance IQ = 68).[3] This represented a drop of approximately 30 points (or 2 standard deviations) from estimated premorbid levels based on educational and occupational attainment. The second examination occurred about 13 months later and revealed significant interval decline in intelligence, which was now in the mildly defective range (WAIS-R, Full Scale IQ = 65, Verbal IQ = 69, Performance IQ = 65). The most significant deficits were in working memory, visuoconstructional ability, and fine manual dexterity. The patient's short-term memory was relatively intact (Wechsler Memory Scale, Logical Memory, Story A = 8.5/24 units recalled immediately and 7/24 units recalled after 30 minute delay; Visual Reproduction 8/14 units recalled immediately and 6/14 after a 30 minute delay). The third assessment took place at age 34, when the patient was a resident in a nursing home, and consisted of the Mini-Mental State Examination (MMSE).[4] His score was 24/30 indicating mild cognitive impairment with more trouble in attention (0/5 on serial subtraction) than memory (2/3 on delayed recall of objects). The fourth examination occurred when the patient was 37-years-old and consisted of the Consortium to Establish a Registry for Alzheimer Disease (CERAD) neuropsychological battery.[5] His MMSE score was fairly stable at 23/30. The most significant deficits on this battery occurred on tests of constructional ability (Constructional Praxis = 1st percentile) and sequential tracking (Trail Making Test Part A = unable to complete); short-term memory was within broad normal limits (3/3 objects recalled after a delay; fully oriented to time and place; CERAD Word List Learning sum recall = 27th percentile, delayed recall = 25th percentile). The fifth examination was done 18 months later, at age 38, again using the CERAD neuropsychological battery. The patient's MMSE score had dropped to 10/30 with marked decline in visuoconstructional ability and expressive language (Animal Fluency < 1st percentile; Boston Naming < 1st percentile) and milder decline in verbal short-term memory (Word List Learning sum recall = 1st percentile).

At the age of 28, three years after the onset of the illness, the patient had already experienced disabling intellectual loss consistent with mild dementia. There was disturbance to his fund of knowledge, but even more marked impairment in novel problem solving. Subsequent examinations revealed progressive deterioration with impairments in visuoconstructional ability more prominent than those to language and short-term memory. By age 38, there was severe generalized impairment consistent with advanced dementia.

Electrophysiology

EEGs, obtained at regular intervals, showed similar results throughout the course of the proband's illness; frequent spikes and spike and wave complexes were particularly prominent in the central and temporal regions bilaterally. An ABR examination, carried out when the patient was 29, suggested a disturbance in the right pontomedullary junction. At the same time, a SEP examination showed normal response to median and tibial nerve stimulation and an EMG showed mildly decreased motor conduction velocity (MCV) and compound muscle action potentials (CMAP) of the left peroneal nerve. Another EMG, obtained at age 37, showed severely decreased MCV and CMAP of the right peroneal and deep tibial nerve. The possibility of a severe peripheral neuropathy was entertained; however, no further studies were carried out.

Skin and Liver Biopsies
A skin biopsy and a liver biopsy were obtained when the patient was 28 and 29, respectively; a repeated skin biopsy was obtained when the patient was 37. The pathologic examination revealed neither Lafora bodies nor cellular deposits consistent with any storage or metabolic disease.

Neuroradiology
At 32 years of age, an MRI showed no abnormal findings; while at age 35, mild cerebellar atrophy was noted. At age 37, cerebral atrophy was evident on CT and MRI scans.

Generalized seizures and myoclonus continued to persist despite pharmacological treatment. At the age of 30, he was slow in mental processing and calculations, but he was still oriented to time and place; his walk was impaired due to severe myoclonus. He was placed in a nursing home at age 32. As the disease progressed myoclonus of the face and extremities worsened as well as cerebellar ataxia. He died from aspiration pneumonia at age 43.

System Pathology
The pathologic findings in the two individuals were similar. The general autopsy revealed normocepahlic, well-developed males. On gross examination, patchy consolidation of the lower lobes of the lungs, mild atheromatous changes of the thoracic aorta and petechial hemorrhages of the mucosa of the urinary bladder were seen.

Light microscopy
The lungs showed an organized aspiration pneumonia and an acute bronchopneumonia. The spleen showed a reduction of the white pulp and the urinary bladder showed an acute cystitis. Tissue samples of the peripheral organs were otherwise histologically unremarkable and the cytological examination did not reveal pathologic intracellular inclusions. Immunohistochemical analysis of skeletal muscles, lung, liver, spleen, and pancreas as well as pituitary, adrenal and thyroid glands, using antibodies against neuroserpin, did not reveal immunopositivity. An examination of the striate muscle revealed mild type II fiber atrophy.

Electron microscopy
Parenchymal cells of the liver did not show intracytoplasmic bodies.

Morphologic and Molecular Neuropathology
The brains of the proband and his brother showed very similar pathologic changes that are reported in a single description. Biochemical studies were carried out on the proband.

Gross neuropathology
In the fresh state, the brain of the proband weighed 980g while that of the brother weighed 958. Both brains showed diffuse atrophy, which was most evident at the level of the frontal lobes. There was no atherosclerosis in the major cerebral arteries. On coronal

sections, the caudate nucleus and cerebellum were mildly atrophic and the brain stem appeared reduced in volume.

Neurohistology

Neuronal loss was moderate in the frontal, cingulate, temporal, parietal, insular, and occipital cortices and the most affected were layers III, IV, V, and VI. Gliosis was present throughout the cortical layers. Mild neuronal loss and gliosis were also seen in the entorhinal and transentorhinal cortices, hippocampus, amygdala, basal ganglia and thalamus. Small vessels with calcified walls were noted in the globus pallidus. Mild gliosis was present in the white matter of the centrum semiovale. In the cerebellum, a mild to moderate loss of Purkinje cells was noted; many of these cell had an eosinophilic cytoplasm consistent with agonal hypoxia. The Golgi epithelial cells appeared more numerous than in control cerebellum and a mild hypertrophy of the Bergmann glia was seen. Furthermore, a mild gliosis was noted in the cerebellar white matter and dentate nucleus. The substantia nigra and locus coeruleus showed moderate neuronal loss and gliosis. Amyloid deposits and neurofibrillary pathology were not seen in thioflavin S and Congo red preparations.

The most striking cytological finding was the presence of intraneuronal eosinophilic homogeneous bodies in the neuronal perikaryon and the neuropil in most gray matter areas of the brain and spinal cord. Within a single neuronal perikaryon, one or more bodies were present; in some instances, they were so numerous and crowded together that they resembled a cluster of grapes. When a major portion of the perikaryon was occupied by one or more intracytoplasmic bodies, the nucleus was eccentric and often deformed. The diameter of these bodies ranged from 1.5 to 25 μm with the smaller more likely to be in a cluster.

In addition to being strongly eosinophilic, these bodies were PAS positive, with and without diastase treatment. In Bodian preparations, large bodies were darkly stained in the core and lightly stained in the outer part, while smaller bodies were diffusely pale throughout; in Heidenhain-Woelcke preparations, the bodies were darkly stained throughout, regardless of their size.

Antibodies against neuroserpin strongly labeled bodies of all sizes. The largest bodies were strongly immunopositive at the periphery with the inner part being less immunoreactive. In some instances, a clear, crescent shaped space was seen on the side of the body with the distal surface of the space being neuroserpin immunopositive. Using single and double immunohistochemistry, it was possible to establish the localization of the bodies in neuronal cell processes. Double immunohistochemistry was particularly useful when antibodies against both non-phosphorylated high molecular weight neurofilament protein and neuroserpin were used in combination. Intracytoplasmic inclusions of various sizes were seen in processes identified as dendrites. These findings were particularly frequent in neurons adjacent to the thalamic fasciculus, substantia nigra and the anterior horn cells. In some instances, the body was seen at a considerable distance from the perikaryon and the diameter of the body was much wider than that of the dendrite. In other instances, the body was in the proximity of the origin of the dendrites, while in other cases they appeared as string of beads.

Immunopositivity, using anti-neuroserpin antibodies, suggested that the intracytoplasmic bodies in the patient of the Indiana family were composed of the protein neuroserpin. These data were then confirmed by biochemical studies. Therefore, these intracellular deposits will be referred to as neuroserpin bodies (NBs) in the rest of the manuscript.

Round NBs measuring two to five μm were observed in the neuropil and it was not possible to determine the cell type with which they were associated; however, in some instances they were seen adjacent to small cells, with round or oval nucleus, resembling glial cells.

NBs appeared more numerous in sections immunolabeled using neuroserpin antibodies[6,7] than in those stained with hematoxylin and eosin or PAS. NBs did not immunoreact with antibodies against GFAP, α-β crystallin, α-synuclein, neurofilament proteins,[8] amyloid β protein, tissue-plasminogen activator, MAP-2,[9] tubulin, tau,[10,11] and ubiquitin.

NBs were numerous in the frontal, cingulate, temporal, parietal, insular and occipital cortices. In the neocortex, NBs were numerous throughout the cortical layers, with the exception of layer I and II. NBs were not seen in layer I and rarely were they found in layer II. In addition, occasionally they could be seen in the subcortical white matter. NBs were seen in most regions of the gray matter, including basal ganglia, thalamus, amygdala, hippocampus, subiculum, entorhinal cortex, substantia innominata, colliculus, periaqueductal gray, substantia nigra, red nucleus, oculomotor nerve nucleus, locus coeruleus, dorsal nucleus of Raphe, pontine nucleus, hypoglossal nerve nucleus and dentate nucleus of the cerebellum. The substantia nigra was the area of the central nervous system most affected with NBs; in fact, they were consistently seen in neurons and cell processes of pigmented cells. In the spinal cord, they were seen in the nucleus of Clark, intermediolateral column nucleus, posterior column and posterior funiculus and anterior horn cells. No NBs were seen in the retina.

As neuroserpin immunoreactivity was seen in association with the round bodies, in some instances, neuronal perikarya and processes were diffusely immunopositive. The latter pattern was observed in neurons of the substantia nigra and the thalamic fasciculus.

In addition to central nervous system neurons, NBs were consistently found in the dorsal root ganglion cells. A significant observation was the moderate loss of these neurons; in the place of a degenerated neuron a cluster of satellite cells was found.

Electron microscopy

In toluidine blue-stained sections, NBs appeared homogeneously blue with a lighter ring in the outer part. Low magnification electron micrographs revealed numerous osmiophilic NBs within neuronal perikarya or neuronal processes. NBs were consistently round, oval or with a slightly irregular contour and their diameter ranged from one to 31 μm. In high magnification electron micrographs, the NBs appeared to be composed of a fine granular material. Frequently, perikarya that contained only one body showed an electron-dense cytoplasm and a deformed nucleus, which was no longer round, but it appeared as a narrow, elongated structure with electron-dense nucleoplasm and clumps of chromatin near the nuclear membrane. In some instances, neurons had a round or oval nucleus and an electron-lucent cytoplasm filled with normal organelles; however, a portion of the cytoplasm was occupied by one or two NBs. These were surrounded by an irregularly shaped, electron lucent space that was limited by a unit membrane, which was most likely the rough endoplasmic reticulum. The space between this membrane and the outer surface of the NB contained different amounts of floccular material. In these neurons, dilated spaces surrounded by endoplasmic reticulum membranes were also seen that contained floccular material only. In some instances, more than one body was surrounded by the electron lucent space containing the floccular material. Often, the electron lucent spaces had a crescent shape on one side of the NB. In electron micrographs that included the entire perikaryon and the NB, the electron dense material surrounded by the electron lucent space formed a compartment that appeared to be separated from the rest of the cytoplasm.

NBs were also found in neuropil elements. In several instances, it was not possible to identify the nature of the cell process; however, the body was always granular, electron dense, and surrounded by an electron lucent space. The latter was limited by a unit membrane. Some NBs appeared as a round, granular structures that contained one or two smaller round and more electron-dense structures. In other instances, the granular electron dense body appeared as though it had incorporated multiple lipofuscin grains within its boundaries. Some NBs could be clearly identified within dendrites that were cut in cross sections. The membranes surrounding the NB were often well preserved and showed ribosomes that were adherent to the outer layer of the membrane. Some dendrites contained granular material that was diffuse throughout the cell process without the presence of dense osmiophilic round NBs.

Protein purification

NBs were isolated from frozen cerebral cortex by homogenization in a buffered sucrose solution and centrifugation. The pellet was then treated with detergent to release the inclusions which were isolated by high speed centrifugation. The inclusions were solubilized in 6 M guanidine HCl in the presence of dithiothreitol and proteins fractionated on a Sepharose CL6B column (2.5 x 90 cm). Only one major retarded peak (Pool III) was found. SDS-PAGE of the solubilized inclusion preparation before fractionation revealed a major protein band migrating at a molecular mass of ~50 Kd. This band was present in Pool III of the fractionated proteins.

Protein characterization

Amino terminal sequence analysis of Pool III gave a major sequence starting with position 20 of human neuroserpin. The first two residues could not be unambiguously identified due to high background in the first few cycles.

The sequence of the isolated protein was obtained from analysis of tryptic peptides, which identified all residues except #1-18 (putative signal peptide), and #285.

Residue 52 was Arg instead of the normal Ser. No peptide with Ser at position 52 was found in the trypsin digest, indicating that normal neuroserpin is not present in the inclusion bodies. While the major N-terminal tryptic peptide was residue 20-36, residue-19-36 peptide was also found. From the recoveries of the peptides, approximately 70% of the mutant neuroserpin in the inclusion bodies starts with residue 20 and 30% with residue 19. No tryptic peptides were found that started with residue 17 or 18. Several carboxyl-terminal tryptic peptides starting with residue 394 and ending with residues 405, 407, 409, and 410 were found indicating that some C-terminal proteolysis of neuroserpin had occurred. Three potential Asn glycosylation sites at residues 157, 321, and 401 were predicted from the neuroserpin cDNA sequence.[12] No amino acid was found at these positions in the tryptic peptides containing these three residues suggesting that all three Asn are glycosylated. Also, peptides containing Asp instead of Asn at residues 83, 95, 116, and 328, and Glu instead of Gln at residue 260 were found indicating some deamidation of Asn and Gln had occurred. Only Asp was found at residues 83 and 116, while residue 95 contained 87% Asp and 13% Asn, and residue 328 contained 70% Asn and 30% Asp. In addition to residue 92-100 peptides with Asp or Asn at residue 95, a peptide yielding only residues 92-94 was found (yield ~ 20% that of #92-100 peptides). Also, an N-terminal residue 20-34 peptide was found in a yield approximately 10% that of the residue 20-36 peptide. The fact that only 4 of 24 Asn and 1 of 16 Gln in neuroserpin have undergone deamidation may indicate these positions are in a tertiary structure especially susceptible to deamidation. A common non-enzymatic mechanism of Asn deamidation is via a cyclic imide formation, which then hydrolyzes to Asp or iso-Asp.[13] The finding of tryptic peptides which on Edman sequence analysis stopped at the residue before Asn35 and Asn95 may indicate the presence of iso-Asp at these positions. An iso-Asp residue would be resistant to Edman cyclization and cleavage.

Several major nontrypsin-like cleavages in neuroserpin were found in the tryptic digest of pool III. The most prominent involved cleavages between adjacent Met residues and on the carboxyl side of Met. Complete cleavage of the Met216-Met217 and Met253-Met254 peptide bonds and approximately 50% cleavage of the Met127-Met128 bond were found. Significant cleavage of the Met254-Leu255 and Met 357-Ile 358 peptide bonds were also observed, as well as cleavage after Asn at residues 149, 182, and 281. Proteolysis after Met is rare by trypsin, but can occur with chymotrypsin. TPCK-treated trypsin was used to minimize chymotryptic-like proteolysis. It is unlikely that these cleavages were due to contaminating chymotrypsin in the trypsin preparation since no usual chymotryptic specific proteolysis after aromatic residues (over 40 in neuroserpin) was observed in the HPLC separated digest. Possibly, the minor residue-20-34-sequence peptide could have resulted from a chymotrypsin-like cleavage of Tyr34-Asn35, or it could be due to cyclization of Asn and termination of Edman degradation as mentioned above. The data would suggest that the rare Met-Met sequence and Met peptide bonds in neuroserpin are unusually susceptible to trypsin cleavage.

Tryptic peptides from human α- and β-tubulin, β- and γ-actin, 2', 3'-cyclic nucleotide - 3'-phosphodiesterase, and creatine kinase B chain were also present in the tryptic digest of Pool III in $\leq 10\%$ of the molar amounts of neuroserpin. All are similar in molecular mass ($\sim$ 40 Kd - 50 Kd) to neuroserpin and would elute from a molecular sieve column close to neuroserpin. It is highly unlikely that these proteins are part of the inclusion bodies, but rather contaminants from the cytosol completely removed during isolation of the inclusion bodies.

DNA Sequence

DNA sequence of neuroserpin exons 3 to 9 of the proband were as published for the normal human cDNA.[12] Sequence of exon 2 revealed both adenine and cytosine at the first position of codon 52 of neuroserpin. This sequence indicates heterozygosity for both the normal serine (AGT) and variant arginine (CGT) at this position in the expressed protein.

RFLP analysis of the 167 bp PCR product from NSE2F and NS$_z$ primers revealed that the propositus and his affected sib both had the AviII recognition site associated with the adenine to cytosine mutation. Electrophoresis of the digested PCR product gave a digestion band of 142 bp in addition to the normal 167 bp band indicating heterozygosity for the mutation. Non-affected individuals (100 unrelated subjects) did not show any digestion of PCR product.

DISCUSSION

Three subjects across two generations of an Indiana family have been diagnosed with progressive myoclonus epilepsy and we have found the *Neuroserpin* Ser52Arg mutation in two of them. Neuropathologic studies in two of these patients revealed that neuroserpin accumulates in most gray matter regions of the central nervous system and in neurons of the dorsal root ganglia. Immunohistochemical and neurocytological studies showed that in most instances, neuroserpin accumulates as round, compact deposits in neuronal perikarya and cell processes, forming bodies that are well defined from the rest of the cytoplasm by the membranes of the endoplasmic reticulum. Less frequently, neuroserpin immunoreactivity may be detected diffusely throughout the neuronal cytoplasm without the formation of well-demarcated bodies.

Four mutations in the *Neuroserpin* gene have been found in five families. These mutations are Ser49Pro, Ser52Arg, His338Arg, and Gly392Glu.[14-16] The disorders caused by these mutations are autosomal dominant and the clinical phenotype associated with each of the *Neuroserpin* mutations differs for the age at onset of the neurological signs. The age at onset of the neurological signs in the Indiana family is as early as 24 or 25 years of age, similar to that seen in patients of the Oregon family were the onset is as early as age 18.[14-15,17] In contrast, in patients carrying the Ser49Pro mutation, the age at onset of the neurological signs occurs as early as age 39 and as late as age 50.[14-15] It is noteworthy that the neurological syndromes in the patients of the families reported show important phenotypic differences. The individuals with the Ser49Pro mutation do not have seizures, but suffer from presenile dementia.[14-15] By contrast, in both the Indiana and Oregon families, subjects with the Ser52Arg mutation have seizures and dementia[17-18] Moreover, the patients from the Indiana family meet the criteria for a diagnosis of progressive myoclonus epilepsy.[19-20] More recently, it has been shown that the

His338Arg and Gly392Glu have a PME clinical phenotype with an onset in the second decade of life.[16]

The neuropathologic data show that neuroserpin accumulation is associated with differing degrees of brain atrophy. In fact, the brain of the patient of the Indiana family with the Ser52Arg weighed 980 g, while in patients with the Ser49Pro mutation, its weight ranged from 1400 to 1530 g.[15] It appears that the severity of neuroserpin accumulation may also vary as we compare the Indiana family with the New York family. In fact, NBs are located mostly in layers III and V of the cortex in the latter, while in the former the deposits are abundant in layers III, IV, V, and VI and only occasionally in layer II and in the subcortical white matter. Further studies may clarify these neuropathologic differences.

Except for a cortical biopsy study in a patient with the Ser52Arg *Neuroserpin* mutation from the Oregon family, no other neuropathologic data have been reported on individuals from this family. In the proband of the Indiana family, NBs are present throughout most gray matter regions and are most numerous in the neocortex and substantia nigra. The severity of neuroserpin deposition in the cortex is greater than that seen in the cortical biopsy of the Oregon patient. It should be emphasized that while the biopsy was carried out on an individual who had symptoms for only three years, the disease had occurred for 19 years in the individuals of the Indiana family.

The severe cortical pathology correlates well with the severe deterioration in cognitive function, documented by repeated neuropsychological testing. In addition, the severe neuroserpin deposition in the substantia nigra may be the cause of the extrapyramidal signs, which developed as the disease progressed. It is significant to note that the spinal cord and the dorsal root ganglia were also affected, a finding that may be correlated with the sensory abnormalities detected clinically. The distribution of NBs involves practically all cortical layers of both association and projection cortices as well as multiple subcortical neuronal populations; therefore, a specific clinicopathologic correlation relevant to the myoclonus cannot be made at this time without the results of a detailed *intra vitam* neurophysiologic analysis. It is of interest, however, that the cerebellar cortex and the dentate nucleus are practically free of NBs.

In diseases caused by *Neuroserpin* mutations, the distribution of NBs may reflect the regional expression of this protein. In fact, in the human brain, neuroserpin is expressed in the neocortex, putamen and spinal cord, but weakly in the cerebellum.[6,12] (Neuroserpin was originally extracted from dorsal root ganglion neurons of chicken embryos.[21] In addition to the central nervous system, neuroserpin is expressed in the pancreas and adrenal gland;[6,22] however, our studies have not revealed neuroserpin bodies in any internal organs.

In the proband of the Indiana family, we have found that the NBs are present in the perikaryon and cell processes in the central nervous system. Within cell processes, they can be seen in dendrites; however, we can speculate that some of them may also be present in axons. These observations may be relevant to the function of the protein in nerve cells. At this time, we cannot establish whether neuroserpin accumulates in glial cells, even though we have occasionally seen neuroserpin immunopositive structures very close to glial cells nuclei.

The immunohistochemical results, using antibodies to human neuroserpin, show strong immunoreactivity of the NBs and are consistent with biochemical data showing that the main constituent of these bodies is neuroserpin.[2,23] Biochemical studies of cortical tissue from the proband have shown that NBs can be isolated in a relatively pure fraction and contain a major protein with a mass of ca. 50 kD. Amino acid sequence of this protein identified it as neuroserpin with a substitution of arginine for serine at residue 52, numbering according to Schrimpf et al., which includes the signal peptide.[12] Further analysis will be needed to determine the changes in molecular structure occurring as the result of this genetic mutation.

Our electron microscopic data show that the accumulation of neuroserpin occurs in association with cellular compartments that can be identified as dilated cisterns of the rough endoplasmic reticulum. The NB, *per se*, is not membrane bound, but it appears to be contained within a space limited by the membranes of the endoplasmic reticulum. The modalities of neuroserpin accumulation in compact homogenous bodies needs to be further investigated in cell models. However, on the basis of the biochemical studies on the patient from the Indiana family, NBs do not appear to be the result of neuroserpin polymerization.[2,23]

The disease caused by the Ser52Arg mutation in the Indiana family may have some analogies with Lafora disease. In both conditions, progressive myoclonus epilepsy is the main clinical feature. However, the age of onset of Lafora disease is most often between 10 and 18 years of age.[24-25] The gene responsible for that condition has be localized on chromosome 6q and the disease is autosomal recessive, however, the enzyme defect in Lafora disease is still unknown.[26] The Lafora bodies are mostly composed of polyglucosans.[27] Their morphological characteristics are only superficially similar to NBs. Both Lafora and NBs are strongly PAS positive and they are approximately in the same size range, i.e. one to 30 µm. Both may be present in perikarya or cell processes. However, electron microscopic examination reveals substantial differences between Lafora and NBs. Lafora bodies are non-membrane bound and are composed of glycogen-like granules interspersed with fine filaments measuring eight to 12 nm in diameter, while NBs are composed of fine granular material and are found within dilated cisterns of the rough endoplasmic reticulum. Furthermore, the distribution of these inclusions in the central nervous system differs, particularly at the level of the cerebellum where Lafora bodies may be numerous and neuroserpin only rarely seen. Lafora bodies may be seen in glial cells but not NBs. Lafora bodies may be found in capillary endothelial cells of the brain, in the retina, skeletal and cardiac muscle, liver and in cells of the sweat ducts of the skin; on the contrary, we found NBs only in the central nervous system and dorsal root ganglia but not in any of the other organs.

Four separate reports[28-31] have described four unrelated patients affected by progressive myoclonus epilepsy associate with intraneuronal deposits referred to as "atypical inclusion bodies" that have histological, histochemical and electron microscopic characteristics similar to those seen in diseases caused by neuroserpin accumulation. The disease in these cases did not appear to be familial.[28-31] These individuals, who had similar signs, suffered from seizures, myoclonus, extrapyramidal signs and mental deterioration or dementia. No pathologic changes were found outside the nervous system in the patients studied at autopsy. Interestingly, Ota et al. reported that the small inclusions were often surrounded by the rough endoplasmic reticulum.[30] Based on the reported studies, it was hypothesized that type II myoclonus bodies are composed of neuroserpin. Indeed, a genetic analysis of tissue from the subject with type II myoclonus bodies, reported by Bergener and Gerhardt, has recently clarified the nature of the disease in that case.[16] In fact, mutation Gly392Glu in the *Neuroserpin* gene was identified.[16]

We have described for the first time the association of progressive myoclonus epilepsy with the deposition of neuroserpin in the central nervous system.[1] We emphasized the phenotypic differences within this recently recognized group of neurodegenerative diseases and highlighted the pathologic differences between progressive myoclonus epilepsy caused by neuroserpin accumulation and Lafora disease. The main morphological findings are: 1) neuroserpin accumulates in both the brain and the spinal cord, 2) outside the central nervous system, neuroserpin accumulates in the dorsal root ganglion neurons, 3) neuroserpin accumulates intracellular within the cisterns of the rough endoplasmic reticulum, and 4) no intracellular accumulation of neuroserpin is found in other organs.[1]

Neuroserpin was originally identified as a protein secreted by cultured chicken dorsal root ganglion cells.[21] Subsequently, isolation and purification from ocular vitreous fluid of 14-day-old chick embryos allowed determination of sufficient amino acid sequence to clone a neuroserpin cDNA from an embryonic chicken brain cDNA library.[32] (The cDNA encoded a 410-residue protein, which by sequence homology was assigned to the serpin superfamily of serine protease inhibitors. Expression of neuroserpin in embryonic neurons and in adult brain regions which exhibit synaptic plasticity supports the hypothesis that this protein is a member of the group of extracellular proteases and protease inhibitors which orchestrate brain development, function, and anatomic integrity.[22-23] As with many proteins expressed by the CNS, the identification of mutant forms of the protein, and diseases associated with these molecular defects, provides a new window to decipher the role of the protein in normal physiology. At the same time the metabolic basis of previously undefined disease is revealed. This is particularly true for the neurodegenerative diseases, which are characterized by dementia. In the past, clinical and anatomic characterizations of these diseases have, by comparing similarities and dissimilarities, resulted in grouping together diseases, which at the molecular level are distinct entities.

The 410-residue neuroserpin deduced from chicken cDNA has a hydrophobic amino terminal sequence of 16 amino acid residues conforming to a consensus signal sequence.[32] The N-terminus of purified chicken neuroserpin protein started with residue 17 of the cDNA encoded protein in agreement with the first 16 residues being the signal peptide.[32] Mouse and rat neuroserpin cDNAs have also been cloned and sequenced.[22,33-34] Both encode for a 410-residue protein, and the N-terminal 16 residues of both were proposed as signal peptides by analogy with chicken neuroserpin. Human neuroserpin cDNA was originally isolated from a fetal retina cDNA library.[12] From analysis of the N-terminal sequence of the encoded 410 residue protein, Schrimpf, et al., concluded that the Ala16-Thr17 and Ala 19-Thr20 peptide bonds had equal probability as signal peptide cleavage sites.[12] By analogy to chicken neuroserpin, they assigned the N-terminal 16 residues as the signal peptide. Davis, et al., have also isolated a mutant neuroserpin from inclusion bodies in the brain of a patient with familial dementia and a *Neuoserpin* mutation.[14-15] The Ser49Pro mutant neuroserpin had an N-terminus starting with Thr20. The Ser52Arg mutant neuroserpin characterized in the present study indicates a heterogeneous N-terminus with the majority starting at Thr20 and approximately 30% at Ala19. Analysis of the human neuroserpin N-terminal sequence by von Heijne's probability matrix indicates that while the Gly18-Ala19 peptide bond has less probability than the Ala16-Thr17 and Ala19-Thr20 peptide bonds as signal peptidase cleavage sites, it does have greater probability than other peptide bonds in the region.[35] This is supported by the finding that a PCR product encoding for residues 1-410 of human neuroserpin inserted into a baculovirus expression vector and expressed in Sf9 insect cells yielded a purified recombinant neuroserpin protein that had equal amounts beginning with Ala19 and Thr20.[6] These results show that the signal peptidase in this system cleaves the expressed normal neuroserpin after Gly18 and Ala19, similar to the results in our characterization of the Ser52Arg mutant neuroserpin.

One distinguishing characteristic of the NBs is that they contain carbohydrate as indicated by their positive staining with periodic acid-Shiff (PAS) reagent.[1] Human, mouse, and rat neuroserpins have three potential carbohydrate attachment sites at Asn residues 157, 321, and 401.[12,22-23] Chicken neuroserpin has only two sites as Asp is at position 321 instead of Asn.[11] All species have carbohydrate attached at least to one site since the size of the protein on SDS-PAGE analysis is greater than its molecular weight calculated from its amino acid sequence.[15,22,32-33] Sequence analysis of the Ser52Arg mutant neuroserpin is consistent with glycosylation of all three Asn. The tertiary structure model, based on the primary structure, positions each of these Asn residues on the surface of the molecule and, therefore, indicates that a carbohydrate moiety can be readily accomodated at all three sites.[36]

The NBs in the brain bear similarity to inclusion bodies in the liver composed of α_1-antitrypsin, another member of the serpin superfamily. While over 70 α_1-antitrypsin variants are known, only three are associated with liver abnormalities.[37] Like the neuroserpin mutants (Ser49Pro and Ser53Arg), two α_1-antitrypsins, Malton (ΔPhe51) and Siiyama (Ser53Phe) have mutations in the shutter region of the molecule.[38-39] The third, α_1-antitrypsin Z (Glu342Lys), involves loss of a salt bridge.[40-42] While inclusion bodies from homozygous variant α_1-antitrypsin patients have been characterized, we are not aware of any studies on inclusion bodies from heterozygous patients investigating if only the variant protein is present as we found with the NBs. Variant α_1-antitrypsin isolated from plasma and liver inclusion bodies has altered carbohydrate compared to the normal protein with no sialic acid and high mannose content.[43-46] The incomplete carbohydrate maturation results in its accumulation in the liver endoplasmic reticulum and reduced secretion into the blood stream. While mutant neuroserpin is glycosylated, its carbohydrate structure is unknown. Elucidation and comparison of the carbohydrate structures on mutant and normal neuroserpin should provide insight on the role of glycosylation in NB formation.

These mutations in α_1-antitrypsin and presumably in neuroserpin result in two effects leading to intracellular inclusion body formation. First, the mutation alters the molecule's structure sufficiently to impair carbohydrate maturation, which results in reduced secretion and increased intracellular concentration. Second, the mutation alters the protein's structure or stability to allow aggregation by the insertion of the reactive loop of one mutant molecule into the β-sheet of a second mutant molecule at the increased intracellular concentration. This aggregation phenomenon is common in the serpin superfamily as certain mutants of antithrombin, C1-inhibitor, and α_1-antichymotrypsin also form inclusion bodies and/or multimers.[47-49]

The finding of only mutant neuroserpin in the inclusions indicates that synthesis and processing of normal neuroserpin is unaltered. It has been postulated that neuroserpin is part of the protease and protease inhibitor complex, which determines neuronal growth and synaptic plasticity, processes which occur extracellularly.[22,33] In the case of mutant neuroserpin, the protein accumulates within neurons of the cerebral cortex, brain stem nuclei and dorsal root ganglia.[1,4] The mutant protein is secreted past the ribosomal membrane with cleavage of the signal peptide; it is post-transcriptionally modified by glycosylation, but is not excreted. If the mutant does retain its function of serine protease inhibition, it is not transported to the location where this function is required. Intracellular accumulation of the abnormally aggregating protein is, therefore, the most likely cause of neuronal dysfunction.

ACKNOWLEDGMENTS

The authors are indebted to "family J," in particular the proband, for their willingness to participate in our studies and for their assistance in gathering information for the preparation of this manuscript. We gratefully acknowledge Francine Epperson for being liaison between family J and our research group and Bradley S. Glazier for his editorial assistance. This study was supported in part by PHS P30 AG10133 and PHS R01 NS14426.

REFERENCES

1. Takao, M., Benson, M.D., Murrell, J.R., Yazaki, M., Piccardo, P. Unverzagt, F.W., Davis, R.L. Holohan, P.D., Lawrence, D.A., Richardson, R., Farlow, M.R., Ghetti, B. (2000) "Neuroserpin mutation S52R causes neuroserpin accumulation in neurons and is associated with progressive myoclonus epilepsy." *Journal of Neuropathology and Experimental Neurology.* 59:1070-1086.

2. Yazaki, M., Liepnieks, J.J., Murrell, J.R., Takao, M., Guenther, B., Piccardo, P., Farlow, M.R., Ghetti, B., Benson, M.D. (2001) "Biochemical characterization of

a neuroserpin variant associated with hereditary dementia." *American Journal of Pathology.* 158:227-233.

3. Wechsler, D. (1981) Wechsler adult Intelligence Scale-Revised manual. San Antonio, TX; The Psychological Corporation.

4. Folstein, M.F., Folstein, S.E., McHugh, P.R. (1975) "Mini-Mental State: A practical method for grading the cognitive state of patients for the clinician." *Journal of Psychiatric Research.* 12:189-198.

5. Morris, J.C., Mohs, R.C., Rogers, H., Fillenbaum, G., Heyman, A. (1988) "Consortium to Establish a Registry for Alzheimer's Disease (CERAD) clinical and neuropsychological assessment of Alzheimer's disease." *Psychopharmacology Bulletin.* 24:641-652.

6. Hastings, G.A., Coleman, T.A., Haudenschild, C.C., Stefansson, S., Smith, E.P., Barthlow, R., Cherry, S., Sandkvist, M., Lawrence, D.A. (1997) "Neuroserpin, a brain-associated inhibitor of tissue plasminogen activator is localized primarily in neurons. Implications for the regulation of motor learning and neuronal survival." *Journal of Biological Chemistry.* 272:33062-33067.

7. Sherman, P.M., Lawrence, D.A., Yang, A.Y., Vandenberg, E.T., Paielli, D., Olson, S.T., Shore, J.D., Ginsburg, D. (1992) "Saturation mutagenesis of the plasminogen activator inhibitor-1 reactive center." *Journal of Biological Chemistry.* 267:7588-7595.

8. Sternberger, L.A., Sternberger, N.H. (1983) "Monoclonal antibodies distinguish phosphorylated and nonphosphorylated forms of neurofilaments in situ." *Proceedings of the National Acadademy of Sciences, USA.* 80:6126-6130.

9. Kaufmann, W.E., Taylor, C.V., Lishaa, N.A. (1997) "Immunoblotting patterns of cytoskeletal dendritic protein expression in human neocortex." *Molecular and Chemical Neuropathology.* 31:235-244.

10. Goedert, M., Jakes, R. Vanmechelen, E. (1995) "Monoclonal antibody AT8 recognises tau protein phosphorylated at both serine 202 and threonine 205." *Neuroscience Letters.* 189:167-169.

11. Carmel, G., Mager, E.M., Binder, L.I., Kuret, J. (1996) "The structural basis of monoclonal antibody Alz50's selectivity for Alzheimer's disease pathology." *The Journal of Biological Chemistry.* 271:32789-32795.

12. Schrimpf, S.P., Bleiker, A.J., Brecevic, L., Kozlov, S.V., Berger, P., Osterwalder, T., Krueger, S.R., Schinzel, A., Sonderegger, P. (1997) "Human neuroserpin (PI12): cDNA cloning and chromosomal localization to 3q26." *Genomics.* 40:55-62.

13. Orpiszewski, J., Schormann, N., Kluve-Beckerman, B., Liepnieks, J.J., Benson, M.D. (2000) "Protein aging hypothesis of Alzheimer disease." *The FASEB Journal.* 14:1255-1263.

14. Davis, R.L., Shrimpton, A.E., Holohan, P.D., Bradshaw, C., Feiglin, D., Collins, G.H., Sonderegger, P., Kinter, J., Becker, L.M., Lacbawan, F., Krasnewich, D., Muenke, M., Lawrence, D.A., Yerby, M.S., Shaw, C.M., Gooptu, B., Elliott,

P.R., Finch, J.T., Carrell, R.W., Lomas, D.A. (1999) "Familial dementia caused by polymerization of mutant neuroserpin." *Nature*. 401:376-379.

15. Davis, R.L., Holohan, P.D., Shrimpton, A.E., Tatum, A.H., Daucher, J., Collins, G.H., Todd, R., Bradshaw, C., Kent, P., Feiglin, D., Rosenbaum, A., Yerby, M.S., Shaw, C.M., Lacbawan, F., Lawrence, D.A. (1999) "Familial encephalopathy with neuroserpin inclusion bodies." *American Journal of Pathology*. 155:1901-1913.

16. Davis, R.L., Shrimpton, A.E., Carrell, R.W., Lomas, D.A., Gerhard, L., Baumann, B., Lawrence, D.A., Yepes, M., Kim, T.S., Ghetti, B., Piccardo, P., Takao, M., Lacbawan, F., Muenke, M., Sifers, R.N., Bradshaw, C.B., Kent, P.F., Collins, G.H., Larocca, D., Holohan, P.D. (2002) "Association between conformational mutations in neuroserpin and onset and severity of dementia." *The Lancet*. 359:2242-2247.

17. Yerby, M.S., Shaw, C.M., Watson, J.M. (1986) "Progressive dementia and epilepsy in a young adult: Unusual intraneuronal inclusions." *Neurology*. 36:68-71.

18. Berkovic, S.F., Carpenter, S., Andermann, F. (1986) "Atypical inclusion body progressive myoclonus epilepsy: A fifth case?" *Neurology*. 36:1275-1276.

19. Berkovic, S.F., Andermann, F., Carpenter, S., Wolfe, L.S. (1986) "Progressive myoclonus epilepsies: Specific causes and diagnosis." *The New England Journal of Medicine*. 315:296-305.

20. Serratosa, J.M., Gardiner, R.M., Lehesjoki, A.E., Pennacchio, L.A., Myers, R.M. (1999) "The molecular genetic bases of the progressive myoclonus epilepsies." *Advances in Neurology*. 79:383-398.

21. Stoeckli, E.T., Lemkin, P.F., Kuhn, T.B., Ruegg, M.A., Heller, M., Sonderegger, P. (1989) "Identification of proteins secreted from axons of embryonic dorsal-root-ganglia neurons." *European Journal of Biochemistry*. 180: 249-258.

22. Hill, R.M., Parmar, P.K., Coates, L.C., Mezey, E., Pearson, J.F., Birch, N.P. (2000) "Neuroserpin is expressed in the pituitary and adrenal glands and induces the extension of neurite-like processes in AtT-20 cells." *The Biochemical Journal*. 345:595-601.

23. Yazaki, M., Lipnieks, J.J., Murrell, J.R., Takao, M., Guenther, B., Piccardo, P., Farlow, M.R., Ghetti, B., Benson, M.D. (2000) "Only mutated neuroserpin protein accumulates in cytoplasmic inclusions of a recently recognized form of progressive myoclonus epilepsy." *Brain Pathology*. 10:682.

24. Lafora, G.R., Glueck, B. (1911) "Beitrag zur Histopathologie der myoklonischen Epilepsie." *Zeitschrift fur die Gesamte Neurologie und Psychiatrie 1911*, 6:1-14.

25. Van Heycop ten Ham MW. (1974) "Lafora disease. A form of progressive myoclonus epilepsy." In: Vinken PJ and Bruyn GW eds. *Handbook of Clinical Neurology* Vol. 15. Amsterdam: North-Holland Publishing Company; pp. 382-422.

26. Minassian, B.A., Lee, J.R., Herbrick, J.A., Huizenga, J., Soder, S., Mungall, A.J., Dunham, I., Gardner, R., Fong, C.Y., Carpenter, S., Jardim, L., Satishchandra, P.,

566

Andermann, E., Snead, O.C. III, Lopes-Cendes, I., Tsui, L.C., Delgado-Escueta, A.V., Rouleau, G.A., Scherer, S.W. (1998) "Mutations in a gene encoding a novel protein tyrosine phosphatase cause progressive myoclonus epilepsy." *Nature Genetics*. 20:171-174.

27. Cavanagh, J.B. (1999) "Corpora-amylacea and the family of polyglucosan diseases." *Brain Research Reviews*. 29:265-295.

28. Dastur, D.K., Singhal, B.S., Gootz, M., Seitelberger, F. (1966) "Atypical inclusion bodies with myoclonic epilepsy." *Acta Neuropathologica*. 7:16-25.

29. Bergener, M., Gerhard, L. (1970) "Myoklonuskörperkrankheit und progressive Myoklonusepilepsie." *Der Nervenarzt*. 41:166-173.

30. Ota, T., Hisatomi, Y., Kashiwamura, K., Otsu, K., Nakamura, Y. (1974) "Histochemistry and ultrastructure of atypical myoclonus body (type II)." *Acta Neuropathologica*. 28:45-54.

31. Dolman, C.L. (1975) "Atypical myoclonus body epilepsy (adult variant)." *Acta Neuropathololologica*. 31:201-206.

32. Osterwalder, T., Contartese, J. Stoeckli, E.T., Kuhn, T.B., Sonderegger, P. (1996) "Neuroserpin, an axonally secreted serine protease inhibitor." *The EMBO Journal*. 15:2944-2953.

33. Krueger, S.R., Ghisu, G.P., Cinelli, P., Gschwend, T.P., Osterwalder, T., Wolfer, D.P., Sonderegger, P. (1997) "Expression of neuroserpin, an inhibitor of tissue plasminogen activator, in the developing and adult nervous system of the mouse." *The Journal of Neuroscience*. 17:8984-8996.

34. Berger, P., Kozlov, S.V., Krueger, S.R., Sonderegger, P. (1998) "Structure of the mouse gene for the serine protease inhibitor neuroserpin (PI12)." *Gene*. 214:25-33.

35. Von Heijne, G. (1983) "Patterns of amino acids near signal-sequence cleavage sites." *European Journal of Biochemistry*. 133:17-21.

36. Huntington, J.A., Pannu, N.S., Hazes, B., Read, R.J., Lomas, D.A., Carrell, R.W. (1996) "A 2.6 A structure of a serpin polymer and implications for conformational disease." *Journal of Molecular Biology*. 293:449-455.

37. Cox, D.W. (1995) "α_1-Antitrypsin deficiency." In *The Metabolic and Molecular Bases of Inherited Disease*, Seventh Edition, Volume III, Chapter 138, Part 18-Connective Tissues. Edited by Scriver CR, Beaudet AL, Sly WS, Valle D, New York, McGraw Hill Book Co., 1995, 4125-4158.

38. Seyama, K., Nukiwa, T., Takabe, K., Takahashi, H., Miyake, K., Kira, S. (1991) "S_{iiyama} (Serine 53 (TCC) to Phenylalanine 53 (TTC)): A new α_1-antitrypsin-deficient variant with mutation on a predicted conserved residue of the serpin backbone." *The Journal of Biological Chemistry*. 266:12627-12632.

39. Curiel, D.T., Holmes, M.D., Okayama, H., Brantly, M.L., Vogelmeier, C., Travis, W.D., Stier, L.E., Perks, W.H., Drystal, R.G. (1989) "Molecular basis of the liver and lung disease associated with the α_1-antitrypsin deficiency allele M_{malton}." *The Journal of Biological Chemistry*. 264:13938-13945.

40. Jeppsson, J-O. (1976) "Amino acid substitution Glu→Lys in α_1-antitrypsin PiZ." *FEBS Letters*. 65:195-197.

41. Yoshida ,A., Lieberman, J., Gaidulis, L., Ewing, C. (1976) "Molecular abnormality of human alpha$_1$-antitrypsin variant (Pi-ZZ) associated with plasma activity deficiency." *Proceedings of the National Academy of Sciences, USA*. 73:1324-1328.

42. Carrell, R.W., Jeppsson, J-O., Laurell, C-B., Brennan, S.O., Owen, M.C., Vaughan, L., Boswell, D.R. (1982) "Structure and variation of human α_1-antitrypsin." *Nature*. 298:329-334.

43. Bell, O.F., Carrell, R.W. (1973) "Basis of the defect in α_{-1}-antitrypsin deficiency." *Nature*. 243:410-411.

44. Eriksson, S., Larsson, C. (1975) "Purification and partial characterization of PAS-positive inclusion bodies from the liver in alpha$_1$-antitrypsin deficiency." *The New England Journal of Medicine*. 292:176-180.

45. Jeppsson, J-O., Larsson, C., Eriksson, S. (1975) "Characterization of α_1-antitrypsin in the inclusion bodies from the liver in α_1-antitrypsin deficiency." *The New England Journal of Medicine*. 293:576-579.

46. Bathurst, I.C., Travis, J., George, P.M., Carrell, R.W. (1984) "Structural and functional characterization of the abnormal Z α_1-antitrypsin isolated from human liver." *FEBS Letters*. 177:179-183.

47. Lindo, V.S., Kakkar, V.V., Learmonth, M., Melissari, E., Zappacosta, F., Panico, M., Morris, H.R. (1995) "Antithrombin-TRI (Ala382 to Thr) causing severe thromboembolic tendency undergoes the S-to-R transition and is associated with a plasma-inactive high-molecular-weight complex of aggregated antithrombin." *British Journal of Haematology*. 89:589-601.

48. Aulak, K.S., Eldering, E., Hack, C.E., Lubbers, Y.P.T., Harrison, R.A., Mast, A., Cicardi, M., Davis, A.E. (1993) "A hinge region mutation in C1-inhibitor (Ala^{436}⇒Thr) results in nonsubstrate-like behavior and in polymerization of the molecule." *The Journal of Biological Chemistry*. 268:18088-18094.

49. Faber, J-P., Poller, W., Olek, K., Baumann, U., Carlson, J., Lindmark, B., Eriksson, S. (1993) "The molecular basis of α_1-antichymotrypsin deficiency in a heterozygote with liver and lung disease." *Journal of Hepatology*. 18:313-321.

THE GENETICS AND EPIDEMIOLOGY OF MULTIPLE SCLEROSIS

JONATHAN L. HAINES, PH.D.

Program in Human Genetics, Department of Molecular Physiology and Biophysics, Vanderbilt University Medical Center, Nashville, TN, USA

EPIDEMIOLOGY OF MULTIPLE SCLEROSIS

Multiple sclerosis (MS) is the prototypic human demyelinating disease. In most Caucasian populations MS is second only to trauma as a cause of acquired neurological disability arising in early to mid adulthood. It has an undetermined etiology affecting the white matter of the central nervous system (CNS) and results in episodic or progressive neurological impairments. The symptoms of MS reflect neurological dysfunction in one or more of the pyramidal pathways, cerebellar efferent or afferent pathways, medial longitudinal fasciculus, optic nerve(s), or posterior columns. MS is most commonly seen in young adults with less than 10% of identified cases beginning after the age of 55 and less than 5% before the age of 14. Females are two to three times more frequently affected than males.[1] Although life span is only slightly shortened the majority of patients experience increasing disability and consequent deterioration in quality of life with passing time. It thus carries a significant morbidity that takes an immeasurable toll on the patients and their family members.

The diagnosis of MS is one of exclusion, and consistent criteria must be used to insure accurate classification.[2] Other possible causes of MS-like symptoms, including B_{12} deficiency, AIDS, rheumatoid arthritis, systemic lupus erythematosus, Sjogrens syndrome, sarcoidosis, Lyme disease, adrenoleukodystrophy, and MELAS and related syndromes, must be eliminated. Physiologically, MS is an inflammatory disorder resulting from an autoimmune response directed against CNS antigens, and myelin proteins in particular, causing selective demyelination with relative sparing of axon cylinders, variable loss of oligodendrocytes, and dense astrogliosis.[3,4] Despite many years of vigorous research, the underlying etiology of MS remains unknown, but it is clear that it is a complex interplay of factors, including genes.

GENETIC EPIDEMIOLOGY OF MULTIPLE SCLEROSIS

There have been many studies measuring the prevalence of MS in various populations.[5] Prevalence rates vary from as low as 0.88 per 100,000 ([6]) to as high as 224 per 100,000.[7] We can come to the general conclusion that the incidence and prevalence of MS is higher in the higher latitudes and lower near the equator. It is also possible that the incidence of MS may be increasing over time. Overall the literature support these conclusions, but it is important to consider the strength of these conclusions since other factors may explain these results. Some of these factors could include the fact that epidemiological methods have progressed substantially over time; that the diagnosis of MS has changed substantially with new advancements in health care; and that the underlying study designs may have been underpowered by the use of small sample sizes. While these conclusions are generally accepted, they should be closely scrutinized and certainly larger epidemiological studies should be undertaken to definitively resolve these issues.

The prevalence of MS differs substantially among different ethnic groups who reside in the same environment and among the same ethnic groups who reside in different environments. One example of the former is the prevalence differences between the Greek and Turkish Cypriots where the reported prevalence is 39 per 100,000 and 6 per 100,000 respectively.[8] Such a result suggests that genetic differences (even small ones) between the populations may well be important. A different example that highlights the latter case is the prevalence rates on the British Isles, which mostly are reported to be greater than 10 per 10,000[7] while the prevalence rates in the similar and derivative population of Australia, are generally reported to be less than 30 per 100,000.[9] Such a result suggests that other (environmental) factors must also be important.

The involvement of genetic factors in MS has been demonstrated by numerous sibling risk, adoption and twin studies. Comparison of the recurrence rates in the relatives of MS patients to the general population prevalence generates a recurrence risk ratio (λ)[10,11] that can be calculated for different degrees of relationship. In most diseases only a sibling recurrence risk (λ_S) is available and in MS the overall λ_S has been estimated to be between 20 and 50.[12,13] While this is substantially less than the λ_S for a Mendelian autosomal dominant disorder such as Huntington disease (where the $\lambda_S = 5000$) or a Mendelian autosomal recessive disorder such as cystic fibrosis (where the $\lambda_S = 500$), it is similar to the risk for other complex genetic disorders such as ALS (where the $\lambda_S = 20\text{-}40$) and autism (where the $\lambda_S = 50\text{-}75$). It is much higher than the λ_S for Alzheimer disease (where 4 genes have already been identified) which is only 4-5.

Twin studies from multiple different populations consistently indicate that a monozygotic (MZ) twin of an MS patient is at higher risk (25-30% concordance) for MS than is a dizygotic (DZ) twin (2-5%).[5,12,14] While the MZ concordance suggests a strong genetic component, the fact that it is not near 100% also suggests that other factors, including possible gene-gene interactions or effects on expression, may also be important.

Adoption studies done in Canada[15] have shown an increased risk of MS only in the biological relatives of adopted MS probands. Half-sibling studies[16] also suggest that genetic, and not environmental, factors are acting in MS since the half-sibs raised apart (different environments) and half-sibs raised together (same environment) have similar risks of developing MS.

MULTIPLE SCLEROSIS AS A COMPLEX GENETIC DISEASE

There are two types of genetic disorders. The first has a simple genetic architecture, and is usually caused by variations in genes that act in a Mendelian manner. That is, these variations actually cause disease by themselves and are inherited in a simple fashion. Because it is clear that MS is not controlled by a single gene, it must have a complex genetic architecture. Complex architectures involve multiple genes, acting individually or together, and possibly interacting with the environment. Most common diseases (e.g. Alzheimer disease, diabetes, cardiovascular disease, MS) have a complex genetic architecture.

There are two ways to explore and dissect the underlying genetic architecture of a complex disease. The first is to use a genomic screening approach. This has the advantage of not needing any knowledge of the function of the gene that is being sought. The gene is localized and identified purely on its location. This is a particularly valuable approach when little is known about the underlying pathophysiology of a disease and when little is known about the function of most genes (as is currently the case in humans).

The second approach is a candidate gene approach. This relies on knowing or supposing the function of one or more genes, and relating this function to the known pathophysiology of disease. In MS, many candidates have been proposed and tested, with a primary focus on genes affecting the immune system. Unfortunately, this approach has, so far, been a dismal failure in MS, with only the MHC (HLA-DR2 allele) having been confirmed.

To analyze the genetic data generated by either of the above approaches, both genetic linkage and allelic association can be used. The linkage analysis approach has its greatest applicability in initial localization of candidate loci. Parametric lod score analysis is the most powerful method of linkage analysis if the genetic model is known. However, we know so little about complex diseases such as AD that accurate model specification is impossible. While lod score methods may be robust to errors underlying assumptions in specific instances, this is not always the case. Non-parametric methods are an attractive alternative. As the interest in mapping complex diseases has blossomed, non-parametric methods have experienced improvements and innovations. Efficient multipoint sibpair analysis using the likelihood approach (MLS)[10,11,17] is now available in several different computer programs. As well, methods that incorporate data on other affected relative pairs (ARP), including the nonparametric linkage (NPL) method implemented in the GENEHUNTER package[18] and extended by Kong and Cox[19,20] in GENEHUNTER+, are now commonly used. Potential gene-gene interactions also may be assessed by using GENEHUNTER-PLUS and ALLEGRO.[19,21] This approach has been successfully used to follow-up the chromosome 12 AD linkage in our laboratories.[22]

To circumvent the difficulties with genetic linkage analysis, we can take advantage of advances in applying allelic association analysis. This has its greatest applicability in the fine localization and identification of disease loci, as it examines directly the effect of a candidate locus, not just a diffused effect spread across a large genomic region.[23] The power and simplicity of allelic association tests depend on the availability of numerous polymorphic markers in any candidate region, a situation only recently realized with the rapid data generation of the human genome project. Evaluation of candidate genes in association studies holds great potential with development of single nucleotide polymorphisms (SNPs). It is estimated that SNPs occur on average every 1000 base pairs and have a low mutation rate, both of which are advantageous in association studies. Nearly 4,000,000 SNPs have already been identified (http://www. ncbi.nlm.nih.gov/SNP/) and more are being identified and confirmed daily. With this large number of available assays, high-throughput approaches toward data generation are necessary. Numerous methods have recently been described[24-26] that can increase genotyping throughput from hundreds of genotypes per day to thousands of genotypes per day.

Analysis of these allelic association data can be done in two ways. A case-control study is a powerful method to investigate the magnitude of association between a polymorphism and risk of disease, as well as the impact of that polymorphism on the prevalence of the disease in the population. The usual case-control design involves representative sampling of cases and controls from the same underlying population, minimization of bias (for example, reducing recall bias by using primary sources of data, etc), and controlling for confounding. In practice, many genetic epidemiology studies of MS have focused on prevalent cases ascertained from academic medical centers and matched to convenience samples of controls collected from other sources (i.e. not drawn from the same underlying population). These case and control samples are poorly matched in several ways: they are not drawn from the same population, are subject to confounding by ethnic background, and may be subject to selection bias by disease severity or selective survival. Thus, in practice the case-control approach can be difficult to apply correctly and the lack of replication for many studies may arise from random statistical variation, from true population-specific genetic effects or from methodological differences.

For these reasons, family-based case-control designs were quickly adopted (and widely promoted) as more efficient, and less biased, methods of investigating candidate genes. One such approach is the transmission/disequilibrium test (TDT).[27] The TDT avoids control-sampling bias by using parental controls, and since it is based on observing transmission of gametes from parents to affected children, it only has power to detect associations between linked loci. Therefore, with a positive result from the TDT, one can infer that the tested allele is both linked and associated with a susceptibility allele. This approach has been applied to a number of disorders, including diabetes and autism.[28,29] One difficulty with the TDT for application to MS is that parents are not always available for genotyping. Several statistics have been proposed to circumvent this problem.[30-35] The Pedigree Disequilibrium Test (PDT) developed by Dr. Eden Martin and colleagues[34] has the most general applicability for studies of MS where pedigree structures can vary substantially. With the large numbers of SNPs available, multi-locus analysis such as that employed in Transmit[35] is essential. Such analyses can take advantage of the emerging information concerning the fine-structure of linkage disequilibrium among SNPs and the description of haplotype blocks spanning 30-60 kb.[36]

THE MHC IN THE GENETICS OF MULTIPLE SCLEROSIS

The association with the HLA class II DR2 haplotype (HLA-DRB1*1501-DQA1*0102-DQB1*0602)[37] been known since the 1970's.[38] While there has been some variation in exactly which allele or haplotype within the MHC is associated with MS, the HLA-DR2 association is the one found primarily in northern Europe and populations of northern European descent.[39,40] The MHC has been estimated to account for 10%[41] and possibly as much as 50%[39] of the genetic component of MS susceptibility, at least in the northern European Caucasian population.

There is some debate whether or not the HLA-DR2 association appears to explain the entire MHC genetic linkage signal in multiplex families.[39,42,43] We previously examined both genetic linkage and allelic association to the HLA-DR2 allele in the multiplex families,[44] and confirmed strong evidence for both. In addition, we determined that the entire linkage signal arose from families segregating the HLA-DR2 allele, suggesting that this allelic association is responsible for the genetic linkage signal in this region. A recent publication from the Canadian group[42] found some residual linkage to the MHC in families that do not segregate the HLA-DR2 allele. They suggest that another gene in the MHC may be responsible for at least some MS risk. However, our most recent analysis confirms that there is no linkage signal in our dataset in the HLA-DR2 negative families (Table 1).[43] These studies are somewhat complicated by the small sample size of HLA-DR2 negative families (the Canadians have 58 mostly small families, we have 34 somewhat larger families).

Table 1. Linkage and association results for HLA-DR.

HLA Genotype	Max Lod Score		Sib Pair Analysis		PDT
	AD*	AR*	MLS	% sharing	p-value
All families	3.80	2.91	2.00	57.4	0.0002
DR2 positive families	4.62	3.95	2.37	58.8	0.0002
DR2 negative families	0.00	0.00	0.00	50.0	0.87

AD=autosomal dominant model; AR=autosomal recessive model

HLA-DR2 and Clinical Expression in Patients

As expected, significant HLA-DR2 associations with disease were present in men and women. We also looked for potential differences in the association by early and late onset, mild and severe disease, and families concordant or discordant for site of onset. No significant differences were observed. There was also no significant correlation between HLA-DR2 and age of onset or progression. Results from other studies have also generally not supported an effect of HLA-DR2 on clinical expression of MS.

<u>The Effect of HLA-DR2 Homozygosity</u>
Previous examinations of the HLA-DR2 effect on MS risk have assumed a dominant action of this allele (e.g. that risk is elevated for both heterozygous or homozygous carriers of the HLA-DR2 allele). In a pilot study, we examined the effect of HLA-DR2 genotype status on MS risk in 549 of our families (187 multiplex, 362 simplex; all Caucasian), with 808 affected family members and 1574 unaffected family members. We observed a very significant difference between the MS risk related to the non-HLA-DR2 carriers (DRX/DRX), the HLA-DR2 heterozygotes (DR2/DRX), and the HLA-DR2 homozygotes (DR2/DR2) (Table 2). This result was observed in both the multiplex and simplex families. These data highlight the need for HLA-DR genotyping and consideration of HLA-DR2 in all analyses.

Table 2. Odds Ratios (OR, 95% CI) for HLA-DR2 genotype and MS Risk.

Test Group	Referent	All Families	Multiplex Only	Simplex Only
DR2/DR2	DRX/DRX	6.7 (4.2 – 10.7)***	6.1 (3.4 – 11.0)***	7.9 (3.7 – 17.0)***
DR2/DRX	DRX/DRX	2.7 (2.1 – 3.6)***	2.6 (1.8 – 3.7)***	3.0 (2.0 - 4.5)***
DR2/DR2	DR2/DRX	2.5 (1.7 – 3.7)**	2.4 (1.4 – 3.9)*	2.7 (1.4 – 5.1)^

***$p<10^{-6}$, **$p<10^{-5}$, *$p<10^{-3}$, ^$p<0.01$

FINDING OTHER RISK GENES IN MULTIPLE SCLEROSIS

<u>Chromosomal Regions with Support for Multiple Sclerosis Genes</u>
To find the genes involved in MS, multiple genomic screens have been performed.[45-50] The strongest and most consistently replicated evidence for an MS susceptibility gene has been found at the major histocompatibility complex (MHC) region on chromosome 6p21.3. This confirmed the known association with the HLA class II DR2 haplotype (HLA-DRB1*1501-DQA1*0102-DQB1*0602).[37,38]

In general, however, there has been little agreement on the chromosomal regions that harbor MS susceptibility genes. Of the 77 regions identified by the first four genomic screens to be published, only 11 overlapped to any substantial degree (Table 3). Of particular interest is the fact that all studies found some evidence of linkage on chromosome 19q.

The variability in the results likely comes from several factors. These include the small initial sample sizes of all the studies, a relatively sparse map of genetic markers, the use of statistical methods that are not very powerful, and the underlying genetic complexity of MS. One attempt to overcome the sample size issue is a combined analysis of the original data from several of the genomic screens.[51] This analysis also has its shortcomings, but pointed to a number of regions, including the MHC on chromosome 6 and another region on chromosome 17q. Evidence for linkage on chromosome 19q was found, but was rather modest.

Table 3. Overlapping Chromosomal Regions in the First Four MS Genomic Screens.

Chromosome	Markers	Studies
1	S201,S255	UK,CA
2	S119,S123	UK,US
3	S1285,S1261	UK,CA
3	S1309,S1744	US,CA,FN
5	S406,S1492	CA,FN
5	S427,S2500	UK,FN
5	S428,S815	UK,US
6	S273,HLA	UK,US
10	S464,S1220	US,FN
17	S942,S1290	UK,FN
19	APOC2,S47	UK,US,CA,FN

The Potential Role of Genes on Chromosome 19q in Multiple Sclerosis

One of the first regions of interest identified in our initial genome screen[45,52] was chromosome 19q13 near the APOC2 and APOE genes. Four other genomic screens[46-48,50] have also shown some support for linkage of an MS risk locus to chromosome 19q (although the regions differ somewhat), as does a recent analysis of Finnish families.[53] The finding is not universal since a small genomic screen in Italian families[49] and an updated analysis of the Canadian families[54] do not find significant evidence for linkage to chromosome 19q. A reanalysis of the primary data of the three largest screens[51] also provided some evidence for chromosome 19q involvement with an NPL score > 1.0. A true meta analysis of the four earlier genomic screens[55] identified 19q13 as the second most significant region of linkage (after the MHC).

Additional evidence for a 19q13 MS risk locus comes from allelic association studies[56,57] and, more recently, from follow-up analyses by our Multiple Sclerosis Genetics Group (MSGG) in both North American[58,59] and San Marino populations,[60] and a study from Denmark.[61] The most recent analysis of the UK data[62] identified an allelic association in a large dataset of multiplex and simplex families, despite earlier negative results.[47,63] However, not all datasets have shown an effect on this region.[46,54,64] These data are summarized in Table 4.

In any complex disease complete consistency of linkage signals and the localization of those signals cannot be expected.[65] The experience in both Alzheimer disease[66,67] and Inflammatory Bowel Disease[68,69] indicate that when the majority of studies identify a signal, it is likely to represent a true effect. Thus the finding of positive linkage results in all but one major multiplex dataset and the multiple allelic association findings in several additional datasets gives us confidence that an MS risk genes lies in chromosome 19q13. However, localization is still difficult. The chromosome 19 MS linkage signals come from positions as proximal as 61 cM (Marshfield map) and as distal as 78 cM (Table 4). The positive allelic associations are similarly dispersed. These studies have all suffered from either small sample sizes and/or a sparse coverage of the region.[62]

Table 4. Location of positive genetic linkage and association signals.

Location (cM)	Type	Score	Dataset	Location	Type	Score	Dataset
61	Lod score	1.8	Finnish	62	P value	0.02	Italian
62	Lod score	1.3	UK	70	P value	0.02	UK
66	Lod score	1.2	US/UK/Can	70	P value	0.03	Danish
68	Lod score	2.1	US	70	P value	0.04	French
70	Lod score	1.2	UK	70	P value	0.02	US/Chinese
70	Lod score	1.2	US/UK/Can	79	P value	0.03	UK
75	Lod score	2.0	US				
78	Lod score	1.6	UK				

Table 5. Results of a Genomic Screen for MS in a San Marinese Dataset.

Marker	Position (Marshfield Cm)	PDT-p-value
D7S3056	7	0.04
D8S1113	78	0.04
D10S1213	148	0.04
D10S212	171	0.03
S12S398	68	0.03
D19S589	88	0.03
D20S477	48	0.04
D20S481	62	0.05
D22S1685	18	0.03

The Use of Special Populations: San Marino

Another possible approach toward finding MS susceptibility genes is to use special populations that may be either genetically, socially, or geographically isolated in some way. One such population exists in the principality of San Marino. We recently studied this population and identified approximately 30 MS individuals in the entire population of 26,000. 25 of these individuals were sampled and 15 were used for a whole-population genomic screen. The results of this screen are given in Table 5. Of particular interest are the results on chromosome 19, which were confirmed when the additional 10 affected individuals were added to the dataset.

THE ROLE OF APOE IN MULTIPLE SCLEROSIS

One of several candidate genes in the 19q13 region is the apolipoprotein E (APOE) gene, which codes for a major lipid carrier protein (apoE) in the brain. The apoE protein has long been associated with regeneration of axons and myelin after lesions in central and peripheral nervous tissue.[70] Decreased apoE concentrations in cerebrospinal fluid in MS patients compared to healthy controls have been reported, and a corresponding decrease in intrathecal apoE synthesis may influence the degree of MS exacerbation over time.[71,72] Therefore, both the APOE coding region and regulatory elements outside of the coding region are plausible candidate genes for MS.

The exact role of APOE in MS has been somewhat controversial. While a few studies have found an effect of APOE on MS Risk,[61,73] most reports have not found an effect.[71,74-78] Conversely, when APOE has been examined for an effect on MS disease expression, most studies have found either increased severity or increased rate of progression associated with the APOE-4 allele,[61,73,74,76-79,82] although a few studies have not documented such an effect.[83,85-87] Despite the large number of studies, only a few clinical variables have been tested and many others (type, symptomatology at onset, progression of specific symptoms) have not been examined. Additionally, only a few studies[73,81,83] examined polymorphisms other than the functional APOE alleles. Given the variable extent of linkage disequilibrium around APOE[88,89] it is possible that a different polymorphism in APOE or a nearby gene is the responsible site. Only a detailed examination of a large well-phenotyped dataset will answer this question.

Examination of APOE in the Risk of MS
We recently analyzed seven SNPs around APOE by genotyping 398 trios and discordant sibpairs (DSPs) from the multiplex and simplex families available to us at that time.[73] We first determined the level of linkage disequilibrium between these markers. All markers were individually in Hardy-Weinberg equilibrium but there was strong linkage disequilibrium between snp992, APOE, snp952, snp873, snp888, and snp988. Thus the individual allelic association results with MS risk cannot be considered independent for these markers, and suggests that examining the data as haplotypes might better characterize any observed associations.

The tests of allelic association identified only snp873 with a possibly interesting P value (0.07) in the overall analysis. However, snp992 and snp952 generated P values <0.05 in the simplex families. To take advantage of the haplotype data around these SNPs, we also performed two locus and three locus analyses. These demonstrated significant associations to MS risk in either two or three locus combinations, centering on SNPs snp952, snp873, and snp888, all of which map distal to APOE. The multi-locus results pointed towards the APOE-snp952-snp873 haplotype as being associated with MS risk primarily in the data set of simplex families (global χ^2 19.00 on 5 df, p=0.002). With a (conservative) Bonferroni correction for 4 types of analyses at each of 8 markers, this p-value is still significant at the global 5% level (0.002=0.05/32). To examine whether the evidence for this haplotype association differed based on HLA-DR2 status of the probands in the simplex families, the three-locus analysis was performed separately in HLA-DR2+ and HLA-DR2- families. Both subgroups supported the above association (P values = 0.01).

These data are consistent with an MS risk gene somewhat distal to APOE, but do not exclude the possibility that such a gene lies elsewhere within the larger region or that multiple MS risk genes might exist. In addition, it is possible that MS risk differs by the type of family (multiplex or simplex), since the association results arise mostly from the simplex dataset. While this could be a result of the larger sample size of the simplex dataset, it could also indicate a true etiologic difference between multiplex and simplex families.

Examination of APOE with Disease Severity and Progression

Our analyses of the relationship between APOE genotype and MS disease severity for the combined data set of multiplex and simplex patients are summarized in Table 6. There was a significantly higher proportion of APOE-4 carriers in the severe disease group (39%), compared to the non-severe group (23%, p=0.03). Most of the evidence for this association came from the group of multiplex patients, where the difference in these proportions was highly significant (7/14=50.0% vs. 73/374=19.5%, respectively; p=0.003). No association of severe disease with APOE-2 carrier status or gender was found. There was no evidence for an association with APOE-4 carrier status and mild disease status (p=0.62), but a higher proportion of patients with mild disease were carriers of the APOE-2 allele (25.5%) than the corresponding proportion of patients with non-mild disease (16.5%, p=0.02).

Table 6. Comparison of APOE Genotypes by Disease Type.

	Disease type			Disease type		
	severe (n=23)	non-severe (n=591)	p-value	mild (n=55)	non-mild (n=559)	p-value
APOE-4: n (%)	9 (39%)	134 (23%)	0.03*	14 (26%)	129 (23%)	0.62
APOE-2: n (%)	6 (26%)	100 (17%)	0.40	14 (26%)	92 (16%)	0.02

* (p=0.003 for multiplex patients only)

We also examined disease progression using time to EDSS ≥ 7. No significant evidence for faster progression to disability, as recently reported,[82] was found for carriers of the APOE-4 allele (hazard ratio 0.84, 95% CI 0.51-1.39, p=0.50), nor did we detect an influence of the APOE-2 allele (hazard ratio 0.84, 95% CI 0.43-1.64, p=0.60). However, the data set currently includes only n=13 carriers of the APOE-2 allele and n=18 carriers of the APOE-4 allele who reached EDSS ≥ 7. Larger sample sizes will be needed to confirm and test these preliminary results.

FUTURE DIRECTIONS

Although there is overwhelming evidence that MS has a strong genetic component, identifying this component has been very difficult. Multiple approaches are now being applied that should help identify these genes. First, many groups are enlarging their sample sizes, and new genomic screen data is being generated. These datasets are being combined into one larger pooled dataset that should render moot the problem of sample size. These analyses are likely to point to just a few chromosomal regions that can then be intensively studied.

To that end, a second approach will take advantage of the vast advances generated by the human genome project. It is now possible, for the first time, to identify most if not all the genes that lie within a critical chromosomal region. This greatly simplifies the search. In addition, much of the common variation in and near these genes is being identified on a global basis. Previously, years of effort would be expended just identifying genes in the various regions and in characterizing the variations within and near those genes. Now it will be easier to test numerous variations quickly.

Another advantage of the human genome project has been the generation of tremendous advances in technology that make it possible to examine large numbers of variations in large numbers of samples. We can anticipate that such advances will continue, and that the time and cost constraints on our current research will be substantially lifted. Finally, we have gained a much greater appreciation for the underlying complexity of MS, and the need for analytical (statistical) approaches that can accommodate this complexity. Such methods are just now becoming available.[90] With all these advances in place, we can anticipate substantial progress in dissecting the complex genetics of MS.

REFERENCES

1. Hauser, S.L., Goodkin, D.E. (1998) In Fauci, A., Braunwald, E., Isselbacher, J., Martin, J., Kasper, D., Hauser, S.L., and Longo, D. (eds), *Harrison's Principle of Internal Medicine*. McGraw Hill:New York, pp. 2409-2419.
2. Goodkin, D.E., Doolittle, H., Hauser, S.S., Ransohoff, R.M., and Roses, A.D. (1991) "Diagnostic criteria for multiple sclerosis research involving multiply affected families." *Arch Neurology*, 48:805-807.
3. Oksenberg, R., Hauser, S.L. (1996) In Goodkin, D.E., Rudnick, R.A. (eds), *Treatments of Multiple Sclerosis: Trial Design, Results and Future Strategies*. Springer-Verlag:London, pp. 17-46.
4. Hemmer, B., Archelos, J.J., and Hartung, H.P. (2002) "New concepts in the immunopathogenesis of multiple sclerosis." *Nat. Rev. Neurosci.*, 3:291-301.
5. Sadovnick, A.D., Armstrong, H., Rice, G., Bulman, D.E., Hashimoto, L., Paty, D.W., Hashimoto, S., Warren, S., Hader, W., and Murray, T.J. (1993) "A population based study of multiple sclerosis in twins: update." *Annal of Neurology*, 33:281-285.

6.   Hauser, L., Fleischnick, E., Weiner, H., Marcus, D., Awdeh, Z., Yunis, E., and Alper, C.A. (1989) "Extended major histocompatibility complex haplotypes in patients with multiple sclerosis." *Neurology*, 39:275-277.

7.   Cook, S.D., MacDonald, J., Tapp, W., Poskanzer, D., and Dowling, P.C. (1988) "Multiple sclerosis in the Shetland Islands: an update." *Acta Neurol. Scand.*, 77:148-151.

8.   Middleton, L.T., Dean, G. (1991) "Multiple sclerosis in Cyprus." *J Neurol. Sci.*, 103:29-36.

9.   Hammond, S.R., McLeod, J.G., Millingen, K.S., Stewart-Wynne, E.G., English, D., Holland, J.T., and McCall, M.G. (1988) "The epidemiology of multiple sclerosis in three Australian cities: Perth, Newcastle and Hobart." *Brain*, 111 (Pt 1):1-25.

10.   Risch, N. (1990) "Linkage strategies for genetically complex traits I. Multilocus models." *Am J Hum Genet*, 46:222-228.

11.   Risch, N. (1990) "Linkage strategies for genetically complex traits II. The power of affected relative pairs." *Am J Hum Genet*, 46:229-241.

12.   Sadovnick, A.D., Ebers, G.C. (1995) "Genetics of multiple sclerosis." *Neurologic Clinics*, 13:99-118.

13.   Robertson, N.P., Fraser, M., Deans, J., Clayton, D., Walker, N., and Compston, D.A. (1996) "Age-adjusted recurrence risks for relatives of patients with multiple sclerosis." *Brain*, 119 (Pt 2),449-455.

14.   Mumford, G.L., Wood, N.W., Kellar-Wood, H.F., Thorpe, J.W., and Miler, D.H. (1994) "The British Isles survey of multiple sclerosis in twins." *Neurology*, 44:15.

15.   Ebers, G.C., Sadovnick, A.D., and Risch, N.J. (1995) "A genetic basis for familial aggregation in multiple sclerosis. Canadian Collaborative Study Group [see comments]." *Nature*, 377:150-151.

16.   Sadovnick, A.D., Ebers, G.C., Dyment, D.A., and Risch, N.J. (1996) "Evidence for genetic basis of multiple sclerosis." *Lancet*, 347:1730.

17.   Risch, N. (1990) "Linkage strategies for genetically complex traits III. The effect of marker polymorphism on analysis of affected pairs." *Am J Hum Genet*, 46:242-253.

18.   Kruglyak, L., Daly, M.J., Reeve-Daly, M.P., and Lander, E.S. (1996) "Parametric and nonparametric linkage analysis: a unified multipoint approach." *Am J Hum Genet*, 58:1347-1363.

19.   Kong, A., Cox, N.J. (1997) "Allele-sharing models: LOD scores and accurate linkage tests." *Am J Hum Genet*, 61:1179-1188.

20.   Cox, N.J., Frigge, M., Nicolae, D.L., Concannon, P., Hanis, C.L., Bell, G.I., and Kong, A. (1999) "Loci on chromosome 2 (NIDDM1) and 15 interact to increase susceptibiltiy to diabetes in Mexican Americans." *Nat Genet*, 21:213.

21.   Gudbjartsson, D.F., Jonasson, K., and Kong, C.A. "Fast multipoint linkage calculation with Allegro." *American Journal of Human Genetics* 65(4), A60. 1999. Ref Type: Abstract.

22. Scott, W.K., Grubber, J.M., Conneally, P.M., Small, G.W., Hulette, C.M., Rosenberg, C.K., Saunders, A.M., Roses, A.D., Haines, J.L., and Pericak-Vance, M.A. (2000) "Fine mapping of the chromosome 12 late-onset alzheimer disease locus: potential genetic and phenotypic heterogeneity [In Process Citation]." *Am J Hum Genet*, 66:922-932.

23. Risch, N., Merikangas, K. (1996) "The future of genetic studies of complex human disorders." *Science*, 273:1516-1517.

24. Chen, X., Levine, L., and Kwok, P.Y. (1999) "Fluorescence polarization in homogeneous nucleic acid analysis." *Genome Research*, 9:492-8.

25. Holloway, J.W., Beghe, B., Turner, S., Hinks, L.J., Day, I.N., and Howell, W.M. (1999) "Comparison of three methods for single nucleotide polymorphism typing for DNA bank studies: sequence-specific oligonucleotide probe hybridisation, TaqMan liquid phase hybridisation, and microplate array diagonal gel electrophoresis (MADGE)." *Human Mutation*, 14:340-7.

26. Hoogendoorn, B., Owen, M.J., Oefner, P.J., Williams, N., Austin, J., and O'Donovan, M.C. (1999) "Genotyping single nucleotide polymorphisms by primer extension and high performance liquid chromatography." *Hum Genet*, 104:89-93.

27. Spielman, R.S., McGinnis, R.E., and Ewens, W.J. (1993) "Transmission test for linkage disequilibrium: the insulin gene region and insulin-dependent diabetes mellitus (IDDM)." *Am J Hum Genet*, 52:506-516.

28. Copeman, J.B., Cucca, F., Hearne, C.M., Cornall, R.J., Reed, P.W., Ronningen, K.S., Undlien, D.E., Nistico, L., Buzzetti, R., Tosi, R. et. al. (1995) "Linkage disequilibrium mapping of a type 1 diabetes susceptibility gene (IDDM7) to chromosome 2q31-q33." *Nature Genetics*, 9:80-85.

29. Martin, E.R., Menold, M.M., Wolpert, C.M., Bass, M.P., Donnelly, S.L., Ravan, S.A., Zimmerman, A., Gilbert, J.R., Vance, J.M., Maddox, L.O. et. al. (2000) "Analysis of linkage disequilibrium in gamma-aminobutyric acid receptor subunit genes in autistic disorder." *Am J Med Genet*, 96:43-48.

30. Curtis, D. (1997) "Use of siblings as controls in case-control association studies." *Annals of Human Genetics*, 61:319-333.

31. Boehnke, M., Langefeld, C.D. (1998) "Genetic association mapping based on discordant sib pairs: the discordant alleles test (DAT)." *Am J Hum Genet*, 62:950-961.

32. Spielman, R.S., Ewens, W.J. (1998) "A sibship test for linkage in the presence of association: the sib transmission/disequilibrium test." *Am J Hum Genet*, 61:450-458.

33. Horvath, S., Laird, N.M. (1998) "A discordant-sibship test for disequilibrium and linkage: no need for parental data." *Am J Hum Genet*, 63:1886-1897.

34. Martin, E.R., Monks, S.A., Warren, L.L., and Kaplan, N.L. (2000) "A test for linkage and association in general pedigrees: the pedigree disequilibrium test." *Am J Hum Genet*, 67:146-154.

35. Clayton, D. (1999) "A Generalization of the Transmission/Disequilibrium Test for Uncertain-Haplotype Transmission." *Am J Hum Genet.*, 65:1170-1177.

36. Daly, M.J., Rioux, J.D., Schaffner, S.F., Hudson, T.J., and Lander, E.S. (2001) "High-resolution haplotype structure in the human genome." *Nat. Genet.*, 29:229-232.

37. Bertrams, J., Kuwert, E. (1972) "HL-A antigen frequencies in multiple sclerosis. Significant increase of HL-A3, HL-A10 and W5, and ecrease of HL-A12." *European Journal of Neurology*, 7:78.

38. Naito, S., Namerow, N., Mickey, M.R., and Terasaki, P.I. (1972) "Multiple sclerosis: association with HL-A3." *Tissue Antigens*, 2:1-4.

39. Haines, J.L., Terwedow, H.A., Burgess, K., Pericak-Vance, M.A., Rimmler, J.B., Martin, E.R., Oksenberg, J.R., Lincoln, R., Zhang, D.Y., Banatao, D.R. et. al. (1998) "Linkage of the MHC to familial multiple sclerosis suggests genetic heterogeneity. The Multiple Sclerosis Genetics Group." *Hum Mol. Genet*, 7:1229-1234.

40. Cocco, E., Marrosu, M.G. (2000) "Is multiple sclerosis severity a genetically influenced trait?" *Neurol. Sci.*, 21:S843-S847.

41. Risch, N. (1987) "Assessing the role of HLA-linked and unlinked determinants of disease." *Am J Hum Genet*, 40:1-14.

42. Ligers, A., Dyment, D.A., Willer, C.J., Sadovnick, A.D., Ebers, G., Risch, N., and Hillert, J. (2001) "Evidence of linkage with HLA-DR in DRB1*15-negative families with multiple sclerosis." *Am J Hum Genet*, 69:900-903.

43. Barcellos, L.F., Oksenberg, J.R., Green, A.J., Bucher, P., Rimmler, J.B., Schmidt, S., Garcia, M.E., Lincoln, R.R., Pericak-Vance, M.A., Haines, J.L. et. al. (2002) "Genetic basis for clinical expression in multiple sclerosis." *Brain*, 125:150-158.

44. Multiple Sclerosis Genetics Group, Haines, J.L., Terwedow, H.A., Burgess, K., Pericak-Vance, M.A., Rimmler, J.B., Martin, E.R., Oksenberg, J.R., Lincoln, R., Zhang, D.Y. et. al. (1998) "Linkage of the MHC to familial multiple sclerosis suggests genetic heterogeneity." *Hum Mol Genet*, 7:1229-1234.

45. Multiple Sclerosis Genetics Group (1996) "A complete genomic screen for multiple sclerosis underscores a role for the major histocompatability complex." *Nature Genetics*, 13:469-476.

46. Ebers, G.C., Kukay, K., Bulman, D.E., Sadovnick, A.D., Rice, G., Anderson, C., Armstrong, H., Cousin, K., Bell, R.B., Hader, W. et. al. (1996) "A full genome search in multiple sclerosis." *Nature Genetics*, 13:472-476.

47. Sawcer, S., Jones, H.B., Feakes, R., Gray, J., Smaldon, N., Chataway, J., Robertson, N., Clayton, D., Goodfellow, P.N., and Compston, A. (1996) "A genome screen in multiple sclerosis reveals susceptibility loci on chromosome 6p21 and 17q22." *Nature Genetics*, 13:464-468.

48. Kuokkanen, S., Gschwend, M., Rioux, J.D., Daly, M.J., Terwilliger, J.D., Tienari, P.J., Wikstrom, J., Palo, J., Stein, L.D., Hudson, T.J. et. al. (1997) "Genomwide scan of multiple sclerosis Finnish multiplex families." *Am J Hum Genet*, 61:1379-1387.

582

49. Broadley, S., Sawcer, S., D'Alfonso, S., Hensiek, A., Coraddu, F., Gray, J., Roxburgh, R., Clayton, D., Buttinelli, C., Quattrone, A. et. al. (2001) "A genome screen for multiple sclerosis in Italian families." *Genes Immun.*, 2:205-210.

50. Coraddu, F., Sawcer, S., D'Alfonso, S., Lai, M., Hensiek, A., Solla, E., Broadley, S., Mancosu, C., Pugliatti, M., Marrosu, M.G. et. al. (2001) "A genome screen for multiple sclerosis in Sardinian multiplex families." *Eur.J Hum Genet*, 9:621-626.

51. Transatlantic Multiple Sclerosis Genetics Cooperative (2001) "A meta-analysis of genomic screens in multiple sclerosis." *Multiple Sclerosis*, 7:3-11.

52. Haines, J.L., Seboun, E., Goodkin, D.E., Usuku, K., Lincoln, R., Rimmler, J., Gusella, JF, Roses, A.D., Pericak-Vance, M.A., and Hauser, S.L. (1993) "Genetic dissection of the multiple sclerosis genotype." *Am J Hum Genet*, 53:A266.

53. Reunanen, K., Finnila, S., Laaksonen, M., Sumelahti, M.L., Wikstrom, J., Pastinen, T., Kuokkanen, S., Saarela, J., Uimari, P., Ruutiainen, J. et. al. (2002) "Chromosome 19q13 and multiple sclerosis susceptibility in Finland: a linkage and two-stage association study." *J Neuroimmunol.*, 126:134-142.

54. Dyment, D.A., Willer, C.J., Scott, B., Armstrong, H., Ligers, A., Hillert, J., Paty, D.W., Hashimoto, S., Devonshire, V., Hooge, J. et. al. (2001) "Genetic susceptibility to MS: a second stage analysis in Canadian MS families." *Neurogenetics.*, 3:145-151.

55. Wise, L.H., Lanchbury, J.S., and Lewis, C.M. (1999) "Meta-analysis of genome searches." *Ann. Hum Genet*, 63 (Pt 3):263-272.

56. Barcellos, L.F., Thomson, G., Carrington, M., Schafer, J., Begovich, A.B., Lin, P., Xu, X., Min, B.Q., Marti, D., and Klitz, W. (1997) "Chromosome 19 single-locus and multilocus haplotype association with multiple sclerosis. Evidence of a new susceptibility locus in Caucasian and Chinese patients." *JAMA*, 278:1256-1261.

57. Zouali, H., Faure-Delanef, L., and Lucotte, G. (1999) "Chromosome 19 locus apolipoprotein C-II association with mutiple sclerosis." *Mult Scler*, 5:134-136.

58. Pericak-Vance, M.A., Rimmler, J.B., Martin, E.R., Haines, J.L., Garcia, M.E., Oksenberg, J.R., Barcellos, L.F., Lincoln, R., Goodkin, D.E., Hauser, S.L. et. al. (2001) "Linkage and association analysis of chromosome 19q13 in multiple sclerosis." *Neurogenetics*, 3,195-201.

59. Multiple Sclerosis Genetics Group. "Multiple Susceptibility Loci for Multiple Sclerosis." *Hum Mol Genet* In Press. 2002. Ref Type: Generic.

60. Haines, J.L., Ashley-Koch, A., Jackson, C.E., Booze, M., Ribble, R.C., Rimmler, J.B., Garcia, M.E., Vance J.M., Barcellos, L.F., Lincoln, R., Hauser, S.L., Oksenberg, J.R., and Pericak-Vance, M. "A genomic screen for multiple sclerosis loci in a San Marino population supports the presence of a locus on 19q." *American Journal of Human Genetics* 67(Supplement 2), 21. 2000. Ref Type: Abstract.

61. Hogh, P., Oturai, A., Schreiber, K., Blinkenberg, M., Jorgensen, O.S., Ryder, L., Paulson, O.B., Sorensen, P.S., and Knudsen, G.M. (2000) "Apoliprotein E and

multiple sclerosis: impact of the epsilon-4 allele on susceptibility, clinical type and progression rate." *Mult. Scler.*, 6:226-230.

62. Sawcer, S., Maranian, M., Setakis, E., Curwen, V., Akesson, E., Hensiek, A., Coraddu, F., Roxburgh, R., Sawcer, D., Gray, J. et. al. (2002) "A whole genome screen for linkage disequilibrium in multiple sclerosis confirms disease associations with regions previously linked to susceptibility." *Brain*, 125:1337-1347.

63. Chataway, J., Feakes, R., Coraddu, F., Gray, J., Deans, J., Fraser, M., Robertson, N., Broadley, S., Jones, H., Clayton, D. et. al. (1998) "The genetics of multiple sclerosis: principles, background and updated results of the United Kingdom systematic genome screen." *Brain*, 121 (Pt 10):1869-1887.

64. D'Alfonso, S., Nistico, L., Zavattari, P., Marrosu, M.G., Murru, R., Lai, M., Massacesi, L., Ballerini, C., Gestri, D., Salvetti, M. et. al. (1999) "Linkage analysis of multiple sclerosis with candidate region markers in Sardinian and Continental Italian families." *Eur. J Hum Genet*, 7:377-385.

65. Altmuller, J., Palmer, L.J., Fischer, G., Scherb, H., and Wjst, M. (2001) "Genomewide scans of complex human diseases: true linkage is hard to find." *Am J Hum Genet*, 69:936-950.

66. Haines, J.L., Bailey, L.R., Grubber, J.M., Hedges, D., Hall, J.L., West, S., Santoro, L., Kemmerer, B., Saunders, A.M., Roses, A.D., Small, G.W., Scott, W.K., Conneally P.M., Vance, J.M., and Pericak-Vance, M.A. (2001) In Iqbal, K., Sisodia, S.S., and Winblad, B. (eds), *Alzheimer's Disease: Advances in Etiology, Pathogenesis and Therapeutics.* John Wiley and Sons, Ltd., pp. 33-43.

67. Farrer, L.A., Bowirrat, A., Friedland, R.P., Warasaka, K., Adams, J.C., Korczyn, A.D., Baldwin, C.T. (2001) "Identification of multiple loci for Alzheimer Disease in an inbred Israeli-Arab community." *Am J Hum Genet* 69 69, 200. 2001. Ref Type: Generic

68. Hugot, J.P., Chamaillard, M., Zouali, H., Lesage, S., Cezard, J.P., Belaiche, J., Almer, S., Tysk, C., O'Morain, C.A., Gassull, M. et. al. (2001) "Association of NOD2 leucine-rich repeat variants with susceptibility to Crohn's disease." *Nature*, 411:599-603.

69. Ogura, Y., Bonen, D.K., Inohara, N., Nicolae, D.L., Chen, F.F., Ramos, R., Britton, H., Moran, T., Karaliuskas, R., Duerr, R.H. et. al. (2001) "A frameshift mutation in NOD2 associated with susceptibility to Crohn's disease." *Nature*, 411:603-606.

70. Ignatius, M.J., Gebicke-Harter, P.J., Skene, J.H., Schilling, J.W., Weisgraber, K.H., Mahley, R.W., and Shooter, E.M. (1986) "Expression of apolipoprotein E during nerve degeneration and regeneration." *Proc. Natl. Acad. Sci. USA*, 83:1125-1129.

71. Gaillard, O., Gervais, A., Meillet, D., Plassart, E., Fontaine, B., Lyon-Caen, O., Delattre, J., and Schuller, E. (1998) "Apolipoprotein E and multiple sclerosis: a biochemical and genetic investigation." *J. Neurol. Sci.*, 158:180-186.

72. Rifai, N., Christenson, R.H., Gelman, .B., and Silverman, L.M. (1987) "Changes in cerebrospinal fluid IgG and apolipoprotein E indices in patients with multiple sclerosis during demyelination and remyelination." *Clin. Chem.*, 33:1155-1157.

73. Schmidt, S., Barcellos, L.F., DeSombre, K., Rimmler, J.B., Lincoln, R.R., Bucher,P., Saunders, A.M., Lai, E., Martin, E.R., Vance, J.M. et. al. (2002) "Association of polymorphisms in the apolipoprotein e region with susceptibility to and progression of multiple sclerosis." *Am J Hum Genet*, 70:708-717.

74. Chapman, J., Sylantiev, C., Nisipeanu, P., and Korczyn, A.D. (1999) "Preliminary observations on APOE epsilon4 allele and progression of disability in multiple sclerosis." *Arch. Neurol.*, 56:1484-1487.

75. Dousset, V., Gayou, A., and Brochet, B. (2001) "APOE polymorphism in multiple sclerosis." *Multiple Sclerosis* 4:357. Ref Type: Generic.

76. Evangelou, N., Jackson, M., Beeson, D., and Palace, J. (1999) "Association of the APOE epsilon4 allele with disease activity in multiple sclerosis." *J. Neurol. Neurosurg. Psychiatry*, 67:203-205.

77. D'Alfonso, S., Nistico, L., Bocchio, D., Bomprezzi, R., Marrosu, M.G., Murru, M.R., Lai, M., Massacesi, L., Ballerini, C., Repice, A. et. al. (2000) "An attempt of identifying MS-associated loci as a follow-up of a genomic linkage study in the Italian population." *J. Neurovirol.*, 6 Suppl 2:S18-S22.

78. Fazekas, F., Strasser-Fuchs, S., Kollegger, H., Berger, T., Kristoferitsch, W., Schmidt, H., Enzinger, C., Schiefermeier, M., Schwarz, C., Kornek, B. et. al. (2001) "Apolipoprotein E epsilon 4 is associated with rapid progression of multiple sclerosis." *Neurology*, 57:853-857.

79. Fazekas, F., Strasser-Fuchs, S., Schmidt, H., Enzinger, C., Ropele, S., Lechner, A., Flooh, E., Schmidt, R., and Hartung, H.P. (2000) "Apolipoprotein E genotype related differences in brain lesions of multiple sclerosis." *J Neurol. Neurosurg. Psychiatry*, 69:25-28.

80. Rubinsztein, D.C., Hanlon, C.S., Irving, R.M., Goodburn, S., Evans, D.G., Kellar-Wood, H., Xuereb, J.H., Bandmann, O., and Harding, A.E. (1994) "Apo E genotypes in multiple sclerosis, Parkinson's disease, schwannomas and late-onset Alzheimer's disease." *Mol Cell Probes*, 8:519-525.

81. Oliveri, R.L., Cittadella, R., Sibilia, G., Manna, I., Valentino, P., Gambardella, A., Aguglia, U., Zappia, M., Romeo, N., Andreoli, V. et. al. (1999) "APOE and risk of cognitive impairment in multiple sclerosis." *Acta Neurol .Scand.*, 100:290-295.

82. Chapman, J., Vinokurov, S., Achiron, A., Karussis, D.M., Mitosek-Szewczyk, K., Birnbaum, M., Michaelson, D.M., and Korczyn, A.D. (2001) "APOE genotype is a major predictor of long-term progression of disability in MS." *Neurology*, 56:312-316.

83. Ferri, C., Sciacca, F.L., Veglia, F., Martinelli, F., Comi, G., Canal, N., and Grimaldi, L.M. (1999) "APOE epsilon2-4 and -491 polymorphisms are not associated with MS." *Neurology*, 53:888-889.

84. Pirttila, T., Haanpaa, M., Mehta, P.D., and Lehtimaki, T. (2000) "Apolipoprotein E (APOE) phenotype and APOE concentrations in multiple sclerosis and acute herpes zoster." *Acta Neurol. Scand.*, 102:94-98.

85. Weatherby, S.J., Mann, C.L., Davies, M.B., Carthy, D., Fryer, A.A., Boggild, M.D., Young, C., Strange, R.C., Ollier, W., and Hawkins, C.P. (2000) "Polymorphisms of apolipoprotein E; outcome and susceptibility in multiple sclerosis." *Mult. Scler.*, 6:32-36.

86. Weatherby, S.J., Mann, C.L., Fryer, A.A., Strange, R.C., Hawkins, C.P., Stevenson, V.L., Leary, S.M., and Thompson, A.J. (2000) "No association between the APOE epsilon4 allele and outcome and susceptibility in primary progressive multiple sclerosis." *J. Neurol. Neurosurg. Psychiatry*, 68:532.

87. Masterman, T., Zhang, Z., Hellgren, D., Salter, H., Anvret, M., Lilius, L., Lannfelt, L., and Hillert, J. (2002) "APOE genotypes and disease severity in multiple sclerosis." *Mult. Scler.*, 8:98-103.

88. Martin, E.R., Lai, E.H., Gilbert, J.R., Rogala, A.R., Afshari, A.J., Riley, J., Finch, K.L., Stevens, J.F., Livak, K.J., Slotterbeck, B.D. et. al. (2000) "SNPing away at complex diseases: analysis of single-nucleotide polymorphisms around APOE in Alzheimer disease." *Am J Hum Genet*, 67:383-394.

89. Nickerson, D.A., Taylor, S.L., Fullerton, S.M., Weiss, K.M., Clark, A.G., Stengard, J.H., Salomaa, V., Boerwinkle, E., and Sing, C.F. (2000) "Sequence diversity and large-scale typing of SNPs in the human apolipoprotein E gene." *Genome Res.*, 10:1532-1545.

90. Ritchie, M.D., Hahn, L.W., Roodi, N., Bailey, L.R., Dupont, W.D., Parl, F.F., and Moore, J.H. (2001) "Multifactor-dimensionality reduction reveals high-order interactions among estrogen-metabolism genes in sporadic breast cancer." *Am J Hum Genet*, 69:138-147.

ALZHEIMER DISEASE: GENES AND ENVIRONMENT; THE VALUE OF INTERNATIONAL STUDIES

HUGH C. HENDRIE, M.B., CH.B., D.Sc.
Department of Psychiatry, Indiana University School of Medicine and The Center for Aging Research, Regenstrief Institute, Indianapolis, IN, USA

KATHLEEN S. HALL, PH.D.
Department of Psychiatry, Indiana University School of Medicine, Indianapolis, IN, USA

ADESOLA OGUNNIYI, M.D.
Department of Medicine, University College Hospital, Ibadan, Nigeria

SUJUAN GAO, PH.D.
Department of Medicine, Indiana University School of Medicine, Indianapolis, IN, USA

INTRODUCTION

Advances in molecular genetics have revolutionized epidemiological research. Epidemiologists are now able to combine the techniques of population genetics with more traditional risk factor research to formulate etiological hypotheses. Cooper and Kaufman,[1] from their studies in hypertension, have proposed a disease model involving the contributions of genes and environment and their possible interactions to explain disease rates in populations.

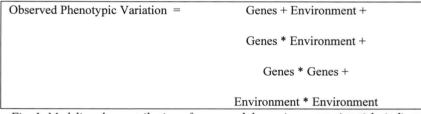

Observed Phenotypic Variation =	Genes + Environment +
	Genes * Environment +
	Genes * Genes +
	Environment * Environment

Fig. 1. Modeling the contribution of genes and the environment. Asterisks indicate interaction between factors.[1]

The resolution of these models, however, is likely to vary between populations. One reason for this variation is that environmental exposures involving putative environmental risk factors for disease are likely to differ between populations.

Comparisons between developing and developed nations offer a unique opportunity for applying this proposed model because such studies provide a much wider diversity of environmental exposures than do studies of populations solely in industrialized countries where important risk factors may be missed because of their very pervasiveness.[2]

However, genetic variation also, clearly influences disease risk. Research involving the human genome project has suggested that while there are few large differences in chromosome structure, there are many differences in small insertions and/or deletions, short tandem repeat sequences, and single nucleotide differences within and between human populations. Any one of these differences may influence disease risk often in conjunction with environmental exposures.[3-5]

Single nucleotide polymorphisms (SNPs) have proven to be an important tool in genetic studies of complex disease. SNPs are single base pair changes in the DNA sequence that can be found in either the coding or noncoding region of the DNA. Estimates suggest that SNPs may occur on average in every 1,000 base pairs; resulting in as many as 3 million SNPs that could be identified.[6-8] Variations in allele frequencies are also common between populations.

Genetic studies in African populations have assumed a particular pertinence. A number of investigators have now studied a wide variety of polymorphic loci to investigate the extent of human genetic diversity and to delineate the relationships between modern human populations. The greatest genetic diversity occurs in Sub Saharan African populations consistent with the anthropological hypotheses that posit an African origin for modern humans.[9-11] It has been established that genetic variations among Nigerian groups appear to exceed the genetic variation among all European populations.[12]

Thus epidemiological research involving African populations, particularly when combined with parallel studies in developed countries, offer the opportunity of evaluating not only wide environmental but also wide genetic diversity in determining disease phenotypes in populations.

The purpose of this chapter is to describe the steps necessary to construct the disease model described by Cooper and Kaufman[1] for Alzheimer disease (AD) with particular reference to the results from our ongoing Indianapolis-Ibadan Dementia Project (I-IDP). These steps include:

- A comparison of the rates of illness (preferably incidence rates) between populations;
- A comparison of the frequency of putative risk factors, both genetic and environmental, between the populations;
- An examination of the association of environmental risk factors with AD within each population;

- An examination of the association of genetic risk factors with AD within each population, including an explanation of possible genetic or genetic/environmental interactions which may account for differences in the strength of genetic (or environmental) risk between populations if it occurs;
- An estimate of the potential significance of these risk factors in explaining the observed differences in illness rates between populations; and
- Development of a risk factor model, which should account for observed phenotypic variation in both (all) populations.

THE INDIANOPOLIS-IBADAN DEMENTIA PROJECT (I-IDP)

Since 1992, research teams from Indiana University and the University of Ibadan have been collaborating on studies of the prevalence and incidence of dementia in elderly African Americans and Yoruba using identical methodology utilizing a two-stage design. So far, a prevalence study followed by two incidence studies at 2 year and 5 year intervals have been conducted. The study, which is supported by the National Institute on Aging, is ongoing.

A COMPARISON OF THE RATES OF ILLNESS (PREFERABLY INCIDENCE RATES) BETWEEN POPULATIONS

It should be emphasized that for the purpose of risk factor research the determination that illness rates in the populations are similar may be just as significant as determining differences in illness rates if the populations are exposed to very different levels of putative environmental or genetic risk factors.

There are many potential methodological pitfalls in comparative studies involving populations in countries at different developmental levels and with different cultures. It is essential; therefore, that the comparative studies be conducted by the same experienced group of investigators familiar with the social and cultural standards of the populations which are being studied and who use test instruments that have been harmonized with adequate normative values. Harmonization is the process of translating and adapting test instruments to be appropriate for the target population's language and culture. Pilot studies are necessary to establish normative values for the target population.

We have reported significantly lower prevalence rates of dementia (8.24% African American, 2.29% Yoruba) and of AD (6.24% African American, 1.41% Yoruba) in Yoruba than in African Americans.[13] Our prevalence rates for African Americans are approximately the same as those reported in the large cross-Canada national prevalence study.[14] Our prevalence rates for Yoruba are at the lower end of previously reported rates.

Prevalence rates, however, are dependent on factors in addition to incidence rates of illness. Differences in life expectancy or in survival of demented and non-demented subjects between sites could also affect prevalence rates. Incidence rates, which are the number of new cases occurring over a fixed period of time, are a better indication of true rates of illness than prevalence rates. In our 5-year incidence study, the age-standardized incidence rates for both dementia and AD were significantly lower for Yoruba than for African Americans (for dementia: Yoruba, 1.35%, and African Americans, 3.24%; for AD: Yoruba, 1.15%, and African Americans, 2.52%).[15] It should be noted that although prevalence and incidence rates were consistently lower among the Yoruba, the association with age was identical between sites; that is, prevalence rates in both sites roughly doubled every 5 additional years of age.

Our reported incidence rates for dementia and AD for African Americans are in the higher range of previously published incidence rates but are similar to other published rates from African American populations. The incidence rates for both dementia and AD for Yoruba are among the lowest of previously reported rates.[16] In the one other study of incidence rates of AD involving a comparison of populations from a developing and developed countries, the Indo-US Cross National Dementia Epidemiology Study, the incidence rates for AD in an Indian population living in Ballabgarh, a rural district of Northern India, was one sixth rate of elderly subjects living in the Monongahela Valley in Pennsylvania.[17]

It is tempting to propose from these studies that dementia rates are lower in developing countries or more traditional societies than in developed countries. However, there are still far too few comparative studies available to make this generalization at this time.

One rather surprising finding from our study was that the increased risk for mortality from dementia was similar in the Yoruba and the African Americans despite very different availability of health care (Ibadan RR=2.83, Indianapolis RR=2.05).[18]

A COMPARISON OF FREQUENCY OF PUTATIVE RISK FACTORS, BOTH GENETIC AND ENVIRONMENTAL, BETWEEN THE POPULATIONS

Genetic Variations

The association between the possession of the Apolipoprotein E (ApoE) ε_4 allele of AD is one of the most consistent findings in AD research being confirmed in many studies throughout the World.[19] Variations in allelic frequency are common between populations and ApoE is no exception. The frequency of the ε_4 allele of ApoE has been reported to vary between 5% in Sardinians to over 40% in Pygmies in Africa.[20] Indeed, ε_4 allele frequency between populations within Sub-Saharan Africa varies as widely as that seen for the rest of the world. It is not clear yet what affect these population frequency allelic variations have on the rates of AD in different countries.

In our study, however, the ApoE allele frequencies were almost identical in the Yoruba and the African Americans (see Table 1).

Table 1. ApoE Allele Frequencies.

	# of Subjects	ε_2	ε_3	ε_4
Indianapolis	396	8.8	67.6	23.6
Ibadan	985	10.1	68.1	21.9

Environmental Risk Factors

Great cultural and socioeconomic differences exist between the impoverished, predominantly Muslim residents of the Idikan wards of Ibadan and the elderly African Americans living in Indianapolis. The elderly Yoruba have relatively limited access to health care and live, for the most part, in large extended families. In contrast, most of the African Americans in our study reported good access to health care and either live in single-family dwellings with members of the immediate family or are widowed and live alone. Fifty percent (50%)of the elderly African Americans report living alone as compared to only 7.4% of Yoruba. One rather intriguing preliminary finding of our study is that there was an overall positive relationship between indices of social involvement and cognitive function for both African Americans and Yoruba; i.e., greater social involvement was associated with better cognitive scores. Educational levels differed between the two populations. In Ibadan, 85% of the subjects received no formal education. In Indianapolis, the mean years of education for our cohort was 9.6.[2]

There are many lifestyle differences between the two populations in our study. For example, dietary intake varies widely: The elderly Yoruba in the Idikan wards consume a low-calorie, low-fat diet consisting mainly of grains, roots, and tubers, supplemented with a small amount of fish. Ascorbic acid levels have been reported to be relatively high among the Yoruba, probably because of the high consumption of peppers. The African-American diet, however, is high in fat and sodium and low in fiber. These lifestyle differences are reflected in significant differences in biological and medical variables (see Table 2) that are often associated with risk of circulatory problems such as heart attack and stroke.[2]

Table 2. Summary of significantly different biological and medical variables between Yoruba and African-American Subjects.

	Yoruba (n)	African American (n)
History of Hypertension	19% (2470)	61% (2204)
History of Diabetes	2.5% (2482)	24% (2206)
History of Stroke	1.3% (2480)	11% (1960)
Ever Smoked	24% (2472)	63% (2205)
Mean Cholesterol (mgs/dl)	166 (71)	221 (117)
Mean Body Mass Index	21.4 (1104)	28.9 (1115)
Mean Systolic BP	135 (1213)	146 (945)

Self reports of diabetes and hypertension may underestimate the extent of these diseases in the elderly. An intensive medical evaluation conducted at the clinical assessment phase of our study in Ibadan reported a higher rate of hypertension (27.8%) than did self reports but still considerably lower than the rates in African Americans. [21] Blood pressure measurements showed only small differences between the two groups. However, approximately 60% of the African Americans with diagnosed hypertension were taking anti-hypertensive medications.

AN EXAMINATION OF THE ASSOCIATION OF ENVIRONMENTAL RISK FACTORS WITH AD WITHIN EACH POPULATION

It would be anticipated that a risk factor, if valid, should modify disease change rates in both populations in the same manner. If this association of the risk factor to disease differs in the two populations, a careful investigation to understand the causes for this discrepancy should be undertaken.

Take, for example, education. Many studies report a high level of education as a protective factor against the development of AD. In Ibadan, 85% of the subjects had received no education. In Indianapolis, the mean number of years of education for our cohort was 9.6. This finding is counterintuitive in view of the low rates of AD in the Yoruba. It might suggest that education level is not directly related to AD risk but instead serves as a marker for other influences in childhood. In the African Americans, for example, it was the combination of low education and childhood residence in the rural South that increased the risk of AD.[22] In Yoruba, education was not significantly associated with AD rates.

There is now increasing evidence that vascular risk factors and vascular disease are not only associated with an increased risk of stroke-related dementia but may also contribute to the development, progression and clinical severity of AD.[23-25] It is noteworthy that the Yoruba had a lower incidence of both vascular disease and vascular risk factors, including hypertension, than did the African Americans.

Many studies, but not all, report that hypertension particularly when occurring in middle age is associated with an increased risk of late onset AD.[26-30] In our study, self-reports of hypertension were not associated with an increased risk for AD in either the Yoruba or the African Americans. However, in both cross-sectional and longitudinal studies, the use of anti-hypertensive medication in African Americans was associated with a reduced risk of dementia and reduced the odds of incident cognitive impairment (poor cognitive performance; cognitive impairment, not dementia; and dementia) by 38% (odds ratio, 0.62; 95% confidence interval, 0.45 – 0.84). Anti-hypertensive medication use was very rare in the Yoruba.[31,32]

Cholesterol levels were much lower in Yoruba than in African Americans, probably dietary related. It has been suggested that lipid-related mechanisms may have a role in the pathogenesis of AD and there is intriguing evidence that statins may reduce the risk of incidence AD.[33] We were unable to confirm a protective effect for statins in our study. However, only a small number of African Americans (n=30) were using them.

There were great differences in diet between the Yoruba and the African Americans. Many reports have suggested a link between certain constituents of diet; e.g., high levels of Vitamin E, low fat, and a reduced risk of dementia.[34-36] While we would anticipate that the Yoruba diet would conform more closely to the hypothetical ideal diet for preservation of brain function than would that of the African Americans, we do not have currently available the detailed nutritional evaluation necessary to support this hypothesis. However, in a small pilot study of lymphoblastoid cell lines from 8 Yoruba subjects, there was little evidence of DNA damage supporting the concept that the low calorie, low fat, high anti-oxidant Yoruba diet produced less evidence of oxidative stress than did the high calorie diets characteristic of Western countries.[37]

AN EXAMINATION OF THE ASSOCIATION OF GENETIC RISK FACTORS WITH AD WITHIN EACH POPULATION, INCLUDING AN EXPLORATION OF POSSIBLE GENETIC OR GENETIC/ENVIRONMENTAL INTERACTIONS WHICH MAY ACCOUNT FOR DIFFERENCES IN THE STRENGTH OF GENETIC (OR ENVIRONMENTAL) RISK BETWEEN POPULATIONS, IF IT OCCURS

In contrast to reports from other countries but consistent with other studies of African Americans, we have found only a relatively weak association between the possession of the ε_4 allele of ApoE and in the elderly African Americans reaching significance only for the ε_4 homozygotes (see Tables 3 and 4). As in other reports, there is a trend for the ε_2 allele of ApoE to be protective in African Americans.[38]

So far, in the elderly Yoruba, we can determine no significant association between the ε_4 allele of ApoE either for a single or a double copy. In fact, in the Yoruba, only possession of the ε_3 allele of ApoE comes close to significance.[39]

Table 3. Allele Frequencies in AD and Normal Subjects: Ibadan and Indianapolis.

Alle le	IBADAN			INDIANAPOLIS		
	AD Subjects (n=66) (%)	Normals (N=326) (%)	P	AD Subjects (n=93) (%)	Normals (n=199) (%)	P
E2	12.9	10.6	0.4414	4.8	11.6	0.0096
E3	59.1	68.1	0.0454	62.4	70.1	0.0627
E4	28.0	21.3	0.0919	32.8	18.3	0.0001

Table 4. Indianapolis–ApoE Genotype and Odds Ratios for AD Subjects Adjusting for Age at Diagnosis and Gender.

ApoE Genotype	AD Subjects (n=93) (%)	Normals (n=199) (%)	OR	95% CL
E2/E2	1 (1.1)	6 (3.0)	0.254	0.026-2.437
E2/E3	4 (4.3)	24 (12.1)	0.249	0.073-0.848
E2/E4	3 (3.2)	10 (5.0)	0.764	0.182-3.210
E3/E3	40 (43.0)	103 (51.8)	1.00	---------------
E3/E4	32 (34.4)	49 (24.6)	1.850	0.990-3.459
E4/E4	13 (14.0)	7 (3.5)	5.051`	1.786-14.287

There are possible genetic mechanisms, which could explain both the lowered risk in African Americans as well as the absence of risk for the ε_4 allele in Yoruba. Perhaps the ApoE ε_4 alleles are not the same from population to population. These alleles may differ by nucleotide changes, which may affect gene function, or nucleotide changes in the non-coding regions, which may affect gene expression.[40,41] In addition, nucleotide changes in other genes that interact with ApoE ε_4, for example apolipoprotein receptors, may affect ApoE ε_4 function and thus how it behaves as a risk factor for AD. We are currently exploring all of these possibilities.[42]

It is also possible that the lack of effect of ApoE ε_4 is due to some gene-environmental interaction. The differences in cholesterol levels between sites and the role that ApoE plays in cholesterol processing make an ApoE-cholesterol interaction resulting in a differential AD risk an obvious possibility. Two prior studies have reported a significant interaction between ApoE and cholesterol in determining risk for AD[43,44] Notkola et al.[44] suggested that cholesterol, in fact, mediates some of the effects of ApoE ε_4 on AD. In a preliminary study in African Americans, we did detect a significant interaction between ε_4 and cholesterol. Increasing levels of cholesterol increased the risk of AD, but only in those subjects who did not possess an ε_4 allele .[45]

Carbo and Scacchi[20] have proposed that ApoE+4 may represent a "thrifty" allele. In early human environments when meeting nutritional needs was an uncertain outcome and diets tended to be very low in fat, the ε_4 allele, which tends to conserve cholesterol, may have conferred an advantage to its possessor thus ensuring its survival. Now, in an environment where obesity is a problem and diets are rich in fat, the original advantage associated with possession of the ε_4 allele became instead a liability.

AN ESTIMATE OF THE POTENTIAL SIGNIFICANCE OF THESE RISK FACTORS IN EXPLAINING THE OBSERVED DIFFERENCES IN ILLNESS RATES BETWEEN THE POPULATIONS

It is likely that the lower incidence of vascular risk factors and vascular disease in the Yoruba as compared to the African Americans accounts for a significant proportion of the differences in incidence rates of AD and dementia between the two populations. However, our measurements of these factors are currently too imprecise to estimate accurately the effect size due to them. In our continuing study we are including biochemical assays of risk factors for vascular disease such as lipid levels, 8-Isoprostanes, homocysteine, insulin, interleukin-6, which together with more comprehensive brain imaging will allow us to determine more precisely the extent and the effect of vascular disease on AD risk in the two populations.

We did attempt to estimate the effect of the difference in the risk associated with the possession of the ε_4 allele between the two populations. However, as can be seen in the table below, ε_4 accounted for only a very small percentage of the variation for developing AD in the African American population, something akin to the risk associated with years of education. So, it is unlikely that the ε_4 related difference in risk accounts for much of the observed differences in incidence rates of AD between the populations.

It is also possible (probable) that other as yet unidentified genetic or environmental risk factors are associated with the observed phenotypic variation of AD between the populations.

Table 5. Explaining Variation for Developing AD in an African American Population Using Generally Recognized Risk Factors.

Variables	Odds Ratio	PEV (%)*	PEV (%)/Model**
Age (yr)	1.12	10.42	69.56
Education (yr)	0.96	1.84	12.28
Female	1.16	0.08	0.53
Any ε_4 vs. $\varepsilon_3/\varepsilon_3$	2.00	2.64	17.66

* A hypothetical model, which assumes that 100% of the variation can be explained.

** A model which assumes that 100% of the variation is explained by the four identified risk factors.

DEVELOPMENT OF A RISK FACTOR MODEL WHICH SHOULD ACCOUNT FOR OBSERVED PHENOTYPIC VARIATION IN BOTH (ALL) POPULATIONS

If we return now to the Cooper and Kaufman[1] disease model, our current knowledge could be characterized as follows. With regard to the genetic contribution to disease risk, if the relationship between ApoE ε_4 is weak in populations of African origin, it strongly suggests that other as yet unidentified genes may be involved in AD in these populations. There are a number of possible candidates but so far none has been identified conclusively.

Our studies and others strongly suggest that vascular risk factors play an important role in the genesis of AD as well as in the other dementias. It is possible that these factors are influenced primarily by diet and that the constituents of the Yoruba diet, low calorie, low fat, and possibly high anti-oxidant levels may lower potential vascular risk factors such as lipid levels and also lower levels of oxidative stress. Vascular risk factors such as high blood pressure also have a significant genetic component, however, and genetic differences in association with environmental factors may account for the variations between the populations. The possibility that other social or cultural influences may account for disease variation between the populations should not be ruled out. The protective value of living in large extended families, with much social interaction and social support available, may be significant.

Our exploration of gene/gene or gene/environmental interaction currently focuses on the attempt to find an explanation for the lowered risk associated with ApoE ε_4 in the two populations either through interaction with lipids or with other contributing genes as described previously.

Table 6. Explanation of Observed Phenotypic Variation of AD in Yoruba and African Americans.

Genes	+Environmental	+ Gene/Gene	+ Gene/Environmental
ApoE ε_4	Vascular Risk	Genes which may	ApoE ε_4/Lipid or other
	Oxidative Stress	affect ApoE ε_4	vascular risk factors
?Other Gene	?Diet	function, expression, or	
	Social and Cultural	its behavior as a risk	
	Factors	factor	

We hope our continuing work in this project will allow us to propose a more comprehensive explanation in the future.

CONCLUSION

International comparative studies, particularly those involving populations from developing and developed countries, offer a unique opportunity for applying the new information regarding population genetics to traditional AD risk factor research to a comprehensive model to explain phenotypic variations in populations. By the year 2005, about 70% of all elderly worldwide will be living in developing countries. The burden of caring for AD patients in these countries is likely to be staggering. It is hoped by including comparisons from the developed and developing words, models of AD etiology may be constructed which are more generalizable than those constructed primarily from investigation into Western populations.

REFERENCE LIST

1. Cooper, R.S., Kaufman, J.S. (1998) "Race and hypertension: science and nescience." *Hypertension*; 32(5):813-816.
2. Hendrie, H.C. (2001) "Exploration of Environmental and Genetic Risk Factors for Alzheimer's Disease: The Value of Cross-Cultural Studies." *Current Directions in Psychological Science*; 10(3):98-101.
3. Barbujani, G., Magagni, A., Minch, E., Cavalli-Sforza, L.L. (1997) "An apportionment of human DNA diversity." *Proc Natl Acad Sci USA*; 94(9):4516-4519.
4. Collins, F.S., Guyer, M.S., Charkravarti, A. (1997) "Variations on a theme: cataloging human DNA sequence variation." *Science*; 278(5343):1580-1581.
5. Collins, F.S., Brooks, L.D., Chakravarti, A. (1998) "A DNA polymorphism discovery resource for research on human genetic variation." *Genome Res*; 8(12):1229-1231.
6. Miller, R.D., Kwok, P.Y. (2001) "The birth and death of human single-nucleotide polymorphisms: new experimental evidence and implications for human history and medicine." *Hum Mol Genet*; 10(20):2195-2198.

7. Gray, I.C., Campbell, D..A, Spurr, N.K. (2000) "Single nucleotide polymorphisms as tools in human genetics." *Hum Mol Genet*; 9(16):2403-2408.

8. Goldstein, D.B. "Islands of linkage disequilibrium." *Nature Genetics*; 29(2):109-111.

9. Tishkoff, S.A., Dietzsch, E., Speed, W., Pakstis, A.J., Kidd, J.R., Cheung, K. et al. (1996) "Global patterns of linkage disequilibrium at the DC4 locus and modern human origins." *Science*; 271(5254):1380-1387.

10. Ingman, M., Kaessmann, H., Paabo, S., Gyllenste,n U. (2000) Mitochondrial genome variation and the origin of modern humans. *Nature*; 408(6813):708-713.

11. Armour, J.A., Anttinen, T., May, C.A., Vega, E.E., Sajantila, A., Kidd, J.R. et al. (1996) "Minisatellite diversity supports a recent African origin for modern humans." *Nature Genetics*; 13(2):154-160.

12. Kidd, J.R., Pakstis, A.J., Zhao, H., Lu, R.B., Okonofua, F.E., Odunsi, A. et al. (2000) "Haplotypes and linkage disequilibrium at the phenylalanine hydroxylase locus, PAH, in a global representation of populations." *Am J Hum Genet*; 66(6):1882-1899.

13. Hendrie, H.C., Osuntokun, B.O., Hall, K.S., Ogunniyi, A.O., Hui, S.L., Unverzagt, F.W. et al. (1995) "Prevalence of Alzheimer's Disease and Dementia in Two Communities: Nigerian Africans and African Americans." *Am J Psychiatry;* 152(10):1485-1492.

14. Canadian Study of Health and Aging Working Group. (1994) "Canadian Study of Health and Aging: Study Methods and prevalence of dementia." *Can Med Assoc J*; 150:899-913.

15. Hendrie, H.C., Ogunniyi, A., Hall, K.S., Baiyewu, O., Unverzagt, F.W., Gureje, O. et al. (2001) "Incidence of Dementia and Alzheimer Disease in Two Communities: Yoruba Residing in Ibadan, Nigeria and African Americans Residing in Indianapolis, USA." *JAMA*; 285(6):739-747.

16. Gao, S., Hendrie, H.C., Hall, K.S., Hui, S. (1998) "The Relationship Between Age, Sex and the Incidence of Dementia and Alzheimer's Disease: a meta-analysis." *Arch Gen Psychiatry*; 55:809-815.

17. Chandra, V., Pandav, R., Dodge, H.H., Johnston, J.M., Belle, S.H., DeKosky, S.T. et al. (2001) "Incidence of Alzheimer's disease in a rural community in India. The Indo-US Study." *Neurology*; 57(6):985-989.

18. Perkins, A.J., Hui, S.L., Ogunniyi, A., Gureje, O., Baiyewu, O., Unverzagt, F.W. et al. (2002) "Risk of mortality for dementia in a developing country: the Yoruba in Nigeria. " *Int J Geriatr Psychiatry*; 17:566-573.

19. Roses, A.D. (1996) "Apolipoprotein E alleles as risk factors in Alzheimer's disease." *Annu Rev Med*; 47:387-400.

20. Carbo, R.M., Scacchi, R. (1999) "Apolipoprotein E (APOE) allele distribution in the world. Is *APOE**4 a 'thrifty' allele?" *Ann Hum Genet*; **63**:301-310.

21. Ogunniyi, A., Baiyewu, O., Gureje, O., Hall, K.S., Unverzagt, F., Oluwole, O.S.A. et al. (2002) "Morbidity patters in a sample of elderly Nigerians resident in Idikan Community, Ibadan. " *West Afr Med J*; In Press.

22. Hall, K.S., Gao, S.J., Unverzagt, F.W., Hendrie, H.C. (2000) "Low education and childhood rural residence: risk for Alzheimer's disease in African Americans." *Neurology*; 54(1):95-99.

23. Ellis, R.J., Olichney, J.M., Thal, L.J., Mirra, S.S., Morris, J.C., Beekly, D. et al. (1996) "Cerebral amyloid angiopathy in the brains of patients with Alzheimer's disease: The CERAD experience, Part XV." *Neurology*; 46(6):1592-1596.

24. Snowden, D.A., Greiner, L.H., Mortimer, J.A., Riley, K.P., Greiner, P.A., Markesbery, W.R. (1997) "Brain infarction and the clinical expression of Alzheimer's disease: The Nun Study." *JAMA*; 227(10):813-817.

25. Skoog, I. (1999) "The interaction between vascular disorders and Alzheimer's disease." *Alzheimer's Disease and Related Disorders*; 58:523-530.

26. Launer, L.J., Masaki, K., Petrovich, H., Foley, D., Havlik, R.J. (1995) "The association between midlife blood pressure levels and late-life cognitive function: The Honolulu-Asia Aging Study." *JAMA*; 274:1846-1851.

27. Kivipelto, M., Helkala, E.L., Laakso, M.P., Hanninen, T., Hallikainen, M., Alhainen, K. et al. (2001) "Midlife vascular risk factors and Alzheimer's disease in later life: longitudinal, population based study." *BMJ*; 322(7300):1447-1451.

28. Desmond, D.W., Tatemichi, T.K., Paik, M., Stern, Y. (1993) "Risk factors for cerebrovascular diasese as correlates of cognitive function in a stroke-free cohort." *Arch Neurol*; 50(2):162-166.

29. Glynn, R.J., Beckett, L.A., Hebert, L.E., Morris, M.C., Scherr, P.A., Evans, D.A. (1999) "Current and remote blood pressure and cognitive decline." *JAMA*; 281(5):438-445.

30. Guo, Z., Viitanen, M., Fratiglioni, L., Winblad, B. (1996) "Low Blood Pressure and dementia in elderly people: the Kungsholmen project." *BMJ*; 312(7034):805-808.

31. Murray, M.D., Lane, K.A., Gao, S., Evans, R.M., Unverzagt, F.W., Hall, K.S. et al. (2002) "Preservation of cognitive function with antihypertensive medications: a longitudinal analysis of a community-based sample of African Americans." *Journal of the American Medical Association*; In Press.

32. Richards, S.S., Emsley, C.L., Roberts .J., Murray, M.D., Hall, K., Gao, S. et al. (2000) "The Association Between Vascular Risk Factor Mediating Medications and Cognition and Dementia Diagnosis in a Community-Based Sample of African-Americans." *J Am Geriatr Soc*; 48:1-7.

33. Jick, H., Zornberg, G.L., Jick, S.S., Seshadri, S. Drachman, D.A. (2000) "Statins and the risk of dementia." *Lancet*; 356:1627-1631.

34. Morris, M.C., Evans, D.A., Bienias, J.L., Tangney, C.C., Bennett, D.A., Aggarwal, N. et al. (2002) "Dietary intake of antioxidant nutrients and the risk of incident Alzheimer disease in a biracial community study." *JAMA*; 287(24):3261-3263.

35. Perkins, A.J., Hendrie, H.C., Callahan, C.M., Gao, S., Unverzagt, F.W., Xu, Y. et al. (1999) "Association of antioxidants with memory in multiethnic elderly

598

sample using the Third National Health and Nutrition Examination Survey." *Am J Epidemiol*; 150(1):37-44.

36.   Butterfield, D.A., Koppal, T., Subramaniam, R., Yatin, S. (1999) "Vitamin E as an antioxidant/free radical scavenger against amyloid beta-peptide-induced oxidative stress in neocortical synaptosomal membranes and hippocampal neurons in culture: insights into Alzheimer's disease." *Rev Neurosci*; 10(2):141-149.

37.   Lahiri, D.K., Xu, Y., Klaunig, J., Baiyewu, O., Ogunniyi, A., Hall, K. et al. (1999) "Effect of Oxidative Stress on DNA Damage and B eta-Amyloid Precursor Proteins in Lymphoblastoid Cell Lines from a Nigerian Population." *Annals of New York Academy of Sciences*; 893:331-336.

38.   Sahota, A., Yang, M., Gao, S., Hui, S.L., Baiyewu, O., Gureje, O. et al. (1997) "Apolipoprotein E - Associated Risk for Alzheimer Disease in the African-American Population is Genotype Dependent." *Ann Neurol*; 42:659-661.

39.   Osuntokun, B.O., Sahota, A., Ogunniyi, A.O., Gureje, O., Baiyewu, O., Adeyinka, A. et al. (1995) "Lack of an Association between the Apolipoprotein E e4 Allele and Alzheimer's Disease in Elderly Nigerians." *Ann Neurol*; 38(3):463-465.

40.   Fullerton, S.M., Clark, A.G., Weiss, K.M., Nickerson, D.A., Taylor, S.L., Stengard, J.H. et al. (2000) "Apolipoprotein E variation at the sequence haplotype level: implications for the origin and maintenance of a major human polymorphism." *Am J Hum Genet*; 67(4):881-900.

41.   Nickerson, D.A., Taylor, S.L., Fullerton, S.M., Weiss, K.M., Clark, A.G., Stengard, J.H. et al. (2000) "Sequence diversity and large-scale typing of SNPs in the human apolipoprotein E gene." *Genome Res*; 10(10):1532-1545.

42.   Hui, D.Y., Innerarity, T.L., Mahley, R.W. (1984) "Defective hepatic lipoprotein receptor binding of beta-very low density lipoproteins from type III hyperlipoproteinemic patients. Importance of apolipoprotein E." *The Journal of Biological Chemistry*; 259(2):860-869.

43.   Jarvik, G.P., Wijsman, E.M., Kukull, W.A., Schellenberg, G.D., Yu, C., Larson, E.B. (1995) "Interactions of apolipoprotein E genotype, total cholesterol level, age, and sex in prediction of Alzheimer's disease: a case-control study." *Neurology*; 45(6):1092-1096.

44.   Notkola, I.L., Sulkava, R., Pekkanen, J., Erkinjuntti, T., Ehnholm, C., Kivinen, P. et al. (1998) "Serum total cholesterol, apolipoprotein E epsilon 4 allele, and Alzheimer's disease." *Neuroepidemiol*; 17(1):14-20.

45.   Evans, R.M., Emsley, C.L., Gao, S., Sahota, A., Hall, K.S., Farlow, M.R. et al. (2000) "Serum Cholesterol, APOE Genotype and the risk of Alzheimer Disease in A Population-based study of African Americans." *Neurology*; 54:240-242.

GENETICS AND THE GLOBAL HEALTH BURDEN OF MOOD DISORDERS

FRANCIS J. MCMAHON, M.D.
National Institute of Mental Health, Bethesda, MD, USA

ABSTRACT

Mood disorders encompass a large and heterogeneous group of mental illnesses ranging from chronic mild depression to manic-depressive disorder, also known as bipolar disorder. Mood disorders account for substantial economic losses due to medical costs, lost productivity, and premature death; and are the main cause of suicide, itself the leading medical cause of death among young people in developed countries. Family, twin, and adoption studies indicate a substantial genetic contribution to mood disorders, particularly the bipolar types, but non-genetic factors still account for 30% to 50% of the variance in individual risk. Molecular studies aimed at identifying the specific genes involved in susceptibility to mood disorders have been underway for close to 20 years, but comparatively few resources have been devoted to this problem and definitive findings have not yet emerged. The identification of all of the important genetic variation that increases individual risk for mood disorders will require a much larger commitment of resources. Such a commitment is needed to support systematic collection of larger study samples, complete characterization of genetic markers covering the entire human genome, and management of the resulting data. The impact of any genetic discoveries is expected to be large, but will depend on the proportion of mood disorders that can be attributed to the discovered genetic variation (attributable risk) and on the degree to which this genetic information can be used to develop novel diagnostic and treatment approaches. Genetically-based improvements in diagnosis, drug development, and preventive strategies, would have major implications for global public health.

INTRODUCTION: MOOD DISORDERS ARE AN IMPORTANT PUBLIC HEALTH PROBLEM

Mood disorders are important for several reasons. They are the most common reason for patients to seek psychiatric care, and are present in about a third of all patients with general medical problems. Mood disorders are the main risk factor for suicide, itself a leading cause of death in young people, and probably contribute to increased mortality also through unhealthy lifestyles, reckless behavior, and poor self-care, particularly in the elderly.[1] On top of all of this, mood disorders are under-recognized and frequently misdiagnosed. This means that many people who would benefit from treatment never get it, too often with grave consequences.

Despite these facts, societies have been slow to recognize that mood disorders are a major global health problem. But in 1990, the World Health Organization launched an international epidemiologic study aimed at quantifying the global burden of all kinds of diseases and injuries, ranging from AIDS to unintentional injuries. The Global Burden of Disease Study developed a new, unified and quantitative method for studying disease burden, one that did not rely on mortality statistics nearly as much as earlier studies. The main measure of disease burden was called the Disability-adjusted-life-year, or DALY, practically equivalent to one lost year of healthy life (http://hsph.harvard.edu/organizations/bdu/summary.html; visited 7/23/02).

The startling result of this new approach was the realization that previous studies, due to their emphasis on mortality, had grossly underestimated the disease burden of mental illnesses, particularly depression. The most recent figures from the Global Burden of Disease study are summarized in Figure 1. Unipolar depressive disorders are the 3rd leading cause of disability worldwide, with only HIV/AIDs and lower respiratory infections accounting for a larger portion of the global health burden. Moreover, if current trends continue, depressive disorders will become the leading cause of disability worldwide by 2020, second only to ischemic heart disease in number of healthy years of life lost.

Years of Healthy Life Lost
Global Burden of Disease 2000

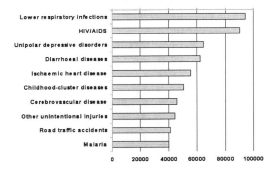

Fig. 1. Top ten causes of disease-related disability, all nations and genders, measured in years of healthy life lost to disease, Global Burden of Disease Study, 2000.

Thus mood disorders constitute a major and growing public health problem around the world. What can we do to address this?

MOOD DISORDERS ARE COMMON DISEASES WITH A GENETIC BASIS

Much of what I will say today depends for its logical foundation on what is called "The Disease Perspective."[2] In this perspective, mood disorders are seen as clinical syndromes–relatively characteristic clusters of signs and symptoms. As with other clinical syndromes in medicine, mood disorders are thus assumed to correspond to some underlying pathological disease entity–some part of the body that is "broken" in either its morphology or physiology, usually both–although such a pathology has yet to be identified for mood disorders in any convincing way. The final component of the disease perspective is the etiologic agent, the events or factors that cause the disease in the usual chemical or physical sense. For mood disorders, these etiologic agents will often correspond to genes, and thus genes and genetics will be the major focus of my talk today.

Mood disorders are typically classified into several categories, reflecting differences in symptoms and course of illness (Table 1). Bipolar I disorder is classic manic-depressive illness, with episodes of severely elevated mood and impaired functioning, known as mania, and episodes of low mood and impaired functioning, known as major depression. People with bipolar II disorder also have major depression, but do not experience mania. Rather, they suffer from distinctive, although less impairing episodes of elevated mood known as hypomania. People with unipolar disorder only have major depressions. There are also milder forms of the illness, known as cyclothymia and dysthymia, that are very common, but less impairing than bipolar or unipolar disorders. Schizoaffective disorder, where the typical symptoms of bipolar I disorder are complicated by persistent hallucinations or delusions, appear to be a severe form of manic-depressive illness, not a form of schizophrenia. Family studies show that all of these forms of manic-depressive illness are seen with increased frequency among the relatives of people with bipolar disorder,[3] but how these forms of the illness correspond to underlying genetic differences is currently unknown.

Bipolar disorder is a common illness, with prevalence estimates ranging from 1-3%, depending on the population and method of study.[4-5] Family, twin, and adoption studies all support a strong contribution of genetic factors to the etiology of bipolar disorder, although specific genes have not yet been identified. Most studies reveal marked anticipation in bipolar disorder, with increasing illness severity and decreasing age at onset seen in successive generations of a family,[6] but the cause of this phenomenon remains unclear. If we look just within families, we see that the risk for developing bipolar disorder is 15-fold higher among the 1st degree relatives of people with bipolar disorder (reviewed in McMahon & DePaulo[7]). However, this increased risk drops off very quickly with each step of relatedness, so that 2nd degree relatives have only a slightly increased risk and 3rd degree relatives have no increased risk at all. This is probably best explained by the theory that about 3 to 5 genes play the major role in bipolar disorder, with no single major gene causing the illness in the vast majority of people.[8] I will show you shortly that this fact, combined with the prevalence estimates for the disease, lead one to the conclusion that each of the gene forms contributing to the illness–what geneticists call susceptibility alleles–must be quite common.

Overall Classification

- Major Mood Disorders
  - Bipolar I
  - Bipolar II
  - Unipolar Disorder (Major Depression)
- Minor Mood Disorders
  - Cyclothymia
  - Dysthymias
- Schizoaffective disorder with mania

Table 1. Typical Classification of Mood Disorders.

Prevalence

The prevalence of mood disorders is not easy to measure. Since the illness inherently makes people withdraw from the outside world, complete case ascertainment is challenging. Since there is no objective clinical test to identify cases, surveyors must rely on peoples' self-report, which is always imperfect. Add to this, difficulties in deciding how best to collect the data and how best to define a case, and you can easily conclude that any prevalence estimates must be rather imprecise.

The most widely cited prevalence study to date, the Epidemiologic Catchment Area Study, was conducted during the 1980's in 5 U.S. cities.[9] Great care was taken to select an epidemiologically valid sample of people, including those in prisons, homeless shelters, and other often-overlooked settings. Clinical assessments were performed by trained laymen, which is not ideal, but a subset of the assessments were later checked by psychiatrists and were found to be reasonably accurate. This study found that mood disorders are very common, with a lifetime prevalence of 6 to 13%[4] (Fig. 2). Bipolar I and Bipolar II disorder each had a prevalence of about 1%, equal for men and women. Major depression was much more common, especially in women, with a lifetime prevalence of 7%, more than twice the prevalence in males. A similar gender difference was observed for dysthymia. Subsequent studies have found even higher rates of mood disorders in the U.S. population,[10] so the ECA data looks conservative by comparison. While similar epidemiologic data is lacking for most of the rest of the world, those data that are available generally agree with the ECA estimates.

Mood disorders have a genetic basis

The case for a genetic basis for mood disorders is built on the three pillars of twin, family, and adoption studies. Most twin studies compare rates of illness in identical (monozygotic) twin pairs with those in fraternal (dizygotic) twin pairs. When a trait is genetically influenced, identical twins who have inherited identical sets of genes will be more alike (concordant) in regard to that trait than fraternal twins, who share only 50% of their genes, on average. The most commonly cited twin data, that from the Danish Twin Registry, shows a 3-fold higher concordance rate for manic depressive disorder in identical compared to fraternal twins.[11] This shows that most of the individual variation in liability to manic depressive disorder is accounted for by genetic factors. In other words, mood disorders are highly heritable.

Lifetime Prevalence of Mood Disorders ECA Data, 1986

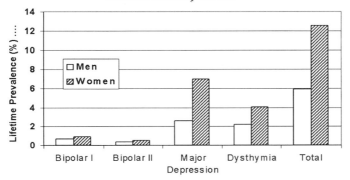

Fig. 2. Lifetime prevalence of mood disorders, all sites, Epidemiologic Catchment Area Study, 1986 (Weissman, et al. 1986).

Twin studies do not shed much light on the ways in which diseases are inherited in families. For this, family studies are needed. In the classic design, rates of various illnesses are compared between relatives of people with a disorder and relatives of those without the disorder. The most widely cited family study of mood disorders was published in 1982 by Gershon and colleagues.[3] They determined the lifetime prevalence of major mood disorders among the relatives of people with bipolar I, bipolar II, unipolar, and schizoaffective disorders, as well as people unaffected by any psychiatric illness. They found an age-adjusted excess of major affective disorders among relatives of probands with mood disorders compared to the relatives of the unaffected controls (Fig. 3). They also found that this excess increased in a graded fashion from the relatives of probands with unipolar disorder to those with schizoaffective disorder. No excess of alcoholism, sociopathy, or drug abuse was found, indicating that the increased familial risk was specific to mood disorders.

Not everything that is familial is genetic, so the final piece of evidence needed to establish the genetic basis of mood disorders is the adoption study. In the classic study design, rates of illness among the biological parents of adoptees and of non-adoptees with a disorder are compared. Two such studies have been performed for bipolar disorder, both with small sample sizes but essentially identical results. The widely-cited study by Mendlewicz and Rainer[12] showed that the rates of mood disorder were similar among the biological parents of adoptees and of non-adoptees with bipolar disorder, and that both were much higher than the rates of mood disorder among the biological parents of adoptees without bipolar disorder. This indicates that the familial risk for mood disorders is due to shared genes, not shared environment. The other adoption study of bipolar disorder reached similar conclusions. The existing data are less clear in studies of unipolar disorder.

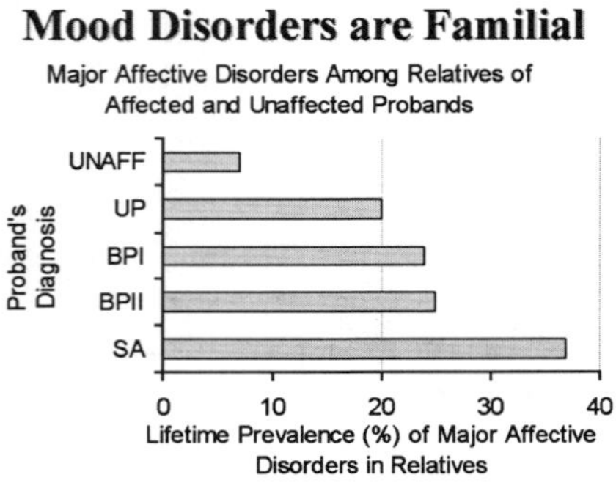

Mood Disorders are Familial

Major Affective Disorders Among Relatives of
Affected and Unaffected Probands

Fig. 3. Lifetime prevalance (age-adjusted) of major mood disorders among the relatives of mood disorder probands and normal control probands (Gershon et al. 1986).

Elucidating the genetic basis of mood disorders

Twin, family, and adoption studies establish a genetic basis, but do not indicate which genes or what kinds of changes within those genes, are responsible. For this, we have a growing range of molecular genetic investigation methods. In linkage studies, the inheritance of disease in families is traced using genetic markers whose location along the chromosomes is known. Thus the co-inheritance of marker and disease indicates that the gene related to that disease is located near that marker. Association studies use genetic markers in populations in order to pinpoint the specific genetic changes associated with a disease. Studies of gene expression look for differences in levels of gene products in tissues taken from people with a disease and those without. Genetic modeling involves the direct manipulation of DNA in a model organism, usually a mouse, and determination of the resulting biochemical and behavioral changes. All of these methods, and doubtless many others, will ultimately be brought to bear on the problem of identifying the genes that influence susceptibility to bipolar disorder. But genetic linkage is the only method that has so far been applied on a large scale in many samples.

A summary of some of the major genetic linkage findings in bipolar disorder to date is shown in Figure 4. Each of the 8 locations indicated has been implicated in more than one study, but each location has also been found to show no evidence of linkage in some studies.[13] This is not unexpected for a disease like bipolar disorder where several genes are involved and each gene individually confers only a small increase in risk.[14] The lack of consistent replication of linkage findings means that it is difficult to distinguish true findings from those that are largely due to chance, however.

MOOD DISORDERS AND THE COMMON DISEASE PARADIGM

We mentioned earlier that one important conclusion that arises from the family study data is that not one but several genes are likely to contribute to mood disorders. This means that instead of dealing with one disease that may be clinically variable, we can actually think of mood disorders as a group of several different diseases, some of which are clinically similar. This also means that some susceptibility alleles will not be seen at all in particular groups of patients, even though these same alleles contribute to disease in other populations. This situation, in which no one gene is necessary or sufficient to cause disease, creates a great challenge for those who would map these genes and establish their contribution to disease. But the problem is not insurmountable, as recent successes in mapping genes that contribute to non-insulin dependent diabetes,[15] inflammatory bowel disease,[16] and schizophrenia[17] illustrate.

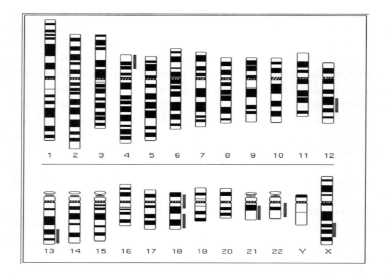

Fig. 4. Genetic linkage findings in bipolar disorder, as of 8/02. Each linkage finding is indicated with an arbitrarily-sized (20 cM) bar next to a cartoon of the implicated chromosomal location. Each of these 8 locations has been implicated in more than one study, but each location has also been found to show no evidence of linkage in some studies.

If we accept the idea that there are several genes that contribute to the risk for bipolar disorder, then it is easy to show that each susceptibility allele must be very common. For example, if 3 genes acting in an equal and additive fashion are needed to manifest an illness with a population prevalence of 2%, then each susceptibility allele must have a frequency equal to the cube root of 0.02, or 27% (Fig. 5). Note that if the disease is as common as 4% and 5 genes (acting equally and additively) are needed to manifest the disease, then susceptibility allele frequencies can climb to more than 50%! This means that the most common form of the gene, the form seen in most people in the population who do not have the disease, will be the form that increases risk for disease. But this increased risk will only be appreciated in that small proportion of the population that happens to inherit all five susceptibility alleles. The assumption of equal and additive effects is of course an oversimplification, but these calculations suggest that the susceptibility alleles for bipolar disorder will certainly be quite common in the population, more common than is widely assumed.

Each Susceptibility Allele Must be Very Common

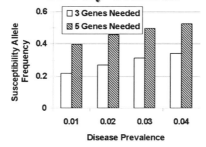

Fig. 5. Theoretical susceptibility allele frequencies under a variety of additive genetic models of bipolar disorder, calculated as $f = p^{(1/n)}$ where f is the susceptibility allele prevalence, p is the disease prevalence and n is the number of equal and additive alleles needed to express disease.

Common Disease-Common Variant Hypothesis

The suggestion that susceptibility alleles for bipolar disorder will be common is consistent with what has come to known in the field of human genetics as the "Common Disease-Common Variant" hypothesis. According to this hypothesis, common diseases are expected to be related to common forms of genetic variation. These common alleles have typically arisen very early in human history and are widespread in all world populations. Biologically, this genetic variation is conservative, causing only subtle changes in gene function. This is in contrast to rare, Mendelian diseases that are caused by rare forms of genetic variation that tend to have arisen recently in human history, occur more often in particular populations, and lead to major disruptions in gene function.

As a corollary to the Common Disease-Common Variant Hypothesis, some have proposed that the higher-order structure of genetic variation in humans–variation that involves groups of related sites along a chromosome–is simple and finite. Genetic variation tends to occur in groups of neighboring sites, leading to the formation of haplotype blocks.[18] While many haplotypes in a given block may exist around the world, only a few haplotypes are maintained in the population at high frequencies. When viewed from this perspective, human beings become much more alike than different, and susceptibility to common diseases becomes something we all share.

CLINICAL IMPLICATIONS OF FUTURE GENETIC FINDINGS

When genetic discoveries do come in psychiatry, they will affect our clinical practice in many ways. The discovery of genes will provide new standards by which to validate psychiatric disease entities. For the first time we will be able to test whether our widely-used disease classification systems actually correspond to underlying biological entities. Mood disorders would still be a disease regardless of any genetic findings, but the distinctions we typically draw between bipolar and unipolar, psychotic and non-psychotic, recurrent and chronic forms of the illness may not hold up when we understand more about the underlying genetic picture.[19]

Genetic discoveries will also improve diagnostic methods, allowing psychiatrists to use genetic testing to confirm clinical diagnoses, even in cases where the presenting symptoms are unusual or too complex. Genetic discoveries will also lead to improved treatment planning. There is also the potential for novel therapies that arise from the deeper understanding of disease physiology genetic discoveries could provide. Genetic discoveries could also provide new insights into the fundamental causes of mood disorders, both those causes that are genetic in nature and those that are not. This is because genetic discoveries may allow us to study individuals who carry high-risk alleles but nevertheless do not develop psychiatric symptoms. How these people differ from those with a similar genetic endowment who do fall ill will provide important clues as to the non-genetic causes of mood disorders.

The study of people who are at high-risk for developing mood disorders could also lead eventually to information about how to prevent mood disorders in susceptible people. Attempts at primary prevention of mental illness have up to now been unsuccessful, but this might be because these attempts were undertaken without the kind of solid information that genetic discoveries could ultimately help provide. Finally, and no less importantly, I believe that genetic discoveries will help to de-stigmatize mental illness.

How genetic findings will affect therapeutics

Although by far the greatest challenge, therapeutic advances are what we are really after in the genetic study of any human disease. But even if they do not provide the kind of understanding of fundamental etiologic mechanisms that will lead to curative treatments, genetic discoveries may still affect therapeutics in many positive ways. To name just a few: Genetic discoveries may lead to greater diagnostic homogeneity, which may in turn lead to more predictable responses to available treatments. Genetic discoveries may illuminate brain pathology at the molecular level, facilitating the development of novel, so-called "designer drugs," aimed at ameliorating the underlying pathology in a targeted manner. The, thus sparing them the risks, is another potential consequence of genetic discoveries with real clinical impact.

But we still have a long way to go. Genetic research progresses only very slowly toward new therapeutic discoveries. The progress of genetic research in humans is shown in Figure 6. The first step is the localization of the genes involved, when multiple studies point to the same chromosomal location in several different groups of patients. This is a stage we have now reached in psychiatry. The identification and positional cloning of the actual genes follows later, sometimes after laborious work with association analysis and genetic modeling. Then comes the first milestone with immediate clinical implications: the identification of disease alleles. Once this is accomplished, it is possible to develop diagnostic tests that identify carriers of susceptibility alleles. Of course, such diagnostic tests may be of little use if the alleles involved are only loosely associated with disease. This is a question of the predictive value of the test that can only be answered when large sets of genetic data are already available. Moving to the determination of gene function is another potentially labor-intensive step, but this step is becoming more efficient as our functional genetics knowledge continues to increase. Knowledge of gene function is only the first step in the elucidation of the pathophysiologic mechanisms involved: how the observed genetic variation actually leads to disease. This is a step that has yet to be fully realized for any genetic disease and is really essential if we are to begin to talk about truly gene-based therapeutics.

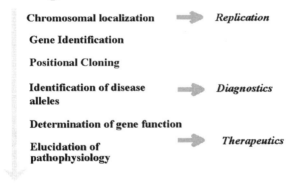

Progress of Genetic Research

Chromosomal localization   →   *Replication*

Gene Identification

Positional Cloning

Identification of disease alleles   →   *Diagnostics*

Determination of gene function

Elucidation of pathophysiology   →   *Therapeutics*

Fig. 6. Progress of genetic research in humans from chromosomal localization through elucidation of pathophysiology.

Genetic Attributable Risk

The concept of genetic attributable risk provides the bridge between the global health burden of mood disorders on the one hand and the clinical impact of genetic discoveries

610

on the other. In epidemiology, attributable risk has to do with the proportion of ill people who would not be ill if it were not for a particular contributing factor. Genetic attributable risk is thus the proportion of ill people who would not be ill if they did not carry a particular susceptibility allele.[20]

I mentioned earlier that several genes are thought to contribute to mood disorders, and that each susceptibility allele is expected to be common, even though each allele may individually increased risk for mood disorder only slightly. The concept of genetic attributable risk shows us that even alleles that have a slight impact on disease risk can have a large attributable risk when the alleles are frequent in the population. Thus the clinical impact of genetic discoveries in mood disorder research is expected to be large, even if the clinical impact of the individual alleles is not.

Stigma: A bottleneck in translating science into public health in psychiatry

Stigma is still the main reason people with mental illness fail to seek treatment. Stigma also contributes to discrimination by employers and insurers against those with mental illnesses. Improvements in the diagnosis and treatment of mental illnesses, along with the clear demonstration to the broader society that mental illnesses are true diseases and not merely the result of poor personal choices will inevitably lead to a broader acceptance of mental illness and the mentally ill and a de-stigmatization of mental illness throughout society. This is very important if the new treatments that come with genetic advances are to become available to all those who could benefit.

CONCLUSIONS

Mood disorders represent a large global health burden of disease, one that is expected to grow over time. We now know that mood disorders have a clear genetic basis, and we are beginning to identify the locations of the genes involved. Genetic discoveries will lead to improved diagnosis, treatment, and understanding of mood disorders. Interventions aimed at the common genetic factors in mood disorders could pay large dividends in reducing the global health burden of these diseases in the future.

REFERENCE LIST

1.   Wyatt, R.J., Henter, I. (1995) "An economic evaluation of manic-depressive illness--1991." *Soc Psychiatry Psychiatr Epidemiol.* 30:213-219.
2.   McHugh, P.R., Slavney, P.R. (1986) *The Perspectives of Psychiatry.* 1st ed. Baltimore: Johns Hopkins.
3.   Gershon, E.S., Hamovit, J., Guroff, J.J., Nurnberger, J.I., Goldin, L.R., Bunney, W.E. (1982) "A Family Study of Schizoaffective, Bipolar I, Bipolar II, Unipolar and Normal Control Probands." *Arch Gen Psychiatry.* 39:1157-1167.

4. Weissman, M.M., Bruce, M.L., Leaf, P.J., Florio, L.P., Holzer, C. (1991) "Affective Disorders." In: Robins L.N., Regier D.A., eds. *Psychiatric Disorders in America: The Epidemiologic Catchment Area Study*. New York: Free Press.

5. Kessler, R.C., Rubinow, D.R., Holmes, C., Abelson, J.M., Zhao, S. (1997) "The epidemiology of DSM-III-R bipolar I disorder in a general population survey." *Psychol Med*. 27:1079-1089.

6. McInnis, M.G., McMahon, F.J., Chase, G.A., Simpson, S.G., Ross, C.A., DePaulo, J.R., Jr. (1993) "Anticipation in bipolar affective disorder." *Am J Hum Genet*. 53:385-390.

7. McMahon, F.J., DePaulo, J.R. Affective Disorders. In: Jamison JL, ed. (1998) *Principles of Molecular Medicine*. Totawa, NJ: Humana; pp. 995-1003.

8. Risch, N. (1990) "Linkage strategies for genetically complex traits." *Am J Hum Genet*. 46:229-241.

9. Robins, L.N., Helzer, J.E., Weissman, M.M., Orvasehel, H., Gruenberg, E., Burke, J.D., Regier, D.A. (1984) "Lifetime prevalence of specific psychiatric disorders in three sites." *Arch Gen Psychiatry*. 41:949-958.

10. Kessler, R.C., McGonagle, K.A., Zhao, S., Nelson, C.B., Hughes, M., Eshleman, S., Wittchen, H-U., Kendler, K.S. (1994) "Lifetime and 12-month prevalence of DSM-III-R psychiatric disorders in the United States: Results from the National Comorbidity Survey." *Arch Gen Psychiatry*. 51:8-19.

11. Bertelsen, A., Harvald, B., Hauge, M. (1977) "A Danish twin study of manic depressive disorders." *Brit J Psychiat*. 130:330-351.

12. Mendlewicz, J., Rainer, J.D. (1977) "Adoption study supporting genetic transmission in manic-depressive illness." *Nature*. 268:327-329.

13. Prathikanti, S., McMahon, F.J. (2001) "Genome scans for susceptibility genes in bipolar affective disorder." *Ann Med*. 33:257-262.

14. Suarez, B., Hampe, C., Eerdewegh, P. (1994) "Problems of replicating linkage claims in psychiatry." In: Gershon ES, Cloninger CR, eds. *Genetic Approaches to Mental Disorders*. Washington, D.C.: American Psychiatric Press.

15. Horikawa, Y., Oda, N., Cox, N.J., Li, X., Orho-Melander, M., Hara, M., Hinokio, Y., Lindner, T.H., Mashima, H., Schwarz, P.E., Bosque-Plata, L., Horikawa, Y., Oda, Y., Yoshiuchi, I., Colilla, S., Polonsky, K.S., Wei, S., Concannon, P., Iwasaki, N., Schulze, J., Baier, L.J., Bogardus, C., Groop, L., Boerwinkle, E., Hanis, C.L., Bell, G.I. (2000) "Genetic variation in the gene encoding calpain-10 is associated with type 2 diabetes mellitus." *Nat Genet*. 26:163-175.

16. Rioux, J.D., Daly, M.J., Silverberg, M.S., Lindblad, K., Steinhart, H., Cohen, Z., Delmonte, T., Kocher, K., Miller, K., Guschwan, S., Kulbokas, E.J., O'Leary, S., Winchester, E., Dewar, K., Green, T., Stone, V., Chow, C., Cohen, A., Langelier, D., Lapointe, G., Gaudet, D., Faith, J., Branco, N., Bull, S.B., McLeod, R.S., Griffiths, A.M., Bitton, A., Greenberg, G.R., Lander, E.S., Siminovitch, K.A., Hudson, T.J. (2001) "Genetic variation in the 5q31 cytokine gene cluster confers susceptibility to Crohn disease." *Nat Genet*. 29:223-228.

17. Straub, R.E., Jiang, Y., MacLean, C.J., Ma, Y., Webb, B.T., Myakishev, M.V., Harris-Kerr, C., Wormley, B., Sadek, H., Kadambi, B., Cesare, A.J., Gibberman, A., Wang, X., O'Neill, F.A., Walsh, D., Kendler, K.S. (2002) "Genetic Variation in the 6p22.3 Gene DTNBP1, the Human Ortholog of the Mouse Dysbindin Gene, Is Associated with Schizophrenia." *Am J Hum Genet.* 71:337-348.
18. Daly, M.J., Rioux, J.D., Schaffner, S.F., Hudson, T.J., Lander, E.S. (2001) "High-resolution haplotype structure in the human genome." *Nat Genet.* 29:229-232.
19. McMahon, F. Chen, Y-S., Simpson, S., McInnis, M., Badner, J., MacKinnon, D., DePaulo, J.R. (2001) "Linkage of Bipolar Disorder to Chromosome 18q and the Validity of Bipolar II Disorder." *Arch Gen Psychiatry* 58:1025-1031.
20. Claus, E.B., Schildkraut, J.M., Thompson, W.D., Risch, N.J. (1996) "The genetic attributable risk of breast and ovarian cancer." *Cancer.* 77:2318-2324.

VIOLENCE AND VIOLENT CONFLICTS: VIEWS FROM AFFECTIVE NEUROSCIENCE

SERGIO PARADISO M.D., PH.D. AND LAUREN SCHROCK, B.S.
The University of Iowa, Roy J. and Lucille A. Carver College of Medicine, Department of Psychiatry, Iowa City, IA, USA

ABSTRACT

Darwin and Freud, who greatly influenced the philosophy of Western civilization, acknowledged the universality of emotion. The purpose of this paper is to discuss the centrality of human affectivity in decision-making and thinking, as well as to highlight its neural basis. The authors draw upon scientific literature and their own studies to illustrate how contemporary neuropsychiatry has delineated the functional connectivity between brain regions that support reasoning and those that support human affectivity. The implications of human reason and emotion interaction and its neurobiological roots are here discussed to understand violent behavior and conflict resolution problems. The disruption of the cross talk between emotion and reason (with respect to violence) and the failure to recognize their relationship (with respect to conflict resolution) have strong consequences that go beyond the individual, the small community, and often become global problems. We hope that the knowledge gained and that development in the years to come in the field of neurosciences will be incorporated in to social and political thinking and interventions.

"The truth of a thing is the feel of it, not the think of it." Stanley Kubrick.

The question as to the primacy of reason or emotion for human thought and action has both epistemic and ethical connotations. However, in the western philosophical tradition, with its strong commitment to rationality, the role of affect in human morality and decision-making has largely been neglected. Few philosophers have felt it necessary or worthwhile to determine the nature of emotion. They would instead take one of two sides in a debate centered on whether or not emotions are an obstacle to moral conduct. Aristotle (384-322 B.C.) viewed affect as similar to belief. To him emotions are not harmful per se, and may be consciously controlled and regulated. The Stoics (322 B.C.- 429 A.D.) on the other hand, believed that emotions happen *to us* and are not controllable. Thus, the only way to be moral is to refrain from acting under their influence. Such radical views continued to be espoused well into the 17th century, culminating with René Descartes (1596-1650), who understood rational thought as the essence of what it means to be human. *Cogito, ergo sum.* I think, therefore I am. It was not until the late 17th century that alternatives to such radical positions on the subject arose. Baruch Spinoza (1632-1677) was strongly influenced by the Stoics' view of affect, but he also argued that we should not reject our emotions but instead should use our reason to correct them. David Hume (1711-1776) expanded upon this, maintaining that morality is based on feelings and can never be based on reason alone. More recently, moral psychologists have argued that affect contributes to morality. In fact, brain imaging studies are now being used to investigate the matter, using the rigorous methods of experimental science. Two functional MRI studies have shown emotion-related brain circuitry to be involved in moral judgment.[1-2]

At the turn of the 20th century Freud demonstrated in his writings an appreciation for the biological basis of affect. Freud considered affects to be manifestations of drives. He saw them as strong and potentially dangerous forces because they are not subject to our conscious control. We may discern in his thinking the Stoic prevailing over the Aristotelian orientation. Charles Darwin understood that human expression of emotion evolved from previous stages of evolution.[3] The neglect of emotions, however, continued for a large part of the past century.

A similar debate to the ethical/philosophical one described above has taken place in the field of psychology. The topic of contention in this case was the origin and nature of emotion. William James postulated that emotions are cognitive perceptions of physiological reactions to the outside world. In 1929, Walter Cannon refuted James' theory and advanced another theory, which was soon modified by Phillip Bard. The Cannon-Bard theory states that, when a person faces an event, a nervous impulse travels to the thalamus, which then acts as a sensory relay station. The thalamus relays one part of this message to the cortex to create a subjective emotional experience, whereas another part is relayed to the hypothalamus, causing peripheral vegetative changes. Thus, independent but simultaneous processes were postulated to explain human emotion.

During the 20th century, largely influenced by the behaviorist paradigm, Silvan Tomkins was isolated in his interest in emotion. He supported the view that emotions are primary biological motivating mechanisms and have a role in human agency.[4] Tomkins argued that there are several basic emotions universal to all human beings. For example, happiness, sadness, anger, fear, and disgust are emotions commonly agreed to be recognized and experienced by all human beings. Tomkins' position is similar to that of the Stoics, in that affect happens *to us*, but they also value human affect as a valuable evolutionary feature contributing to survival. In the early 1980s the debate continued with a dialogue between Lazarus[5] and Zajonch[6] about the importance of cognition in human emotion. Zajonch maintained that it is possible to have affects without any accompanying cognition.

The value of the neuroscientific approach to the study of emotion lies in its ability to further elucidate the relative value of reason (i.e., conscious thought) and body (i.e., visceral autonomic phenomena) in matters of emotion. Neuroanatomy and neurobiology offer a basis for integration. The neuroanatomy underlying emotion processing can help explain why we perceive emotions as happening *to us,* as the Stoics believed. A neural level analysis shows that most of the process of emotion production occurs without the participation of brain structures believed necessary for conscious awareness. For example, in the case of the emotion of fear, the amygdala receives sensory inputs from the sensory cortices via the thalamus before they reach the associative cortex. It is only at the level of the association cortex that we become aware of feeling fear. This explains why it is possible to react to danger even before knowing it exists. Conscious feelings are generated only when the signal reaches the prefrontal regions of the brain. We then find out after a delay (and sometimes not at all) about emotional states that our nervous system has generated. Thus, we are under the impression that emotions happen to us, since the visceral components of emotional states are already in place by the time that we are aware of them. Involvement of the prefrontal cortex not only determines the conscious feelings of an emotion but it also refines our ability to respond to environmental stimuli by integrating a cognitive component into our selection of an appropriate response.

"Nature appears to have built the apparatus of rationality not just on top of the apparatus for biological regulation but also from and with it."[7] Rationality is shaped and modulated by body signals. Studies of brain injured patients have shown that impairment in the mechanisms of emotion impinges on their capacity to reason. As we will see more in detail later, a neuroscientific approach reframes the ethical-philosophical dilemma concerning the "goodness or badness of emotion." From both a psychological and evolutionary viewpoint, emotions are neither good nor bad. Emotion evolved from homeostatic mechanisms meant to increase our chances for survival. In Damasio's view, emotions are intimately associated with rationality itself and form the basis of what we refer to as the self.[8]

In the remainder of this paper we will apply the neuro-affective approach to global issues such as violence and terrorism, the consequences of trauma and political oppression, and conflict negotiations. We posit that a reformulation of our thinking concerning these phenomena will benefit from the novel contributions of affective brain science. Specifically, we will examine the neural circuitry related to aggression and violence, the brain changes associated with trauma in children, and how the neuroscientific approach, which highlights the importance of both reason and emotion, can help us to understand conflict negotiations.

Affective science is the interdisciplinary field of science that deals with the description and understanding of phenomena related to emotion and feeling (and by extension their interaction with cognition). Affective neuroscience deals specifically with the brain circuitry and neurobiological systems underlying emotion. Integrated models combining the contributions of the social, political, and neural sciences may foster more targeted solutions to complex global issues such as terrorism and conflict resolution. An analogy to this integrated approach comes from current thinking about psychiatric disorders. Psychiatrists have learned to appreciate the complexity of the causes of psychiatric illness and their effects using integrated models, and often observe that interventions at the microscopic level (biological and molecular) have an effect on the macroscopic (personal or social environment) level. Furthermore, research in areas such as the neurobiology of child abuse has shown that the macroscopic impacts upon the microscopic.[9]

VIOLENCE AND TERRORISM

"The answer (to terrorism) may depend upon the strength of our resolve to understand the mind – and ultimately the brain – of the suicidal terrorists." (R. Restak).[10]

Most brain research on violence comes from animal studies or studies of victims of brain injury. These models have allowed us to study the neural underpinnings of impulsive aggression. Research on the relation between impulsive and premeditated aggression is in it infancy. To study premeditated aggression researchers have employed the antisocial personality disorder or the criminal model. However, data on this population is difficult to interpret since subjects with impulsive and premeditated aggression have often been studied as part of the same group. Another important area of study that can contribute to our understanding of violent behavior involves the growing body of data on abused children. This topic will be addressed separately below.

Affective neuroscience offers the possibility to integrate the phylogenetic and neurodevelopmental point of view in order to study violence, even those actions that seem so atrocious as to be inexplicable. For affective neuroscience aggression is the precursor to violence. Aggression is an ubiquitous phenomenon in the animal kingdom that stems from a basic will to survive. Stimuli that may give rise to a potential aggressive response are directed to the brain system that oversees and regulates emotional behavior, which includes the brain circuitry that provides an evaluation and an answer to threats. The choice of fleeing or fighting in the face of danger is the result of an affective appraisal of the situation. Violence occurs when an aggressive response is out of proportion to the threat encountered.[a] Before performing an aggressive action, the danger evaluation system examines the environmental stimuli and sends information to systems apt to select a possible response. The neural system that allows animals to respond to threat has been broadly identified as the limbic system.

The limbic system has been defined as "an interrelated group of . . . structures that are involved in the regulation of the emotional state, with the accompanying behavioral, physiologic, and psychologic responses."[11] Originally described by Papez,[12] the limbic system has since broadened its boundaries based on results from anatomical and functional studies. Currently structures in the midbrain, temporal and frontal lobes, and basal ganglia have been linked to "limbic functions" (Fig. 1).

---

[a] In animals, aggression may be also a form of exploratory behavior. Young chimpanzees in the Arnhem Zoo chimpanzee colony are frequently observed throwing sticks and stones at adult group members, slapping or punching them. This behaviour becomes noticeable at the age of two and continues until adolescence at about the age of nine. Even occasional punishment does not discourage the youngsters from persisting in this type of annoying behaviour, also referred to as teasing, pestering, harassment, provocative behaviour, etc. (taken from website of Arnhem Zoo).

Medial prefrontal cortex
Orbital frontal cortex
Cingulate gyrus
Insular cortex

Amygdala
Hippocampal formation

Nucleus accumbens
Ventral pallidum
Ventral striatum

Thalamus
Hypothalamus
Basal forebrain
Limbic midbrain
Limbic forebrain
Pituitary gland
Septal region

Olfactory system

Fig. 1. Limbic structures.

Two limbic structures are of particular relevance for our understanding of aggression: the amygdala and the frontal lobes. Several animal and human studies suggest that the amygdala has a specific role in the detection of aversive phenomena and in the attribution of an affective flavor to remembered material. The expression of anger in normal individuals activates the orbital frontal cortex, the right anterior cingulate and bilateral temporal lobes.[13] In a study we performed at the University of Iowa, 17 normal healthy subjects were asked to judge the affective value of pleasant or unpleasant pictures presented to them while the functioning of their brains was recorded using positron emission tomography. We found that subjects engaged the left amygdala when viewing and appreciating the unpleasant nature of aversive stimuli.[14] Studies of brain function in normal healthy subjects are supported by observations of subjects with brain damage to specific brain regions. For example, a woman who had lost the functioning of her left and right amygdala as a result of a chronic brain disease was unable to appreciate fear in the faces of individuals, whereas her ability to recognize all other emotions was unchanged.[15] This young woman was known for her pleasant attitude and her ability to easily make friends. She was not aggressive or violent. Animal studies confirm that lesions of the mesial temporal lobe including the amygdala reduce aggressiveness.

In stark contrast to lesions involving the amygdala and mesial temporal lobe, damage to the frontal cortex, particularly the medial and ventral sectors, may give raise to *de-novo* violent behavior. The most famous case is that of Phineas Gage, who survived a horrific accident in 1848 that destroyed a large part of his frontal lobe. Following the accident his personality was transformed despite having no impairment of motor and cognitive functioning. Prior to the accident Phineas had been polite, and was a model employee. After the accident, however, he turned into a violent and irresponsible man, unable to hold a job.

Another patient, J.S., was 56 year old man who sustained damage to the right orbital prefrontal cortex and left amygdala, after which he began having problems with unpredictable episodes of unpredictable impulsive aggression and violence. He exhibited a striking deficit in his ability to recognize danger signals and he could no longer infer the emotions of others in situations where a response involving anger, disgust and embarrassment would be expected.[16] There have been several such accounts in the literature describing drastic personality changes following damage to the ventral medial sectors of the frontal lobe (other refs Harlow, Benton see Decartes' Error). The case of J.S. is particularly revealing because he sustained a combined frontal/amygdala lesion. Not only was J.S. prone to violence, as persons who incur frontal lobe damage often are, but he also was unable to recognize social cues that would be apt to incite anger or aggressive behavior in normal individuals.

Large-scale studies have confirmed the role of the ventral medial prefrontal cortex in the regulation of aggressive behaviors. In a study of 279 Vietnam veterans who were victims of brain injury and 57 normal controls, using data from family observations and self-reports, frontal ventromedial lesions were consistently associated with aggressive behavior. Verbal confrontations were more frequent than physical assaults.[17] Aggression is also frequently observed in the acute period following stroke (about 5% of all cases). In study of 309 consecutive admissions to a stroke unit at the University of Iowa, we found that significantly more subjects with left frontal damage admitted to aggressive behavior than subjects with lesions in any other location.[18] A unique functional neuroimaging study of normal volunteers without a history of violent behavior, which used visual imagery as a means to assess the neural correlates of aggression, found reduced function in the ventral medial prefrontal cortex during imagined aggressive action against a violent offender.[19] This raises important questions about the etiology of aggression and its neural correlates, the role of cognition and conscious control in the modulation of emotion and behavior, and hints at the complexities involved in the study of emotion and motivated behavior.

Damage to the ventral medial prefrontal cortex during childhood may have more profound implications than simply reduced inhibition of aggressive behavior. The ventral medial prefrontal cortex has been found to have a role in the acquisition of social maturation and cognition. Lesions at a very young age have been observed to lead to an impairment in the development of moral judgment.[20]

Allan Shore,[21] in a review of the literature, concluded that adult patients with damage to the right frontal lobe (as opposed to the left) have deficient moral judgment and empathy. This is consistent with the role of right frontal lobe in the processing emotion (particularly negative emotion). The two subjects in the study of Anderson at al. (cited above) had lesions that disrupted large portions of the right prefrontal cortex. The inappropriate aggressive behavior of J.S., who presented with "acquired sociopathy" following damage to the right orbital frontal cortex and left amygdala, may now be understood to be related to his inability to generate a mental image of others' negative emotional reactions, a skill thought necessary for moral behavior and judgment.[16] The role of the right prefrontal cortex in affective moral judgment was again highlighted in a recent functional imaging study.[2]

STUDY OF CRIMINALS

The neural biology of murderers and subjects with antisocial personality disorder is fairly consistent with the lesion literature. Frontal lobe and limbic system abnormalities play a major role in the current thinking about the neuropathology of criminality.

Early studies using functional neuroimaging showed patients with a history of personal and property aggression to have decreased functionality (SPECT) of the prefrontal cortex, increased activity in the left basal ganglia and/or limbic system, and an increased frequently of left temporal lobe abnormalities as compared to non-aggressive psychiatric control subjects.[22]

Psychopaths have been shown to have abnormalities of emotion processing. They were found to need more blood flow in areas such as the medial frontal and associated sub-cortical regions (e.g., the thalamus) for emotional word processing compared with control subjects.[23] Antisocial males may also have reduced size frontal lobes. One study[24] found 11% less prefrontal gray matter in subjects with antisocial personality disorder compared with non-clinical control subjects, men with substance dependence, or male psychiatric control subjects. The frontal lobe size correlated with autonomic activity during a stressor.[24] Thus, subjects with antisocial personality disorder appear to have a poorly responsive autonomic nervous system, making them less able to appropriately adapt to their environment.

Murderers who have pleaded not guilty by reason of insanity were found to have reduced metabolism in the medial prefrontal cortex and hyperactivity in the left amygdala in while doing a continuous performance task.[25] A secondary analysis of these data showed that those individuals who had committed premeditated murder showed normal frontal lobe metabolism but abnormal subcortical limbic metabolism compared to those who had committed an impulsive murders.

In summary, decreased ability of the orbital frontal cortex to control a hyper-responsive limbic system may be at the neuroanatomical basis for impulsive aggression. Premeditated violence and criminal behavior may have as a neuroanatomical underpinning an increased reactivity of the subcortical limbic system. The data reviewed below will shed light on the pathway leading to abnormal limbic function in children exposed to trauma.

BIOLOGICAL CONSEQUENCES OF TRAUMA, POLITICAL OPPRESSION, AND WARFARE IN CHILDREN

The data showing brain changes associated with early traumatic experiences is very relevant to the topic of violence. The consequences of child abuse at the neurological level are varied. The behavioral consequences span from depression and anxiety or post-traumatic stress disorder to aggression impulsivity/hyperactivity and delinquency.

An environment promoting empathy and communication, a sense of right and wrong and of causality, and the ability to overcome stereotypes and frustration, usually fosters the development of appropriate critical and moral powers. Adolescents who have not benefited from such a nurturing environment are more vulnerable to the influence of ideologies, including ideologies of intolerance and hate. During adolescence connections are reinforced between the brain's cognitive and emotional systems, and a healthy replacement of family bonding with group identity occurs. The adolescent seeks new ideas, attempts to find his or her own values. The proper maturation of brain systems allows for a balanced integration of cognition and emotion.

A major achievement of brain science is the discovery that the negative consequences of a disruption in the above process through psychological or physical abuse can be found at the level of the nervous system. The resultant nervous system abnormalities begin to account for the behavioral changes that follow abuse and trauma. Physical and emotional exposure to trauma and a violent environment (warfare, famine or pestilence) can set off a ripple of neurobiological and emotional changes that permanently alter the mechanisms underlying the perception of threat and response to stress, wiring a child's brain to cope with a malevolent world.[26]

While the neurobiology of violence is complex, it appears that stress mechanisms play an important role. Animal studies suggest that maltreatment stress including maternal deprivation and peer rearing in early life alters norepinephrine, serotonin and dopamine neurotransmitter systems in ways that can persist into adulthood and influence aggressive behavior.[27-30] Alterations in norepinephrine and serotonin activity is linked to aggressive behavior in humans.[31] The mesial temporal lobe, with its many limbic structures (e.g. amygdala, hippocampus) is especially vulnerable to damage because it is a major brain target of stress and catabolic hormones.[32] Structured interviews measuring temporal lobe symptomatology and EEG recordings of electrical brain activity reveal an over-excitability of the limbic temporal regions in subjects exposed to early trauma. Additionally, young adults who were exposed to sexual abuse showed on average a 10% reduction in the size of the left amygdala, regardless of the severity of current symptoms. A possible mechanism has been posited to explain these findings, involving the molecular reorganization of GABA receptor protein subunit in the amygdala in response to early stress.[33] GABA is a neurotransmitter that inhibits neuronal activity. Reduction of the function of the GABA receptors at the level of the amygdala as a result of early stress may lead to an overreactivity in response to threat. There is also evidence that deficient MAOA activity, leading to increased levels of monoamines, predisposes one to a neurogical hyperactivity to threat.[34]

Another anatomical change that can result from early trauma is a reduction in the size of the corpus callosum.[35] The corpus is a collection of white matter tracks that allows the communication between left and right hemispheres. This structural observation is consistent with findings of decreased hemispheric functional integration in abused children during recall of early disturbing memories.[36]

Another structure found to be selectively damaged in victims of childhood trauma is the cerebellar vermis. This is the middle aspect of the cerebellum and has an even higher density of receptors for stress hormones than the hippocampus. It is thought to regulate the electrical activity in the limbic system. In individuals exposed to trauma, the amount of blood flow (and hence the activity) in the cerebellar vermis is decreased.[37] Thus, it has been postulated that the decreased function of the cerebellar vermis leads to dysregulation of the limbic system, which may explain the abnormal EEG findings in abused children.

We are learning with the help of neuroscience research that the poor cognitive affective balance observed in disturbed children may have its anatomic underpinnings in the alterations of neurodevelopment. These molecular and neurobiological mechanisms secondary to early trauma subsequently may cause left-right hemisphere (functional or anatomical) disconnection.[38] The result of a disrupted cross-talk between hemispheres is a disintegrated ability to reconcile emotional and cognitive material for effective decision making. Limbic dysfunction as a result of poor control by a dysfunctional cerebellar vermis, combined with decreased cross-hemispheres information exchange, may predispose these individuals to have an exaggerated and overactive fight or flight response. They are on heightened alert for danger and will be more likely to react aggressively to challenge without hesitation. A similar model (high limbic activity – poor regulatory functions) may help explain the episodes of impulsive aggression that are sometimes observed in patients with temporal lobe epilepsy. Patients who display such episodes have been found to have a highly significant reduction of left prefrontal gray matter as compared to patients with no history of aggression.[39]

Studies over the past two decades have shown that genes influence many traits associated with violent behavior, including impulsivity and an oppositional temperament. About 50% of the variation in aggressive violence can be attributed to genes. Maltreatment and poor parenting are other important factors.[40] Whatever malignant combination of events happen, it seems to have a lasting effect into the teenage years and perhaps into adulthood.[41] A trait seen across age groups that is thought to increase one's risk for psychopathy is hyporeactivity of the peripheral nervous system to stressful situations. This trait can be found as early as the age of three.[42]

More recently research suggests that an individual's genetic makeup may moderate the influence of a damaging environment. High levels of the neurotransmitter metabolizing enzyme monoamine oxidase A (MAOA) regulated by a functional polymorphism due to a specific genotype, make it less likely that a person will develop antisocial problems.[43] The MAOA gene is located on the X chromosome and encodes for enzymes that metabolize norepinephrine, serotonin and dopamine. This study supports what was known about the genetic deficiencies in MAOA activity and their relationship to violence in mice and humans.[44] A polymorphism in the gene that codes for tryptophan hydroxylase, a regulatory enzyme for serotonin synthesis, correlates with serotonergic function and aggressive behavior differences.[45] Various serotonin abnormalities have been found in several groups of individuals with affective disorders and other psychiatric pathologies and have been associated with impulsivity and violence (including to self).

Serotonin has been hypothesized to exert inhibitory control over impulsive aggression.[46] Subjects with aggressive impulsive personality disorder are unable to increase the glucose metabolism in the prefrontal cortex, a region with a high density of serotonin type II receptors, following a serotonergic challenge (normal subjects respond with increased metabolism in the prefrontal cortex and anterior cingulate regions).

SUMMARY ON MECHANISMS OF AGGRESSION

Although there are many mechanisms in which aggression becomes impulsive violence,[47] impulsive affective aggression is often the product of failure of emotion regulation. Normal humans are able to voluntarily regulate their negative affect and also profit from environmental cues that act as modulators of their affective response. Individuals predisposed to aggression and violence have an abnormality in the emotional brain circuitry responsible for an adaptive behavioral changes in response to threats and cannot make the appropriate use of affective environmental cues. The balance between threats and response is achieved through the interaction between prefrontal circuitry (mostly ventral medial – or orbital frontal cortex-highly innervated by serotonin), and amygdala. As we can observe, the neuroscientific approach allows an understanding of emotions that does not require casting judgment whether the emotions are bad or good. Affectivity is observed as a mechanism to protect the individual and ultimately the species. It is the lack of harmony between emotion and reason that can lead to prejudice and violence.

A summary of the findings from lesion method, studies of functional neuroimaging in normals and criminals, and accounts of brain abnormalities in children exposed to early trauma highlight the fronto-amygdalar disconnection for impulsive aggression. Whereas the data for premeditated aggression and violence is less clear, data suggest a disregulation sub-cortical limbic system with hyperactivity at the level of central structures generating inappropriate responses to perceived noxious stimuli and a hyporesponsivity of the limbic governed autonomic nervous system.

THE TERRORIST MIND – THE TERRORISTS BRAIN

"The commitment to terrorism is largely produced, intensified and sustained through learning."[48]

Although much needs to be known about the neurobiology of the mind/brain of the terrorists, these models of violence currently available are heuristic in nature. We are only at the beginning in our understanding of the differences of violent phenomena with features of premeditation and complete disregard for human life including the personal life of the perpetrators of such an event as the massacre of September 11th.

Insults of psychological or biological nature, as in the case of children exposed to trauma, act with a biological mechanism changing brain systems. These systems are then very resilient to *restitutio ad integrum* (Latin for return to normalcy). We may posit that the behavior of the terrorists is a result of brain changes occurring throughout childhood and adolescence. In addition to changes secondary to trauma, changes may be obtained as a result of strong and sustained affective indoctrination that laid out bad associations and memories in a system formed by amygdala, hippocampus, entorhinal cortex and the frontal cortex. Indoctrination may or may not start from childhood. Charismatic leaders who set out to do evil have certain ways of inducing a suspension of reason through brainwashing and instigation to the ultimate violence. How this may be obtained is suggested by the work of the Russian physiologist Ivan Pavlov. In his work with dogs Pavlov found by accident that dogs subjected to extremely stressful situations lost all conditioning behavior that they had acquired (by extrapolation all habits and beliefs of humans). They appeared to undergo permanent changes in temperament and emotion sensitivity. Later Pavlov was able to re-condition these dogs with entirely new behavior opposite to that they had lost. The work of Josef LeDoux [49] has demonstrated that the basis for affective conditioning can be studied in the animal model. There is a suggestive overlap between the structure LeDoux recognized as the structures for necessary conditioning (e.g. fear conditioning–the amygdala) and the neurobiology of aggressive and violent behavior.

Data on children exposed to early trauma suggest that the world views in the mind of a terrorist become hard-wired. We may not expect to recondition suicide bombers especially when they inducted and trained when very young.

CONFLICT NEGOTIATIONS

A fundamental contribution that affective neuroscience can give to conflict negotiations is connected with its ability to conceptually integrate reason and emotion.[8] A neural level analysis shows that most of the process of emotion production occurs without the participation of the conscious, since the amygdala receives sensory inputs from the sensory cortices via the thalamus before these reach the associative cortex. This explains why it is possible to react to danger even before knowing exactly what is going on. Conscious feelings are generated when the signal reaches the prefrontal regions of the brain. The capacity of the frontal cortex brain to pay attention to the stimuli in the environment including the changes occurring in brain regions (such as the subcortical limbic system) engaged in emotion is (fortunately) limited. This means that only a discrete number of images are formed in the prefrontal cortex and determine the conscious feelings of an emotion. Often emotions have behavioral consequences without subjective awareness. There is neurological and neuropsychological evidence for this phenomenon but examples drawn from political science are strikingly consistent.

It would be foolish to attempt to bring "two nations in conflict" to reason and hence to peace without understanding how affectivity and reason are integrated in human decision making. Multiple lines of research have confirmed the not only emotions are integral part of human decision making. Most importantly emotions participate in human decision-making without the awareness of the individual.[8] To the untrained eye political negotiations are pure cognitive processes of reason. The negotiator who is in the position to regulate and understand his own and the emotions of his counterpart will play an effective role in the process.

Further insight into the role of affect in conflict negotiations can be gained from observational studies of primate aggression and reconciliatory behavior in conditions resembling their natural habitat (http://chimpansee.homestead.com/arnhemzoo.html). Prior to the 1970s, the study of aggression was approached as a phenomenon that occurred at the level of the individual. The focus was on the influences, both internal and external, that determine an individual's propensity to become aggressive. The individual model did not conceptualize aggressive behavior as a social phenomenon. It failed to address the societal context of aggression. Because this model did not look at how families or societies dealt with the disruptive consequences of aggression, it made no contribution to our understanding of conflict resolution.

Primatologists were the first to move toward a more integrated paradigm, in which aggression was understood as a socially embedded behavior involving familiar individuals the vast majority of the time. This implied that, for the integrity of social groups to be maintained, primates, let alone humans, must have devised mechanisms to resolve conflict.

Surprisingly, it was a simple observation in the 1970s of an incident in the world's largest chimpanzee colony at the Arnhem Zoo in the Netherlands that made it clear that a new paradigm for the understanding of aggression was necessary. The fortuitous observation of this single incident then spurred the study of aggression forward to a societal paradigm that examined not only how aggression starts, but, as in the real world, how it ends or is kept under control in the context of social groups. The observation at the Arnham Zoo was as follows: an alpha male fiercely attacked a female, causing other apes to come to her defense, at which time a scene of prolonged screaming and vicious chasing in the group ensued. After a while, when the chimpanzees had calmed down, a tense silence overcame the group. Then suddenly, the silence was broken and the chimps burst out in a wild uproar of hooting. In the center of this pandemonium, it turned out, was the male and female chimpanzee who had been involved in the previous fight, and they were kissing with their arms wrapped around each other. From this observation the phenomenon of primate reconciliation came to be defined as a friendly reunion between former opponents not long after an aggressive confrontation. Since that time, data on hundreds of instances have shown this pattern of reconciliatory behavior to be a regular, conspicuous part of social life in the Arnhem chimpanzee colony.

Aggression was thereafter conceptualized as a societal issue, a natural phenomenon integral to social behavior, but at the same time it was understood to pose an everpresent threat to the very structure of the society from which it arose. A solid framework for the study of conflict resolutions had thus been laid.

Although this model is not directly applicable to conflict resolution in societies where the individuals do not have strong ties with each other, results of subsequent studies, which have shown that reconciliatory behavior among primates can be positively modified, are encouraging. For instance, in an experiment involving macaques investigated whether tying a food reward to reconciliatory behavior would increase the frequency of reconciliation following conflict, it was found that increasing the value of the macaques' relationships through this conditioning significantly increased their tendency to reconcile following conflict. In this experiment, pairs of macaques were trained to obtain rewards by acting in a coordinated fashion: The only way to obtain a food reward would be for two monkeys to sit side-by-side at a dispenser, a procedure that attached significant benefits to their relationship. After this training, the paired monkeys showed a three times greater tendency to reconcile after an induced fight than monkeys that had not been trained to cooperate.

The results of this and other studies have buttressed the *valuable relationship model* of aggressive and reconciliatory behavior among primates, according to which reconciliation is most likely to occur after conflict between parties that represent a high social or reproductive value to each other. Instead of treating aggression as an instinct or an automatic response triggered by frustration, this model sees it as one of several options for the resolution of conflicts of interest.

Further studies have also demonstrated that the reconciliatory behavior of monkeys can be modified by social experience. The learned nature of peace-making behavior is highlighted by studies of experimental cohabitation of different primate species with large differences in their tendency for reconciliatory behavior. In these studies the specie less inclined to reconciliation learns through modeling of the more peaceable specie of monkey to increase its tendency to reconcile following conflict.

There is always concern when data from non-human primates are extrapolated for the purpose of understanding human behavior. In this case, however, observations of children in unstructured environments (e.g., the school yard) have shown similar patterns of aggressive and reconciliatory behavior as that seen in primates. In accordance with the *valuable relationship model* of aggression, positive contact between children before the eruption of conflict has been found to be one of the best predictors of peacemaking. Research has demonstrated that these peacemaking skills are acquired through interactions with peers and siblings. An impoverished social environment, such as that seen in conditions of war, deprives children of this essential aspect of socialization, causing deficits in conflict management and moral development.

Similar themes can be seen in the history of human societies, where many political interactions appear to recognize the tenets of the *valuable relationship model* of aggression and conflict management. We can see this in the reconstruction of Europe following World War II, wherein the European community was founded with the premise that the best way to bring all parties together was to ensure a peaceful future through economic ties. Thus, like the macaque pairs trained to cooperate for a food reward, the cost of damage to the relationship between nations was raised.

This model cannot explain certain forms of aggression, such as random shootings, suicide bombings, or warfare, but it does set up a framework for possible means of prevention through conflict resolution, by increasing ties among the individual members of communities in conflict. Further basic research is needed to increase our understanding of the integral role that affect plays in both the creation and resolution of individual and group conflict. New insights will open possibilities for the development of new models of understanding that might promote reconciliation in the complex arena of human political conflict.[50]

As research in the affective neurosciences is making it clear that the perception of threat by an individual can be distorted (possibly even permanently) by exposure to a stressful environment, both past and present, it behooves us to consider the implications of this knowledge as we examine the relationship between perceived threat and decision-making. In a study exploring the relationship between feelings of threat in the context of a political conflict and policy choices of the public regarding the conflict, Gordon and Arian [51] found there to be a strong correlation between the level of perceived threat and public policy choice.

Using public opinion survey data from Israel and the Palestinian Authority, Gordon and Arian sought specifically to determine the relationship between perceived threat and policy choice for Israelis and Palestinians with regard to the Arab/Israeli conflict. According to their survey data, in 1986 more than 70% of Israeli Jews felt very threatened by the Arabs. It is not surprising, therefore, that when asked if they support the creation of a Palestinian state, 80% of Israeli Jews were opposed. Over the following years, both feelings of threat and support for a Palestinian state changed within the Israeli public in almost a mirror-image pattern. As Israelis felt less threatened, their support for a Palestinian state grew.

The results of surveys among Palestinians in the West Bank and Gaza collected between 1994 and 1999 suggest a similar pattern. No direct question was asked about threat, but a clear pattern was observed using the fluctuations in the responses of Palestinian public regarding armed attacks and the peace process against a timeline of actual events perceived as threatening or reassuring to Palestinians. For example, before 49 Palestinians were massacred in February 1994 in a Hebron mosque by a Jewish Israeli, 51% of Palestinians supported the peace process; whereas after the massacre, only 17% did so.

The results from this study suggest that the more threatened people feel, the more their policy choice tends to maintain or intensify the conflict—that is, the more incendiary the policy choice is, and vice versa—the lower the threat the more conciliatory the policy choice is. These findings may seem so obvious as to be trivial, however, public policy decision-makers often act as if they believe the opposite were true.

In conflicts at a national level, in the final analysis it is individuals who make the final decisions and individuals come to the process with a complex history of personal and national attitudes and beliefs and they also come with affects, feelings and emotions. In prolonged social conflicts where the parties always feel threatened the new data are rarely interpreted at face value. Perceptions are based on stereotypes of the parties to the conflict. Who is the victim, who is the oppressor, who is truthful and who lies, who is morally justified and who is evil. In many theories that attempt to explain the process of information processing and decision-making, emotion is not part of the calculation and does not enter the equation.

In summary, what can affective neuroscience offer to the understanding of violence? Can it offer a way to combat violence and terrorism? And, further, can neuroscientific views help to devise more effective conflict resolution strategies? Whereas in the present paper we have underlined what has been accomplished in the area of impulsive aggression, the field is in its infancy with regard to understanding the neurobiology of premeditated violence and terrorism. It should be noted, however, that a method has been laid out for future work. The common thread between various forms of violent behavior is the emotional and limbic bases of these phenomena. Emotions influence reason and therefore behavior. The disruption of the cross talk between emotion and reason (with respect to violence) and the failure to recognize their relationship (with respect to conflict resolution) have strong consequences that go beyond the individual, the small community and often become global problems. We hope that the knowledge gained and that developing in the years to come will be incorporated in to social and political thinking and interventions.

REFERENCES

1. Green, J.D., Nystrom, L.E., Darley, J.M., Cohen, J.D. (2001) "An fMRI investigation of emotional engagement in moral judgment." *Science*, volume 293.
2. Moll, J., de Oliveira-Souza, R., Eslinger, P.J., Bramati, I.E., Mourao-Miranda, J., Andreiuolo, P.A., Pessoa, L. (2002) "The neural correlates of moral sensitivity: a functional magnetic resonance imaging investigation of basic and moral emotions." *Journal of Neuroscience. 22(7):2730-6.*
3. Darwin, C. (1872) *The Expression of Emotion in Man and Animals*, New York Philosophical Library.
4. Tomkins, S. (1995) *Exploring Affect: The Selective Writings of Silvan Tomkins*, Cambridge UK, Cambridge University Press.
5. Lazarus. (1984) "On the Primacy of Cognition," in *American Psychologist* 39:124-129.
6. Zajonch, R.B. (1984) "On the Primacy of Affect," *American Psychologist*, 39:117-123.
7. Damasio, A. (1994) *Descartes' Error: Emotional Reason and the Human Brain*, page 128: London, McMillian.
8. Damasio, A, (1999) *The Feeling of What Happens: Body and Emotion in the Making of Consciousness*, New York, Harcort Brace.
9. Andreasen, N.C., Black, D.W.: (2001) *Introductory textbook of psychiatry*, 3rd Edition- Washington, DC: American Psychiatric Pub.
10. Restak, R. (2002) "Cerebrum." *The Dana forum on Brain Science*, p.37.
11. Hendelman, Walter J. (1994) *Student's Atlas of Neuroanatomy*. Philadelphia: W.B. Saunders Company: A Division of Harcourt Brace and Company.
12. Papez, J.W. (1937) "A proposed mechanism of emotion," *Arch Neurol Psychiatr* 79:217-224.
13. Dougherty, D.D., Shin, L.M., Alpert, N.M., Pitman, R.K., Scott, P., Orr, M., Lasko, M.L., Macklin, A., Fischman, J., and Rauch, S.L. (1999) "Anger in

healthy men: a PET study using script-driven imagery." *Biological Psychiatry,* 46: 466-472.

14. Paradiso, S., Johnson, D.L., Andreasen, N.C., O'Leary, D.J., Watkins, G.L., Boles, Ponto, L.L., Hichwa, R.D. (1999) "Cerebral blood flow changes associated with attribution of emotional valence to pleasant, unpleasant and neutral visual stimuli in a PET Study of normal individuals," *American Journal of Psychiatry* 156:1618-29.

15. Adolphs, R., Tranel, D., Damasio, H., Damasio, (1995) "A. Fear and the human amigdala." *J Neurosci* 15 5879-91.

16. Blair, R.J., Cipolotti, L. (2000) "Impaired social response reversal. A case of 'acquired sociopathy'." *Brain.* 123 :1122-41.

17. Grafman, J., Schwab, K.. Warden, D., Pridgen, A., Brown, H.R,. Salazar. A,M. (1996) "Frontal lobe injuries, violence, and aggression: a report of the Vietnam Head Injury Study." *Neurology.* 46:1231-8.

18. Paradiso, S., Robinson, R.G., Arndt, S. (1996) "Self-reported aggressive behavior in patients with stroke." *Journal of Nervous & Mental Disease. 184(12):746-53.*

19. Pietrini, P., Guazzelli, M., Basso, G., Jaffe, K., Grafman, J. (2000) "Neural correlates of imaginal aggressive behavior assessed by positron emission tomography in healthy subjects." *American Journal of Psychiatry.* 157:1772-81.

20. Anderson, S.W., Bechara, A., Damasio, H., Tranel, D., Damasio, A.R. (1999) "Impairment of social and moral behavior related to early damage in human prefrontal cortex." *Nature Neuroscience. 2(11):1032-7.*

21. Shore, A. (1994) *Affect regulation in the origin of the self.* Erlbaum Associates Publisher, Hillsdale New Jersey and Hove UK.

22. Amen, D.J., Stubblefield, M., Carmichael, B., Thisted, R. (1996) "Brain SPECT findings and aggressiveness," *Ann Clinical Psychiatry*, 8:129-137.

23. Intrator, J., Hare, R., Stritzke, P., Brichtswein, K., Dorfman, D., Harpur, T., Bernstein, D., Handelsman, L., Schaefer, C., Keilp, J., Rosen, J., Machac, J.(1997) "A brain imaging (single photon emission computerized tomography) study of semantic and affective processing in psychopaths." *Biological Psychiatry.* 42:96-103.

24. Raine, A., Lencz, T., Bihrle, S., LaCasse, L., Colletti, P. (2000) "Reduced prefrontal gray matter volume and reduced autonomic activity in antisocial personality disorder." *Archives of General Psychiatry* 57(2):119-27.

25. Raine, A., Buchsbaum, M., LaCasse, L. (1997) "Brain abnormalities in murderers indicated by positron emission tomography." *Biological Psychiatry* 42:495-508.

26. Meaney, M.J. (1996) *Dev Neurosci* 18:49; Kreamer G.W. Ann NY *Acad Sci* 794:125 1996.

27. Bremner, J.D. and Vermetten, E. (2001) *Developmental psychopathology*, 13473.

28. Francis, D.D. and Meany, M.J. (1999) in Current Opinion in *Neurobiology*, 9128.

29. A.J. Bennett et al., (2002) *Molecular psychiatry*, 7188; G.W. Kraemer (1989) in *Neuropsychopharmacology* 2175.

3 0.   S.J. Swomi in the Handbook of Developmental Psychopathology, A.J. Summeroff, M. Lewis and S. Miller (eds.), Plenum New York, in press

31.   M.E. Berman, R.J. Kavoussi, N.E.F. Coccaro, in Handbook of Antisocial Behavior, D.M. Stauff, M. Breiling, and J.D. Mazur (eds.), Wiley, New York 1997.

32.   Neihoff, D.L., (1999) *The Biology of Violence: How Understanding the Brain Behavior and Environment can Break the Vicious Cycle of Aggression.* New York, Free Press.

33.   Caldji, C., Francis, D., Sharma, S., Plotsky, P.M., Meaney, M.J. (2000) "The effects of early rearing environment on the development of GABA and central benzodiazepine receptor levels and novelty-induced fearfulness in the rat." *Neuropsychopharmacology.* 22(3):219-29.

34.   V. Morell (1993) *Science*, 260, 1722.

35.   De Bellis, M.D, Keshavan, M.S., Clark, D.B., Casey, B.J.N., Frustaci, K., Ryan, N.D. (1999) "Developemental traumatology part II: Brain Development," *Biol Psychiatry* 45:1271-84.

3 6.   Schiffer, F., Teicher, M.H., Papanicolaou, A.C. (1995) "Evoked potential evidence for right brain activity during the recall of traumatic memories." *Journal of Neuropsychiatry & Clinical Neurosciences.* 7:169-75.

37.   Anderson, C.M., Teicher, M.H., Polcari, A., Renshaw, P.F. (2002) "Abnormal T2 relaxation time in the cerebellar vermis of adults sexually abused in childhood: potential role of the vermis in stress-enhanced risk for drug abuse." *Psychoneuroendocrinology.* 27(1-2):231-44.

38.   M.H. Teicher. (2002) "Scars that won't heal: The neurobiology of child abuse." *Scientific American* pp. 69-75, March 2002

39.   F.G. Borman et al. (2000) *Journal of Neurology, Neurosurgery, and Psychiatry*, 36 81-62.

40.   Widem, C.S. (1997) *Handbook of Antisocial Behavior*, D.M. Stauff, M. Breiling, J.D. Mazur (eds.), Wiley, New York.

41.   Raine, A., Reynolds, C., Venables, P.H., Mednick, S.A., Farrington, D.P., (1998) "Fearlessness, stimulation-seeking, and large body size at age 3 years as early predispositions to childhood aggression at age 11 years." *Archives of General Psychiatry.* 55(8):745-51.

42.   Raine, A., Venables, P.H., Mednick, S.A. (1997) "Low resting heart rate at age 3 years predisposes to aggression at age 11 years: evidence from the Mauritius Child Health Project." *Journal of the American Academy of Child & Adolescent Psychiatry.* 36(10):1457-64.

43.   Caspi, A., McClay, J., Moffitt, T.E., Mill, J., Martin, J., Craig, I.W., Taylor, A., Poulton, R. (2002) "Role of Genotype in the Cycle of Violence in Maltreated Children." *Science* 297 851-54.

44.   Rowe, D.C. (2001) *Biology and Crime*. Roxbury Publishers, Los Angeles.

630

45. Manuck, S.B., Flory, J.D., Ferrell, R.E., Dent, V.M., Mann, J.J., Muldoon, M.T. (1999) "Aggression and anger-related traits associated with a polymorphysm of the tryptophan hydroxylase gene." *Biol Psychiatry* 45- 603.
46. Volavka, J., (1999) *Journal of Clinical Psychiatry* 60 (suppl 1243).
47. Davidson, R.J., Putnam, K.M., Larson, C.L. (2000) *Science*, 289, 591-4.
48. Bernard, B., Asper, (1988) "On learning terrorism," *Terrorism* 11(1):13-27.
49. LeDoux, J. (1994) "Emotion, memory and the brain." *Scientific American*, June 50-57.
50. de Waal, F.B.M. (2000) "Primates - A natural heritage of conflict resolution." *Science* 289 586-590.
51. Gordonm C., Asherm A. (2001) "Threat and Decision Making." *Journal of Conflict Resolution*, 45:196-215.

THE GENETICS OF ALZHEIMER DISEASE

MARGARET A. PERICAK-VANCE, PH.D.
James B. Duke Professor of Medicine, Director, Center for Human Genetics,
Duke University Medical Center, Durham, NC, USA

Alzheimer disease (AD) is the leading cause of dementia in the elderly. There are over 4 million affected individuals in the U.S., a number projected to quadruple over the next 50 years as the population ages.[1] Numbers in other developed countries parallel that of the U.S. In Italy, for example, over 90,000 new cases of AD are recognized each year. AD has a complex etiology with strong genetic and environmental determinants. Pathologically AD is characterized by neurofibrillary tangles found in the neurons of the cerebral cortex and hippocampus and the deposition of amyloid within senile plaques and cerebral blood vessels.[2] Clinically AD is slowly progressive, resulting in memory loss and alterations of higher intellectual function and cognitive abilities.[3]

Although AD was first described in 1907[4] definitive clues to its etiology have emerged only recently. Evidence that AD has a genetic component has come from several sources. First, large families were discovered with multiple affected individuals in several generations. Families with small aggregates of affecteds were also reported. Second, twin studies found greater concordance of affection status in monozygotic than in dizygotic twins. Third, siblings of affected individuals have a higher recurrence risk then siblings of unaffected individuals.[5]

Using the powerful tools of genetic analysis, four AD genes have been identified to date. Three of these (the amyloid precursor protein [APP],[6] and the presenilin 1 and 2 [PS1 and PS2] genes[7-9] were identified using standard positional cloning methods facilitated by simple autosomal dominant inheritance in early-onset AD families. While these three genes account for the majority of early-onset familial AD and their identification represents a tremendous accomplishment, collectively they only account for less than 2% of all cases of AD.

The genetic architecture underlying the far more common late-onset type of AD[10] is much more complex. Comparison of the recurrence rates in the siblings of AD patients to the general population prevalence (λs)[11-13] for AD give surprisingly constant results across studies[5,14,15] with a range of 4 to 5. Power studies[12,16] show that the genes responsible for λs as low as 1.5 can be detected with sample sizes of affected sib pairs equivalent to what we have assembled.

In 1991, we[17] reported evidence for linkage of late-onset AD to chromosome 19q13. Apolipoprotein E (APOE), with three functional alleles (-2, -3, -4),[18,19] also maps to this region. The confluence of biology[20,21] and genetic mapping facilitated our identification of the association between the APOE-4 allele in both familial late-onset and sporadic AD patients[19,22]. Subsequent analyses[23] showed that the APOE-4 allele acts in a dose-dependent manner to increase risk and decrease age of onset in both late-onset familial and sporadic and early-onset sporadic AD.[23-26] The APOE-2 allele affords protection against late-onset AD[27] (see Fig. 1).[28,29] APOE represents the fourth confirmed genetic factor for AD and is the single most significant genetic risk factor thus far identified. Figure 2 shows the confirmed genes identified for AD.

Figure 1. Affect of APOE-4 on Alzheimer Disease

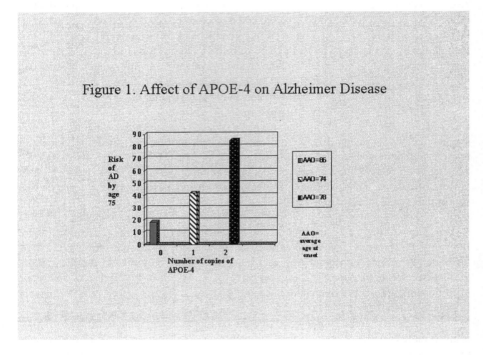

Fig. 1. Affect of APOE-4 on Alzheimer Disease.

Several lines of evidence indicate that APOE does not account for all of the genetic variation seen in AD. While the heritability of AD has been estimated at about 80%[30], more than one-third of AD cases do not have a single APOE-4 allele. The APOE-4 associated risk of AD appears to differ among ethnic groups, suggesting ethnicity may influence genetic risk of AD.[29,31,32] In addition we have estimated the λs for the APOE locus[33] to be approximately 2. Since the overall λs is estimated to be between 4 and 5, APOE is likely to account for at most 50% of the total genetic effect in AD.

Efforts to identify these additional AD loci have taken two forms: whole-genome scans for linkage in multiplex families followed by association studies on locational candidate genes, and association tests of functional candidate genes. The association studies in both approaches have been done in case-control and/or (more recently) family based association samples.[34]

Figure 2. Confirmed Genes in AD

GENES IN AD
1995-PRESENT

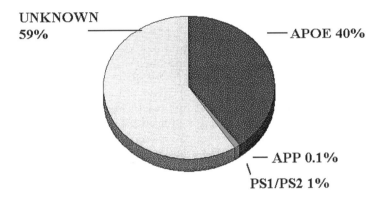

Fig. 2. Confirmed Genes in AD.

Lod score analysis is the most powerful method of linkage analysis if the genetic model for a disease is known, but this approach can suffer significantly if the model is unknown. For a complex disease such as AD, where multiple genes of moderate effect may be acting independently or together, accurate model specification is impossible. While lod score methods may be robust to errors underlying assumptions in specific instances, this is not generally the case. Model-free methods are an attractive alternative. As our interest in mapping complex diseases has increased, non-parametric methods of linkage analysis have been developed and extended, including multipoint sib pair analysis using the likelihood approach (MLS),[11-13] now available in several different computer programs. In addition, methods that incorporate data on other affected relative pairs (ARP), including the nonparametric linkage (NPL) method implemented in the GENEHUNTER package[35] and extended by Kong and Cox,[36,37] are now commonly used.

The association approach ultimately is more powerful than the linkage approach, as it directly examines the effect of a candidate locus, not just a diffused effect spread across a large genomic region.[38] The power and success of association tests depend on the availability of numerous polymorphic markers in any candidate gene. Evaluation of candidate genes in association studies holds great potential with development of single nucleotide polymorphisms (SNPs). SNPs occur approximately one every 1000 base pairs and have a low mutation rate, which may confer advantages in association studies. Over 4.2 million SNPs have been identified by the Human Genome Project.[39]

Numerous investigators have taken the approach of focusing on candidate genes selected because of their known biological functions. These case-control association studies of candidate genes have been far less successful. Sample size and methodological issues likely play a major role in generating the inconsistent results and underscore the need for well-designed association studies of AD candidate genes. These association studies of candidate genes have also been less successful because our knowledge of gene function is still very limited.

Many genes have been reported as being associated with late-onset AD. At best, the evidence for any of these loci is mixed, and some associations have never been replicated. These functional candidate genes include α_1-antichymotrypsin (AACT),[40] low-density lipoprotein-like receptor (LRP)[41], presenilin-1 (PS1),[42] ubiquitin,[43] the HLA complex,[44-45] butyrylcholinesterase K variant (BCHE-K),[46] non-amyloid component of plaques/α-synuclein (NACP/α-synuclein)[47], and mitochondrial mutations.[48] Successful examination of these and other candidate genes requires sufficiently large samples to detect modest genetic effects and appropriately matched cases and controls to avoid spurious associations due to biased sampling. Over 40 genes have been reported as being associated with late-onset AD. At best, the evidence for any of these loci is mixed, with the majority of studies refuting any association. Some associations have never been replicated.

Other researchers have taken the alternative approach to candidate gene analysis and have performed genomic screens to identify regions of linkage interest before choosing candidates. Two recent genome scans have implicated several chromosomes (1, 4, 6, 9, 10, 12, 19, and 20) as potential locations of additional AD loci.[49-50] The chromosome 12 linkage[50] has since been supported by results from an independent sample[51,52]. Candidate genes on chromosome 12 have been examined, but none have yet been confirmed (e.g. LRP1,[41,53] A2M,[54] the transcriptional factor lLBP-1.[55-58] Additional effort has been focused on chromosome 12 in an attempt to better define the chromosome 12 candidate gene region. New markers were genotyped across the region. In analyzing these data, the question of heterogeneity was addressed by performing a conditional linkage analysis using methods described by Cox et al.[37] Scott et al.[59] performed multipoint linkage analysis of chromosome 12 markers using GENEHUNTER-PLUS,[35,36] weighting by sibship size, APOE genotype, and by clinical and neuropathologic features to evaluate potential interactions. Statistical significance of conditional analyses was assessed by shuffling family-specific weights to create a null distribution, as originally described by Cox and colleagues.[37]

To explore potential interactions between chromosome 12 linkage and APOE, LOD* were calculated conditional on the proportion of affected individuals in each family possessing (APOE4+ weighting; modeling additive or epistatic interaction) or lacking (APOE4- weighting; modeling heterogeneity) an APOE-4 allele. Consistent with a heterogeneity model, linkage results were strongest when using APOE4- weighting (peak LOD* = 2.43, at D12S1632). With APOE4+ weighting, LOD* remain low throughout the region (peak LOD* = 0.48 at D12S368). Simulations determined that the increase in LOD* using APOE4- weighting was statistically significant (p= 0.04).

In addition, neuropathologic findings are a second potential indicator of genetic heterogeneity. Families were stratified into two groups, based on the presence of at least one family member with autopsy findings consistent with consensus criteria for dementia with Lewy bodies (DLB).[60] The peak LOD* of 2.18 obtained in the eight DLB families occurs in between D12S1042 and D12S1090, while the remaining 46 families generate a peak LOD* of 0.58 at D12S1632. Simulation also determined that the increase in LOD* using the DLB criteria was statistically significant (p = 0.035). Not surprisingly, these two sets of results are not independent. Six of the eight families with DLB also had affected individuals lacking an APOE-4 allele, representing the two groups with the highest lod scores. To examine this in more detail, the results in the 8 DLB families and the 46 other families were weighted by the proportion of affected individuals lacking an APOE-4 allele. In the DLB families, the results were not significantly different from stratification on DLB alone: a peak LOD* of 2.02 occurs between D12S1042 and D12S1090. However, in the remaining 46 families, the LOD* increases to 1.63 at D12S1632, indicating that evidence for linkage remains in this subset and is stronger in APOE4- families. The data also support the hypothesis that there may be two genes on chromosome 12 involve in AD risk. One gene is on chromosome 12p and another on 12q. The evidence for a gene in dementia associated with Lewy bodies is further supported by the recent report by Funayama[61] that showed linkage of a gene for Parkinson disease with Lewy bodies (PARK8) to 12p11.2-q13.1. This linkage directly overlaps the area reported in Scott et al.[59]

The linkage region for AD risk identified on chromosome 10 has also proven to be interesting and controversial (Fig. 5). The initial linkage reported by Kehoe et al.[49] was later confirmed by Myers et al.[62] At the same time Ertekin-Taner[63] reported linkage to the same region of chromosome 10 in families with high levels of Aβ42. They suggested that Aβ42 was a surrogate phenotype for AD and that examining these families would help in identifying the chromosome 10 AD gene. Independently Bertram et al.[64] found linkage on chromosome 10 in a region slightly distal to that of Myers et al.[62] They suggested that the insulin degrading enzyme (IDE) was the chromosome 10 risk gene as it mapped right at their peak linkage result. These data, however, have not been confirmed.[65] Recently, again using Aβ42 as the phenotype, Ertekin-Taner et al.[66] suggested that α-T Cathenin was the chromosome 10 risk gene.[65,66] These data are also unconfirmed.

One of the most promising new regions is on chromosome 9 identified by the recent genomic screen by our group.[67,68] They used a total of 455 families with late-onset AD (family mean age of onset ≥ 60 years) and 334 microsatellite markers, producing an approximate 10 cM grid. We designated as interesting any marker that resulted in a two-point lod score (MLS or parametric heterogeneity lod score [MLOD]) ≥ 1.00. 14 regions met this criterion. The region on chromosome 9p gave the highest lod score with an MLS of 3.31 and an MLOD of 3.43 for D9S741 (Table 2). Positive results were also found for the markers flanking the chromosome 9p peak. Analysis of this marker in the subset of families with at least one autopsy confirmed AD patient resulted in an increase in the MLS for 9p to 4.42 and the MLOD to 3.97. Multipoint analyses in these regions confirmed the two-point findings. For example, the peak multipoint MLS for 9p in the overall dataset is 3.73, somewhat higher than the two-point scores. The peak multipoint MLS for 9p in the CONF subset is 3.43, somewhat lower than the two-point peak. Recently Dr. Allison Goate at the National Institute of Aging Genetics Symposium at the 2001 Neurosciences Meeting in San Diego presented a reanalysis of their genomic screen data[49]. Their reanalysis also found evidence for linkage on chromosome 9 in the same region. However, there is substantial overlap in the families genotyped by groups from the NIMH and IU datasets and though a testament to accurate genotyping in the independent laboratories, this cannot be seen as an independent replication.

Table 2. Genomic Screen Results

LOCATION	MLS	MLOD	LOCATION	MLS	MLOD
2q36	0.94	1.25	9p22	3.32	3.45
4q32	2.01	2.01	10p11	0.70	1.31
5p15	0.74	1.87	10q22	2.12	2.65
6q26	0.92	1.39	11q25	0.33	1.41
7q31	2.21	2.51	12p11	0.26	1.42
7q35	0.02	1.17	13q11	0.83	1.15
8q13	0.80	1.61	19q13	2.71	4.24
8q24	0.76	1.71	APOE	5.87	12.10

Of critical import, however, is another, totally independent, replication of the chromosome 9p finding. Farrer et al.[52] at the American Society of Human Genetics Annual Meeting in San Diego (October 12-17, 2001) in an independent data set of inbred Arab-Israeli families confirmed our previous report of linkage to chromosome 9.[67,68] Their most significant result was at D9S171 (p=0.0005). Their area of linkage completely overlaps the area of reported linkage, as bioinformatics efforts now confirm that D9S171 and D9S741, the marker with the peak lod score (MLS=4.41 and MLOD=3.94 in autopsy confirmed families), are the same microsatellite marker. The importance of this report[52] cannot be overemphasized, as it is extremely unusual in complex diseases for two independent and significant localizations to fall exactly on top of each other. This gives added confidence that this region needs immediate and detailed molecular genetic analysis.

Characterization of chromosome 9 has begun in the AD candidate gene region as well as specific candidate genes on chromosome 9p. Figure 3 shows the locations of SNPs that have been analyzed and Figure 4 shows the summary of association results.

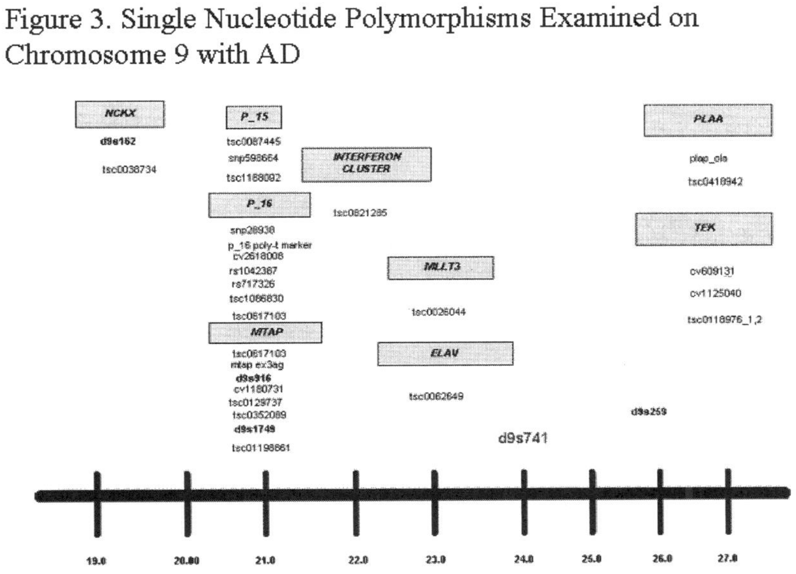

Figure 3. Single Nucleotide Polymorphisms Examined on Chromosome 9 with AD

Fig. 3. Single Nucleotide Polymorphisms Examined on Chromosome 9 with AD.

The region from the p16 (CDKNA2)/p15(CDKN2B) complex to (MTAP) encompasses approximately 200,000 bp with p15 proximal and MTAP distal relative to the centromere. p16 is located between p15 and MTAP and is an approximately 7kb tumor suppressor gene that produces a 987 bp transcript and has three exons. It utilizes a different promoter but shares portions of its exon 1, exon 2, and part of exon 3 with an overlapping p14 isoform/gene. Of interest to this proposal is that p16 has been shown to highly co-localize with nNOS and p21[ras] in pyramidal neurons in Alzheimer's disease.[69] P15 is also a closely related three exon gene that is believed to be involved in growth regulation. Other potential alternate p-gene transcripts are predicted. In addition to the p complex this region contains the susceptibility protein NSG-X and MTAP. Little is known about NSG-x, but MTAP has been characterized[70] and shown to play a major part in the salvage of adenine and methionine and polyamine metabolism. ELAV1 is also an interesting candidate as it maps near the peak of the lod score results at D9S741.

Figure 4.

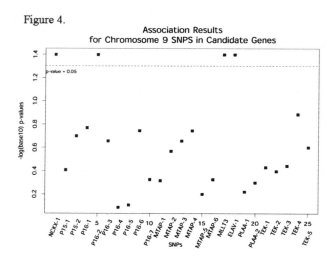

Fig. 4. Association Results for Chromosome 9 SNPS in Candidate Genes.

Another approach to examining genetics in AD is to look at expression in AD. Most studies have modeled the risk of AD as a simple qualitative dichotomous trait. However, examining age-at-onset (AAO) as a quantitative trait can provide novel information and more directly model modulation of onset.

Li et al.[71] recently performed a genome scan of 455 families for AD risk and analyzed AAO as a truncated quantitative trait using the variance-components approach (SOLAR)[72] to identify quantitative trait loci (QTL). 1121/2821 individuals were affected (mean AAO: 72.77±6.81 years), 742 were unaffected at the time of exam (mean age at examination: 70.18±13.04 years) and the rest were unknown. Two polygenic models were considered: one included sex as a covariate, the other included sex and apolipoprotein E (APOE) genotypes as covariates. Interestingly, these analyses identified two novel regions and only one region that overlapped with any proposed region harboring risk genes for AD (see Table 3 for a summary of linkage results). The three identified regions were found on chromosomes 4 (LOD=2.41 and 2.20 for each model, respectively); 8 (LOD=2.24 and 2.62); and 10 (Figure 5) (LOD=2.36 and 2.55). The known effect of APOE on AAO was detected only when the polymorphism itself was tested (LOD=2.92). Further analysis of the region on chromosome 10 extended the age of onset effect to include families with idiopathic Parkinson disease[71]. Analysis of potential candidates in the region is in progress.

Table 3. AAO Linkage Results

Marker Region	Map Position (cM)	Multipoint LOD Model 1	Model 2
Chromosome 4:			
Peak (D4S1652)	208	2.29	1.84
Chromosome 8:			
Peak(D8S592)	126		2.09
D8S1128	140		
Peak	142/150	2.09(150cM)	1.73(142cM)
D8S373	165		
Chromosome 10:			
Peak (D10S1237)	139	2.39	2.58
Chromsome 19:			
Peak(APOE)	70	0.78	

Figure 5. Chromosome 10q
Linkage Summary

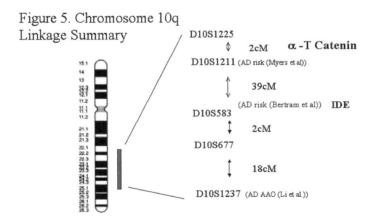

Fig. 5. Chromosome 10q Linkage Summary.

In summary, the deconstruction of the complex genetic architecture of Alzheimer disease despite our many advances has only begun. AD has become a paradigm for the identification and understanding of susceptibility alleles in diseases of the elderly, and thus is an ideal candidate for the application of new approaches and paradigms. The ability to develop a single, unified, and efficient sampling design to exploit new statistical and molecular technologies is the key to identifying the remaining genes involved in AD. The rich resources and progress of the Human Genome Project will provide the anchor for these studies. Over the next decade we will see great advances in our understanding of this complex problem with the potential for its application to treatment and prevention on the horizon.

REFERENCE LIST

1.   Brookmeyer, R., Gray, S., Kawas, C. (1998) "Projections of Alzheimer's disease in the United States and the public health impact of delaying disease onset." *American Journal of Public Health.* 88:1337-1342.

2.   Wisniewski, T., Golabek, A., Matsubara, E., Ghiso, J., Frangione, B. (1993) "Apolipoprotein E: binding to soluble Alzheimer's beta-amyloid." *Biochem. Biophys. Res. Commun.* 192:359-365.

3.   Guttman, R., Altman, R.D., Nielsen, N.H. (1999) "Alzheimer disease: report of the Council on Scientific Affairs." *Archives of Family Medicine* 8:347-353.

4.   Alzheimer A. Ueber eine eigenartige Erkrankung der Himrinde. Allg Z Psychiat Med 1907;64:146-148.

5.   Hirst, C., Sadovnick, A.D., Yee, I.M.L. (1994) "Familial risks for Alzheimer disease: data from an Alzheimer clinic population." *Genet Epidemiol.* 11:365-374.

6.   Goate, A., Chartier-Harlin, M.C., Mullan, M., Brown, J., Crawford, F., Fidani, L., Giuffra, L., Haynes, A., Irving, N., James, L., et al. (1991) "Segregation of a missense mutation in the amyloid precursor protein gene with familial Alzheimer's disease." *Nature* 349:704-706.

7.   Levy-Lahad, E., Wasco, W., Poorkaj, P., Romano, D.M., Oshima, J., Pettingell, W.H., Yu, C.E., Jondro, P.D., Schmidt, S.D., Wang, K., et al. (1995) "Candidate gene for the chromosome 1 familial Alzheimer's disease locus." *Science* 269:973-977.

8.   Rogaev, E.I., Sherrington, R., Rogaeva, E.A., Levesque, G., Ikeda, M., Liang, Y., Chi, H., Lin, C., Holman, K., Tsuda, T. (1995) "Familial Alzheimer's disease in kindreds with missense mutations in a gene on chromosome 1 related to the Alzheimer's disease type 3 gene." *Nature* 376:775-778.

9.   Sherrington, R., Rogaev, E.I., Liang, Y., Rogaeva, E.A., Levesque, G., Ikeda, M., Chi, H., Lin, C., Li, G., Holman, K., et al. (1995) "Cloning of a gene bearing missense mutations in early-onset familial Alzheimer's disease." *Nature* 375:754-760.

10.   Pericak-Vance, M.A., Yamaoka, L.H., Haynes, C.S., Speer, M.C., Haines, J.L, Gaskell, P..C, Hung, W.Y., Clark, C.M., Heyman, A.L., Trofatter, J.A., et al.

(1988) "Genetic Linkage Studies in Alzheimer's Disease Families." *Exp.Neurol* 102:271-279.

11. Risch, N. (1990) "Linkage strategies for genetically complex traits I. Multilocus models." *Am.J.Hum.Gen.* 46:222-228.

12. Risch, N. (1990) "Linkage strategies for genetically complex traits II. The power of affected relative pairs." *Am.J.Hum.Gen.* 46:229-241.

13. Risch, N. (1990) "Linkage strategies for genetically complex traits III. The effect of marker polymorphism on analysis of affected pairs." *Am.J.Hum.Gen.* 46:242-253.

14. Breitner, J.C., Silverman, J.M., Mohs, R.C., Davis, K.L. (1988) "Familial aggregation in Alzheimer's disease: comparison of risk among first degree relatives of early- and late-onset cases, and among male and female relatives in a successive generation." *Neurol.* 38:207-212.

15. Sadovnick, A.D., Irwin, M.E., Baird, P.A., Beattle, B.L. (1989) "Genetic studies on an Alzheimer clinic population." *Genet Epidemiol.* 6:663-643.

16. Hauser, E.R., Boehnke, M., Guo, S.W., Risch, N. (1996) "Affected-sib-pair interval mapping and exclusion for complex genetic traits: sampling considerations." *Genet Epidemiol.* 13:117-137.

17. Pericak-Vance, M.A. Bebout, J.L., Gaskell, P.C., Yamaoka, L.H., Hung, W.Y., Alberts, M.J., Walker, A.P., Bartlett, R.J., Haynes, C.S., Welsh, K.A., et al. (1991) "Linkage studies in familial Alzheimer's disease: Evidence for chromosome 19 linkage." *Am.J.Hum.Gen.* 48:1034-1050.

18. Menzel, H.J., Kladetzky, R.G., Asman, G. (1983) "Apolipoprotein E polymorphism and coronary artery disease." *Arteriosclerosis* 3:310-315.

19. Saunders, A.M., Strittmatter, W.J., Schmechel, D., Pericak-Vance, M.A., Joo, S.H., Rosi, B.L., Gusella, J.F., Crapper-MacLachlan, D.R., Alberts, M.J., et al. (1993) "Association of apolipoprotein E allele e4 with late-onset familial and sporadic Alzheimer's disease." *Neurol.* 43:1467-1472.

20. Namba, Y., Tamonaga, M., Kawasaki, H., Otomo, E., Ikeda, K. (1991) "Apolipoprotein E immunoreactivity in cerebral amyloid deposits and neurofibrillary tangles in Alzheimer's disease and cru plaque amyloid in Creutzfeldt-Jakob disease." *Brain Res.* 541:163-166.

21. Wisniewski, T., Frangione, B. "Apolipoprotein E: A pathological chaperone protein in patients with cerebral and systemic amyloid." *Neurosci Let* 135:235-238.

22. Strittmatter, W.J., Saunders, A.M., Schmechel, D., Pericak-Vance, M.A., Enghild, J., Salvesen, G.S., Roses, A.D. (1993) "Apolipoprotein E: High-avidity binding to b-amyloid and increased frequency of type 4 allele in late-onset familial Alzheimer disease." *Proceedings of the National Academy of Sciences of United States of America* 90:1977-1981.

23. Corder, E.H., Saunders, A.M., Strittmatter,W.J., Schmechel, D.E., Gaskell, P.C., Small, G.W., Roses, A.D., Haines, J.L., Pericak-Vance, M.A. (1993) "Gene dose

of apolipoprotein E type 4 allele and the risk of Alzheimer's disease in late onset families." *Science* 261:921-923.

24. Okuizumi, K., Onodera, O., Tanaka, H., Kabayaski, H., Tsuji, S., Takahashi, H., Oyanagi, K., Seki, K., Tanaja, M., Naruse, S. (1994) "ApoE-epsilon 4 and early-onset Alzheimer's disease." *Nat.Genet.* 7:10-11.

25. Van Duijn, C.M., deKnijff, P., Cruts, M., Wehnert, A., Havekes, L.M, Hofman, A., Van Broeckhoven, C. (1994) "Apolipoprotein E4 allele in a population-based study of early-onset Alzheimer's disease." *Nat.Genet.* 7:74-78.

26. Roses, A.D., Pericak-Vance, M.A., Rimoin, D.L., Connor, J.M., Pyeritz, R.E., editors. (1997) Emery and Rimoin's Principles and Practice of Medical Genetics. 3rd ed. New York: Churchill Livingston Publishing Co., 83, Alzheimer's disease and other dementias. p. 1807-25.

27. Corder, E.H., Saunders, A.M., Risch, N., Strittmatter, W.J., Schmechel, D.E., Gaskell, P.C. Rimmler, J.B. Locke, P.A., Conneally, P.M., Schmader, K.E., et al. (1994) "Apolipoprotein E type 2 allele decreases the risk of late onset Alzheimer disease." *Nat.Genet.* 7:180-184.

28. Locke, P., Conneally, P.M., Tanzi, R.E., Gusella, J., Haines, J.L. (1995) "APOE and Alzheimer's disease: examination of allelic association and effect on age at-onset in both early and late-onset cases." *Genet Epidemiol.* 12:83-92.

29. Farrer, L.A., Cupples, L.A., Haines, J.L., Hyman, B., Kukull, W.A., Mayeux, R., Myers, R.H., Pericak-Vance, M.A., Risch, N., Van Duijn, C.M. (1997) "Effects of age, sex, and ethnicity on the association between apolipoprotein E genotype and Alzheimer disease. A meta-analysis. APOE and Alzheimer Disease Meta Analysis Consortium." *JAMA* 278:1349-1356.

30. Bergen, A.L. (1994) "Heredity in dementia of the Alzheimer type." *Clin Genet* 46:144-149.

31. Tang, M.X., Maestre, G., Tsai, W.Y, Liu X.H,, Feng, L., Chung, W.Y., Chun, M., Schofield, P., Stern,Y., Tycko, B., et al. (1996) "Relative risk of Alzheimer disease and age-at-onset distributions, based on APOE genotypes among elderly African Americans, Caucasians, and Hispanics in New York City." *Am. J. Hum. Gen.* 58:574-584.

32. Maestre, G., Ottman, R., Stern, Y., Gurland, B., Chun, M., Tang, M.X., Shelanski, M., Tycko, B., Mayeux, R. (1995) "Apolipoprotein E and Alzheimer's disease: ethnic variation in genotypic risks." *Ann Neurol* 37:254-259.

33. Roses, A.D., Saunders, A.M., Alberts, M.A., Strittmatter, W.J., Schmechel, D., Gorder, E., Pericak-Vance, M.A. (1995) "Apolipoprotein E E4 allele and risk of dementia [letter; comment]." *JAMA* 273:374-375.

34. Martin, E.R., Monks, S.A., Warren, L.L., Kaplan, N.L. (2000) "A test for linkage and association in general pedigrees: the pedigree disequilibrium test." *Am. J. Hum. Gen.* 67:146-154.

35. Kruglyak, L., Daly, M.J. Reeve-Daly, M.P., Lander, E.S. (1996) "Parametric and nonparametric linkage analysis: a unified multipoint approach." *Am. J. Hum. Gen.* 58:1347-1363.

36. Kong, A., Cox, N.J. (1997) "Allele-sharing models: LOD scores and accurate linkage tests." *Am. J. Hum. Gen.* 61:1179-1188.

37. Cox, N.J., Frigge, M., Nicolae, D.L., Concannon, P., Hanis, C.L., Bell, G.I., Kong, A. (1999) "Loci on chromosomes 2 (NIDDM1) and 15 interact to increase susceptibility to diabetes in Mexican Americans." *Nat. Genet* 21:213-215.

38. Risch, N., Merikangas, K. (1996) "The future of genetic studies of complex human disorders." *Science* 273:1516-1517.

39. Collins, F.S., Brooks, L.D., Chakravarti, A. (1998) "A DNA polymorphism discovery resource for research on human genetic variation." *Genome Res.* 8:1229-1231.

40. Kamboh, M.I., Sanghera, D.K., Ferrell, R.E., DeKosky, S.T. (1995) "APOE*4-associated Alzheimer's disease risk is modified by alpha 1-antichymotrypsin polymorphism." *Nat. Genet.* 10:486-488.

41. Lendon, C.L., Talbot, C.J., Craddock, N.J., Han, S.W., Wragg, M., Morris, J.C., Goate, A.M. (1997) "Genetic association studies between dementia of the Alzheimer's type and three receptors for apolipoprotein E in a Caucasian population." *Neurosci Let* 222:187-190.

42. Wragg, M., Hutton, M., Talbot, C., Alzheimer's Disease Collaborative Group. (1996) "Genetic association between an intronic polymorphism in the presenilin 1 gene and late onset Alzheimer's disease." *Lancet* 347:509-512.

43. Van Leeuwen, F.W., Dekleijn, D.P.V., Vandenhurk, H.H., Neubauer, A., Sonnemans, M.A.F., Sluijs, J.A., Koycu, S., Ramdjielal, R.D.J., Salehi, A., Martens, G.J.M., et al. (1998) "Frameshift mutants of beta amyloid precursor protein and ubiquitin-b in Alzheimers and Down patients." *Science* 279:242-247.

44. Payami, H., Schellenberg, G.D., Zarepars,i S., Kaye, J., Sexton, G.J., Head, M.A., Matsuyama, S.S., Jarvik, L.F., Miller, B., McManus, D.Q., et al. (1997) "Evidence for association of HLA-A2 allele with onset age of Alzheimer's disease." *Neurol.* 49:512-518.

45. Curran, M., Middleton, D., Edwardson, J., Perry, R., McKeith, I., Morris, C., Neill, D. "HLA-DR antigens associated with major genetic risk for late-onset Alzheimer's disease." *Neuroreport* 8:1467-1469.

46. Lehmann, D.J., Johnston, C., Smith, A.D. (1997) "Synergy between the genes for butyrylcholinesterase K variant and apolipoprotein E4 in late-onset confirmed Alzheimer's disease." *Hum. Mol. Genet.* 6:1933-1936.

47. Xia, Y., da Silva, R., Rosi, B.L., Yamaoka, L.H., Rimmler, J.B., Pericak-Vance, M.A., Roses, A.D., Chen, X., Masliah, E., DeTeresa, R., et al. (1996) "Genetic studies in Alzheimer's disease with an NACP/alpha-synuclein polymorphism." *Ann Neurol* 40:207-215.

48. Hutchin, T., Cortopassi, G. (1995) "A mitochondrial DNA clone is associated with increased risk for Alzheimer disease." *Proc. Natl. Acad. Sci.(USA)* 92:6892-6895.

49. Kehoe, P., Wavrant-De Vrieze, F., Crook, R., Wu, W.S., Holmans, P., Fenton, I., Spurlock, G., Norton, N., Williams, H., Williams N., et al. (1999) "A full genome scan for late onset Alzheimer's disease." *Hum. Mol. Genet.* 8:237-245.

50. Pericak-Vance, M.A., Bass, M.P., Yamaoka, L.H., Gaskell, P.C., Scott, W.K., Terwedow, H.A., Menold, M.M., Conneally, P.M., Small, G.W., Vance, J.M., et al. (1997) "Complete genomic screen in late-onset familial Alzheimer disease: evidence for a new locus on chromosome 12." *JAMA* 278:1237-1241.

51. Rogaeva, E., Premkumar, S., Song,Y., Sorbi, S., Brindle, N., Paterson, A., Duara, R., Levesque, G., Yu, G., Nishimura, M., et al. (1998) "Evidence for an Alzheimer disease susceptibility locus on chromosome 12 and for further locus heterogeneity." *JAMA* 280:614-618.

52. Farrer, L.A., Bowirrat, A., Friedland, R.P., et al. (2001) "Identification of multiple loci for Alzheimer Disease in an inbred Israeli-Arab community. [Abstract]" *Am J Hum Genet* 69 (supp):200

53. Scott, W.K., Yamaoka, L.H., Bass, M.P., Gaskell, P.C., Conneally, P.M., Small, G.W., Farrer, L.A., Auerbach, S.A., Saunders, A.M., Roses, A.D., et al. (1998) "No genetic association between the LRP receptor and sporadic or late-onset familial Alzheimer disease." *Neurogenetics* 1:179-183.

54. Blacker, D., Wilcox, M.A., Laird, N.M., Rodes, L., Horvath, S.M., Go, R.C.P., Perry, R., Watson, B., Bassett, S.S., McInnis, M.G., et al. (1998) "Alpha-2 macroglobulin is genetically associated with Alzheimer disease." *Nat. Genet.* 19:357-360.

55. Lambert, J.C., Goumidi, L., Vrieze, F.W., Frigard, B. Harris, J.M., Cummings, A., Coates, J., Pasquier, F., Cottel, D., Gaillac, M., et al. (2000) "The transcriptional factor LBP-1c/CP2/LSF gene on chromosome 12 is a genetic determinant of Alzheimer's disease." *Hum. Mol. Genet.* 9:2275-2280.

56. Rogaeva, E.A., Premkumar, S., Grubber, J., Serneels, L., Scott, W.K., Kawarai, T., Song, Y., Hill, D.L., Abou-donia, S.M., Martin, E.R., et al. (1999) "An alpha-2-macroglobulin insertion-deletion polymorphism in Alzheimer disease [letter]." *Nat. Genet.* 22:19-22.

57. Dow, D.J., Lindsey, N., Cairns, N.J., Brayne, C., Robinson, D., Huppert, F.A., Paykel, E.S., Xuereb, J., Wilcock, G., Whittaker, J.L., et al. (1999) "Alpha-2 macroglobulin polymorphism and Alzheimer disease risk in the UK" [letter] [see comments]. *Nat. Genet.* 22:16-17.

58. Rudrasingham, V., Wavrant-De, V.F., Lambert, J.C., Chakraverty, S., Kehoe, P., Crook, R., Amouyel, P., Wu, W., Rice, F., Perez-Tur, J., et al. (1999) "Alpha-2 macroglobulin gene and Alzheimer disease" [letter] [see comments]. *Nat. Genet.* 22:17-19.

59. Scott, W.K., Grubber, J.M., Conneally, P.M., Small, G.W., Hulette, C.M., Rosenberg, C.K., Saunders, A.M., Roses, A.D., Haines, J.L. Pericak-Vance, M.A. (2000) "Fine mapping of the chromosome 12 late-onset Alzheimer disease locus: potential genetic and phenotypic heterogeneity." *Am. J. Hum. Gen* 66:922-932.

60. McKeith, .I.G., Galasko, D., Kosaka, K., Perry, E.K., Dickson, D.W., Hansen, L.A., Salmon, D.P., Lowe, J., Mirra, S.S., Byrne, E.J., et al. (1996) "Consensus guidelines for the clinical and pathologic diagnosis of dementia with Lewy bodies (DLB): Report of the consortium on DLB International Workshop." *Neurol.* 47:1113-1124.

61. Funayama, M., Hasegawa, K., Kowa, H., Saito, M., Tsuji, S., Obata, F. (2002) "A new locus for Parkinson's disease (PARK8) maps to chromosome 12p11.2-q13.1." *Ann. Neurol.* 51:296-301.

62. Myers, A., Holmans, P., Marshall, H., Kwon, J., Meyer, D., Ramic, D., Shears, S., Booth, J., DeVrieze, F.W., Crook, R., et al. (2000) "Susceptibility locus for Alzheimer's disease on chromosome 10." *Science* 290:2304-2305.

63. Ertekin-Taner, N., Graff-Radford, N., Younkin, L.H., Eckman, C., Baker, M., Adamson, J., Ronald, J., Blangero, J., Hutton, M., Younkin, S.G. (2000) "Linkage of plasma Abeta42 to a quantitative locus on chromosome 10 in late-onset Alzheimer's disease pedigrees." *Science* 290:2303-2304.

64. Bertram, L., Blacker, D., Mullin, K., Keeney, D., Jones, J., Basu, S., Yhu, S., McInnis, M., Go, R.C.P., Vekrellis, K., et al. (2000) "Evidence for genetic linkage of Alzheimer's disease to chromosome 10q." *Science* 290:2302-2305.

65. Abraham, R., Myers, A., Wavrant-DeVrieze, F., Hamshere, M.L., Thomas, H.V., Marshall, H., Compton, D., Spurlock, G., Turic, D., Hoogendoorn, B., et al. "Substantial linkage disequilibrium across the insulin-degrading enzyme locus but no association with late-onset Alzheimer's disease." *Hum. Genet* 109:646-652.

66. Ertekin-Taner, N., Ronald, J., Jain, S., et al. (2002) "Identification of a novel late onset AD gene on chromosome 10." [Abstract] *The 8th International Conference on Alzheimer's Disease and Related Disorders* Hot Topics-Abstract.

67. Pericak-Vance, M.A., Bailey, L.R., Nicodemus, K., et al. (2001) "Genomic Screen of 726 sibpairs with late-onset Alzheimer disease (AD)." [Abstract] *European Journal of Human Genetics* 9:(1)361

68. Haines, J.L., Pericak-Vance, M.A., Iqbal, K., Sisodia, S.S., Winblad, B., editors. (2001) *Alzheimer's Disease: Advances in Etiology, Pathogenesis and Therapeutics.* London: John Wiley & Sons; "A Genomic Search for Alzheimer's Disease Genes." p. 33-43.

69. Luth, H.J., Holzer, M., Gertz, H.J., Arendt, T. (2000) "Aberrant expression of nNOS in pyramidal neurons in Alzheimer's disease is highly co-localized with p21ras and p16INK4a." *Brain Res.* 852:45-55.

70. Ragione, F.D., Takabayashi, K., Mastropietro, S., Mercurio, C., Oliva, A., Russo, G.L., Della, P., Borriello, A., Nobori, T., Carson, D.A., et al. (1996) "Purification and characterization of recombinant human 5'-methylthioadenosine phosphorylase: definite identification of coding cDNA." *Biochem. Biophys. Res. Commun.* 223:514-519.

71. Li, Y.J., Scott, W.K., Hedges, D.J., Zhang, F., Gaskell, P.C., Nance, M.A., Watts, R.L., Hubble, J.P., Koller,W.C., Pahwa, R., et al. (2002) "Age at onset in two

common neurodegenerative diseases is genetically controlled. " *Am. J. Hum. Gen.* 70:985-993.

72.   Almasy, L., Blangero, J. (1998) "Multipoint quantitative-trait linkage analysis in general pedigrees." *Am.J.Hum.Gen.* 62:1198-1211.

TAU GENE MUTATIONS IN FRONTOTEMPORAL DEMENTIA AND PARKINSONISM LINKED TO CHROMOSOME 17

MARIA GRAZIA SPILLANTINI

Cambridge Centre for Brain Repair and Department of Neurology, University of Cambridge, Cambridge, UK

SUMMARY

Microtubule-associated protein tau is involved in microtubule assembly and stabilisation. Abnormal filamentous tau deposits constitute a major defining characteristic of several neurodegenerative diseases collectively known as "tauopathies". Alzheimer's Disease is considered a "secondary tauopathy" due to the additional presence of β-amyloid plaques. Until recently there was no genetic evidence linking tau to neurodegeneration. Since 1998, the identification of 28 mutations in the *tau* gene associated with frontotemporal dementia and parkinsonism linked to chromosome 17 has demonstrated that tau dysfunction can lead to neurodegeneration and development of clinical symptoms.

TAU PROTEIN

Tau is a microtubule-associated protein that promotes microtubule assembly and stability and plays a role in maintaining neuronal integrity and axonal transport.[1,2] In adult human six tau isoforms are produced through alternative splicing from a single gene present in chromosome 17.[3,4] These isoforms differ in the presence or absence of 29 or 58 amino acid inserts in the amino-terminal half and the presence of 3 or 4 tandem repeats in the carboxy-terminal region of the protein (Fig. 1). In adult human brain similar levels of 3R and 4R tau are found while in fetal brain only the shortest tau isoform with 3R is present, demonstrating developmental regulation of tau expression. The repeats, encoded by exons 9-12, together with some adjoining sequences, constitute the microtubule-binding domain of tau. Tau is a phosphoprotein predominantly expressed in neurons, where it is largely localised to axons. Phosphorylation is developmentally regulated such that fetal tau is more phosphorylated than adult brain tau.[5] Phosphorylation inhibits the ability of tau to bind to microtubules making them less stable. This is a favorable condition during development when plasticity of the nervous system is needed.

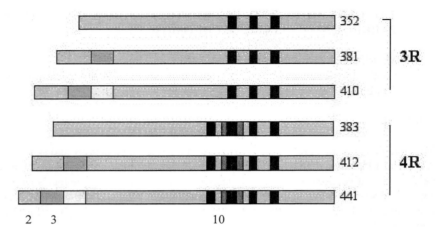

Fig.1. Six tau isoforms expressed in adult human brain. Boxes representing alternatively spliced exons 2, 3 and 10 are indicated. Microtubule-binding repeat are shown as black boxes. The number of amino acids in each isoform is indicated.

The "tauopathies" are a group of neurodegenerative disorders characterised by the presence of filamentous deposits in neurons and glia consisting of hyperphosphorylated tau protein.[6] This term, which was first used to describe a family with frontotemporal dementia and abundant tau deposits,[7] is now used to identify a group of diseases with widespread tau pathology, in which tau accumulation is believed to be directly associated with neuronal death and disease development. This group of diseases includes Pick's disease/frontotemporal dementia (FTD), corticobasal degeneration (CBD), progressive supranuclear palsy (PSP) and frontotemporal dementia and parkinsonism linked to chromosome 17 (FTDP-17). The term "tauopathies" can also be extended to include several other neurodegenerative diseases, such as Alzheimer's disease, where tau pathology is found in conjunction with other abnormal protein lesions. Such disorders may be considered "secondary tauopathies" and in these diseases, although tau is probably not the initial pathological factor, tau aggregates are the cause of the neurodegeneration.

Frontotemporal dementias occur in both familial and sporadic forms. FTDP-17 is inherited as an autosomal dominant condition characterised initially by behavioural and motor disturbances that are later associated with cognitive impairment. At autopsy, FTDP-17 patients usually display predominant frontotemporal atrophy with neuronal loss, gliosis and cortical spongiform changes in layer 2. Neuropathological analysis reveals the presence of abundant intraneuronal tau inclusions, with glial inclusions observed in several families. In 1998 the identification of exonic and intronic mutations in the *tau* gene associated with FTDP-17 established that tau dysfunction can cause neurodegeneration.[8-10] These findings and subsequent reports have to date identified more than 25 such tau mutations that can be classified according to their positions in the *tau* gene, their effects on tau mRNA and protein, and the type of tau pathology they lead to. Furthermore, polymorphisms have been identified within the *tau* gene that appear to be associated with progressive supranuclear palsy.[11]

TAU GENE MUTATIONS

Tau mutations can be classified according to their position in the *tau* gene. The vast majority are missense, deletion or silent mutations in the coding region, or intronic mutations located close to the splice-donor site of the intron following the alternatively spliced exon 10 (Fig. 2). Most coding region mutations are located in the microtubule-binding region (exons 9-12) of *tau* or close to it (exon 13). Recently, however, the R5H and R5L mutations in exon 1 of *tau* have been reported.[12-13] Mutations in exon 1 (R5H, R5L), exon 9 (K257T, L266V, G272V), exon 11 (S320F), exon 12 (V337M, E342V, K369I) and exon 13 (G389R, R406W) affect all six tau isoforms. In contrast, mutations in exon 10 (N279K, ΔK280, L284L, ΔN296, N296H, N296N, P301L, P301S, S305N, S305S) affect only 4R tau isoforms or their expression. The mutations can also be categorised functionally according to whether their primary effect is exerted directly at the protein level and/or upon RNA splicing.

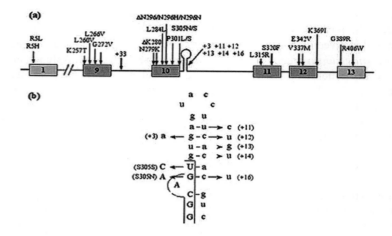

Fig. 2. Mutations in the tau gene associated with FTDP-17. (a) Exons 1 and 9-13 of the tau gene are shown with mutations indicated. (b) Stem-loop pre-mRNA structure downstream of exon 10 and following intronic sequence. Eight mutations that reduce the stability of this structure increasing splicing in of exon 10 are indicated. Exon sequences are shown in upper-case letters and intronic sequences in lower-case.

MISSENSE MUTATIONS AFFECTING TAU-MICROTUBULE INTERACTIONS

In vitro studies have demonstrated that coding region mutations in exons 9, 11, 12 and 13 of *tau* disrupt tau-microtubule interactions, reducing the ability of mutant tau to promote microtubule assembly. This effect is also seen with the P301L and P301S mutations in exon 10.[14-16] Furthermore, a number of missense mutations (K257T, G272V, P301L, P301S, V337M, K369I) have a direct stimulatory effect on heparin-induced tau filament assembly *in vitro*, with some mutations leading to the aggregation of specific tau isoforms only.[17-20] A reduction in microtubule assembly and a promotion of tau filament formation have also recently been reported for the R5H mutation.[12-13] Located in exon 1 of *tau*, far from the microtubule-binding domain, the mechanism by which the R5H and R5L mutations exert their effects is currently unclear. It is possible that the amino acid substitution causes a conformational change in the tau molecule altering both its interactions with microtubules and with other tau molecules.

MUTATIONS AFFECTING EXON 10 SPLICING

The vast majority of identified intronic mutations are located in the intron following exon 10, at positions +3, +11, +12, +13, +14 and +16, with the first nucleotide of the splice-donor site taken as +1 (9,10,21,22) (Fig. 2). Secondary structure analysis has predicted the presence of a stable, folded RNA stem-loop at the boundary of exon 10 with the intron that follows.[23] Intronic mutations analysed to date have been demonstrated to reduce the thermodynamic stability of this structure, to various extents, thereby disrupting the stem-loop.[23] In addition, the +3 mutation is predicted to result in increased binding of the U1 snRNP to the 5' splice site.[10] Exon trapping studies have shown that these intronic mutations increase splicing in of exon 10.[9,21-25] This increase is reflected by a preponderance of 4R soluble tau in the brains of patients carrying these mutations[10,15,21,26-27] Besides mutations in the intron following exon 10, further pathogenic mutations may exist in other introns of the *tau* gene.

The pattern described thus far is one in which missense mutations lead to a reduced ability of tau to promote microtubule assembly and increased tendency to stimulate filament aggregation, and in which intronic mutations exert their effects at the RNA level, resulting in an overproduction of 4R tau. However, several other mutations within exon 10 (N279K, L284L, N296N, S305N, and S305S) also have the primary effect of increasing splicing of exon 10. The N279K missense and L284L silent mutations strengthen an exon splicing-enhancer element located in the 5' region of exon 10, resulting in an increase in exon 10 containing RNA and 4R soluble tau protein.[24,28-29] A second silent mutation, N296N leads to increased levels of exon 10 containing transcripts. It is proposed that this increase results either from the disruption of an exon splicing-silencer (30), or from the creation of an exon splicing-enhancer sequence in exon 10.[31] Two exonic mutations at codon 305, the missense mutation S305N and the silent mutation S305S each alters the predicted stem-loop structure. The S305N mutation changes the last amino acid of exon 10, reducing the thermodynamic stability of the stem-loop[23,32] and, as for the +3 intronic mutation, increasing binding of U1 snRNP to the 5' splice site. This leads to increased splicing of exon 10.[29] The silent S305S mutation is not expected to lead to an increase in U1 snRNA binding, but to a disruption of the stem-loop structure alone.[33]

MUTATIONS AFFECTING TAU-MICROTUBULE INTERACTIONS AND EXON 10 SPLICING

The mutations discussed so far have had the primary effect either of disrupting tau-microtubule interactions, or of affecting exon 10 splicing and therefore the ratio of 4R:3R tau protein. However, a third group of mutations exists which could potentially exert its effects at both the protein and RNA levels. This group includes the ΔK280 and ΔN296 deletion mutations, and the N296H mutation, all located in exon 10 of *tau* (Fig. 2). *In vitro* studies have demonstrated that like many other coding sequence mutations, these three exon 10 mutations greatly reduce the ability of tau to promote microtubule assembly.[31,34] Their impact on heparin-induced tau filament assembly, however, is currently under debate, with both stimulatory effects[31,35] and no effect[18,34] reported. In addition to decreasing microtubule assembly, the N296H mutation has been demonstrated to increase splicing in of exon 10,[31,34] with accumulation of sarkosyl-insoluble 4R tau observed in the brain of an individual carrying this mutation.[36] (The ΔN296 mutation has been reported to lead to an increase[34] or no change[31] in exon 10 splicing, this issue could be resolved when soluble tau will become available. The ΔK280 mutation, in contrast, leads to reduced splicing in of exon 10, suggesting that its primary effect may be the overproduction of 3R tau, rather than the reduced ability of 4R tau to interact with microtubules.[24] If, however, some 4R, i.e. ΔK280-containing tau is produced, its effect on microtubule polymerisation may contribute to pathogenesis. Once again clarification must await the availability of frozen brain tissue. It is possible that the E342V mutation may also affect tau at both the RNA and protein levels. Lippa and coworkers[37] have reported an increase in 4R tau with no amino-terminal inserts and a decrease in 4R tau containing these inserts in the brain of a patient with this mutation. This suggests that the E342V mutation may alter splicing of exons 2, 3 and 10 of *tau*. Although, this remains to be determined, it is possible that this mutation, located in exon 12, would also be able to reduce tau's ability to promote microtubule assembly.

CHARACTERISTICS OF TAU DEPOSITS IN FTDP-17

All cases of FTDP-17 analysed to date have been characterised by the presence of an abundant filamentous pathology consisting of hyperphosphorylated tau protein. However, the morphology, isoform composition and distribution of tau filaments and tau deposits appear to vary according to the type of mutation.

Missense mutations located outside exon 10 with a primary effect of reducing microtubule assembly lead to a tau pathology that is largely neuronal, without a significant glial component. Some of these mutations, such as V337M (exon 12), found in the Seattle family A, lead to the formation of paired helical filaments (PHF) and straight filaments (SF) that contain all six tau isoforms identical to those found in Alzheimer's disease.[38] Similar findings have been reported for the R406W (exon 13) mutation.[39-40] In contrast, another exon 13 mutation, G389R, leads to a pathology more closely resembling Pick's disease, with large number of tau-immunoreactive Pick body-like and axonal inclusions (41). While the majority of filaments have the appearance of the SF of Alzheimer's disease, a minority is twisted. Both filaments are labelled by anti-tau antibodies and closely resemble the filaments of sporadic Pick's disease. Pick bodies are also a shared characteristic of brains from patients carrying the K257T, L266V and G272V mutations (exon 9;[6,19,42]), the S320F mutation (exon 11;[43]) and of those with the E342V and K369I mutations (exon 12;[20,37]). However, when analysed by electron microscopy, variations in the composition and structure of tau filaments produced by these mutations are observed. The S320F and K396I mutations both lead to filaments composed of 3R and 4R tau. However, while the majority of filaments resulting from the S320F mutation resemble the SF of Alzheimer's disease (with a minority being irregularly twisted), the K369I mutation leads to small, irregular twisted filaments and rare PHF. Filaments produced by the K257T mutation are irregularly twisted, but are composed predominantly of 3R tau.[19] Differing again is the E342V mutation that results in filaments similar in structure to the PHF of Alzheimer's disease, but composed mostly of 4R tau with no amino-terminal inserts and only low levels of 3R tau.[37] The lack of fresh tissue from individuals with the G272V mutation has precluded biochemical analysis of tau and tau filaments. However, as for the other missense mutations affecting microtubule binding, immunohistochemistry has revealed a largely neuronal tau pathology.[6] One mutation that does not conform to this general pattern is the R5H mutation in exon 1, in which glial tau deposits predominate and consist of PSP-like straight filaments[12] and PSP-like tau pathology is found in R5L.[13] Together these findings indicate that the positions of these mutations in the coding region of the *tau* gene, and perhaps the nature of the amino acid changes, appear to determine whether the ensuing tau pathology resembles Alzheimer's disease, Pick's disease, PSP or CBD.

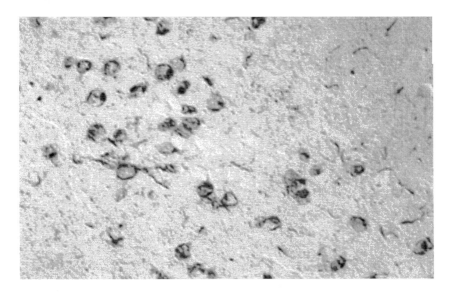

Fig.3. Tau pathology observed in frontal cortex from a case with P301L. Tau pathology is present in both neurons and glia.

The P301L and P301S missense mutations within exon 10 lead to a pathology that is both neuronal and glial[6,44-45] (Fig. 3). Analysis of insoluble tau from brains from the many families carrying the P301L mutation has revealed the presence of narrow twisted filaments composed of 4R tau, with a small amount of the most common 3R isoform.

Electron microscopy of tissue sections suggests that similar filaments are present in those with the P301S mutation.

Intronic tau mutations that increase splicing in of exon 10 lead to a widespread neuronal and glial pathology, with the glial component being more significant than that for the P301L and P301S mutations. Ultrastructurally, wide twisted ribbons are produced, containing only 4R tau isoforms. This has been shown in individuals with the +3, +11, +12, +13, and +16 intronic mutations.[7,21-22,26-27,46] Similar filaments are present in an individual with the +14 mutation (unpublished personal observation).

Neuronal and glial pathology has also been reported for several of the coding region mutations increasing exon 10 splicing (N279K, L284L, N296N, S305N, S305S). Some variability in the morphology of tau filaments has, however, been reported for such mutations. While electron microscopy of tissue sections with the S305N mutation demonstrates the presence of straight filaments,[32] the silent S305S mutation results in both straight and twisted structures.[33] As for the intronic mutations, the N279K mutation produces twisted ribbons, predominantly composed of 4R tau.[47-48] The N296H mutation differs once again by having a mainly glial pathology with coiled bodies composed of straight filaments, as detected in tissue sections.[36] The lack of available tissue has meant that ultrastructural and/or biochemical analysis of several exon 10 mutations affecting splicing (ΔK280, L284L, ΔN296, N296N, S305N, S305S) has not yet been possible.

CLINICAL FEATURES OF FTDP-17

Although different tau mutations can lead to quite specific tau pathologies, this is not the case for clinical phenotype. Clinical presentation can differ not only between mutations but also within individual families depending on the brain region where the tau pathology develops initally. For example, in one family carrying the P301S mutation, the proband presented with FTD, whereas CBD in the absence of dementia was diagnosed in the proband's son.[45] In some cases, such as those with the N279K and S305S mutations, the symptoms instead proved similar to PSP.[33.48] In contrast, Pick's disease without motor dysfunction was the diagnosis for mutations such as G272V, K257T, G389R.[18,41,49] Another interesting observation has been that, in general, parkinsonism is more frequently present in families with *tau* mutations that alter tau splicing, while Pick's disease is more common for missense mutations in exon 9 and to some degree, exons 12 and 13. Mental retardation has also been observed in one family with the +11 mutation.[22] Psychoses have been diagnosed in some patients, such as those carrying the V337M mutation. However to date, no clear definite diagnosis of Alzheimer's disease has been made in any family with mutations in the *tau* gene. This is probably due to the fact that cognitive impairment tends to appear later than abnormal behaviour or parkinsonism, which are the most frequently presenting features.

CONCLUSIONS

The question of how a mutation in the *tau* gene leads to neurodegeneration is, as yet, not fully clear. The primary effect of most missense mutations appears to be the reduced ability of tau to interact with microtubules. This may equate to a partial loss of function, resulting in microtubule destabilisation and deficits in cellular processes such as axonal transport. However, mice lacking the tau gene are fully viable, demonstrating that the microtubule-binding of tau is not an essential function.[50] Furthermore, missense tau mutations do not seem to alter axonal transport.[51] As FTDP-17 is characterised by filamentous accumulations of hyperphosphorylated tau, perhaps a more plausible explanation for the effect of mutations is that they lead to a 'toxic gain of function'. Decreased binding of mutated tau to microtubules could result in an excess of 'free' tau available for hyperphosphorylation and filament assembly. Work by Goode and Feinstein[52] has suggested that 3R and 4R tau may bind to different sites on microtubules. Intronic and exonic mutations that increase exon 10 splicing leading to overproduction of 4R tau isoforms may therefore, result in an excess of tau over available binding sites, once again with unbound tau available for hyperphosphorylation and assembly into filaments. Since known mutations in *tau* do not create additional phosphorylation sites (with the possible exceptions of the K257T and P301S mutations), hyperphosphorylation probably occurs downstream of the primary effects of the mutation. However, some missense mutations may indirectly affect tau phosphorylation. For example in cells transfected with the R406W mutation, tau is less phosphorylated at T231, S396 and S404 than wild-type tau and tau with the P301L or V337M mutations.[16,53] Currently, there is no experimental evidence linking tau hyperphosphorylation to filament assembly, and whether hyperphosphorylation is either necessary or sufficient for filament assembly *in vivo* is unknown. Assembly is energetically unfavourable and is a nucleation-dependent process relying on a critical concentration of tau.[54,55] Some cells may have tau levels below this threshold. Others cells may have proteolytic degradation pathways that prevent tau aggregation. Tau concentrations and the extent of protective mechanisms may determine the selective degeneration of certain neurons and glial cells observed in FTDP-17. Nevertheless the exact nature and sequence of events underlying this degeneration remain to be elucidated.

REFERENCES

1.   Hirokawa, N. (1994) "Microtubule organization and dynamics dependent on microtubule-associated proteins." *Curr. Opin. Cell. Biol.* 6:74-81.
2.   Ebneth, A. et al. (1998) "Overexpression of tau protein inhibits kinesin-dependent trafficking of vesicles, mitochondria, and endoplasmic reticulum: implications for Alzheimer's disease." *J. Cell Biol.* 143:777-794.
3.   Goedert, M. et al. (1989) "Cloning and sequencing of the cDNA encoding an isoform of microtubule-associated protein tau containing four tandem repeats:

differential expression of tau protein mRNAs in human brain." *EMBO J.* 8:393-399.

4. Goedert, M. et al. (1989) "Multiple isoforms of human microtubule-associated protein tau: sequences and localization in neurofibrillary tangles of Alzheimer's disease." *Neuron* 3:519-526.

5. Goedert, M. et al. (2001) "From genetics to pathology: tau and alpha-synuclein assemblies in neurodegenerative diseases." *Phil. Trans. R. Soc. Lond. B. Biol. Sci.* 356:213-227.

6. Spillantini, M.G. et al. (1998) "Tau pathology in two Dutch families with mutations in the microtubule-binding region of tau." *Am. J. Pathol.* 153:1359-1363.

7. Spillantini, M.G. et al. (1997) "Familial multiple system tauopathy with presenile dementia: a disease with abundant neuronal and glial tau filaments." *Proc. Natl. Acad. Sci. U S A* 94:4113-4118.

8. Poorkaj, P. et al. (1998) "Tau is a candidate gene for chromosome 17 frontotemporal dementia." *Ann. Neurol.* 43:815-825.

9. Hutton, M. et al. (1998) "Association of missense and 5'-splice-site mutations in tau with the inherited dementia FTDP-17." *Nature* 393:702-705.

10. Spillantini, M.G. et al. (1998) "Mutation in the tau gene in familial multiple system tauopathy with presenile dementia." *Proc. Natl. Acad. Sci. U S A* 95:7737-7741.

11. Conrad, C. et al. (1997) "Genetic evidence for the involvement of tau in progressive supranuclear palsy." *Ann. Neurol.* 41:277-281.

12. Hayashi, S. et al. (2002) "Late-onset frontotemporal dementia with a novel exon 1 (Arg5His) tau gene mutation." *Ann. Neurol.* 51:525-530.

13. Poorkaj P. et al. (2002) "An R5L mutation in a subject with a progressive supranuclear palsy phenotype." *Ann Neurol*, in press.

14. Hasegawa, M., Smith, M.J. and Goedert, M. (1998) "Tau proteins with FTDP-17 mutations have a reduced ability to promote microtubule assembly." *FEBS Lett.* 437:207-210.

15. Hong, M. et al. (1998) "Mutation-specific functional impairments in distinct tau isoforms of hereditary FTDP-17." *Science* 282:1914-1917.

16. Dayanandan, R. et al. (1999) "Mutations in tau reduce its microtubule binding properties in intact cells and affect its phosphorylation." *FEBS Lett.* 446:228-232.

17. Nacharaju P. et al. (1999) "Accelerated filament formation from tau protein with specific FTDP-17 missense mutations." *FEBS Lett.* 447:195-199.

18. Goedert, M., Jakes, R. and Crowther, R.A. (1999) "Effects of frontotemporal dementia FTDP-17 mutations on heparin-induced assembly of tau filaments." *FEBS Lett.* 450:306-311.

19. Rizzini, C. et al. (2000) "Tau gene mutation K257T causes a tauopathy similar to Pick's disease." *J. Neuropathol. Exp. Neurol.* 59:990-1001.

20. Neumann, M. et al. (2001) "Pick's disease associated with the novel Tau gene mutation K369I." *Ann. Neurol.* 50:503-513.

21.   Yasuda, M. et al. (2000) "A novel mutation at position +12 in the intron following exon 10 of the tau gene in familial frontotemporal dementia (FTD-Kumamoto)." *Ann. Neurol.* 47:422-429.

22.   Miyamoto, K. et al. (2001) "Familial frontotemporal dementia and parkinsonism with a novel mutation at an intron 10+11-splice site in the tau gene." *Ann. Neurol.* 50:117-120.

23.   Varani, L. et al. (1999) "Structure of tau exon 10 splicing regulatory element RNA and destabilization by mutations of frontotemporal dementia and parkinsonism linked to chromosome 17." *Proc. Natl. Acad. Sci. USA* 96:8229-8234.

24.   D'Souza, I. et al. (1999) "Missense and silent tau gene mutations cause frontotemporal dementia with parkinsonism-chromosome 17 type, by affecting multiple alternative RNA splicing regulatory elements." *Proc. Natl. Acad. Sci. USA* 96:5598-5603.

25.   Grover, A. et al. (1999) "5' splice site mutations in tau associated with the inherited dementia FTDP-17 affect a stem-loop structure that regulates alternative splicing of exon 10." *J. Biol. Chem.* 274:15134-15143.

26.   Goedert, M. et al. (1999) "Tau gene mutation in familial progressive subcortical gliosis." *Nat. Med.* 5:454-457.

27.   Hulette, C.M. et al. (1999) "Neuropathological features of frontotemporal dementia and parkinsonism linked to chromosome 17q21-22 (FTDP-17): Duke Family 1684." *J. Neuropathol. Exp. Neurol.* 58:859-866.

28.   Clark, L.N. et al. (1998) "Pathogenic implications of mutations in the tau gene in pallido-ponto-nigral degeneration and related neurodegenerative disorders linked to chromosome 17." *Proc. Natl. Acad. Sci. USA* 95:13103-13107.

29.   Hasegawa, M. et al. (1999) "FTDP-17 mutations N279K and S305N in tau produce increased splicing of exon 10." *FEBS Lett.* 443: 93-96.

30.   Spillantini, M.G. et al. (2000) "A novel tau mutation (N296N) in familial dementia with swollen achromatic neurons and corticobasal inclusion bodies." *Ann. Neurol.* 48:939-943.

31.   Grover, A. et al. (2002) "Effects on splicing and protein function of three mutations in codon 296 of *tau* in vitro." *Neurosci. Lett.* 323:33-36.

32.   Iijima, M. et al. (1999) "A distinct familial presenile dementia with a novel missense mutation in the tau gene." *Neuroreport* 10:497-501.

33.   Stanford, P.M. et al. (2000) "Progressive supranuclear palsy pathology caused by a novel silent mutation in exon 10 of the tau gene: expansion of the disease phenotype caused by tau gene mutations." *Brain* 123:880-893.

34.   Yoshida, H., Crowther, R.A. and Goedert, M. (2002) "Functional effects of tau gene mutations deltaN296 and N296H." *J. Neurochem.* 80:548-551.

35.   von Bergen, M. et al. (2001) "Mutations of tau protein in frontotemporal dementia promote aggregation of paired helical filaments by enhancing local beta-structure." *J. Biol. Chem.* 276:48165-48174.

36. Iseki, E. et al. (2001) "Familial frontotemporal dementia and parkinsonism with a novel N296H mutation in exon 10 of the tau gene and a widespread tau accumulation in the glial cells." *Acta Neuropathol.* 102:285-292.

37. Lippa, C.F. et al. (2000) "Frontotemporal dementia with novel tau pathology and a Glu342Val tau mutation." *Ann. Neurol.* 48:850-858.

38. Spillantini, M.G., Crowther, R.A. and Goedert, M. (1996) "Comparison of the neurofibrillary pathology in Alzheimer's disease and familial presenile dementia with tangles." *Acta Neuropathol.* 92:42-48.

39. Reed, L.A. et al. (1997) "Autosomal dominant dementia with widespread neurofibrillary tangles." *Ann. Neurol.* 42:564-572.

40. van Swieten, J.C. et al. (1999) "Phenotypic variation in hereditary frontotemporal dementia with tau mutations." *Ann. Neurol.* 46:617-626.

41. Murrell, J.R. et al. (1999) "Tau gene mutation G389R causes a tauopathy with abundant pick body-like inclusions and axonal deposits." *J. Neuropathol. Exp. Neurol.* 58:1207-1226.

42. Bigio, E. et al. (2002) "L266V tau mutation produces a tauopathy clinically and pathologically analogous to sporadic Pick Disease." *J. Neuropathol. Exp. Neurol.* 61:A168.

43. Rosso, S.M. et al. (2002) "A novel tau mutation, S320F, causes a tauopathy with inclusions similar to those in Pick's disease." *Ann. Neurol.* 51:373-376.

44. Mirra, S.S. et al. (1999) "Tau pathology in a family with dementia and a P301L mutation in tau." *J. Neuropathol. Exp. Neurol.* 58:335-345.

45. Bugiani, O. et al. (1999) "Frontotemporal dementia and corticobasal degeneration in a family with a P301S mutation in tau." *J. Neuropathol. Exp. Neurol.* 58:667-677.

46. Pickering-Brown, S.M. et al. (2002) "Inherited frontotemporal dementia in nine British families associated with intronic mutations in the tau gene." *Brain* 125:732-751.

47. Reed, L.A. et al. (1998) "The neuropathlogy of a chromosome 17-linked autosomal dominant parkinsonism and dementia ("pallido-ponto-nigral degeneration")." *J. Neuropathol. Exp. Neurol.* 57:588-601.

48. Delisle, M.B. et al. (1999) "A mutation at codon 279 (N279K) in exon 10 of the Tau gene causes a tauopathy with dementia and supranuclear palsy." *Acta Neuropathol.* 98:62-77.

49. Heutink, P. et al. (1997) "Hereditary fronto-temporal dementia is linked to chromosome 17q21-22: a genetic and clinico-pathological study of three Dutch families." *Am. J. Pathol.* 153:1359-1363.

50. Harada, A. et al. (1994) "Altered microtubule organization in small-calibre axons of mice lacking tau protein." *Nature* 369:488-491.

51. Utton, M.A. et al. (2002) "The slow axonal transport of the microtubule-associated protein tau and the transport rates of different isoforms and mutants in cultured neurons." *J. Neurosci.* 22:6394-6400.

52. Goode, B.L. and Feinstein, S.C. (1994) "Identification of a novel microtubule binding and assembly domain in the developmentally regulated inter-repeat region of tau." *J Cell Biol.* 124:769-782.

53. Matsumura, N., Yamazaki, T. and Ihara, Y. (1999) "Stable expression in Chinese hamster ovary cells of mutated tau genes causing frontotemporal dementia and parkinsonism linked to chromosome 17 (FTDP-17)." *Am. J. Pathol.* 154:1649-1656.

54. Goedert, M. et al. (1996) "Assembly of microtubule-associated protein tau into Alzheimer-like filaments induced by sulphated glycosaminoglycans." *Nature* 383:550-553.

55. Friedhoff, P. et al. (1998) "A nucleated assembly mechanism of Alzheimer paired helical filaments." *Proc. Natl. Acad. Sci. USA* 95:15712-15717.

PSYCHIATRIC DISORDERS AS VECTORS FOR HIV AND OTHER BEHAVIORALLY TRANSMITTED INFECTIOUS EPIDEMICS.

GLENN JORDAN TREISMAN M.D., PH.D.
Department of Psychiatry and Behavioral Sciences, Johns Hopkins University School of Medicine, Baltimore, MD, USA

Identification of the transmission routes for the human immunodeficiency virus (HIV) and of behaviors that promote transmission has led to a shift in the population becoming infected. In the face of widespread public awareness of the risk factors, people have changed their behavior to prevent infection. People who are unable to modify their behavior and who become infected are now more likely to have a psychiatric disorder that prevents behavioral change and makes them vulnerable. Disorders such as depression, demoralization, substance abuse, impulsive personality, and cognitive impairment can all contribute to vulnerability.

This shift has shown up in the population we treat at The Johns Hopkins Hospital. Just over half of the patients who seek medical care at the Moore Clinic have a major psychiatric disorder other than substance abuse or personality disorder, 75% have a substance abuse disorder, and almost 20% have significant cognitive impairment. This psychopathology affects all elements of patient care in HIV clinics. Untreated psychiatric disorders reduce patients' compliance with medication regimens, trigger behaviors that spread HIV, and "burn out" health care workers.

FOUR CATEGORIES OF PSYCHIATRIC DISORDERS

In general, psychiatric disorders may be viewed as falling into 4 categories: brain diseases, personality disorders, disorders of motivated behavior (addictions), and problems that emerge from life circumstances. The majority of patients seen by the Hopkins AIDS Psychiatry Service suffer from disorders in more than one of these categories.

Diseases

This first category is the most familiar to medical professionals. A psychiatric disease is a syndrome caused by a lesion in the brain. The most common psychiatric disease that we see in the HIV Clinic is major depression. The differential diagnosis of a patient who complains of depression or with suspected depression includes at a minimum Major

Depression, Demoralization, AIDS dementia (or other subcortical dementias) and delirium.

Major depression usually presents with anhedonia, a loss of ability to derive pleasure or satisfaction from the activities that usually provide it. Most patients also have a change to a prevailing sad mood, although some feel "flat" or "empty of feelings." Many patients report a diminished sense of well-being, a sense of being ill, and a sense of guilt or self-loathing. Some patients suffer from delusions or hallucinations, usually with a guilty or depressive theme reflecting their mood. Almost all patients have a sleep disturbance, often with early morning wakening. Many patients have a diurnal variation in mood, with mornings usually worse than evenings. Many patients lose their appetite. Cognitive impairment (the so-called "pseudo-dementia" of depression) may mimic AIDS dementia. These changes are usually episodic, lasting a few months and then resolving spontaneously, only to recur again a few months later; however, depression can also be continuous and chronic.

Unfortunately, complicating the diagnosis of depression in HIV-infected patients is the tendency for both patients and clinicians to attribute all the depressive symptoms to the psychological effects of having HIV. Patients "explain" their mood changes and other difficulties as a product of their illness, and their caregivers accept their assessment and miss the underlying depression. In a patient like ours, the diagnosis can be challenging.

One-fifth of our patients are suffering from a major depressive episode at the time of their first HIV medical evaluation, and we estimate that about 60% of HIV-infected patients have a depressive episode sometime during their illness. Depression increases hopelessness, demoralization, and impulsiveness. Depressed patients have poor compliance, are more likely to have substance abuse disorders, and are less likely to be able to meet the demands of managing their chronic illness. Because depression increases the risk of behaviors that lead to acquiring HIV infection, we believe that depression itself has become a factor in the HIV epidemic.

At the Moore Clinic, as many patients present with demoralization as with major depression. The psychiatric term "adjustment disorder" is used in the DSM-IV to describe this state, in which the patient has a pervasive sense of sadness, low mood, or hopelessness that can go so far as to interfere with usual activities. This reaction is almost always precipitated--and can be explained--by recent events, but again it can co-exist with major depression and can complicate the diagnosis. Demoralized patients with HIV feel sad because of the overwhelming loss, stigma, and helplessness associated with a chronic, progressive, and potentially fatal illness. This is a form of the grief reaction seen in patients with all kinds of illnesses. Like other demoralized patients suffering from grief or bereavement, demoralized patients with HIV respond well to support, encouragement, education, and time.

AIDS dementia is a "subcortical" dementia producing a flat, apathetic state that can be hard to distinguish from major depression and can co-exist with it, again complicating the diagnosis.

Delirium, an impairment of consciousness produced by global derangement of brain function, often masquerades as depression by altering patients' emotions. While the workup of delirium in HIV-infected patients is complex, this state may be best characterized—and distinguished from depression—by two consistent features: an alteration in level of consciousness and a waxing and waning of the problem. Delirious patients appear intermittently hypervigilant and stuporous, and their disorder episodically worsens and improves over hours or a day.

In the Moore Clinic, aggressive treatment of major depression with both pharmacotherapy and psychotherapy helps 85% of patients and restores half of them to baseline. Aggressive treatment is critical to giving patients a sense of hopefulness about the treatment of their HIV infection. Despite accumulating evidence that depression is a recognizable and treatable disease, it remains the most under-recognized and under-treated psychiatric disorder in patients with chronic medical illness.

Personality, Character, and Temperament

Disorders of temperament and character often baffle and frustrate the most well-meaning and patient of clinicians. While hard-to-treat diseases can frustrate and anger physicians, the focus of their anger is directed at the disease. With disorders of character, clinicians often find themselves frustrated and angry at the patients because of their seemingly irrational and deliberately self-destructive behavior.

Descriptions and measurements of temperament are directed at describing people's nature--their natural response to a given problem or situation. An overly simplistic but useful approach to modeling personality has become essential to our ability to help patients in the HIV Clinic. Patients can be characterized in many ways. A simple but useful approach reduces patients to two dimensions: stability-instability and introversion-extroversion. In the general population, the distribution of these traits roughly follows a normal curve (Fig. 1). Instability describes the degree of excursion of emotion in response to a stimulus, and the maximal excursion (Fig. 1). Patients with high levels of instability have changeable natures and are difficult to predict; they have large emotional responses to modest experiences.

The second dimension is the extroversion-introversion axis. Extroverts tend to seek rewards rather than avoid consequences, focus on now rather than the future, and respond to feelings rather than cognition. Extroverts are more likely to act than not to act.

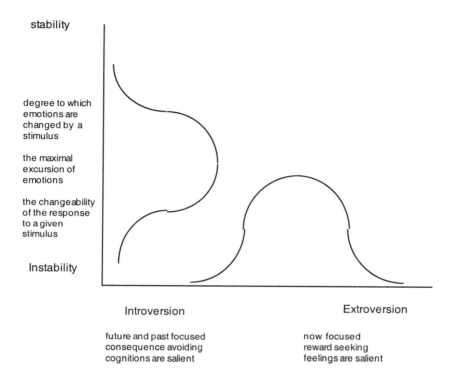

stability

degree to which
emotions are
changed by a
stimulus

the maximal
excursion of
emotions

the changeability
of the response
to a given
stimulus

Instability

Introversion

Extroversion

future and past focused
consequence avoiding
cognitions are salient

now focused
reward seeking
feelings are salient

Fig. 1. Patient characterizations.

Patients at the extremes of the curve are not sick. Rather, they have an excess of a trait that makes them excel in certain situations and be vulnerable in others. Extreme extroverts are vulnerable when it is important for them to avoid consequences and focus on the future, as when managing chronic HIV infection and continuing treatment to prevent full-blown AIDS. Such patients are vulnerable allowing their feelings to direct their behavior, and they may leave the hospital against medical advice, demand unreasonable or poorly conceived treatments, and even impulsively injure themselves.

Most people fall in the middle of the curve. They can use both extroverted and introverted styles. Medical students study for exams to avoid failing; given a choice between an evening on the town and studying for an exam, they drive themselves to study by imagining failure. In contrast, dancing is more fun when one just enjoys it rather than being preoccupied by "trying not to look stupid." Extremely extroverted or introverted people get "stuck" in one style. They run into trouble when faced with situations that are not suited to their style. Most health-care workers tend to be on the introverted side, i.e., consequence-avoidant, so they are puzzled by extroverts' insensitivity to consequences. Providers sometimes find the communications gap impossible to bridge as they stress the long-term negatives while patients focus only on their immediate goals.

I have found 3 approaches particularly useful in managing unstable extroverted patients:

- *Reframe all consequence avoidance so it becomes a reward.* For example, "If you don't stop shooting drugs, you'll get sicker," can be reframed as, "If you get off drugs, you'll feel better."
- Whenever possible, *appeal to the patient's cognitive side.* Even though emotions are more salient to extroverts, many have cognitive skills with which you can divert them when you have their attention. Through long-term treatment, a patient's intellectual recognition that it is ineffective to lose one's temper may make them more aware of their temper and triggers for losing it. This cognitive skill can be used to "walk away" from potential disaster.
- Most important, *the treatment plan should be written down clearly and should set firm limits.* This gives all the clinicians a unified set of goals and expectations, and eventually persuades patients to consider the clinicians' goals.

The goal of treating personality problems is to change the patient's style through a series of gradual behavior changes sustained over several years. Patients make slow, incremental changes rather than an abrupt "conversion." To adapt successfully to life with HIV, extremely extroverted patients must change how they respond to problems. Their goals must become directed at health and function. Patients are still quite vulnerable and will have some setbacks, but over time patients make steady progress toward changing their lives.

Addictions: Disorders of Motivated Behavior

Many HIV-infected people have substance abuse disorders (addictions) that both play a role in disseminating HIV infection and complicate its treatment. In patients whose HIV risk factor is injection drug use, the etiologic role of addiction is obvious. Substance abuse plays a broader role in HIV transmission by increasing the risk to the heterosexual partners of injection drug users. Substance abuse is related to other risk behaviors, possibly through disinhibition and poor judgment. Independent of injection use, intoxication with drugs or alcohol has been linked to high-risk sexual activity and high rates of sexually transmitted diseases.

A simplified model of substance use disorders requires an understanding of both patient's abnormal biological drive and the volitional component that gives rise to the term "behavioral disorder." McHugh has suggested the term "motivated behavior" to encompass these disorders. Twelve-step programs cannot ease the symptoms of schizophrenia, but they help plenty of alcoholics stop drinking. This difference distinguishes alcoholism from disease; alcoholism has a clearly volitional component. At the same time, alcoholics have an abnormal and difficult-to-control "biological" drive or craving that is clearly different from the desire to take a walk or choosing a tie.

To try to understand this behavior, we may look to animal models of "self-administration." In these experiments, an animal pulls a lever a specified number of times to obtain a "drug reward." There is a tight correlation between a drug's addictiveness and how hard an animal will work to get a dose of it. For example, an animal may pull the lever thousands of times to get a single dose of cocaine and may endure electric shocks rather than give up the attempt. This is in keeping with the misery and risk tolerated by addicted humans.

The treatment of substance abuse requires a team of determined clinicians with a common plan. Because these disorders are chronic and relapsing, they require a long-term plan rather than a short-term "cure."

Extreme Reactions to Life Circumstances

Patients with HIV infection can sustain numerous personal losses, many of them catastrophic. Despite public education, the stigma attached to HIV and AIDS remains enormous. Misconceptions about transmission sometimes lead to HIV-infected persons being treated as outcasts, rejected even by family and friends. Some patients keep their serostatus secret, even from their most intimate partners. Many HIV-infected persons suffer frequent losses as loved ones die from AIDS. Bereavement and reaction to losses often take the form of demoralization--grief and post-traumatic stress reactions.

Patients can suffer severe reactions when they first learn that they are infected with HIV, and again throughout their course when they learn that their disease has progressed or their T-cell counts have fallen. Patients are temporarily at higher-than-normal risk for suicidal thoughts and actual suicide during the acute response to these events. Many people also feel self-pity, victimization, guilt, and imminent mortality, and some just feel overwhelmed. As with any devastating news, initial shock and denial can turn to sadness, anger, and hopelessness. As their illness advances, most patients struggle with pain and inability to care for themselves. Many grieve over loss of employment and other features of independence, as well as impoverishment and social disenfranchisement. All of these factors understandably lead to some degree of demoralization. Demoralized patients can be helped by counseling, support groups, family groups, family education programs, drop-in centers, and advocacy programs.

Treatment by compassionate caregivers can greatly improve patients' sense of hope and quality of life. Most essential is that caregivers enable patients to plan for changes in their medical condition, discuss treatment options, and understand the goals of treatment.

SUMMARY

It is important to emphasize the ever more complex and intense needs of HIV-infected patients. With the increasing emphasis on cost saving and fiscal management, patients are often denied care because of high cost and intensive use of medical resources. Despite the expense of treatment, it is still far cheaper to make patients better than to allow them to remain ill.

I have suggested that psychiatric disorders increase risk behaviors for HIV infection, a position supported by many studies. The data also suggest that HIV causes psychiatric disorders, not just by direct subcortical injury but also through psychological and sociological repercussions of infection. Many HIV-infected patients have psychiatric disorders, including affective disorders (major depression and mania, dementia, addiction, personality disorders, and demoralization. These disorders not only directly impair patients' quality of life, but they interfere with compliance with medical treatment and with modifying risk behaviors. Antiretroviral therapies will have no benefit for patients who are too disturbed by mental illness to take them correctly. These patients may even come to be a reservoir of resistant virus.

Caregivers' empathic understanding can become a kind of clinical nihilism in which all psychological distress is interpreted as deserving of comfort measures such as support, sedatives, and narcotics, while treatable mood disorders are missed. It can be difficult to diagnose these disorders in HIV-infected patients, and in particular to distinguish major depression from the demoralization caused by the burdens of living with HIV; however, this distinction is crucial so that each disorder can be treated correctly.

Treatment improves mood disorders in HIV-infected patients, even those with advanced AIDS, dementia, or comorbid conditions such as addiction or personality disorder. Substance abuse also responds to treatment. Personality disorders, though chronic, can be managed so that life can proceed less chaotically and treatment more fruitfully. Life's most trying events can be overcome with support, counseling, and care.

HIV-infected patients benefit from therapeutic optimism and aggressive treatment of the whole person. Their management requires consultation and liaison relationships between specialties, and must include those directed at mental health. With comprehensive care, the toughest patients can surprise clinicians with dramatic recovery.

REFERENCES

1.   Treisman, G., Fishman, M., Lyketsos, C., McHugh, P.R. (1994) "Evaluation and Treatment of Psychiatric Disorders Associated with HIV Infection." In: *HIV, AIDS and the Brain*, R.W. Price and S.W. Perry (Eds) pp. 239-250. New York, Raven Press, Ltd.
2.   McHugh, P.R., Slavney, P.R. (1983) *The Perspectives of Psychiatry.* Baltimore, Maryland, The Johns Hopkins University Press.

3.   Lyketsos, C.G., Hanson, A.L., Fishman, M., et al. (1994) "Screening for Psychiatric Morbidity in a Medical Outpatient Clinic for HIV Infection: the need for a psychiatric presence." *International Journal of Psychiatry and Medicine*. 24:103-113.

4.   Lyketsos, C.G., Fishman, M., Treisman, G., et al. (1995) "Effectiveness of psychiatric treatment for HIV-infected patients." *American Neuropsychiatric Association 6th Annual Meeting*. Abstract.

5.   "Continued sexual risk behavior among HIV-seropositive, drug-using men—Atlanta; Washington, D.C.; and San Juan, Puerto Rico." *Morbidity and Mortality Weekly Report*. 1996; 45:151-152.

6.   Booth, R.E., Watters, J.K., Chitwood, D.D. (1993) "HIV risk-related sex behaviors among injection drug users, crack smokers, and injection drug users who smoke crack." *American Journal of Public Health*. 83:1144-8.

7.   Goodkin, K., Blaney, N., Tuttle, R., et al. (1996) "Bereavement and HIV infection." *International Review of Psychiatry*. 8:267-76.

8.   Perry, S.W., Jacobsberg, L., Fishman, B. (1990) "Suicidal ideation and HIV testing." *Journal of the American Medical Association*. 263:679-682

9.   Lyketsos, C.G., Treisman, G.J. (1995) "Psychiatric Disorders in HIV-infected patients: Epidemiology and issues in drug treatment." *CNS Drugs*. 4:195-206

10.   Fishman, M., Lyketsos, C., Schwartz, J., Treisman, G. (1998) "Psychiatric Disorders in HIV Infection," In: *The Neurology of AIDS*, H. Gendelman, S. Lipton, L. Epstein, S. Swindells (Eds), pp 524-535 Chapman and Hall, New York.

VARIANT CREUTZFELDT-JAKOB DISEASE AND BOVINE SPONGIFORM ENCEPHALOPATHY: CURRENT STATUS

R.G. WILL

National Creutzfeldt-Jakob Disease Surveillance Unit, Western General Hospital, Edinburgh, UK

The transmission of bovine spongiform encephalopathy (BSE) from cattle to the human population has resulted in a new form of human prion disease, variant Creutzfeldt-Jakob disease (vCJD). This is the first known zoonotic transmisssion of animal prion diseases and has resulted in widespread concern about the possible risks to public health. In the past year there have been worrying developments, including the identification of cases of vCJD and BSE in countries that were previously unaffected. This article reviews the current status of prion diseases.

VARIANT CJD

Cases of vCJD continue to occur in the United Kingdom and since 2000, following the publication of diagnostic criteria for case classification,[1] the monthly reported figures include surviving cases classified on clinical grounds as diagnostically 'probable.' Current data (August 2002) are shown in Table 1, which lists deaths from vCJD and sporadic CJD and provides the number of surviving 'probable' cases in a subscript.

Trends in the occurrence of cases of vCJD are analysed quarterly and the latest review indicates an annual increase of 18% for onsets and 20% for deaths, taking into account a decrease in the delay from onset to diagnosis of about 5% per annum.[2] The increasing trend is most apparent in those cases with vCJD born after 1970. However, it is not possible from these analyses to make long-term predictions, because it is not known whether the increasing trend will continue and, if so, for how long. A number of mathematical groups have attempted to predict the eventual size of the epidemic of vCJD in the UK and the most recent estimates are more conservative than in the past,[3,4,5] ranging from hundreds to thousands of cases. All these predictions depend on a range of assumptions and a commentary accompanying two of these articles was entitled 'Predicting the unpredictable.'[6] A significant future epidemic cannot yet be excluded.

Cases of vCJD have been identified in a number in a number of countries other than the UK, including most recently two cases in North America (Table 2). It is important to stress that there is a consensus that cases of vCJD will be classified geographically by the country of normal residence at the time of disease onset. This does not indicate that there is necessarily human exposure to BSE in the country of attribution. The cases of vCJD in the USA and Canada had a history of significant periods of residence in the UK during the 1980s, when there is likely to have been extensive exposure of the human population to high titre BSE tissues in the food chain. It is therefore highly probable that the causal exposure to BSE took place in the UK rather than in North America. The case of vCJD in Ireland also had a history of residence in the UK during the relevant period and may have been infected by BSE in Britain rather than by indigenous BSE in Ireland. The fact that the first cases of vCJD in the USA and Canada have a history of extended residence in the UK is consistent with the hypothesis that exposure to BSE is causally related to the development of vCJD.

Table 1. Creutzfeldt-Jakob Disease in ihe UK.

REFERRALS OF SUSPECT CJD		DEATHS OF DEFINITE AND PROBABLE CJD						
Year	Referrals	Year	Sporadic	Iatrogenic	Familial	GSS	vCJD	Total Deaths
1990	[53]	1990	28	5	0	0	-	33
1991	75	1991	32	1	3	0	-	36
1992	96	1992	44	2	5	1	-	52
1993	78	1993	37	4	3	2	-	46
1994	116	1994	51	1	4	3	-	59
1995	87	1995	35	4	2	3	3	47
1996	134	1996	40	4	2	4	10	60
1997	161	1997	59	6	4	1	10	80
1998	154	1998	63	3	4	1	18	89
1999	169	1999	61	6	2	0	15	84
2000	178	2000	48	1	2	1	28	80
2001	172	2001	51	3	2	2	20	78
2002*	89	2002	13	0	1	0	11	25
Total Referrals	1562	Total Deaths	562	40	34	18	115	769

* As at 19 August 2002

Summary of vCJD cases
   Deaths
   Deaths from definite vCJD (confirmed):   92
   Deaths from probable vCJD (without neuropathological confirmation):   22
   Deaths from probable vCJD (neuropathological confirmation pending):   1
   Number of deaths from definite or probable vCJD (as above):   115
   Alive
   Number of probable vCJD cases still alive: 11
   Total number of definite or probable vCJD (dead and alive):   126

Table 2. Cases of vCJD In UK and Elsewhere.

Country	Number of Cases
UK	126
France	6
Republic of Ireland	1
Italy	1
USA	1
Canada	1

Five of the cases of vCJD in France and the Italian case did not have a history of travel to the UK, nor a significant travel history to other BSE affected countries, and must have been exposed to BSE in their own countries. The risk of BSE infection in these cases may relate to exposure to indigenous cattle infection or to risk of BSE infection from the UK in the form of exported bovine food products, cattle feed or cattle incubating BSE. A risk analysis in France, combing these potential sources of human exposure, estimated that the extent of human BSE exposure in France was about 10% of that in the UK.[7] There has been only a very limited and recent observed BSE epidemic in Italy, but it is of interest that about 10 years ago 2 cases of BSE in cattle imported from the UK were identified in the same region in Italy where the case of vCJD was identified earlier this year.

BOVINE SPONGIFORM ENCEPHALOPATHY

The epidemic of BSE in the UK continues to decline, from a peak of 36,682 confirmed cases in 1992 to 781 in 2001. These figures relate to cases identified through the passive surveillance system and a further 332 cases were identified through an active testing programme. Within the European Union, Sweden is the only country that remains BSE free and the numbers of cases are increasing in many countries, including France, Germany, Ireland and the Netherlands. It is important to stress that despite this the absolute numbers of cases annually in these countries are still currently lower than in the UK and much less than the UK rates in the 1990s. A summary of the total number of cases of BSE per country is shown in Table 3 and includes cases identified by both passive surveillance and the testing programme.

Since 1999 a number of countries which were previously thought to be free of BSE have identified cases, often through active testing of cattle at abattoirs or of fallen stock. These countries include Denmark, Finland, Germany, Greece, Israel, Italy, Japan, Liechtenstein, Luxembourg, Poland, Slovakia, Slovenia and Spain. It is apparent that the risk of developing BSE in cattle populations is far more widespread than previously assumed. Although it may not be possible to identify the specific source of infection in individual countries, there is a likelihood that seeding of infection from past exports from BSE affected countries may be implicated, probably in the form of cattle feed or incubating bovines. Infection may have been amplified in countries that, in the past, recycled cattle for the production of cattle feed with a resultant dissemination of exposure.

A joint meeting of the WHO, FAO and OIE in June 2001 on 'Bovine spongiform encephalopathy: public health, animal health and trade' reached the following conclusions:[8]

a) the disease (BSE) is transmissible to humans; scientific consensus confirms that food is the main avenue of exposure
b) bovines, bovine products and by-products potentially carrying the BSE agent have been traded worldwide, giving this risk a global dimension
c) the exchanges mentioned above have or can have repercussions on public health, animal health and trade.

The Scientific Steering Committee of the European Union have carried out an assessment of the geographical risk of BSE (GBR), which is regularly updated. The GBR relates to the 'Presence of one or more cattle clinically or pre-clinically infected with the BSE agent in a geographical region or country' and the levels are classified as follows:

I.   Highly unlikely
II. Unlikely but not excluded
III. Likely but not confirmed or confirmed, at a lower level
IV. Confirmed, at a higher level

Only two countries are currently classified as level IV, Portugal and the UK. Countries in level III, excluding those in which BSE has already been identified (see Table 3), were (as of 11 January 2001) Albania, Cyprus, Estonia, Hungary, Lithuania and Romania. Category II included Canada, Colombia, India, Kenya, Mauritius, Nigeria, Pakistan and Sweden. It is of note that a formal GBR risk assessment has not been completed for many countries. In the past some countries previously categorised as level II have subsequently been reclassified as level III when BSE was identified.

CONCLUSION

BSE and vCJD are novel diseases, which have had profound political and economic implications. The geographical distribution of both diseases is extending. Prion diseases pose complex problems for public and animal health because of extended incubation periods and the absence of a diagnostic marker for infection prior to the onset of clinical disease. There continues to be a need to closely monitor the epidemiology of all prion disease and an important scientific objective is the development of an effective therapy.

Table 3. Reported Cases of BSE (Including Cases Detected During Testing Programmes).

Country	Total BSE cases since 1987	Total in 2002 reported 28 July
Great Britain**	179,325	515
Northern Ireland**	1,986	54
GB and NI total	*181,311*	*569*
Isle of Man***	437	0
Guernsey***	699	0
Alderney	2	0
Jersey***	149	0
Azores	1	--
Austria	1	0
Belgium**	85	20
Canada	1	0
Czech Republic	2	0
Denmark	9	1
Falkland Islands	1	0
Finland	1	0
France*	675	159
Germany**	193	55
Greece	1	0
Ireland*	1030	209
Israel**	1	1
Italy**	70	18
Japan***	4	1
Liechtenstein	2	0
Luxembourg	1	0
Netherlands**	40	12
Oman	2	0
Poland	1	1
Portugal***	674	31
Slovakia**	10	5
Slovenia***	2	1
Spain*	150	70
Switzerland***	416	8
Ukraine**	1 possible	1 possible

*=national authority;   **=news sources, including Braakman;

***=European Commission

(Adapted from the Consumer's Association BSE Report 2002)

REFERENCES

1. Will, R.G., Zeidler, M., Stewart, G.E., Macleod, M.A., Ironside, J.W., Cousens, S.N. et al. (2000) "Diagnosis of new variant Creutzfeldt-Jakob disease." *Ann Neurol*; 47:575-582.
2. Andrews, N.J. (2002) Incidence of variant Creutzfeldt-Jakob disease: onsets and deaths in the UK: January 1994 - June 2002. National CJD Surveillance Unit Website www.cjd.ed.ac.uk, July 2002.
3. Huillard d'Aignaux, J.N., Cousens, S.N., Smith, P.G. (2001) "Predictability of the UK variant Creutzfeldt-Jakob disease epidemic." *Science*; 294:1729-1731.
4. Valleron, A-J., Boelle, P-Y., Will, R., Cesbron, J-Y. (2001) "Estimation of epidemic size and incubation time based on age characteristics of vCJD in the United Kingdom." *Science*; 294:1726-1728.
5. Ghani, A.C., Ferguson, N.M., Donnelly, C.A., Anderson, R.M. (2000) "Predicted vCJD mortality in Great Britain." *Nature*; 406:583-584.
6. Medley, G.F. (2001) "Predicting the unpredictable." *Science*; 294:1663-1664.
7. Alperovitch, A., Will, R.G. (2002) "Predicting the size of the vCJD epidemic in France." *CR Biologies*; 325:33-36.
8. Proceedings of the Joint WHO/FAO/OIE Technical Consultation on BSE: public health, animal health and trade. OIE Headquarters, Paris, 11-14 June 2001.

NEUROPSYCHIATRIC ASPECTS OF VARIANT CREUTZFELDT-JAKOB DISEASE

R.G. WILL, R.S.G. KNIGHT, M.D. SPENCER
National Creutzfeldt-Jakob Disease Surveillance Unit, Western General Hospital, Edinburgh, UK

INTRODUCTION

Variant Creutzfeldt-Jakob disease (vCJD) is a novel form of human prion disease, which was identified by the UK National Creutzfeldt-Jakob Disease Surveillance Unit in 1996.[1] The original hypothesis that vCJD was caused by transmission of bovine spongiform encephalopathy to the human population has been supported by subsequent epidemiological evidence and by laboratory research, including transmission experiments in rodent models. Suspicion that a new form of CJD had developed in the UK was initially raised by the identification of a small number of cases of CJD with unusual clinical characteristics, which included a young age at death and a predominantly psychiatric presentation. Analysis of the clinical features of larger numbers of cases has confirmed the common occurrence of early psychiatric symptoms,[2] but this is not uniform.[3] This article reviews the neuropsychiatric features of vCJD.

DEMOGRAPHICS OF vCJD

Diagnostic criteria for vCJD were first published in 2000[4] and have been partially validated (Table1). Cases can be classified as 'definite' with neuropathological confirmation, as 'probable' on the basis of clinical features and investigations or 'possible', again based on clinical characteristics. The current sensitivity of a 'probable' diagnosis exceeds 80% and the specificity is 100%; there have been no cases of 'probable' vCJD with an alternative final neuropathological diagnosis. 'Possible' cases are infrequent and are not included in reported figures or scientific analyses because of diagnostic uncertainty. In the UK to date (August 2002) 92 definite and 34 probable cases have been identified, with 11 of these 'probable' cases still alive. Cases of vCJD have been confirmed in other countries (Table 2), but it is important to stress that cases are classified geographically by the country of normal residence at the time of disease onset. This does not necessarily imply the country in which exposure to BSE took place. For example, the cases of vCJD in the USA and Canada both had a history of extended residence in the UK during the 1980s when human dietary exposures to BSE were likely to have been extensive. Although attributed to the USA and Canada, these cases are more likely to have been infected by BSE in the UK than in the country of residence at the time of diagnosis.

Table 1. Diagnostic Criteria for vCJD.

I	A	Progressive neuropsychiatric disorder
	B	Duration of illness > 6 months
	C	Routine investigations do not suggest an alternative diagnosis
	D	No history of potential iatrogenic exposure
	E	No evidence of a familial form of TSE
II	A	Early psychiatric symptoms[a]
	B	Persistent painful sensory symptoms[b]
	C	Ataxia
	D	Myoclonus or chorea or dystonia
	E	Dementia
III	A	EEG does not show the typical appearance of sporadic CJD[c] (or no EEG performed)
	B	Bilateral pulvinar high signal on MRI scan
IV	A	Positive tonsil biopsy[d]
DEFINITE:		I A **and** neuropathological confirmation of vCJD[e]
PROBABLE:		I **and** 4/5 of II **and** III A **and** III B
		OR
		I **and** IV A[d]
POSSIBLE:		I **and** 4/5 of II **and** III A

a   depression, anxiety, apathy, withdrawal, delusions.

b   this includes both frank pain and/or dysaesthesia.

c   generalised triphasic periodic complexes at approximately one per second.

d   tonsil biopsy is **not** recommended routinely, nor in cases with EEG appearances typical of sporadic CJD, but may be useful in suspect cases in which the clinical features are compatible with vCJD and MRI does not show bilateral pulvinar high signal.

e   spongiform change and extensive PrP deposition with florid plaques, throughout the cerebrum and cerebellum.

676

Table 2. Cases of vCJD in the UK and elsewhere.

COUNTRY	NUMBER OF CASES	YEAR FIRST IDENTIFIED
UK	126	1995
France	6	1996
Republic of Ireland	1	1999
Italy	1	2002
USA	1	2002
Canada	1	2002

NEUROPSYCHIATRIC FEATURES OF vCJD

The most striking characteristics of vCJD are the relatively young age at death and long duration of illness in comparison to sporadic CJD (Figs. 1 and 2), but the clinical presentation of vCJD is also relatively distinctive.

The initial symptoms in vCJD are usually psychiatric, most frequently depression, anxiety and withdrawal, although a minority of cases exhibit first-rank symptoms suggestive of a psychotic illness. After a median of 6 months clear-cut neurological features develop, including cognitive impairment, ataxia and involuntary movements. Chorea and dystonia occur as well as the myoclonic movements which are a common characteristic of sporadic CJD. The clinical course is relentlessly progressive with the development of dementia and diffuse cortical deficits. Terminally patients are usually mute, bed-bound and helpless. Death occurs a median of 14 months from the onset of symptoms and is often due to an intercurrent infection such as bronchopneumonia.

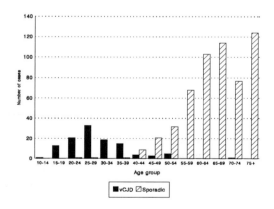

Fig. 1. Age at Death in vCJD AND sCJD (1990-2002).

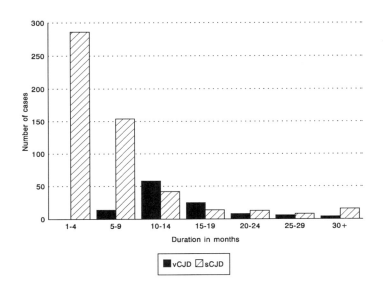

Fig. 2. Duration of Illness in vCJD AND sCJD (1990-2002).

An analysis of the neurological and psychiatric features of the first 100 cases of vCJD has been published recently[3] with the aim of clarifying the early clinical characteristics of vCJD. One important conclusion of this study is that the clinical presentation of vCJD is heterogeneous: 63% of cases present with psychiatric symptoms alone, 15% with isolated neurological symptoms and 22% with mixed features (Fig. 3). In the group with initial neurological symptoms 11/15 cases developed associated psychiatric symptoms within 4 months of onset and all cases had mixed neurological and psychiatric symptoms by 9 months of onset.

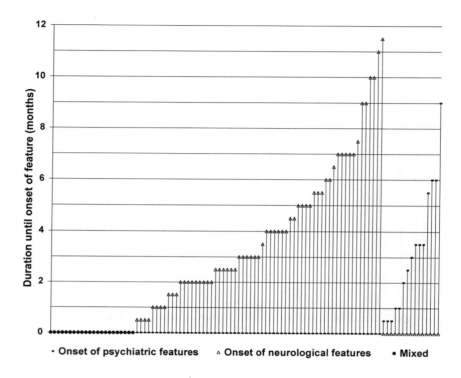

Fig. 3. Case by Case Plots of Onset of Psychiatric and Neurological Features (Cases Sorted by Times to Onset).

The specific symptoms at onset found in each group are shown in Table 3 (it should be noted that some patients exhibited multiple symptoms at onset). In the cases with a purely psychiatric mode of onset the most frequent features were behavioural change, dysphoria, irritability, anergia, withdrawal and anxiety. However, a significant minority of cases (10/63) had poor memory as an early symptom. In the cases with a neurological onset there were a range of symptoms, but sensory features were predominant and included pain, paraesthesia, numbness, hypersensitivity, coldness and 'odd sensation.' Four cases exhibited gait disturbance as an initial symptom and two slurring of speech. In the mixed category there were a wide range of neurological and psychiatric symptoms, but again pain or sensory symptoms were prominent in a significant proportion of cases. Gait disturbance was a feature in six, poor memory in three and slurring of speech in one.

Table 3. Analysis of Initial Features in 100 Cases Categorized by Mode of Onset of Illness (Psychiatric, Neurological or Mixed) - Figure in Brackets Represents Number of Cases With That Initial Feature.

Psychiatric onset N=63	Neurological onset N=15	Mixed onset N=22
Behavioural change (27)	Pain (4)	Behavioural change (8)
Dysphoria (21)	Paraesthesia (4)	Dysphoria (8)
Irritability (16)	Numbness (4)	Insomnia (7)
Anergia (15)	Gait disturbance (4)	Anxiety (4)
Withdrawal (14)	Hypersensitivity (2)	Withdrawal (4)
Anxiety (12)	Coldness (2)	Irritability (3)
Loss of interest (11)	Slurring of speech (2)	Poor memory (3)
Aggression (10)	Odd sensation (1)	Impaired concentration (3)
Poor memory (10)	Impaired coordination (1)	Appetite change (3)
Tearfulness (9)	Sweatiness (1)	Paranoid delusions (3)
Insomnia (8)		Aggression (2)
Hypersomnia (8)		Poor performance (2)
Poor performance (7)		Impaired self-care (2)
Impaired concentration (5)		Hypersomnia (2)
Appetite change (5)		Weight loss (2)
Weight loss (5)		Tearfulness (2)
Agitation (4)		Loss of interest (1)
Paranoid delusions (3)		Anergia (1)
Bizarre behaviour (2)		Suicidal ideation (1)
Panic attacks (2)		Agitation (1)
Obsessive features (2)		Panic attacks (1)
Losing things (2)		Bizarre behaviour (1)
Loss of confidence (2)		Paranoid ideation (1)
Suicidal ideation (1)		Disorientation (1)
Paranoid ideation (1)		Confusion (1)
Confusion (1)		Pain (8)
Diurnal mood variation (1)		Gait disturbance (6)
Recognition impairment (1)		Tremor (3)
		Coldness (3)
		Paraesthesia (2)
		Slurring of speech (1)
		Swallowing impairment (1)
		Handwriting impairment (1)
		Numbness (1)
		Odd sensation (1)
		Taste disturbance (1)
		Myoclonus (1)
		Hyperacusis (1)
		Dizziness (1)
		Headaches (1)
		Loss of consciousness (1)

This analysis together with a previous study of the subsequent evolution of psychiatric and neurological symptoms[4] suggests that, although the diagnosis of vCJD may be impossible in the early stages, the combination of an affective or psychotic disorder with persistent pain, sensory symptoms, gait ataxia or dysarthria may at least raise the suspicion of the diagnosis of vCJD. This is particularly the case in younger patients in view of the age distribution of vCJD.

The variation in clinical presentation is reflected in the range of speciality at initial referral. 38% of cases were first seen by a psychiatrist, 30% by a neurologist, 21% by a physician in general medicine and 11% by other specialists. Accurate diagnosis of vCJD was impossible prior to the description of the clinical phenotype in 1996. However, the range of initial diagnoses in the first 100 cases, the great majority of which presented after the publication of the first series of cases of vCJD, emphasises the difficulty of early diagnosis (Table 4).

Table 4. Clustering by Diagnosic Category.

DIAGNOSTIC CLUSTER	INITIAL DIAGNOSES	n
PSYCHIATRIC		
Depression	Depressive episode, agitated depression, depression with psychotic symptoms, depression with anxiety symptoms, depression with anorexia nervosa	42
Paranoid psychosis	Paranoid psychosis, schizophreniform psychosis	3
Post natal depression	Post natal depression, maternity blues	4
Post-viral fatigue	Post-viral fatigue, post-viral infection	4
Anxiety	General anxiety disorder, anxiety-related collapse	2
Other neurotic	Hysterical, situational reaction, acute stress reaction, due to stress, psychological dysfunction	5
NEUROLOGICAL		
CJD	vCJD, CJD, spongiform encephalopathy	6
Encephalopathy	Encephalopathy	3
Progressive disorder	Rapidly progressive neurological disorder, progressive neurodegenerative disorder, degenerative or parainfectious aetiology, progressive neurological condition involving frontal lobe pathology, serious diffuse intercranial [sic] pathology possible degenerative or inflammatory in nature, neurodegenerative disorder, progressive disorder of cognition and ataxia	7
MS	Multiple sclerosis, demyelination, MS with anxiety state	7
Cerebral lesion	Cerebral lesion, tunour	2
Cerebellar lesion	Cerebellar lesion, cerebellitis, chronic cerebellar alcoholic degeneration	3
Other organic	Organic cause, organic brain state, "?dementia ?viral"	4

Table 4. Clustering by Diagnosic Category (continued).

DIAGNOSTIC CLUSTER	INITIAL DIAGNOSES	n
MIXED PSYCHIATRIC AND NEUROGICAL		
Mixed	Anxiety and post-herpetic neuralgia, anxiety and depression and neurological symptoms	2
ORTHOPAEDIC		
Orthopaedic	Meniscal cyst, nerve root entrapment	2
NO DIAGNOSIS		
None		4

The diagnosis of vCJD is likely to become suspected with the evolution and progression of frank neurological deficits. There are a range of potential differential diagnoses, including structural lesions, inflammatory disease and metabolic disorders, for example Wilson's disease. Appropriate investigation is essential to exclude alternative diagnoses and this requires referral to a specialist neurological centre. In vCJD the most helpful investigation is MRI brain scan,[5] which shows symmetrical high signal in the posterior thalamus on T2, PD or FLAIR images in about 90% of cases. The EEG does not show the typical triphasic periodic complexes that are characteristic of sporadic CJD, but may show generalised slowing. The 14-3-3 cerebrospinal fluid immunoassay is positive in about 50% of cases and has a low specificity, because of the high positive rate in sCJD. In cases that die the most frequent differential diagnosis is sporadic CJD and Table 5 summarises the clinical and investigative differences between vCJD and sporadic CJD.

Table 5. Differences between Sporadic and Variant CJD.

	Sporadic	Variant
Mean age at death	66 years	29 years
Median duration of illness	4 months	14 months
Thalamic MRI high signal	Caudate/Putamen 60%	Pulvinar 90%
EEG	'Typical' 70%	'Typical' 0%
Neuropathology	Plaques 10%	Florid plaques 100%

CONCLUSION

Early diagnosis of vCJD is important for the patient and their relatives and may have implications for the timeliness of public health measures to reduce the risk of secondary iatrogenic transmission. However, analysis of the clinical characteristics of vCJD emphasises the non-specific nature of the early features in the majority of cases and explains the resultant difficulty in early diagnosis. There is an imperative to develop techniques to allow prompt diagnosis and this will become pressing if effective treatments are developed.

REFERENCES

1. Will, R.G., Ironside, J.W., Zeidler, M., Cousens, S.N., Estibeiro, K., Alperovitch, A. et al. (1996) "A new variant of Creutzfeldt-Jakob disease in the UK." *Lancet* 347:921-5.

2. Will, R.G., Stewart, G., Zeidler, M., Macleod, M.A., Knight, R.S.G. (1999) "Psychiatric features of new variant Creutzfeldt-Jakob disease." *Psychiatric Bulletin* 23:264-7.

3. Spencer, M.D., Knight, R.S.G., Will, R.G. (2002) "First hundred cases of variant Creutzfeldt-Jakob disease: retrospective case note review of early psychiatric and neurological features." *BMJ* 324:1479-82.

4. Will, R.G., Zeidler, M., Stewart, G.E., Macleod, M.A., Ironside, J.W., Cousens, S.N. et al. (2000) "Diagnosis of new variant Creutzfeldt-Jakob disease." *Ann Neurol* 47:575-82.

5. Collie, D.A., Sellar, R.J., Zeidler, M., Colchester, A.F.C., Knight, R., Will, R.G. (2001) "MRI of Creutzfeldt-Jakob disease: imaging features and recommended MRI protocol." *Clinical Radiology* 56:726-39.

18. INFORMATION SECURITY WORKSHOP

NEW FORMS OF CONFRONTATION: CYBER-TERRORISM AND CYBER-CRIME

AHMAD KAMAL

Senior Fellow, United Nations Institute of Training and Research, New York, NY, USA

There are many reasons why we must analyse new forms of confrontation, but the impending threats of cyber-terrorism and cyber-crime are two of the most important ones.

Cyber-terrorism lurks around the corner, as everybody warns us, but its dangers have to be placed in context.

Even though many countries around the world had faced terrorism through history, the attack of 11 September 2001 brought home, with brutal force, a new face of terrorism in the world. It marked a sea change in our thinking, and shook the complacency, which had marked the times prior to that tragedy. Its ripple effect has been felt far and wide around the world, and will continue to be felt for years to come.

The event signaled two profound changes in terrorism; first, the motivation of the attackers; and second, the extensive use of information technology, primarily the Internet, in planning and communicating the attacks.

In a sense, the event was unique, because of this quantum jump that it signaled in the technique of terrorism. Almost all our analyses in the past had been based on the theory that traditional weapons – daggers, poisons, guns, bombs, etc. – were the only means to be used by terrorists. As a result, almost all our counter-measures were focused on detecting and preventing the possession and movement of these weapons.

Now, for the first time, the weapon used was "motivation," or a willingness to die in whatever causes these perpetrators were fighting.

As we know all too well, it is difficult enough to detect and prevent the possession and movement of weapons, but it is virtually impossible to do the same with motivations. The latter are universal and invisible, and largely undetectable. This difficulty in detecting the undetectable underlies the fact that sophisticated intelligence services were unable to set off warning bells despite the extended periods of preparation that were spent in the planning and execution of the events of 11 September 2001.

It is necessary, of course, to try to examine the root causes of this new terrorism. Most of them are known, and most of them arise from problems to which there are no easy solutions. Bottom-up solutions, which address the root causes, are not likely to be followed, and it is the top-down approach that will determine the actual course of action in the foreseeable future.

Nevertheless, the motivation has to be analysed, and its psychology dissected. It is after all highly abnormal for relatively educated individuals to lay their lives on the line for suicidal missions. The inherent frustrations cannot be easily explained away by facile talk of "brain-washing," as many of these individuals do not fit into that profile.

A problem lies also in the fact that motivated individuals are highly creative. That creativity remains visible even in their motivations. That is why the motivation of the thief is always greater than the motivation of the detective. The criminal is always a couple of jumps ahead of the policeman. As and when the law plugs any of its numerous loopholes, the motivated criminal will always discover new cracks in the armor.

In the case of terrorism, it is essential to note that the objective of the terrorist is not so much to create damage, as to create panic. The damage is really collateral, and comes from the panic, the loss of confidence, the injection of doubts and hesitations, and the absence of trust, all of which are the primary factors on which the fabric of modern society is constructed. The success of the terrorist's effort comes from the fact that the damage caused is totally out of proportion to the effort expended in the planning and execution of the terrorist act.

Terrorism, as with any war, is not won by simply overwhelming the enemy with superior force. If the absolute size of forces were the only deciding factor, the more powerful would always win, and that is not so. It is the intelligent and accurate analysis of ones own assets and the other's vulnerability, and then of concentrating one's own forces on that vulnerability, that wins wars. History is replete with examples of how smaller forces have won wars by using this obvious technique.

The most important defense, therefore, is one, to begin with a correct analysis of one's own vulnerabilities, because this is where cyber-terrorists will attack, and two, try to determine the opponents motivations.

Vulnerability and motivation are then the two keys to a correct understanding of and reaction to the dangers of cyber-terrorism.

The wide and pervasive integration of computers and embedded chips into modern society is what makes it vulnerable to cyber-attacks. Computers are now deeply integrated in the management and processing of our daily actions, and embedded chips are so omni-present today that it is virtually impossible to determine even their actual numbers and locations. This became abundantly clear during the Y2K exercise, when businesses and governments spent billions to make sure computer systems would work when the year 2000 began.

This profound integration of computers and information technology is obviously the strength of modern life, but it is also its vulnerability. The greater the vulnerability the greater the ease with which it can be exploited. Vulnerability also arises from the finite number of nodal exchange points on the Internet network. While the permutations and combinations of routes that they offer is infinite, the exchange points themselves rank no more than a hundred or so, and their existence and location is public knowledge.

The motivation to commit cyber-crime is also increasing exponentially. The number of reported incidents has gone up from just 8 in 1988 to almost 53,000 in 2001, and the graph shows a constantly steepening increase. The first half of the year 2002 shows a 26 percent increase over the same period of the previous year.

Add to that the simple fact of its tempting results. Where the average bank hold-up brings in no more than $14,000, the average computer technology theft is of the order of magnitude of no less than $2 million. The temptation is just too great.

The status of how much is lost annually as the result of cyber-crime is unclear. Only a minute portion of computer crime gets reported. Most corporations have a well-defined tendency to conceal the manner and depth of the attacks on their facilities, for fear of the panic effect that this information would create on their image and stock prices.

In short, reported incidents are just the tip of the iceberg. The true cyber-criminal has no interest in advertising his successes, and the victims are afraid of reporting them. So the environment is entirely propitious for further damage.

A distinguishing feature of cyber-crime lies in the fact that the single unattached criminal – the hacker, or the virus spreader, or even the disgruntled insider – is really not the main danger. That is of course what hits the tabloids, partly because of the Robin Hood syndrome, and partly because it is considered "fun" among the software-literate youth. The actual minefield lies, however, in "organized" cyber-crime and cyber-terrorism, where the technical competence of youth is exploited and channeled by organised elements towards criminal and politically motivated ends.

Whereas the single hacker can work alone, organised crime requires proper networking through lines of communication between component elements. The essential need for those lines of communication are its vulnerability in turn, so that is where the counter-terrorism efforts will have to concentrate.

It is therefore essential to spotlight the techniques that cyber-criminals are likely to use as their primary means of communication in the current state of the technology. Most of them are known – untraceable emails, encryption, digital compression, steganography – but others will turn up as the technology evolves, as it inevitably will. All these loop-holes will have to be plugged.

The response of the law-abiding society will not be easy. The cyber world is ethereal in its nature, and largely uncontrollable in its anarchy. The Internet was after all designed initially as a non-linear means of communication that would survive any nuclear attack. That is what makes it indestructible. By the same token, that is what makes it uncontrollable, and thus a tempting asset for criminal exploitation.

Although many nations have written legislation against crimes committed over the Internet, such as hacking, illegal transfers of funds, identity theft, etc., the laws just cannot keep up with the technological advancements. The lure of the criminal mind and the opportunities are just too great. Add the fact that in many recent cases, the sentences have been minimal. It would be useful to remember that the young hacker who caused billions of dollars of damage around the world with the "I love you" virus, spent no more than a few months in jail. Cyber-space is virgin territory for the individual criminal, and even more attractive territory for the organized criminal.

Then there is the disturbing fact that intelligent cyber-crime is virtually undetectable. This is, in many ways, a "stealth" activity, where the motivated and organized criminal can slowly and painstakingly plant "sleeper" corruptions and viruses into critical databases and systems, and not pull the plug until much later. In fact, the plug does not need to be pulled at all; the mere threat of exploding such a "logical bomb" may be enough to disrupt all peace of mind and create mass panic.

Every technical advance in human history has been mirrored in the techniques used by criminals. The expansion of human effort into the cyber-sphere will be no different. Cyber-crime and cyber-terrorism will be an inevitable part of our future landscape.

The question then is, where do we go from here. Are we condemned to a future of fear and uncertainty, or can something be done about this new danger to society.

We are not completely without tools and solutions. There are some steps that need to be taken immediately.

The first, and by far the most important, is to begin to correctly analyze the vulnerability. This would be best done by using a team of trustworthy "ethical hackers", who would be given the job of conducting war-games aimed at penetrating existing systems. Many of our vulnerabilities, and many of the solutions to these vulnerabilities would be identified by this simple methodology.

The second would be to encourage all governments around the world to allot due priority to the need for deterrent legislation, not just against software piracy, but against the larger danger of cyber-crime and cyber-terrorism. At the moment, despite some tentative movement in the Council of Europe, such legislation is either sadly lacking, or completely insufficient. In fact, almost no information exists or is available about the "ownership" or responsibilities of cyber-space, or about the rights and obligations of countries, or about the rights and obligations of individuals. Sooner or later, and sooner rather than later, action will have to be taken to draft and enact a Law of Cyber-Space, as was the case in the negotiation and passage of the nearest equivalent, namely, the Law of the Sea.

The third would be to identify and establish a forum for this universal effort. This is not a task that can be undertaken by individual countries working in isolation, as any weak link in any one part of the world would be immediately exploited by the determined criminal. It cannot be left to private societies either, as the latter have no legal jurisdiction and sanction over transgressions. It must, therefore, be a global effort at a global forum in the search for a global consensus.

It can be done. It may take time, but it can be done. We just have to start the ball rolling. That message can usefully be initiated here in Erice.

19. KANGAROO MOTHER CARE WORKSHOP

A TOOL FOR THE FOLLOW-UP OF YOUR KANGAROO MOTHER CARE: BABY FROM BIRTH TO ONE YEAR OF CORRECTED AGE

NATHALIE CHARPAK, O. GUIFO, CHRISTIANE HURAUX, S. MENDOZA
Kangaroo Mothers Foundation, Bogota, Colombia

A fair humankind shall protect the children's right regardless of their origin. Rights of the LBW infants are the same all over the world. KMC is a concept of Integral Care for the Low Birth Weight Infant (premature infant or intra uterine growth retardation less than 2000g).

1. IDENTIFICATION OF THE BABY HISTORY

Year	2
History Code	4
Center	2

The number of the center code has to be decided in agreement with the KMC network so that the number will not be doubled

2. FAMILY HISTORY

Maternal Surname	20	
Maternal Name	10	
Civil Status		
Alone with support		
Alone without support		
Stable couple		
Level of Education:	Mother	Father
Reader		
Not Reader		
Working Status	Mother	Father
Working		
Unemployed		
Housewife		
Number of meals per day		
Access to safe water		

Number of infants less than 5 years in house

3. PREGNANCY

Gravity (including this pregnancy)
Parity (including this delivery)
Number of prenatal controls
Ultrasound: yes   no
Detection of infectious diseases
    No
    Syphilis
    Toxoplasmosis
    Hepatitis B
    HIV
    Malaria
    Urinary Tract Infection (UTI)
    Others
Pathology
    Acute hepatitis
    Toxemia
    AIDS
    Multiple pregnancy
    Anemia
Tuberculosis or other acute respiratory diseases
UTI
Threatened Premature Labor
Other
Substance Abuse (must be defined)
    Cigarette
    Alcohol
    Others
Treatments
    Antenatal corticoids   Number of doses
    Iron
    Malaria Prevention
    HIV prevention
        AZT
        Nevirapine
        Others
    Antibiotics
    Others
Pregnancy desired

4. BIRTH

Date: Day   Month Year
Gender
Female
Male
Ambiguous
If multiple pregnancy, rank in birth
Place of Birth:
Inborn
Outborn in Hospital
Outborn in primary health center
Outborn in home
Outborn in vehicle
Others
Attendance at birth
    Professional attendant
    Trained birth attendant
    Others
Weight
Length
Head Circumference
Gestational age
Method of evaluation
Lubchenco
    PTAGA
    PTSGA
    PTLGA
    TSGA
Method of birth
    Vaginal
    Elective cesarean section
    Cesarean Section
Apgar 1'   5'   10'
Fetal Distress
    Abnormal fetal heart rate
    Abnormal monitoring
    None
Resuscitation
Prevention of HIV
    Nevirapine
    AZT
    Others

Management of the baby
   NICU
   Stay with the mother
   Neonatal Unit

5. NEONATAL COURSE

Total Hospital Stay in Days
   NICU
   Neonatal Unit
   KMC ward
Days of assisted ventilation
Days of CPAP
Days of Oxygen
Days of exclusive parenteral nutrition
Age (day) of the first administration of the own mother milk
Diagnosis
   Respiratory Distress Syndrome
   Pathologic Jaundice
   Intraventricular Hemorrhage (IVH)
      Unknown
      No
      Yes
         Clinical Diagnosis
         Ultrasound Diagnosis   Degree of IVH
   Symptomatic Hypoglycemia
Infections
      Primary   Localization Sepsis
                                        Meningitis
                                        Omphalitis
                                        Arthritis
   Necrotizing enterocolitis
                                        Others
      Secondary   Localization Sepsis
                                        Meningitis
                                        Omphalitis
                                        Arthritis
   Necrotizing enterocolitis
                                        Others
         Nosocomial   Localization   Sepsis
                                        Meningitis
                                        Omphalitis
                                        Arthritis

Necrotizing enterocolitis

Others

Neurological Dysfunction
Abnormal tonus
Seizures
Apneas
  Primary
  Secondary
  Oxygen dependency

Vital status of the baby up to one year of follow up
  Alive
Dead before enrolment in KMC
  Dead between enrolment and discharge from the hospital
Dead between discharge and 40 weeks of post conceptional age
  Dead between 40 weeks and 3 months of corrected age
  Dead between 3 and 6 months of corrected age
  Dead between 6 and 9 months of corrected age
  Dead between 9 and 12 months of corrected age
Age (days) of death
Mother status
  Adult intensive cares
  Recovering
  Well
  Died
  Disappeared

6. KMC ENROLLMENT

Reasons of no KMC Enrollment
  Mother not willing or not here
  Staff not willing
  Others
Age (day) at enrollment
Localization of the baby
  NICU
  Neonatal Ward
  KMC Ward
Weight
Length
HC
Breastfeeding

Possible
Not recommended permanently
Not recommended temporarily
Supply by others
    Pasteurized
    Not pasteurized (not recommended)
Alimentation
    Mother milk
    Artificial milk and mother milk
    Artificial milk
Method of administration
    Breast
    Continuous gavage
    Discontinuous gavage
    Bottle
    Others
Parenteral nutrition
Use of fortifiers
Persistence of pathology
    Respiratory
    Infectious
    Neurologic
KMC providers
    Mother
    Other

KMC Adaptation and Application in the Hospital:

	NICU	Neonatal Unit	KMC ward
Total days			
Maximum of hours per day in KMC (KPosition or Mother with baby and gavage or breastfeeding)			
Weight gain per Kg per Day during the stay (using the last weight available)			
Aminofilina			
Number of blood transfusion			

Alimentation
    Human Milk
    Human and artificial milk
    Artificial Milk			

Parenteral Nutrition			

Method of administration
    Breast
    Continuous gavage
    Discontinuous gavage
    Bottle
    Others			

Training of other provider			
At how many days after enrollment the mother is becoming confident			

KMC DISCHARGE AT HOME

       Age of discharge
       Alimentation
           Human Milk
           Human and artificial milk
           Artificial Milk
       Method of administration
           Breast
           Bottle
           Tube
           Other
       Oxygen dependency
       Neurological dysfunctions at discharge
       Aminofilina
       Iron
       Multivitamins

Commitment of the family with the KMC follow up

7. KMC AMBULATORY PROGRAM AND FOLLOW UP TO ONE YEAR OF CORECTED AGE

Screening at 40 Weeks of Post Conceptional Age
    Status of the baby
        Inpatient
        Outpatient
    Weight
    Length
    HC
    Alimentation
        Human Milk
        Human and artificial milk
        Artificial Milk
    Method of administration
        Breast
        Bottle
        Other
    Mother accompanied at the consultation
    KMC providers
    Mother
    Father
    Others
    Age (days) and weight when the baby is taken off the kangaroo position
    Number of consultations since discharge
    Number of antibiotic treatment
    Number of readmission
    Total readmission stay in days
    Diagnosis of readmission
        Infectious diseases
        Aspirative pneumonia
        Anemia
    Hypoglycemia
        Failure to thrive
        Hemorraghic illness of the new born
        Others
    Neurological status
        Abnormal tone
        Abnormal primitive reflexes
    Others
    ROP

No
Yes   Degree Right eye   Degree Left eye
Ongoing pathology
    Respiratory illness
Neurological illness
    Others

Screening at 3 Month of Corrected Age:
    Weight
    Length
    HC
    Alimentation
        Human Milk
        Human and artificial milk
        Artificial Milk
    Method of administration
        Breast
        Bottle
    Introduction of other alimentation
    Mother accompanied at the consultation
    Number of consultations since 40 weeks
    Number of antibiotic treatment
    Number of readmission
    Total readmission stay in days
    Diagnosis of readmission
        Acute respiratory diseases
        Acute gastro intestinal disease
        Others
    Neurological status
        Abnormal
        Transient
    Ophthalmologic refraction assessment
        Myopia
        Astigmatism
        Hypermetropia
        Other
    Audition screening
    Ongoing pathology
        Respiratory illness
    Neurological illness
        Others
    Primary care givers:

Mother
Father
Grandparents
Others
Number of doses
DPTPolio
Hemophilus
Hep B
BCG
Measles

Screening at 6 Months of Corrected Age:
Weight
Length
HC
Alimentation
Human Milk
Human and artificial milk
Artificial Milk
Method of administration
Breast
Bottle
Adequate diversification
Number of consultations since 3 months
Number of antibiotic treatment
Number of readmission
Total readmission stay in days
Diagnosis of readmission
Acute respiratory diseases
Acute gastrointestinal disease
Others
Neurological status
Normal
Abnormal
Transient
Psychomotor development
Normal
Mild delay
Moderate delay
Severe delay
Ongoing pathology
Respiratory illness
Neurological illness

Others
Primary care givers:
    Mother
    Father
    Grandparents
Others
Number of doses
    DPTPolio
    Hemophilus
    Hep B
BCG
Measles

Screening at 9 Months of Corrected Age

Weight
Length
HC
Alimentation
    Human Milk
    Human and artificial milk
    Artificial Milk
Method of administration
    Breast
    Bottle
Adequate diversification
Number of consultations since 6 months
Number of antibiotic treatment
Number of readmission
Total readmission stay in days
Diagnosis of readmission
    Acute respiratory diseases
Acute gastrointestinal disease
    Others
Neurological status
    Normal
Abnormal
    Transient
Ongoing pathology
    Respiratory illness
Neurological illness
    Others
Primary care givers:
    Mother

Father
Grandparents
Others
Number of doses
DPTPolio
Hemophilus
Hep B
BCG
Measles

Screening at 12 Months of Corrected Age
Weight
Length
HC
Alimentation
Human Milk
Human and artificial milk
Artificial Milk
Method of administration
Breast
Bottle
Adequate diversification
Number of consultations since 9 months
Number of antibiotic treatment
Number of readmission
Total readmission stay in days
Diagnosis of readmission
Acute respiratory diseases
Acute gastrointestinal disease
Others
Neurological status
Normal
Abnormal
Transient
Risk of Cerebral Palsy
Psychomotor development
Normal
Mild delay
Moderate delay
Severe delay
Ongoing pathology
Respiratory illness
Neurological illness

Others
Primary care givers:
    Mother
    Father
    Grandparents
Others
Number of doses
    DPTPolio
    Hemophilus
    Hep B
BCG
Measles

SEMINAR PARTICIPANTS

SEMINAR PARTICIPANTS

Dr. Anatoly Adamishin

Ambassador of Russia (ret.)
Foreign Affairs
Moscow, **Russia**

Dr. Nafia Al-Shalabi

Meteorological Department
Civil Aviation
Damascus, **Syrian Arab Republic**

Dr. Donald M. Anderson

Biology Department
Woods Hole Oceanographic Institution
Woods Hole, **USA**

Professor William A. Barletta

Accelerator & Fusion Research Division
Lawrence Berkeley National Laboratory,
Berkeley, **USA**

Dr. Anne S. Bassett

Clinical Genetics Research Program
Centre for Addiction & Mental Health
Toronto, **Canada**

Professor André Beauchamp

Commission on the Ethics of Science and
Tecnology, Government of Quebec
Quebec, **Canada**

Professor Leonid A. Bolshov

Nuclear Energy Safe Development Institute
Russian Academy of Sciences
Moscow, **Russia**

Professor J. M. Borthagaray

Instituto Superior de Urbanismo
University of Buenos Aires
Buenos Aires, Argentina

Dr. Olivia Bosch — International Institute for Strategic Studies
London, UK

Professor Joseph Chahoud — Physics Department
Bologna University
Bologna, **Italy**

Dr. Nathalie Charpak — Kangaroo Mothers Foundation
Bogota, **Colombia**

Professor Dmitry Chereshkin — Institute of Systems Analysis
Russian Academy of Sciences
Moscow, **Russia**

Professor Robert Clark — Hydrology and Water Resources
University of Arizona
Tucson, **USA**

Dr. Robert Cloninger — Department of Psychiatry
Washington University School of Medicine
St Louis, **USA**

Dr. P. Michael Conneally — Department of Medical & Molecular Genetics
Indiana University of School of Medicine
Indianapolis, **USA**

Dr. Christopher Daase — University of Kent at Canterbury
Brussels School of International Studies
Brussels, **Belgium**

Dr. Socorro de Leon-Mendoza	Neonatology Unit Jose Fabella Memorial Hospital Manila, **Philippines**
Dr. Charles DeCarli	Department of Neurology University of California at Davis Davis, **USA**
Dr. Carmen Difiglio	Energy Technology Policy Division International Energy Agency Paris, **France**
Dr. Mbareck Diop	Science & Technology Advisor to the President of Senegal Dakar, **Senegal**
Professor Christopher Ellis	Landscape Architecture & Urban Planning Texas A&M University College Station, **USA**
Professor Lorne Everett	The IT Group Santa Barbara, **USA**
Dr. Marshal Folstein	NEMC/Tufts University of School of Medicine, Boston, **USA**
Dr. Susan E. Folstein	Tufts/New England Medical Center Boston, **USA**
H. E. Francesco P. Fulci	Ambassador - Former Permanent Representative of Italy to the United Nations New York, **USA**

Dr. William Fulkerson	Joint Institute for Energy and Environment University of Tennessee Tennessee, **USA**
Dr. Andrei Gagarinski	PRC "Kurchatov Institute" Moscow, **Russia**
Dr. Bertil Galland	Writer and Historian Buxy, **France**
Dr. Richard L. Garwin	Thomas J. Watson Research Center IBM Research Division New York, **USA**
Professor Bernardino Ghetti	Pathology & Laboratory Medicine Indiana University Indianapolis, **USA**
Professor Michel Gourdin	Physique Théorique et Hautes Energies Université Pierre et Marie Curie Paris, **France**
Dr. Alfred Grieder	Bank Julius Baer & Co. Ltd Lucerne, **Switzerland**
Dr. Alfred T. Grove	Geography Department University of Cambridge Cambridge, **UK**
Dr. Odette Guifo	Department of Pediatrics Hopital La Quintinie Douala, **Cameroon**

Dr. Jonathan L. Haines

Vanderbilt University Medical Center
Program in Human Genetics
Nashville, **USA**

Dr. Hugh C. Hendrie

Regenstrief Institute
Indiana University Centre for Aging Research
Indiana, **USA**

Professor Reiner K. Huber

Universität der Bundeswehr München
Neubiberg, **Germany**

Dr. Christiane Huraux

Mother-infant HIV Transmission
Consultant
Paris, **France**

Dr. P.K. Iyengar

Indian Atomic Energy Commission
Mumbai, **India**

Senator Josef Jarab

Czech Senate
Olomouc, **Czech Republic**

Dr. Ahmad Kamal

Ambassador (ret.) - United Nations Institute of
Training and Research, New York Office, New
York, **USA**

Dr. Ibrahim Karawan

Middle East Center
University of Utah
Salt Lake City, **USA**

Dr. Norbert Kroo

Hungarian Academy of Sciences
Budapest, **Hungary**

Dr. Andrei Krutskih

Department of Science & Technology
Russian Foreign Ministry
Moscow, **Russia**

Professor Valery Kukhar	Institute for Bio-organic Chemistry Academy of Sciences Kiev, **The Ukraine**
Professor Tsung Dao Lee	Department of Physics Columbia University New York, **USA**
Professor Axel Lehmann	Universität der Bundeswehr München Neubiberg, **Germany**
Dr. Peter Lock	European Association for Research on Transformation, EART r.V. Hamburg, **Germany**
Professor Pilar López	National Council for Scientific Research Instituto de Historia , CSIC Madrid, **Spain**
Professor Sergio Martellucci	Faculty of Engineering University of Rome "Tor Vergata" Rome, **Italy**
Professor R. A. Mason	University of Birmingham Birmingham, **UK**
Dr. Francis J. McMahon	Jules F. Knapp Research Centre Department of Psychiatry Chicago, **USA**
Professor Farhang Mehr	University of Boston Boston, **USA**

Dr. Anton Micallef	Euro-Mediterranean Centre on Insular Coastal Dynamics Valletta, **Malta**
Professor Gretty M. Mirdal	Department of Psychology University of Copenhagen, Copenhagen, **Denmark**
Professor Jürgen Mittelstrass	University of Konstanz Konstanz, **Germany**
Dr. Akira Miyahara	National Institute for Fusion Science Tokyo, **Japan**
Dr. W. Müller-Seedorf	Center for Analyses and Studies German Armed Forces Waldbröl, **Germany**
Dr. Slobodan Nickovic	Euro-Mediterranean Centre on Insular Coastal Dynamics Valletta, **Malta**
Dr. Micheal Ó Cinnéide	Marine Environment & Health Services Division Galway, **Ireland**
Dr. Jef Ongena	Ecole Royale Militaire Laboratoire Plasmaphysics Brussels, **Belgium**
Professor Gennady Palshin	ICSC World Laboratory Branch Ukraine Kiev, **The Ukraine**
Professor Donato Palumbo	World Laboratory Fusion Centre Brussels, **Belgium**

Dr. Sergio Paradiso	The University of Iowa College of Medicine Psychiatry Research Iowa City, **USA**
Dr. Tatyana Parkhalina	Moscow European Security Centre Moscow, **Russia**
Professor Stefano Parmigiani	Evolutionary and Functional Biology University of Parma Parma, **Italy**
Dr. Margaret A. Pericak-Vance	Duke University Medical Center Durham, **USA**
Professor Margaret Petersen	Dept. of Hydrology & Water Resources University of Arizona Tucson, **USA**
Professor Alain Peyraube	Directorate of Research Ministry of Higher Education and Research Paris, **France**
Professor Andrei Piontkovsky	Strategic Studies Centre Moscow, **Russia**
Professor Juras Pozela	ICSC World Laboratory Branch Vilnius, **Lithuania**
Professor Richard Ragaini	Lawrence Livermore National Laboratory Dept. of Environmental Protection Livermore, **USA**
Professor Vittorio Ragaini	Chemical Physics and Electro-Chemistry University of Milano Milan, **Italy**

Professor Karl Rebane

Department of Physics
University of Tallinn
Tallinn, **Estonia**

Professor Emanuele Ricotta

Experimental Medicine Department
Institute of Biophysics and Biochemistry
Rome, **Italy**

Professor Zenonas Rudzikas

Theoretical Physics & Astronomy Institute
Lithuanian Academy of Sciences
Vilnius, Lithuania

Professor Eda Sagarra

Irish Research Council for the Humanities and
Social Sciences
Dublin, **Ireland**

Dr. Mohamed Sankhare

Education, Planning and Training
Government of the Republic of Senegal
Dakar, **Senegal**

Dr. Ashot Sarkisov

Nuclear Energy Safe Development Institute
Russian Academy of Sciences
Moscow, **Russia**

Dr. Don Scavia

National Centers for Coastal Ocean Service
National Oceanic & Atmospheric Administration
Silver Spring, **USA**

Professor Hiltmar Schubert

Fraunhofer Institute for Chemical Technology
Pfinztal, **Germany**

Professor Daniel V. Segre

Institute for Mediterranean Studies
Università della Svizzera Italiana
Lugano, **Switzerland**

Professor Geraldo Gomes Serra

NUTAU
São Paulo State University
São Paulo, **Brazil**

Professor William R. Shea

Committee for the Humanities
European Science Foundation
Strasbourg, **France**

Professor Kai M. B. Siegbahn

Institute of Physics
University of Uppsala
Uppsala, **Sweden**

Professor K.C.
Sivaramakrishnan

Centre for Policy Research
New Dehli, **India**

Dr. Maria Grazia Spillantini

Centre for Brain Repair
University of Cambridge
Cambridge, **UK**

Professor William A. Sprigg

Institute for the Study of Planet Earth
University of Arizona
Tucson, USA

Dr. Bruce Stram

WFS Energy Permanent Monitoring Panel
Houston, **USA**

Dr. V.J. Sundaram

National Design & Research Forum
The Institute of Engineers (India)
Bangalore, **India**

Professor Kamran Talattof

Department of Near Eastern Studies
University of Arizona
Tucson, **USA**

Dr. Pieter Tans

National Oceanic and Atmospheric
Administration
Boulder, **USA**

Dr. Terence Taylor

International Institute for Strategic Studies-USA
Washington, **USA**

Dr. Larry Tieszen

International Programs
EROS Data Center, USGS
Sioux Falls, **USA**

Dr. Andrew F.B. Tompson

Geosciences and Environmental Technologies
Lawrence Livermore National Laboratory
Livermore, **USA**

Dr. Glenn Triesman

Psychiatry and Behavioral Sciences
John Hopkins Hospital
Baltimore, **USA**

Professor Vitali Tsygichko

Institute for System Studies
Russian Academy of Sciences
Moscow, **Russia**

Dr. Bob van der Zwaan

Energy Research Centre of the Netherlands
ECN - Policy Studies
Amsterdam, **The Netherlands**

Professor Jan Veizer

Ruhr-Universitaet Bochum and
Department of Earth Sciences
University of Ottawa
Ontario, **Canada**

Professor Marcel Vivargent

CERN
Geneva, **Switzerland**

Dr. Frederick vom Saal

Division of Biological Sciences
University of Missouri
Columbia, **USA**

Professor François Waelbroeck

Juelich Fusion Centre
St. Amandsberg, **Belgium**

Professor Hui-jun Wang

Institute of Atmospheric Physics
Chinese Academy of Sciences
Beijing, **P.R. China**

Professor Tao Wang

Lanzhou Institute of Cold and Arid
Regions Environmental & Engineering Research
Lanzhou, **P.R. China**

Dr. Andrew W. Warren

Department of Geography
University of London
London, **UK**

Dr. Henning Wegener

Ambassador of Germany (ret.)
Madrid, **Spain**

Dr. Jody Westby

The Work-It Group
Denver, **USA**

Professor Robert G. Will

Western General Hospital
National CJD Surveillance Unit
Edinburgh, **UK**

Professor Richard Wilson

Department of Physics
Harvard University
Cambridge, MA, **USA**

Dr. Lowell Wood — Lawrence Livermore National Laboratory
Livermore, **USA**

Professor Aaron Yair — Department of Geography
The Hebrew University
Jerusalem, **Israel**

Professor Donald A. Yerxa — The Historical Society
Boston, **USA**

Professor Antonino Zichichi — CERN & University of Bologna
Geneva, **Switzerland**